# Intracerebral Hemorrhage

# Intracerebral Hemorrhage

## Carlos S. Kase, M.D.

Professor of Neurology, Department of Neurology, Boston University
School of Medicine, Boston, Massachusetts

## Louis R. Caplan, M.D.

Professor and Chairman, Department of Neurology, Tufts University
School of Medicine, and Neurologist-in-Chief and Chairman, Department
of Neurology, New England Medical Center, Boston, Massachusetts

With 7 Contributing Authors

## Butterworth–Heinemann

Boston   London   Oxford   Singapore   Sydney   Toronto   Wellington

Dedicated to José A. Kase, and to
the memory of Vlasta S. Kase and
Carl and Bess Caplan

Every effort has been made to ensure that the drug dosage schedules within this text are
accurate and conform to standards accepted at time of publication. However, as treatment recommendations vary in the light of continuing research and clinical experience,
the reader is advised to verify drug dosage schedules herein with information found
on product information sheets. This is especially true in cases of new or infrequently
used drugs.

 Recognizing the importance of preserving what has been written, it is the policy of
Butterworth-Heinemann to have the books it publishes printed on acid-free paper, and
we exert our best efforts to that end.

**Library of Congress Cataloging-in-Publication Data**

Kase, Carlos S.
    Intracerebral hemorrhage / Carlos S. Kase, Louis R. Caplan; with
7 contributing authors.
      p.  cm.
    Includes bibliographical references and index.
    ISBN 0-7506-9308-8 (alk. paper) :
    1. Brain—Hemorrhage.  I. Caplan, Louis R.  II. Title.
    [DNLM:  1. Cerebral Hemorrhage.  2. Hematoma.  WL 355 K19i 1994]
RC394.H37K37 1994
616.8'1—dc20
DNLM/DLC
for Library of Congress                                    93-43303
                                                                CIP

**British Library Cataloguing-in-Publication Data.**

A catalogue record for this book is available from the British Library.

Butterworth–Heinemann
313 Washington Street
Newton, MA 02158

10  9  8  7  6  5  4  3  2  1

Printed in the United States of America

# Contents

# Foreword

The lineage of medical thought about apoplectic brain hemorrhages is long and tortuous. The topic has attracted the attention of some of the most eminent figures in medical history. Their ideas and interpretations, some now appearing quite bizarre and fanciful, are set forth in an entertaining fashion in the first part of this monograph.

Only in the past few decades, however, have the methods of medical science been brought to bear on this subject. Once the sphygmomanometer was used to measure blood pressure, replacing the compressibility of the pulse, prominence of the aortic heart sounds, and size of the heart, hypertension became accepted as a causative factor. Indeed, the term was incorporated in the name of the condition, namely, hypertensive brain hemorrhage. Age and atherosclerosis were found to be contributing factors. Saccular aneurysms, vascular malformations, and hematologic diseases became recognized causes.

Certainly the most significant advance in the study of brain hemorrhage was the invention of computed tomography and magnetic resonance imaging devices. For the first time clinicians had a way of visualizing hemorrhages during life. This has resulted in rapid advances in the field of cerebrovascular disease. Small hemorrhages could now be differentiated from infarcts, and this has altered clinical investigations of therapies and outcomes. The clinical manifestations of hemorrhages confined to particular regions of the brain (caudate nucleus, putamen, thalamus, tegmentum of the brainstem, cerebellum) could now be reevaluated.

Despite the advances made possible by neuroimaging, problems of a more fundamental nature, concerning the origin of the lesion(s) causing rupture of the brain vessels, have not been resolved. What causes brain vessels to rupture whereas those of other organs remain intact? If hypertension is a factor, why are nearly half the patients normotensive when the hemorrhage occurs? Since the presence of atheroma does not correlate with the occurrence of hemorrhage, what is the basic lesion leading to rupture? Fisher's lipohyalinosis is linked to the lacunar state, miliary aneurysm formation, and hemorrhage; is it merely an effect of the atheromatous process acting on smaller vessels in hypertensive and diabetic patients? What part does amyloidosis play in parenchymal hemorrhage?

These questions have piqued the curiosity and exercised the minds of Professors Louis Caplan and Carlos Kase. And they have been prompted to write this book, which reviews the present state of knowledge of the neurology and neuropathology of brain hemorrhage.

The reader, I am sure, will find their observations and those of their colleagues highly instructive. They have spent much time thinking about some of the most perplexing and unsettled aspects of this subject.

Raymond D. Adams

# Contributing Authors

**Darío V. Caccamo, M.D.**
Senior Staff Pathologist, Department of Pathology, Henry Ford Health Sciences Center, Detroit, Michigan

**Robert M. Crowell, M.D.**
Formerly, Director, Aneurysm Center, Department of Neurosurgery, Massachusetts General Hospital, Boston, Massachusetts, Berkshire Associates for Neurological Diseases, Pittsfield, Massachusetts

**Burton P. Drayer, M.D.**
Director, Magnetic Resonance Imaging and Research, Department of Neuroradiology, and Radiologist-in-Chief, Department of Radiology, Barrow Neurological Institute and St. Joseph's Hospital and Medical Center, Phoenix, Arizona

**Kevin Dul, M.D.**
Fellow, Department of Neuroradiology, Barrow Neurological Institute, Phoenix, Arizona

**Julio H. García, M.D.**
Professor, Department of Pathology, Case Western Reserve University, Cleveland, Ohio, and Head, Division of Neuropathology, Department of Pathology, Henry Ford Hospital, Detroit, Michigan

**Khang-Loon Ho, M.D.**
Department of Pathology, Henry Ford Hospital, Detroit, Michigan

**Philip A. Wolf, M.D.**
Professor of Neurology, Department of Neurology, Boston University School of Medicine, and Senior Visiting Neurologist, Boston University Medical Center/University Hospital, Boston, Massachusetts

# Preface

Hemorrhages in the brain have been known for more than two hundred years, but only recently have modern medicine and technology permitted recognition of their causes and localization during life. Since the advent of computed tomography in the mid-1970s and magnetic resonance imaging in the late 1980s, precise localization of brain hemorrhages has been possible in living patients. Correlation of the clinical symptoms and signs with the focal lesions shown on computed tomography or magnetic resonance imaging provides insight into how lesions at various locations affect the functions of the nervous system. Recognition of the usual findings, for example, in patients with left ventrolateral thalamic hemorrhages teaches clinicians what to look for in patients with abscesses, tumors, infarcts, and other focal lesions in the same area. Also, since hematomas arise from identifiable, usually deep-penetrating arteries, and since both infarcts and hemorrhages arise from degenerative changes in the same arteries, identification of a site frequently involved by hemorrhage allows alert clinicians to look for and recognize infarcts in the same location. Lateral pontine tegmental hematomas and caudate hemorrhages were recognized long before infarcts in the same locations, and provided the blueprint for their later identification.

Our teacher, C. Miller Fisher, whose work is often cited in this text, is fond of saying that neurology is learned "stroke by stroke." Hematomas have literally taken us and many neurologists "to school" on the subject of clinicoanatomical correlations and cerebral localization of function. For these reasons, we want to share the richness of the subject of the topography of hematomas and their clinical phenomenology with younger physicians who are beginning to explore this exciting area of clinical medicine.

During the past decade and a half, much information has become available about the clinical, epidemiological, radiological and pathological findings in large groups of patients with brain hemorrhages at various sites and of various causes. Yet no detailed monographs have been published that make this information available to clinicians caring for stroke patients. We believe that the time is ripe to organize, coordinate, and summarize this large body of information. We have collaborated in this monograph in order to bring the topic of intracerebral hemorrhage into the modern era. The book emphasizes the historical background and context of the new information, tracing the origins of notions about brain hemorrhage, and reviewing prior concepts and theories. This work is concerned only with intracerebral hemorrhage in the adult, since neonatal intracranial hemorrhage and intracerebral hemorrhage in children relate to different pathophysiological mechanisms, and they are outside our area of interest and expertise as adult clinical neurologists. The major portion of the book consists of detailed discussions of the clinical, radiological and pathological findings in patients with hemorrhages at various locations and of various causes. We have personally written all the chapters on mechanisms, location, and treatment of intracerebral hemorrhage. In the areas outside our expertise, we have been fortunate to have contributions by Philip A. Wolf, M.D. on epidemiology, by Julio H. García, M.D., Khang-Loon Ho, M.D., and Darío V. Caccamo, M.D. on pathology, and by Kevin Dul, M.D. and Burton P. Drayer, M.D. on neuroimaging. In the area of treatment of intracerebral hemorrhage, we had the generous collaboration of Robert M. Crowell, M.D., who provided the neurosurgical point of view on the subject. We are grateful to them for joining us in the production of this book.

We would like to acknowledge the guidance, example, and help of many people who made this monograph possible. For Dr. Caplan, a considerable debt is owed to Drs. Walle Nauta, Derek Denny-Brown, Flaviu Romanul, Raymond Adams, Miller Fisher, and Pierson Richardson who taught him basic neurology and neuropathology. Colleagues at Harvard, the University of Chicago, and Tufts who have been particularly helpful are Chaim Mayman, J. P. Mohr, Nicholas Zervas, Barry Arnason, Daniel Hier, Michael Pessin, Dana DeWitt, Dushyant Patel, and Samuel Wolpert. Former and present neurology residents and stroke fellows, especially Thomas Brott, Philip Gorelick, Cathy Helgason, Michael Sloan, Marc Chimowitz, Conrado Estol, Barbara Tettenborn, Philip Teal, Robert Wityk, Axel Rosengart, Joan Breen, and Chin-Sang Chung, and our Tufts nurse coordinator, Loretta Barron, have been esteemed coworkers of Dr. Caplan.

For Dr. Kase, this is an appropriate time to gratefully acknowledge the early guidance and generous teaching of Dr. Camilo Arriagada, of Santiago, Chile, along with Drs. Jaime Court and Fernando Díaz. They provided the clinical foundation in neurology, and Dr. Arriagada demonstrated the irreplaceable value of neuropathology for the understanding of neurologic disease. In the United States, at the Massachusetts General Hospital, Drs. Raymond D. Adams, C. Miller Fisher, and E. P. Richardson were exemplary teachers of the rigorous methods of clinical observation and clinicopathological correlations. Their ability to learn from the in-depth analysis of individual patients has been an inspiring model throughout a career in the study of the neurology of stroke. Special recognition goes to J. P. Mohr, M.D. who was able to carry over in the tradition of our mentors at the Massachusetts General Hospital, excelling as a clinician and teacher, and having become for Dr. Kase an esteemed mentor and friend. At Boston University, the guidance and support of Philip A. Wolf, M.D. have been a constant stimulus to pursue various aspects of cerebrovascular research.

We also thank a multitude of other clinicians and researchers who have generously provided us with clinical data and stimulating discussions. Our co-investigators in the Stroke Data Bank have been most cooperative in sharing unpublished data. We have particularly benefited from our interactions and discussions on the subject of intracerebral hemorrhage with Drs. Takenori Yamaguchi of Osaka, Japan, Hansjörg Schütz of Frankfurt, Germany, and Fernando Barinagarrementería of Mexico City. They have considerable experience on the subject, and we have often drawn from their expertise in the production of this monograph. The generous sharing of their time and materials with us is gratefully acknowledged. We are also indebted to the many colleagues who supplied us with data on special patients with intracerebral hemorrhage, which helped us in the illustration of a particular clinical or radiological aspect of the condition.

We are grateful to Pauline Dawley and Elise Bardsley, who worked long and hard at transcribing, correcting, nursing, and mothering the manuscript to completion. The staff at Butterworth-Heinemann, especially Debbie S. MacDonald (Assistant Editor) and Susan F. Pioli (Publisher of Medical Books), have been very helpful and patient in finally giving birth to this work.

Finally, we give special thanks to our patient and devoted families, especially our wives and children, who endured the many hours we spent away from them, while at the library or at the hospital, in order to complete this work. In great measure, whatever merits this work has, are to be credited to them as we could have never accomplished the task without their generous support and understanding.

Carlos S. Kase
Louis R. Caplan

# PART ONE
## General Features

# Chapter 1
# Historical Aspects

## Louis R. Caplan

Regarding any disease or condition, clinicians and researchers alike will be better able to tell where they are and where they should be going if they know where they and their predecessors have been. History adds a dimension that broadens knowledge. For this reason, we begin this book on intracerebral hemorrhage with this chapter, which sketches a broad outline of the history of the development of ideas, information, and opinions about brain hemorrhage and stroke. Within subsequent chapters that discuss specific etiologies and locations of hemorrhage, we will elaborate more on the historical aspects of these special areas.

### Early Writings

*Hippocrates* (460–370 B.C.) was probably the first to write about the medical aspects of stroke.[1,2] His followers were keen observers and recorders of phenomenology, especially as it related to prognosis.[3] In his aphorisms on apoplexy, Hippocrates noted that "persons are most subject to apoplexy between the ages of 40 and 60"[4] and that attacks of numbness might reflect "impending apoplexy."[1] He knew of mild and severe forms of apoplexy. Hippocrates astutely observed "when persons in good health are suddenly seized with pains in the head, and straightway are laid down speechless and breathe

with a stertor, they die in seven days when fever comes on."[2,5] This is surely a description of subarachnoid hemorrhage in which the dire prognosis and major clinical features were recognized by Hippocrates. He also described what was probably the first reported account of intracerebral hemorrhage. The patient was a woman who "lived on the seafront" who developed headache, right arm weakness, and an inability to articulate during the third month of pregnancy.[2] Hippocrates observed that there were many blood vessels connected to the brain, most of which were thin, and two (presumably the carotid arteries) were stout. The Greeks knew that interruption of these blood vessels to the brain resulted in unconsciousness and so named the arteries carotid, from the Greek word *karos* meaning deep sleep.[2]

*Aurelius Celsus* writing during the time of Christ (25 B.C. to A.D. 50) described "apoplexy," differentiating it from paralysis.[2] In apoplexy the body weakness was sudden and localized, while in paralysis "the whole body was affected." *Areteus of Cappadocia* noted that paralysis in apoplexy was on the side of the body opposite the affected side of the head. He wrote "but if the head be primarily affected on the right side, the left side of the body will be paralyzed; and the right, if on the left side."[2] *Paul of Aegina* (A.D. 625–690) was probably the first to use the term "hemiplegia."[2]

In these early writings, the authors described mostly the outward manifestations, those that could be noted by talking to the sufferer, or observing him or her while fully dressed. Epidemiological and geographical features were also studied. The main interest was prognosis, for the mark of a wise physician was to accurately predict outcome. Treatment involved mostly general health measures. Little was known or written about the nature or cause of the illness described.

*Galen* (A.D. 131–201) with his observations, analysis, and voluminous writings dominated the thirteen hundred years that followed his death.[3] His first writings emphasized observation and experimentation. Galen made very important contributions to knowledge about anatomy, mostly through his dissection of animals. He described the anatomy of the brain and its blood vessels as well as the body's other viscera and vasculature. Unfortunately, all else was theorizing and speculation. Galen attributed disease to chemical factors—a disequilibrium between various body humors and secretions, such as water, phlegm, blood, bile, and so forth. During the years of the Dark Ages and Middle Ages, persons who represented themselves as physicians gained their knowledge from poring over the Latin in the Galenic texts considered to be the epitome of all medical wisdom. Dissection, experimentation, and personal observations were discouraged. Of course, these were centuries in which authority— God, Church, and King—dominated. Not until the Renaissance was there real interest in or encouragement for new ideas, new observations, and new thoughts and insights.

## Sixteenth, Seventeenth, and Eighteenth Centuries

*Andreas Vesalius* (1540–1564) challenged tradition by dissecting humans and relying on his own observations instead of Galenic pronouncements. Vesalius was also blessed with a very talented artist as a collaborator and illustrator and a great flair for lecturing and teaching.[3] The *Fabrica* contained fifteen detailed anatomical plates on the brain[6] and greatly advanced knowledge of human brain and cerebrovascular anatomy. Vesalius could not find the rete mirabile vessels that Galen described. *Thomas Willis* (1621–1675) added more detail on the anatomy and branching of the intracranial arteries. Willis suggested that the anatomical configuration of the arterial circle of anastomosis at the base of the brain had an influence on the presence and severity of apoplectic paralysis.[2]

Beginning in the early seventeenth century, there were several monographs on apoplexy. The first such book was written by *Gregor Nymman* (1594–1638) at Wittenberg in 1619. Nymman dissected the blood vessels and recognized that closure of the cerebral vessels or passageways could cause apoplexy. Hemorrhage was not recognized as a cause of apoplexy. Nymman harkened back to Galen in his interpretation of abnormal movement of vital spirits as a cause of the brain derangement.[1] *Johann Jacob Wepfer* (1620–1695), also a German from Schaffhausen, wrote a more popular and betterknown treatise on apoplexy in 1658.[7] This monograph had five editions, the last issued in 1724. Wepfer performed meticulous examinations and dissections of the brain and arteries of patients with apoplexy. He described the appearance of the carotid siphon and the course of the middle cerebral artery in the Sylvian fissure. Obstruction of the carotid or vertebral arteries was recognized as a cause of apoplexy, the blockage preventing sufficient entry of blood into the brain.

Wepfer was the first to clearly show that bleeding into and around the brain was an important cause of apoplexy. In his treatise, he included the findings in four patients with either subarachnoid or intracerebral bleeding. Wepfer recognized that the clinical picture and severity of apoplexy varied greatly. He noted that those most susceptible to apoplexy were those who were obese, those whose face and hands were livid, and those whose pulse was constantly unequal.[1,2] These observations presaged the recognition that hypertension and cardiac disease were important causes of stroke. *Domenico Mistichelli* (1675–1715), a professor in Pisa, also wrote a monograph on apoplexy published in 1709.[8] His major contribution was an anatomical explanation for crossed representation, the pyramidal decussation, although apparently his anatomical description was later shown to be inaccurate.[1,2] Earlier, *Francois Bayle* (1672–1709) had also written a tractate on apoplexy[9] in French and had described calcification in plaques within cerebral arteries.

## Morgagni and the Eighteenth Century

The publication of a single work, *De Sedibus* (*De Sedibus et Causis Morborium per Anatomen Indagatis*)[10] by Morgagni in 1761 stimulated a monumental change in the direction of thought in medicine and neurology. *Giovanni Battista Morgagni* (1682–1771) was a distinguished professor of anatomy at the renowned University of Padua. He was a very careful scholar who worked his entire career to collect material for his epic work, which was finally published when he was 79 years old.[3] Morgagni had a vision that the secret to the understanding of disease was to carefully study at necropsy humans with illnesses and to correlate the findings with symptoms during life. Though we now take the clinicopathological method for granted, it was a new approach for physicians in the eighteenth century. Morgagni's work did not arise de novo. In 1679 *Theophilus Bonetus* of Genoa had written a book called *Sepulchretum Sive Anatomica Practica*, which was a literature review of prior pre- and postmortem observations on the same individuals. Translation of the full title gives insight into Bonetus's goals—"Repository of Anatomy, Practice on Corpses deceased of disease, which reports the history and observations of all alterations of the human body and reveals the hidden causes." Indeed it (anatomy) deserves to be called the foundation of real pathology and a proper treatment of disease, even the inspi-

ration of old and recent medicine." Bonetus reviewed the writings of 470 authors who described nearly 3,000 cases in the 1700 pages of the *Sepulchretum*.[3] Unfortunately, Bonetus was not up to the monumental task. The studies were often inadequate, and misquotations, misinterpretations, and complete lack of indexing made the book virtually useless to scholars and practitioners alike. The young Morgagni poured over the *Sepulchretum* because he believed in the concept. He vowed to write his own work on clinicopathological correlation but to do it prospectively by collecting his own case material. This process took many years.

*De Sedibus* is a work in five volumes, which is organized in the form of 70 letters written to a young man describing the cases in the collection. The first book is called *Diseases of the Head*. Morgagni's descriptions of the patients are very vivid as are his descriptions of the circumstances surrounding the onsets of their illnesses. One case of intracerebral hemorrhage deserves to be cited: "N. Ferrarini, a priest of Vienna, who had formerly been supposed consumptive at Venice, and had been treated for one-sided headache ten years before at Padua, having now completed his 43rd year, the hair of his head was gray, and his face was sometimes too red; his habit of body was slender, yet not lean; and though he seem'd spritely and joyful, he was very anxious with dissembled cares, and was very prone to anger."[3] Father Ferrarini apparently died suddenly one day and was found at autopsy to have an intracerebral hemorrhage, no doubt due to his hypertension.

Morgagni demonstrated that the paralysis was on the side opposite the brain lesion. He thought that the extravasation of blood was from an aneurysmic dilatation of the arteries and enlargement of the delicate coats of the brain arteries.[1] The soft substance of the brain yielded to the impulse of the blood causing apoplexy. Blood-filled cavities could rupture into the ventricles or onto the outer surface of the brain.[1]

Morgagni also described traumatic extradural hemorrhage in a case quite reminiscent of patients now often seen in Emergency Rooms of urban hospitals. "A certain man, who was a native of Genoa, blind in one eye and lived by begging, being drunk and quarreling with other drunken beggars, received two blows by their sticks; one on his hand, which was slight and another violent one at the left temple; so that blood came out of the left ear. Yet soon after, the quarrel being made up, he sat down at the fire with them at the same place, and again filled himself with a great quantity of wine by way of pledge of friendship being renewed; and not long after, on the very same night, he died."[3] At necropsy he had a large epidural hematoma.

Before Morgagni, there were no systematic detailed pathological studies or atlases. Wepfer's studies of apoplexy came close, but much of that text was blind speculation and theory rather than systematic data collection and analysis. The way was now open for observation, pathological examination, and data analysis. The emphasis shifted from the study of normal anatomy to inquiry about disease, and its appearance, causes, and clinical manifestations during life.

## Nineteenth Century—Cheyne, Cooke, and the Atlas Makers

*John Cheyne* (1777–1836), an Irish physician, wrote an important treatise on apoplexy in 1812. Cheyne's book entitled *Cases of Apoplexy and Lethargy with Observations upon the Comatose Diseases* sought to separate the phenomonology of lethargy from apoplexy.[11] Clinical descriptions were detailed and "morbid appearances" of the brain were emphasized following the lead of Morgagni. After reviewing the history of apoplexy and the issues of treatment (bloodletting, emetics, and purges, and external applications), Cheyne reported 23 cases and then commented upon them. Plates were included at the end illustrating some of the necropsy findings. Figure 1.1 is Plate 4 from Cheyne with his own description of the findings.[11] Cheyne described

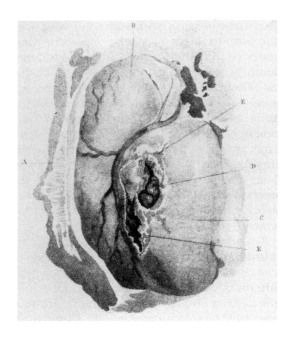

**Figure 1.1.** This plate represents the effect of an extravasation of blood between the corpus striatum and thalamus nervi optici, which the patient survived for some time. (A) Corpus callosum. (B) Corpus striatum. (C) Thalamus nervi optici. (D) Coagulum of blood contracted and in part absorbed. (E) The extent of the irregular cavity formed by the extravasation, now chiefly containing serum. (From Cheyne J. Cases of apoplexy and lethargy with observations upon the comatose diseases. London: J Moyes, Printer, 1812.)

brain softenings and both intracerebral and subarachnoid hemorrhage. He wrote of vascular congestion as "excitement of the arteries of the brain."[1] In those who survived an apoplexy for some time, Cheyne found in the brain a cavity filled with rusty, yellowcolored serum which also stained the neighboring brain tissue. He postulated that the cavities were lined by a membrane that could absorb red particles of the blood.

Excerpts from two of the case reports should illustrate Cheyne's contribution. Case IV, J.A., was a 32-year-old woman who was nearing the end of pregnancy. After a premonitory headache she became less responsive. Cheyne found when he examined her that "she preserved the power of voluntary motion of the left side, but the right was completely paralytic. She seemed perfectly conscious when raised, attempted to speak, but could not articulate. She signified by pointing with her left hand that she desired to drink."[11] After death, "on dissection of the cerebrum I found a coagulum of blood in the left lateral ventricle; and in withdrawing it, the plexus of vessels at the bottom of the ventricle was torn." This was presumably a vascular malformation or an eclamptic hemorrhage.

A pontine hemorrhage was also described for the first time. The patient (Case IX) was a "carpenter, 35 years of age, phlegmatic, pale, muscular, not habitually intemperate . . . who died on the first of June 1868."[11] He suffered from severe headaches, probably from hypertension. After one such nearly intolerable headache, he vomited and "soon after became insensible."[11] About an hour later, his breathing became irregular, he was deeply comatose, and died. "In dissecting the base of the brain, there was discovered, formed by a rupture in the substance of the pons varolii, a collection of dark clotted blood, in an irregular cavity, having a ragged surface and communicating with the fourth ventricle, which was full of blood."[11]

*John Cooke* (1756–1838), a physician to the London Hospital, wrote a treatise on nervous disease that was compiled between 1820 and 1823.[2] The first volume *On Apoplexy* was presented in 1819 as the Croonian Lecture of that year to the Royal College of Physicians.[12] This work included a lengthy review of the history of neurology and apoplexy up to his time and a summary of the contemporary view of apoplexy. There were no new observations or insights offered. The work was primarily a scholarly review of neurological thought at the time.

Following the lead of Morgagni and Cheyne, the second quarter of the nineteenth century saw an outpouring of atlases illustrating the morbid appearance of organs.

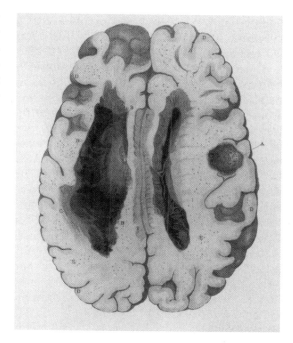

**Figure 1.2.** This plate exhibits the usual appearances which the brain presents when blood is extravasated from the spontaneous rupture of a vessel in its substance. (A) An apoplectic cell, in the centre of the right hemisphere, between the middle of the corpus striatum and the external and lateral surface of the brain. The contents were a sanguineous fluid, partly coagulated. The sides of the cell have become more dense than is natural, and formed into a membranous-like surface, of a brownish color, which gradually vanishes in the surrounding medullary substance. (B) The left lateral ventricle, as it appeared when a great quantity of coagulated blood was removed. (C) The part where the blood vessel ruptured. (D) The cineritious or cortical substance of the brain. (E) The medullary substance. (F) The corpus callosum. (From Hooper R. The morbid anatomy of the human brain. London: Longman, Hurst, Rees, Orme, Brown, and Green, 1828.)

Some also contained illustrations of patients with various maladies. The first of these was published in 1828 by *Robert Hooper*.[13] The atlas contained plates of brain lesions. Figure 1.2 is from Hooper's atlas and clearly illustrates a large intracerebral and probably putaminal hemorrhage.[13] Pontine hemorrhage and a subdural hematoma were also illustrated. *Gruveilhier* (1835–1842),[14] *Carswell* (1838),[15] and *Richard Bright*,[16] also published atlases of general pathology and neuropathology using detailed lithographs. Bright (1789–1858) was a physician at Guy's Hospital and one of the leading consultants in London. He had become very well known for his work on kidney disease. Volume II of his *Reports of Medical Cases* was published in 1831 and was called *Diseases of the Brain and Nervous System*.[16] Bright had collected over 200 neuropathological cases and illustrated 25 in color plates in this volume. Vascular cases were included, and in fact, Bright also published in 1836 a paper on the clinical and necropsy findings in patients with abnormalities of the arteries of the brain, including the internal carotid artery.[1,17]

Now that the basic rudimentary pathological and clinical features had been described, clinicians and morphologists turned during the remainder of the nineteenth century to an elaboration of the clinical and necropsy features.

## Further Clinical, Anatomical, and Pathological Definition and Interest in Etiology in the Nineteenth Century

Following the lead of Morgagni and Cheyne and the interest in pathology, physicians in the middle years of the nineteenth century became interested in the clinical features of apoplexy. What symptoms or findings might predict the presence of brain softening or hemorrhage (meningeal or intracerebral)? *Antoine Etienne Renaud Augustin Serres* (1787–1868) was an anatomist by training and a physician to the Hôpital de la Pitié in Paris. In a series of publications, he tried to classify and characterize the apoplexies into meaningful subdivision. Serres used a rather simple schema: he separated apoplexies into two types depending on the presence of paralysis. Paralytic cases predominated in a ratio of 4:1.[1,18] Serres noted that in those with paralysis, the brain was involved (softening or intracerebral hemorrhage) but in those without paralysis, the disorder was meningeal (subarachnoid hemorrhage). Clinically, those without paralysis had general lassitude, obtundation, slow pulse, and slow respirations. Serres, an anatomist, was interested primarily in the anatomical structures affected rather than the cause. He also described cerebellar and pontine apoplexy.[1,19]

*John Abercrombie* offered a more detailed clinical classification of apoplexy in his book on neurology published in 1828.[1,20] Abercrombie used several different clinical features to separate apoplectic sufferers into three groups. His classification depended on the presence of headache, stupor, paralysis, and on outcome. In the first group, called primary apoplexy by Abercrombie, the onset was sudden, stupor and unilateral paralysis and/or rigidity were present, and the prognosis was poor. Patients either died or remained hemiplegic. Some recovered surprisingly well. In the second group, the disorder began with sudden head pain, vomiting, and faintness or falling. The patient was usually not paralyzed. This group is identical to the nonparalytic group of Serres and undoubtedly referred to subarachnoid hemorrhage. In the third group, patients were suddenly deprived of the power on one side of the body, and often of speech, but they were not stuporous and headache often was not prominent. Large intracerebral hemorrhages and infarcts probably accounted for the findings in Abercrombie's first group, while small infarcts and hemorrhages explained the third group, for which there were little necropsy data since they survived. Rapid recovery in group one, we would now ascribe to embolism or so-called vascular insufficiency.

Abercrombie also was interested in the cause of apoplexy. He noted opaque osseous-like constrictions of arteries, and suggested as possible mechanisms of apoplexy: spasm of vessels, interruption of circulation, narrowing of arteries, and rupture of diseased vessels causing hemorrhage.[1] Others, for example *Serres, Foville, and Pinel* were inter-

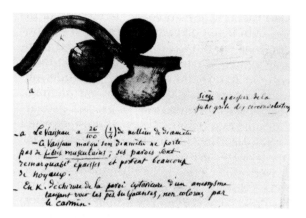

a

Siège épargné de la
substance des circonvolutions

a Le Vaisseau a $\frac{26}{100}$ $\left(\frac{1}{4}\right)$ de millim. de diamètre.
— Ce Vaisseau malgré son diamètre ne porte
pas de fibres musculaires; ses parois sont
remarquablement épaisses et portent beaucoup
de noyaux.

— En K. Déchirure de la paroi extérieure d'un anéurysme
laissant voir les pts lacunaires, non colorés par
le carmin.

**Figure 1.3.** Drawings and notes by Bouchard on Charcot-Bouchard aneurysms. (From Gautier JC. Accidents vasculaires. Rev Neurol 1982;138:939–951. With permission of the publisher.)

ested in cerebral localization and the probable location of the lesions shown by the pathologists in their atlases.[1]

In the later portion of the century, interest turned to the causes and locations of hemorrhages. *Jean Martin Charcot* (1825–1893), the great French neurologist, was clearly one of the pioneers in this interest and study.[1,21] In 1868, working with his protegé, *Charles Bouchard* (1837–1915), Charcot found small aneurysms within large intracerebral hemorrhages in three of eighty-four brains of patients dying of stroke.[2,21,22] They also found these small lesions, which resemble tiny globules of grain, along many arteries. The lesions were described in great detail and were liberally illustrated. Figure 1.3 is a picture of an original sketch by Bouchard from a review of Gautier,[21] of three miliary aneurysms along one vessel. Bouchard later published a volume about his ideas and findings in the pathology of cerebral hemorrhage.[23] Bouchard emphasized the uniqueness of intracerebral hemorrhage: ". . . hemorrhage into the substance of the brain presents itself as a distinct and separate disease characterized by changes percular to itself, and really meriting a special place in nosology."[23] Although best known for this discovery of mil-

iary aneurysms, Bouchard made some other important points. Bouchard reviewed the evidence that left ventricular hypertrophy and "a state of rigidity of the main arterial trunks or some obstacle to the flow of blood" often was found in patients with intracerebral hemorrhage. This meant that "increased tension of the fluid" probably played a role in some cases of intracerebral hemorrhage. This data of course preceded measurement of blood pressure clinically. Also, evidence was cited against the idea that atheromatous changes caused bleeding and that most intracerebral hemorrhages occurred in areas of prior softening.

*Henry Duret* (1849–1921), a prominent French neurosurgeon, was stimulated by the work of Charcot and began to study the cerebral vasculature and brain hemorrhage, especially that due to trauma. Duret was the first to illustrate secondary hemorrhages (now called Duret hemorrhages) in the upper brainstem in brain trauma specimens.[24] Duret, more importantly, was one of the first to become interested in the vascular and brain anatomy of patients with brain softenings and hemorrhages. Studying more than 200 specimens in Charcot's laboratory, Duret recognized the common distribution of these brain lesions and mapped the distribution of the anterior, middle, and posterior cerebral arteries and the distribution of deep branches to the basal gray, thalamus, and brainstem.[1,25,26] With Charcot, he described the lenticulostriate artery and dubbed it appropriately "the artery of cerebral hemorrhage."[1] In the ensuing years, *Stopford* in England[27] and *Foix* in France[28] carefully studied the anatomy, distribution, and supply zones of the large and small cerebral arteries.

In 1873, *Lidell*, a surgeon and anatomist, wrote a treatise on apoplexy and included a section on cerebral hemorrhage.[29] Lidell's description of the pathology covers most of the main features even as they are known today. "The size of the clot varies from that of a hemp-seed to that of the fist. If the extravasation occurs in the vicinity of a ventricle, it often breaks through the wall of the latter, and flows therein. Extravasations forming near the surface of the brain not unfrequently break through the cortical substance and escape into the subarachnoid space. Usually there is only one hemorrhagic effusion in the whole brain, occasionally several. The most frequent seat of these effusions is the corpus striatum, the thalamus opticus, and the large medullary masses of the cerebral hemispheres; less frequently they occur in the cortical substance of the cerebrum, in the cerebellum, and in the pons Varolii. Extravasations in the corpora quadrigemina, and in the medulla oblongata are rare; and they hardly ever occur in the corpus callosum and fornix."[29]

## State of Knowledge at the Turn of the Twentieth Century

English-speaking physicians in 1900 and in the ensuing half century who sought the latest clinical information about stroke or other neurological matters would have probably referred to William Osler's very popular textbook of medicine,[30] or to Gowers's textbook of neurology.[31] Gowers began his text on cerebral hemorrhage with a discussion of cause, unlike prior generations of writers who would doubtless have begun with symptoms or morbid anatomy. "Hemorrhage is always due to rupture of a vessel. The rupture may be the result of injury or may occur spontaneously, that is as a result solely of internal causes. The vessel that bursts is usually an artery, very rarely a vein. Capillaries may also rupture, but only minute extravasations result."[31] Gowers spoke of predisposing causes and immediate "exciting causes" at the time of bleeding. He apparently knew about hypertension. (Sphygmomanometers were not in use until 1896 and not generally available until after 1905.[2]) Gowers noted "when the wall of an artery is weakened, it yields before the blood pressure and becomes bulged."[31] He quoted the studies of Charcot and Bouchard and stated that "miliary aneurysms, as they are termed, are therefore al-

ways to be found in cases of 'spontaneous cerebral hemorrhage.' "[31] Gowers wrote of atheroma but did not think it was causally related to hemorrhage; the two merely coexisted as "senile changes." Alcoholism, gout, kidney disease, and general diseases with bleeding tendencies (purpura, scurvy, and leukemia) were all recognized to be potential predisposing factors to intracerebral hemorrhage. Writing about exciting causes, Gowers said "the actual rupture sometimes occurs during some temporary increase in the blood pressure from muscular effort, such as straining at stool, lifting a heavy weight, during coitus . . . or from excited action of the heart, consequent on emotion."[31] But sometimes, the artery gives way during sleep or seeming tranquility. Gowers wrote in some detail about the usual sites of intracerebral hemorrhage. He divided hemorrhages into the corpus striatum in three groups: anterior, middle, and posterior. Anterior lesions were caudate hemorrhages, which usually broke into the ventricle and came from the anterior cerebral artery branches. Those of the middle group were putaminal ("lenticular nucleus") and came from the lenticulostriate branches of the middle cerebral artery. Those of the posterior group were into the anterior part of the optic thalamus and Gowers falsely attributed the source to "lenticulo-optic" branches of the middle cerebral artery. Foix, a quarter of a century later, would describe the posterior cerebral artery branches to the thalamus.[28,32,33] Gowers also wrote of the pattern of dissection of these supratentorial hemorrhages and also wrote of primary ventricular, pontine, and cerebellar hemorrhages.

The description of symptoms and signs was less complete than the discussion of cause or pathology. Gowers wrote of two types of symptoms, "the one general and transient, the other local and more or less permanent. Of the general cerebral symptoms, the most common is loss of consciousness; of the local symptoms, hemiplegia."[31] He described the prototypic intracerebral hemorrhage as follows: "the patient may fall senseless without any subjective symptoms. More commonly, giddiness, pain in the head, weakness in one side, or difficulty in speaking is the first indication of the attack; and in the course of a few minutes or longer, the patient becomes unconscious and seems to go to sleep, but it is a sleep from which he can not be roused—the sleep of coma."[31] In most cases, two or three days after onset, the patient developed "febrile disturbances," for example, headaches, loss of appetite, quickening or slowing of the pulse, and a temperature rise, and might die. If and when the general symptoms subsided and the patient survived, the local symptoms would remain. Gowers knew of conjugate eye deviation as a common sign in intracerebral hemorrhage. Prognosis was usually very poor, especially if there were coma or bilateral palsies that indicated a pontine lesion. Treatment was always supportive and Gowers did not favor blood-letting.

Gowers pondered the clinical differentiation of intracerebral hemorrhage and infarction. "The attacks of simple apoplexy that occur in the old, mysterious in their nature, may resemble closely the apoplexy of cerebral hemorrhage, and it is doubtful whether the distinction between the two is possible in practice."[31] Further discussing differential diagnosis, he wrote "the most important indications are those drawn from the state of the heart in circulation, the presence of conditions favoring the bursting of an artery, especially a pulse of high tension and a strongly acting hypertrophied heart. The opposite conditions favoring the formation of a clot in a degenerated vessel, and therefore thrombotic softening."[31] Irregularity of the pulse and "degeneration" of the arteries to the limbs favored infarction. Gowers came down on the side of risk factors rather than clinical signs.

Osler's discussion of cerebral hemorrhage closely adheres to that of Gowers, and is not presented in detail here.[30] Osler emphasized morbid anatomy and phenomenology rather than cause. He stated that more than 60% of cases of intracerebral hemorrhage were from the "lenticulo-striate artery of Duret" and the "lenticulo-thalamic" artery, and involved the corpus striatum and thalamus. Osler cited rheumatic endarteritis as the cause of apoplexy causing embolism and "aneurysms" of the vessels to the brain."[30] Osler, differing from Gowers, did not always blame Charcot-Bouchard aneurysms as the cause of the intracerebral hemorrhage. He cited as an alternate cause endarteritis and periarteritis and posited that "increased permeability of the walls of the vessels may account for hemorrhages by diapedesis without actual rupture. Such hemorrhages are not uncommon in cases of contracted kidney, grave anemia, and various infections and intoxications."[30] Osler devoted considerable space to discussions of the resulting hemiplegia and conjugate eye deviation. He recognized that the side of eye deviation was opposite in cerebral and pontine lesions. Prognosis was poor. "In any case of cerebral apoplexy, the following symptoms are of grave omen: persistence or deepening of the coma during the second and third day; rapid rise in temperature within the first 48 hours . . . the rapid formation of bed sores . . . and the occurrence of albumin and sugar if abundent in the urine." Osler, agreeing with Gowers, found the differentiation between infarction and hemorrhage to be very difficult. Osler was concerned that physicians should differentiate either cause of apoplexy from a variety of other diseases, especially alcoholism.

## Aring and Merritt— Differential Diagnosis

Gowers[31] and Osler[30] had each emphasized the difficulty in clinically differentiating brain infarction from intracerebral hemorrhage. In 1935, Charles Aring and Houston Merritt reported a detailed analysis of 245 stroke cases studied clinically and at necropsy at the Boston City Hospital.[34] The stated goal of the study was "to determine the significant findings in the history and ex-

**Table 1.1.** Differential Diagnosis: Brain Hemorrhage versus Thrombosis or Embolism (Aring and Merritt[34])

| Strongly Favoring Hemorrhage | Favoring Hemorrhage | Favoring Thrombosis | Favoring Embolism | Not Helpful |
|---|---|---|---|---|
| Loss of consciousness | Younger age | Cardiac abnormalities | Cardiac abnormalities | Seasonal incidence |
| Seizures | Conjugate eye deviation | Peripheral atherosclerosis | | Activity at onset |
| Vomiting | Quadriplegia | | | Prior strokes |
| Headaches at onset | Bilateral Babinski signs | | | Premonitory symptoms |
| Higher blood pressure | Albuminuria | | | Temperature |
| Stiff neck | Leukocytosis | | | Pulse |
| Progression | Hyperglycemia | | | Hemiplegia |
| Shorter survival | Glycosuria | | | CSF protein |
| Higher CSF pressure | | | | CSF colloidal gold curve |
| Bloody CSF | | | | |

amination that will aid in the differential diagnosis between cerebral hemorrhage and cerebral thrombosis."[34] After discarding cases in which the clinical details were sparse, they studied 116 cases of cerebral hemorrhage, 106 cases of cerebral thrombosis and 23 cases of cerebral embolism. Most patients were personally examined by one of the authors. The authors analyzed the data to see which demographical, epidemiological, and historical features differentiated thrombosis from hemorrhage. They also analyzed differences in physical signs, course, prognosis, and laboratory findings. Table 1.1 lists those features that favored one or another condition and those that did not aid in the distinction. The key features favoring hemorrhage were the presence of decreased level of consciousness on admission, headache, vomiting, seizures, stiff neck, bilateral Babinski signs, conjugate eye deviation, progression of the deficit after onset, increased cerebrospinal fluid (CSF) pressure and bloody CSF. Only the presence of cardiac abnormalities and evidence of peripheral atherosclerosis favored thrombosis. All patients with embolism had cardiac abnormalities probably by definition since the diagnosis of embolism was not made unless the patient had cardiac disease. The authors

concluded that the key data items came from a thorough and detailed history and from lumbar puncture. Perhaps even more important than the findings and conclusions was the method. Aring and Merritt showed that careful, personal study of series of patients with detailed data analysis can be very useful. Their study presaged the stroke registries and data banks that became popular and productive in the second half of the twentieth century.

## The Mid-Twentieth Century—Wilson and Necropsy Series

The textbook of *Neurology*, written initially by Kinnier Wilson (1878–1937) and later by Wilson and Bruce, was certainly the most influential and widely used text in the mid-twentieth century.[35] Wilson was a master at observation and his lively prose was descriptive and unusually entertaining for a text. Wilson included some statistical data citing an incidence of 3.5% of intracranial bleeding in large necropsy series. He was less convinced than Osler and Gowers of the importance of the miliary aneurysms of Charcot and Bouchard in causing intracerebral hemorrhage.

Wilson noted the importance of transient fluctuations of blood pressure, presaging more recent observations. "Prolonged or severe muscular effort is a conventional excitant as in straining at stool, lifting weights, coughing, sneezing, vomiting, laughing, running, during coitus, and so on. . . . Emotional experience, joy, anger, fear or apprehension may disturb the action of the heart, trivial though the incident may be—an address at a public meeting, trouble with the cook, and so on."[35] Wilson recognized that subcortical hemorrhages frequently "cause fits," and pointed out that "capsular" hematomas were associated with diverse symptoms depending on whether the anterior "geniculate" or posterior divisions were involved. The syndrome of pontine hemorrhage was better defined than by Osler and Gowers due to citation of several necropsy series in the years between 1905 and 1951. Wilson, rather accurately, listed the symptoms of "less tragic cases" of cerebral hemorrhage: "pain at the back of the head, nausea, vomiting, acute vertigo, sense of rotation of objects, ataxia, inability to stand upright, stiffness of the neck."[34] Wilson reviewed the sites of hemorrhages in prior pathological series.

Though Wilson discussed his own rules for diagnosing intracerebral hemorrhage, he was skeptical of their value. "Distinctions between hemorrhage and thrombosis . . . often appear more impressive on paper than during anxious moments at the bedside." Wilson, as had his predecessors, wrote of the poor prognosis of intracerebral hemorrhage. "The immediate and more distant outlook is anxious. Initial attacks are seldom followed by complete and lasting cure." He further commented, "as tokens of the gravity of the condition the observer will regard 1) depth and duration of coma, 2) embarassment of heart and breathing, 3) bilaterality of symptoms, 4) fall or pronounced rise of body temperature." These features would similarly be considered today as predicting a grave outlook. Little was said of treatment of intracerebral hemorrhage.

During the early and middle portions of the twentieth century, a number of necropsy series defined better the pathological findings and usual loci of bleeding as well as the frequency of the various etiologies. Among 235 cases of massive intracerebral hemorrhage, Mutlu et al. found that 60% were hypertensive, 20% aneurysmal, 13% due to blood dyscrasias, and 3% due to angiomas.[36] The basal ganglia region was the site of bleeding in 70% of cases (including a mesial group that included the caudate and thalamus), the cerebral lobes in 24%, and brainstem in 6%.[36] In a larger series of 393 fatal hemorrhages studied by Lindenberg and Freytag, 42% were in the "striate body," 10% pontine, 15% thalamic, 12% cerebellar, and 10% cerebral white matter.[37] This series came from the medical examiner's office in Baltimore, Maryland. Freytag noted that blacks were particularly susceptible to intracerebral hemorrhage, and hemorrhages in blacks often occurred at an earlier age than in whites.[37]

## C. Miller Fisher

In considering the historical development of ideas concerning any area of cerebral vascular disease, it would be difficult to omit the contributions of C. Miller Fisher (Figure 1.4). This is especially true with respect to cerebral hemorrhage since Fisher made sentinel contributions to knowledge about both pathological and clinical aspects. Fisher's earliest most complete observations and thoughts about the pathology, pathogenesis, and clinical aspects of intracerebral hemorrhage were presented at a meeting of the Houston Neurological Society in 1959. The presentations and discussions were subsequently compiled and edited by William Fields in 1961.[38,39] Fisher and his colleagues subsequently included much of their didactic thinking in the very popular editions of *Harrison's Principles of Internal Medicine*.[40]

Fisher made some important pathological observations. He pointed out that small hem-

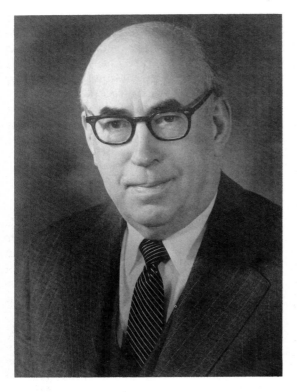

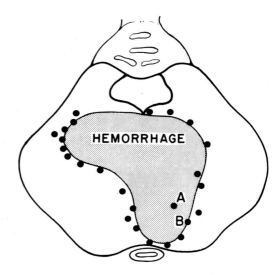

**Figure 1.5.** Diagram of fibrin globe bleeding spots in a pontine hematoma. A and B are areas of large fibrin globes. (From Fisher CM. Pathological observations in hypertensive cerebral hemorrhages. J Neuropathol Exp Neurol 1971;30:536–550. With permission of the publisher.)

**Figure 1.4.** C. Miller Fisher.

orrhages (less than 0.5 cm) were found most often in association with recent or old hematomas. He commented "the fact that hypertensive hemorrhages can be of such restricted size is often lost sight of at the bedside."[38] He then cited two personally examined specimens with twenty to thirty 1-mm and fifteen 1-mm to 6-mm hemorrhages. Fisher also discussed "old hemorrhages" found in the brains of persons dying at a chronic disease hospital, commented on their "slit"-like shape and pointed out that although "not harmless" some patients made good recoveries. "That almost all intracerebral hemorrhages are necessarily fatal or accompanied by a deep coma is a clinical dictum that needs drastic modification."[38] Fisher noted in that early presentation and in much more detail later[41] that along the periphery of the hematoma there were many, small, globoid caps that represented small

bleeding capillaries or arterioles. He believed that the hemorrhage probably developed gradually with pressure effects leading to secondary pressure on small vessels on the periphery that then led to further bleeding. The hematoma enlarged on its periphery like a snowball picking up snow as it rolls downhill. Figure 1.5 is from Fisher's study of pontine hemorrhage,[41] illustrating the loci of bleeding sites at the periphery of a pontine hematoma studied in serial section. Fisher was also not impressed that the Charcot-Bouchard concept of miliary aneurysms satisfactorily accounted for most cases of intracerebral hemorrhage. He described two examples of atypically located hematomas that developed while the patients were being given vasopressors in the operating room. "Since the disaster occurred immediately, it is almost certain that a miliary aneurysm, a hyalin change, and fibrinoid impregnation could not have been factors."

Though Fisher considers himself a pathologist, most would agree that his major contributions were clinical. He made some sentinel observations in discussing the clinical findings in intracerebral hemorrhage.[39] He noted that the deficit most often did not develop instantly. "When the hemorrhage occurs when the patient is under observation, it will be found that the deficit comes not instantaneously, but gradually and steadily over an appreciable length of time, possibly ten minutes or a few hours, or even a few days (rarely 7–14 days)."[39] He contrasted this course with fluctuating signs in thrombosis and lightning-like onset in embolism. He pointed out that headache was not invariable. "It is commonly stated that headache is a prominent feature in intracerebral hemorrhage but this is by no means the rule and indeed in our clinical material, somewhat fewer than half of the patients have complained of headache."[39] He also emphasized that not all patients had reduced alertness or stiff neck. Fisher discussed the clinical signs in hematomas at the various common sites. He was the first to discuss in this and a prior report[42] the signs in thalamic hemorrhage. Previously, authors had grouped thalamic and putaminal hemorrhages together clinically. Especially emphasized were the eye signs, abnormalities of pupillary and oculomotor function. Eyes looking down and in, vertical gaze palsies, "wrong way eyes" with congugate deviation opposite to that usually seen in supratentorial lesions, and "pseudosixth palsy" were all described first by Fisher.[39,42,43] The speech and behavioral manifestations were also mentioned.[39,44] In pontine hemorrhage, Fisher noted the presence of a bobbing motion ("ocular dance").[40,44] Fisher and his colleagues described the clinical syndrome of cerebellar hemorrhage.[45] Previous authors had concluded that this disorder was not readily diagnosable clinically. In cerebellar hemorrhages, ipsilateral conjugate gaze paralysis without a hemiplegia was considered diagnostic of a cerebellar localization of a hematoma.[40,45]

Fisher later was very active in early computed tomography–clinical correlations. By his meticulous observations and careful analysis, he stimulated many of his protegés and students, including J. P. Mohr and the present authors, to make contributions in the areas of intracerebral hemorrhage. He said that "neurology is learned stroke by stroke" and that learning all about the findings in hematomas at various locations would go a long way toward understanding brain localization.

## Neuroimaging Technology and Angiography

And then came computed tomography (CT). No other discovery in any field of medicine or neurology has led to as much change in knowledge and practice as that of the introduction of CT. With regard to brain hemorrhage, the change in the evaluation and management of patients was so dramatic that historians in retrospect might easily divide care into BCT (before CT) and ACT (after CT). Godfrey Hounsfield of the research laboratories of EMI Ltd. in Great Britain originated the concept of CT and the instrument was first tried at the Atkinson-Morley Hospital in London.[2] CT scanners were first introduced into North America in 1973. Scans from first generation scanners were very primitive when compared with the present films. The technology quickly advanced and by the late 1970s second and third generation scanners were available in most large academic medical centers. By the mid 1980s, CT was readily available throughout North America.

CT proved to be nearly an ideal technology for the diagnosis of intracerebral hemorrhage. Hemorrhages appeared as white, hyperdense lesions in stark distinction from neighboring tissues, which imaged gray or black. Lesions were distinct and easily seen even by the novitiate. Not only could CT clearly distinguish among hemorrhage, infarction, and normal brain, but CT also showed the size of the lesion, the presence of surrounding edema, the path of the spread of the lesion, drainage into the ventricular system, and mass effects on the adjacent brain and on the ventricular system.[46]

Prior to CT, clinical distinction between infarction and hemorrhage was clearly inaccurate. Daslgaard-Nielsen examined the accuracy of clinical diagnosis in his necropsy series: of 239 strokes diagnosed clinically as hemorrhage, only 155 (65%) were hemorrhages at necropsy and only 58% of infarcts were diagnosed accurately.[47,48] More recently, studies in patients whose hemorrhages were confirmed by CT, rather than necropsy, showed that the clinical features often do not allow accurate separation of infarction from hemorrhage.[49,50]

The capability of diagnosing intracerebral hemorrhage with certainty in patients with stroke was a great advance. Ideas, concepts, and teachings about intracerebral hemorrhage had been derived from careful study of series of patients studied at necropsy. Clinico-pathological series were biased toward larger hemorrhages that led to death. New clinical-CT correlations could include even small and moderate-sized lesions from which patients survived, sometimes with very minor residual deficits.[51] The rules about the general findings in patients with intracerebral hemorrhage, derived so carefully by Osler, Gowers, Wilson, and Fisher, had to be revised to include smaller lesions. The frequency of headache, seizures, loss of consciousness, vomiting, and other general signs in patients with intracerebral hemorrhage had to be revised. The present authors were fortunate to be actively investigating stroke and intracerebral hemorrhage and to have available CT early in its introduction. CT allowed analysis of the general features of patients with intracerebral hemorrhage collected in the Harvard Stroke Registry in the mid-1970s and the findings were in sharp contrast to earlier teachings.[52,53,54] By defining more throughly the location of hematomas, CT also allowed considerable clarification of the usual symptoms and signs found in patients with hemorrhages at various brain sites. New syndromes, such as caudate hemorrhage[55,56] and lateral tegmental brainstem hemorrhage,[57,58] were reported. The process of the development and resolution of hematomas could also be now studied in some detail.

The advent of nuclear magnetic resonance (first called NMR and now called magnetic resonance imaging [MRI]) into clinical brain imaging in the mid-1980s was a further advance. MRI, by showing hemosiderin-containing regions, allowed detection of older hemorrhages. MRI was superior to CT in showing lesions that abutted on bony areas, for example, traumatic contusions and hematomas on the orbital surface of the frontal lobes and in the anterior and inferior temporal lobes. MRI allowed better definition of posterior fossa hemorrhages and vascular malformations such as cavernous angiomas and arteriovenous malformations (AVM). MRI also allowed easier viewing of the lesions in multiple planes: horizontal, coronal, sagittal, and so forth.

Though angiography was introduced into clinical neurology in 1927 by Moniz,[59] early studies were rather primitive. A cutdown or surgical procedure was required to introduce rather toxic dyes and the films were suboptimal. Even in 1969 when one of us (LRC) was a stroke fellow at the Massachusetts General Hospital, films were still hand pulled and only one view was obtainable at a time. Advances in technology led to safer angiography in the 1960s and 1970s. Cerebral angiography was very important in providing information and knowledge about the causes of intracerebral hemorrhage. Opacification of arteries usually led to the detection of aneurysms, AVM, and extracerebral collections of blood. Aneurysmal hemorrhage could be separated from spontaneous intracerebral hemorrhage. AVM could be better studied. Angiography for a long time was the best way to detect the location and mass effects of space-occupying lesions such as hematomas. Displacement of arteries and ventricular enlargement could be defined and were helpful in diagnosis and prognosis.[60] The introduction of CT and MRI has led to reduced need for angiography in evaluating patients with suspected or known intracerebral hemorrhage.

## Stroke Registries, Data Banks, and Series of Cases

Fisher and his predecessors emphasized the importance of detailed history and meticulous general and neurological examinations and data recording. Now that the pathological and clinical features were generally known, interest began to focus on the acquisition of more quantitative data. How often did intracerebral hemorrhage and the other subtypes of stroke occur? How often did each of the features occur in each of the subtypes of stroke? Aring and Merritt had led the way by showing the value of collecting a large series of cases that were well studied. But clinicians recognized that true frequency data could not be obtained if the series included only fatal cases. Clearly, to yield valid, statistically meaningful results, series had to be large and include all representative patients. Large series of cases, and formal registries and data banks were collected to provide the quantitative data sought. The advent of computers greatly facilitated the storage and analysis of large quantities of data, and the introduction of neuroimaging and ultrasound technology in the 1970s and 1980s facilitated more accurate stroke diagnoses. Many of the participants in the collection of series, particularly the authors of this monograph, were students or fellows of Fisher, or were taught by Fisher's protegés.

The initial studies, like that of Aring and Merritt, were retrospective. Dalsgaard-Nielsen in 1955[47] and 1956[48] reviewed one thousand cases of apoplexy admitted to the Neurological Department of the Fredericksburg Hospital in Denmark. There were 432 cases (43%) of hemorrhage, 500 patients with thromboses (50%), and 68 cases of embolism (6.8%). Much of the data were demographical and epidemiological. Dalsgaard-Nielsen combined all cases of hemorrhage and did not separate subarachnoid from intracerebral hemorrhage. Neurologists and epidemiologists studied the natural history of stroke in Rochester, Minnesota, taking advantage of the extensive data collection system of the Mayo Clinic. First, patients seen between 1945 and 1954 were analyzed,[61] and later the data from 1955 through 1969 were studied and the groups were compared.[62] During the later period, 71% of strokes were judged thrombotic, 8% embolic, 10% intracerebral hemorrhage, and 6% subarachnoid hemorrhage. Incidence and prevalence rates were estimated for the population, and outcome and recurrence of strokes were the major features analyzed.[61,62]

In 1972, a different type of case collection was begun at two hospitals in Boston. This series, called the Harvard Cooperative Stroke Registry by its founders, differed in three important ways from its predecessors.[54] The collaborators decided on the information that they would record and collected all data *prospectively*, ensuring that the desired information would be available. The major focus was not epidemiological but was the nuances and details of the risk factors, historical features, course, and physical findings. A large computer was used to store and retrieve data. Also, in the later years of the Harvard Stroke Registry, CT data were included, making the ascertainment of intracerebral hemorrhage more reliable. Ten percent of the 694 patients had intracerebral hemorrhage,[54] a figure nearly identical to that found in Rochester, Minnesota.[61,62] Later, a number of other registries and data banks including the Pilot Stroke Data Bank,[63] the Stroke Data Bank,[64] the Michael Reese Stroke Registry,[65] the Austin Hospital Registry,[66] and the Lausanne Stroke Registry[67] reported their series of hospital-based stroke cases. All were prospective, included CT results, and utilized computers for storage and analysis of data. A number of population-based series also appeared because stroke epidemiologists recognized that series of cases studied at academic hospitals were probably biased and not representative of the community at large. South Alabama,[68] Framingham,[69,70] Oxfordshire,[71,72] Lehigh Valley,[73] and a consortium from North Carolina, Oregon, and New York[74,75] were the sites of the community projects, many of which are still

**Table 1.2.** Percentage of Patients with ICH in Various Series

| Series | % ICH |
|---|---|
| Denmark (Dalsgaard-Nielsen)[47] | 43 |
| Rochester, MN 1945–1954[61] | 10 |
| Rochester, MN 1955–1969[62] | 10 |
| Harvard Stroke Registry[54] | 10 |
| Pilot Stroke Data Bank[63] | 8.8 |
| Stroke Data Bank[64] | 16 |
| Michael Reese Registry[65] | 14 |
| Austin Stroke Unit[66] | 6 |
| Lausanne Stroke Registry[67] | 11 |
| South Alabama[68] | 8 |
| Framingham Study[69,70] | 5 |
| Oxfordshire Community Stroke Project[71,72] | 10 |
| Lehigh Valley[73] | 8 |
| Community Hospital-based Stroke Programs[74,75] | 10 |

active. The frequency of intracerebral hemorrhage in these various studies is listed in Table 1.2. Mohr[76] and Caplan[77] have reviewed the functions and utilities of stroke registries. The only feature of intracerebral hemorrhage that has not been systematically studied has been treatment.

## References

1. McHenry LC. Garrison's history of neurology. Revised and Enlarged. Springfield: Charles C Thomas, 1969.
2. Fields WS, Lemak AN. A history of stroke: its recognition and treatment. New York: Oxford University Press, 1989.
3. Nuland, S. Doctors, the biography of medicine. Birmingham: Libraries of Gryphon Editions, 1988.
4. Adams F. The genuine works of Hippocrates. Translated from the Greek. Baltimore: Williams & Wilkins, 1939.
5. Clark E. Apoplexy in the hippocratic writings. Bull Hist Med 1963;37:301–314.
6. Vesalius A. De humani corporis fabrica. Basiliae: J. Oporini, 1543.
7. Wepfer JJ. Observationes anatomicae ex cadaveribus eorum, quos sustulit apoplexia cum exercitatione de ejus loco afecto. Schaffhausen: John Caspari Suteri, 1658.
8. Mistichelli D. Trattato dell apoplessia. Roma: A de Rossi alla Piazza di Ceri, 1709.
9. Bayle F. Tractatus de apoplexia. Toulousse: B Guillemette, 1677.
10. Morgagni GB. The seats and causes of diseases investigated by anatomy. Translated by B Alexander. London: Millar and Cadell, 1769. Birmingham Classics of Medicine Library.
11. Cheyne J. Cases of apoplexy and lethargy with observations upon the comatose diseases. London: J Moyes, Printer, 1812.
12. Cooke J. A treatise on nervous diseases. Vol. I. On apoplexy. London: Longman, Hurst, Rees, Orme and Brown, 1820.
13. Hooper R. The morbid anatomy of the human brain, illustrated by coloured engravings of the most frequent and important organic diseases to which that viscus is subject. London: Longman, Hurst, Rees, Orme, Brown, and Green, 1828. (Special edition, the classics of neurology and neurosurgery library. Birmingham: Gryphon Editions, 1984.)
14. Cruveilhier J. Anatomie pathologique du corps humain: description avec figures lithographiques et colorées des diverses altérations morbides dont le corps humain est susceptible. Paris: J. B. Bailliére, 1835–1842.
15. Carswell R. Pathological anatomy: illustrations of the elementary forms of disease. London: Longman, 1838.
16. Bright R. Reports of medical cases, selected with a view of illustrating the symptoms and cure of diseases by a reference to morbid anatomy. Vol. II. Disease of the brain and nervous system. London: Longman, Rees, Orme, Brown, and Green, 1831.
17. Bright R. Cases illustrative of the effects produced when the arteries and brain are diseased. Guy's Hosp Rep 1836;1:9.
18. Serres AER. New divisions of apoplexies. Phil J Med Phys Sci 1823;7:227; 1824;8:89,53,304.
19. Serres AER. Sur les maladies organiques du cervelet. Des apoplexies cérébelleuses. J Physiol Exp Path 1822;2:172, 249.
20. Abercrombie J. Pathological and practical researches on diseases of the brain and spinal cord. Edinburgh: Waugh and Innes, 1828.
21. Gautier JC. Accidents vasculaires. Rev Neurol 1982;138:939–951.
22. Charcot JM, Bouchard C. Nouvelles recherches sur la pathogénie de l'hémorragie cé-

rébrale. Arch Physiol Norm Path 1868;1:110–127, 643–665, 725–734.

23. Bouchard C. A study of some points in the pathology of cerebral haemorrhage. London: Simpkin, Marshall, 1872.

24. Duret H. Études experimentales et cliniques sur les traumatismes cérébraux. Paris: V Adrien Delahayes, 1878.

25. Duret H. Sur la distribution des artères nourriciéres du bulbe rachidien. Arch Physiol Norm Pathol 1873;2:97–113.

26. Duret H. Recherches anatomiques sur la circulation de l'encéphale. Arch Physiol Norm Pathol 1874;60–91, 316–353, 664–693, 919–957.

27. Stopford JS. The arteries of the pons and medulla oblongata. J Anat Physiol 1928;50:255–280.

28. Caplan LR. Charles Foix—the first modern stroke neurologist. Stroke 1990, 21:348–356.

29. Lidell JA. A treatise on apoplexy, cerebral hemorrhage, cerebral embolism, cerebral gout, cerebral rheumatism and epidemic cerebro-spinal meningitis. New York: Wm. Wood, 1873. (Reprinted as part of the classics of neurology and neurosurgery library. Birmingham: Gryphon Editions.)

30. Osler W. The principles and practice of medicine. Fifth Edition. New York: D Appleton, 1903;997–1008.

31. Gowers WR. A manual of diseases of the nervous system. London: J and A Churchill, 1893;384–413.

32. Foix C, Masson A. Le syndrome de l'artère cérébrale postérieure. Presse Med 1923;31:361–365.

33. Foix C, Hillemand P. Les syndromes de la région thalamique. Presse Med 1925;33:113–117.

34. Aring CD, Merritt HH. Differential diagnosis between cerebral hemorrhage and cerebral thrombosis: A clinical and pathologic study of 245 cases. Arch Intern Med 1935;56:435–456.

35. Wilson SAK, Bruce AN. Neurology. Second Edition. London: Butterworth, 1955;1367–1383.

36. Mutlu N, Berry RG, Alpers BJ. Massive cerebral hemorrhage: clinical and pathological correlations. Arch Neurol 1963;8:644–661.

37. Freytag E. Fatal hypertensive intracerebral haematomas: a survey of the pathological anatomy of 393 cases. J Neurol Neurosurg Psychiatry 1968;31:616–620.

38. Fisher CM. The pathology and pathogenesis of intracerebral hemorrhage. In Fields WS, ed.

Pathogenesis and treatment of cerebrovascular disease. Springfield: Charles C Thomas, 1961;295–317.

39. Fisher CM. Clinical syndromes in cerebral hemorrhage. In Fields WS, ed. Pathogenesis and treatment of cerebrovascular disease. Springfield: Charles C Thomas, 1961;318–342.

40. Mohr JP, Fisher CM, Adams RD. Cerebrovascular diseases. In Thorn GW, et al. eds. Harrison's principles of internal medicine. Eighth Edition. New York: McGraw-Hill, 1977;1832–1868.

41. Fisher CM. Pathological observations in hypertensive cerebral hemorrhage. J Neuropathol Exp Neurol 1971;30:536–550.

42. Fisher CM. The pathologic and clinical aspects of thalamic hemorrhage. Trans Am Neurol Assoc 1959;84:56–59.

43. Fisher CM. Some neuro-ophthalmological observations. J Neurol Neurosurg Psychiat 1967;30:383–392.

44. Fisher CM. Ocular bobbing. Arch Neurol 1964;11:543–546.

45. Fisher CM, Picard EH, Polak A, et al. Acute hypertensive cerebellar hemorrhage: diagnosis and surgical treatment. J Nerv Ment Dis 1965;140:38–57.

46. Scott WR, New PFJ, Davis KR, et al. Computerized axial tomography of intracerebral and intraventricular hemorrhage. Radiology 1974;112:73–80.

47. Dalsgaard-Nielsen T. Survey of 1000 cases of apoplexia cerebri. Acta Psychiatr Neurol Scand 1955;30:169–185.

48. Dalsgaard-Nielsen T. Some clinical experience in the treatment of cerebral apoplexy (1000 cases). Acta Psychiatr Neurol Scand (Suppl) 1956;108:101–119.

49. Allen CMC. Clinical diagnosis of the acute stroke syndrome. Quart J Med 1983;52:515–523.

50. Harrison MJ. Clinical distinction of cerebral haemorrhage and cerebral infarction. Postgrad Med J 1980;56:629–632.

51. Weisberg LA. Computerized tomography in intracranial hemorrhage. Arch Neurol 1979;36:422–426.

52. Caplan LR, Mohr JP. Intracerebral hemorrhage: an update. Geriatrics 1978;33:42–52.

53. Caplan LR. Intracerebral hemorrhage: new clues to an old entity. Med Times 1978;106:55–61.

54. Mohr JP, Caplan LR, Melski JW, et al. The Harvard Cooperative Stroke Registry: a prospective registry. Neurology 1978;28:754–762.

55. Stein RW, Kase CS, Hier DB, et al. Caudate hemorrhage. Neurology 1984;34:1549–1554.

56. Weisberg LA. Caudate hemorrhage. Arch Neurol 1984;41:971–974.

57. Caplan LR, Goodwin JA. Lateral tegmental brainstem hemorrhages. Neurology 1982;32:252–260.

58. Kase CS, Maulsby GO, Mohr JP. Partial pontine hematomas. Neurology 1980;30:652–655.

59. Moniz E. L'encéphalographie artérielle, son importance dans la localisation des tumeurs cérébrales. Rev Neurol 1927;2:72–90.

60. Mizukami M, Araki G, Mihara H. Angiographic sign of good prognosis for hemiplegia in hypertensive intracerebral hemorrhage. Neurology 1974;24:120–126.

61. Whisnant JP, Fitzgibbons JP, Kurland LT, et al. Natural history of stroke in Rochester, Minnesota, 1945 through 1954. Stroke 1971;2:11–22.

62. Matsumoto N, Whisnant JP, Kurland LT, et al. Natural history of stroke in Rochester, Minnesota, 1955 through 1969: an extension of a previous study, 1945 through 1954. Stroke 1973;4:20–29.

63. Kunitz SC, Gross CR, Heyman A, et al. The Pilot Stroke Data Bank: definition, design and data. Stroke 1984;15:740–746.

64. Foulkes MA, Wolf PA, Price TR, et al. The Stroke Data Bank: design, methods and baseline characteristics. Stroke 1988;19:547–554.

65. Caplan LR, Hier DB, D'Cruz I. Cerebral embolism in the Michael Reese Stroke Registry. Stroke 1983;14:530–536.

66. Chambers BR, Donnan GA, Bladin PF. Patterns of stroke: an analysis of the first 700 consecutive admissions to the Austin Hospital Stroke Unit. Aust NZ J Med. 1983;13:57–64.

67. Bogousslavsky J, Van Melle G, Regli F. The Lausanne Stroke Registry: analysis of 1,000 consecutive patients with first stroke. Stroke 1988;19:1083–1092.

68. Gross CR, Kase CS, Mohr JP, et al. Stroke in South Alabama: Incidence and diagnostic features—a population based study. Stroke 1984;15:249–255.

69. Kannel WB, Dawber TR, Cohen ME, McNamara PM. Vascular disease of the brain—epidemiologic aspects: the Framingham Study. Am J Publ Hlth 1965;55:1355–1366.

70. Wolf PA, Kannel WB, Dawber TR. Prospective investigations: the Framingham Study and the epidemiology of stroke. Adv Neurol 1978;19:107–120.

71. Oxfordshire Community Stroke Project. Incidence of stroke in Oxfordshire: first year's experience of a community stroke register. Br Med J 1983;287:713–717.

72. Bamford J, Sandercock P, Dennis M, et al. A prospective study of acute cerebrovascular disease in the community: the Oxfordshire Community Stroke Project—1981–96: 2. Incidence, case fatality rates and overall outcome at one year of cerebral infarction, primary intracerebral and subarachnoid haemorrhage. J Neurol Neurosurg Psychiatry 1990;53:16–22.

73. Alter M, Sobel E, McCoy RL, et al. Stroke in the Lehigh Valley: incidence based on a community-wide hospital register. Neuroepidemiology 1985;4:1–15.

74. Yatsu FM, Becker C, McLeroy KR, et al. Community hospital-based stroke programs: North Carolina, Oregon and New York: I: goals, objectives, and data collection procedures. Stroke 1986;17:276–284.

75. Becker C, Howard G, McLeroy K, et al. Community hospital-based stroke programs: North Carolina, Oregon and New York: II: description of study population. Stroke 1986;17:285–293.

76. Mohr JP. Stroke data banks. Stroke 1986;17:171–172 (editorial).

77. Caplan LR. Stroke data banks, then and now. In Courbier R, ed. Basis for a classification of cerebrovascular disease. Amsterdam: Excerpta Medica, 1985;152–162.

# Chapter 2

# Epidemiology of Intracerebral Hemorrhage

## Philip A. Wolf*

## Background and Magnitude of the Problem

Cerebral apoplexy, stroke as a consequence of spontaneous bleeding into the brain, has been known since antiquity and is referred to in writings attributed to Hippocrates. Modern imaging has facilitated the differentiation of hemorrhage from infarction and is widely available in most developed countries. Nevertheless, questions about disease mechanisms, risk factors, and, therefore, prevention and treatment persist. Differentiation of intracerebral hemorrhages (ICH) resulting from amyloid angiopathy, cryptic vascular malformations, arteritis, or hypertension is not easily accomplished, even with magnetic resonance imaging (MRI) and computed tomography (CT), and this diagnostic uncertainty seriously impedes the study of the epidemiology and natural history of ICH.

There are a number of unresolved issues and unexplained phenomena in the epidemiology of ICH. These include a wide variation in hemorrhage rates in different racial groups. The incidence is highest in Asians,

*Supported in part by Grants 2-RO1-NS-17950-11 (National Institute of Neurological Disorders and Stroke), 1-R01-AG-08122-05 (National Institute on Aging) and Contract NIH-NO1-HC-38038 (National Heart, Lung, and Blood Institute).

intermediate in blacks and lowest in whites; rates in Asians are many times higher than in whites. The mechanisms underlying these differing racial susceptibilities are unknown. Although the disease has often been referred to as "hypertensive" ICH, and there is little doubt that elevated blood pressure promotes it, other factors that influence and modify the impact of increased blood pressure are still being identified. Recent attention has focused on the association of low serum total cholesterol and an increased incidence of ICH; the mechanism underlying this relationship is unclear. Heavy alcohol consumption, cigarette smoking, dietary patterns, and use of oral contraceptives have also been implicated as risk factors for ICH. Also reported are seasonal variations in hemorrhage occurrence— winter and cold weather are times of highest hemorrhage incidence. Illicit drugs, including cocaine and amphetamines, by oral, nasal, and intravenous routes, have been associated with ICH. There have been a number of anecdotal reports of hemorrhage associated with phenylpropanolamine, a frequent ingredient in widely available over-the-counter appetite suppressants and nasal decongestants.

Death rates from ICH have fallen dramatically during the past twenty years in parallel with the overall decrease in stroke deaths. It seems likely that this is a result of a decline in incidence of the disease, due to modification of risk factors, particularly improved control of hypertension. In recent years, substantial strides have been taken in reaching an understanding of the frequency and determinants of ICH. It seems ironic that this understanding of pathogenetic mechanisms is occurring as death rates and incidence of the disease are plummeting worldwide. Some of these findings are also applicable to subarachnoid hemorrhage, and both forms of intracranial hemorrhage are major contributors to death and disability in middle-aged adults. There is no convincing evidence, however, that major advances in surgical or medical treatment have played any substantive role in reducing case-fatality rates or in improving useful recovery from ICH. An understanding of the risk factors promoting hemorrhage may lead to further strategies for prevention of this frequently fatal and disabling disease. Review of the current state of knowledge of the frequency and determinants of all causes of intracranial hemorrhage is beyond the scope of this chapter, which focuses on the epidemiology of primary spontaneous ICH.

## Epidemiology

### Incidence

Reliable estimates of the incidence of ICH and identification of predisposing factors have been hampered by the relative infrequency of well-documented cases in defined populations. The small numbers of cases occurring in most United States and European series make such efforts difficult.[1] Intracranial hemorrhage in the United States and Western Europe accounts for less than 20% of all strokes. After thirty-six years of follow-up of the general population sample of 5070 men and women, ages 30 to 62 years at entry, at Framingham, Massachusetts, 541 completed strokes had occurred. Of the total, 81 were due to intracranial hemorrhage: 35 intracerebral, and 46 subarachnoid, the latter largely due to ruptured berry aneurysm (Table 2.1).[2] Thus, ICH accounted for a small fraction of total strokes, representing 7.5% of all stroke cases in men and 5.6% in women.

Similarly, during thirty years of case collection in Rochester, Minnesota, 180 cases of spontaneous ICH occurred: 142 were categorized as primary, 19 arose from aneurysm, 7 from arteriovenous malformation, and 22 were a consequence of other illness, particularly bleeding diatheses.[3] Between 1955 and 1979, incidence of hemorrhage was low in the Rochester, Minnesota, population.[4] During this period, 83 *primary* ICH occurred in the entire Rochester, Minnesota, population (Table 2.2). Average annual age-adjusted incidence of primary ICH above age 35 was 6 per 100,000 in men, and 7 per 100,000 in women. Incidence more than doubled with each decade of age after age 35 (see Table 2.2).

In a population of 103,358 persons residing in a circumscribed region of southern Alabama, intensive surveillance was conducted to achieve complete stroke ascertainment and systematic categorization according to stroke type.[5] In the calendar year 1980, 13 parenchymatous and 9 subarachnoid hemorrhages were identified.

Hospital record review of all residents of the Cincinnati metropolitan area admitted for spontaneous ICH during the calendar year 1982 yielded 154 cases fulfilling the authors' criteria[6] (Table 2.3). On the basis of these 154 ICH, incidence rates were computed. The rate per 100,000 was 17.5 for blacks, 13.5 for whites, 15.1 for women, and 12.6 for men. Twenty-seven of these cases would not properly be categorized as primary ICH since the hemorrhages were associated with leukemia, anticoagulant medication, arteriovenous malformation, and neoplasm.

A more comprehensive assessment of hemorrhage in the Cincinnati metropolitan area, in 1988, yielded 186 cases, and included 25 "secondary" hemorrhage cases among the 1,267,924 residents (Table 2.4).[7] Of the 25 episodes of ICH resulting from known mech-

**Table 2.1.** Frequency of Stroke by Type, 36-Year Follow-up. The Framingham Study, Ages 35–94[2]

| Stroke Type | Men No. | Men Percent | Women No. | Women Percent | Total No. | Total Percent |
|---|---|---|---|---|---|---|
| ABI | 141 | 59.0 | 164 | 54.3 | 305 | 56.4 |
| CE | 59 | 24.7 | 86 | 28.5 | 145 | 26.8 |
| ICH | 18 | 7.5 | 17 | 5.6 | 35 | 6.4 |
| SAH | 19 | 7.9 | 27 | 8.9 | 46 | 8.5 |
| Other | 2 | 0.8 | 8 | 2.6 | 10 | 1.8 |
| Total stroke | 239 | | 302 | | 541 | |
| Isolated TIA | 74 | | 73 | | 147 | |
| Total cerebro-vascular events | 313 | | 375 | | 688 | |

Abbreviations: ABI = atherothrombotic brain infarction, CE = cerebral embolus with a cardiac source, ICH = intracerebral hemorrhage, SAH = subarachnoid hemorrhage, TIA = transient ischemic attack.

anisms, 10 were due to ruptured arteriovenous malformation, 3 occurred as hemorrhage into a tumor, 11 were from bleeding diatheses, and 1 as a result of cocaine ingestion. Including all 186 cases, these data disclose an overall age- and sex-adjusted incidence of hemorrhage in blacks that is 1.4-fold greater than in whites. Below age 75, however, the incidence was 2.3 times higher in blacks, perhaps a consequence of the increased prevalence of hypertension among blacks.[7]

In striking contrast, population-based series from Asia, specifically from Japan, included thousands of stroke cases. Hemorrhage accounted for approximately 25% of all strokes, and intraparenchymatous hemor-

rhage comprised two-thirds of the total.[8,9] Hemorrhage was a frequent mechanism of stroke in the 8,006 Japanese men living in Hawaii who were participants in the Honolulu Heart Study.[10,11] After eighteen years of follow-up, 490 strokes had occurred, of which 116 were hemorrhages.[11] Much of the information concerning the epidemiology of ICH has been determined from study of this and other Asian populations.

Incidence of ICH in the Japanese community of Hisayama was 310 per 100,000 among men age 40 or older in 1961 to 1970.[9] With time, incidence fell dramatically; in 1974 to 1983 incidence was 120 per 100,000. Even this reduced later incidence was eight times higher than the incidence in the greater Cin-

**Table 2.2.** Average Annual Age- and Sex-specific Incidence Rates of Intracerebral Hemorrhage in Rochester, Minnesota per 100,000 Population for 1955–1979

| Age in Years | Males No. | Males Rate | Females No. | Females Rate | Total No. | Total Rate |
|---|---|---|---|---|---|---|
| <34 | 1 | 0.3 | 1 | 0.3 | 2 | 0.3 |
| 35–54 | 4 | 3 | 3 | 2 | 7 | 3 |
| 55–64 | 8 | 20 | 9 | 17 | 17 | 18 |
| 65–74 | 16 | 64 | 13 | 31 | 29 | 44 |
| >75 | 6 | 39 | 22 | 65 | 28 | 57 |
| Total >35 | 34 | 6 | 47 | 7 | 81 | 7 |

(Adapted from Drury I, Whisnant JP, Garraway WM. Primary intracerebral hemorrhage: impact of CT on incidence. Neurology 1984;34:653–657.)

**Table 2.3.** Incidence of Spontaneous Intracerebral Hemorrhage, Men and Women Combined, Greater Cincinnati 1982

| Age in Years | Number | Incidence/100,000 | % Hypertensive |
|---|---|---|---|
| 20–39 | 10 | 1.9 | 30 |
| 40–49 | 12 | 5.7 | 33 |
| 50–59 | 29 | 17.2 | 48 |
| 60–69 | 31 | 25.0 | 65 |
| 70–79 | 42 | 53.0 | 50 |
| 80+ | 30 | 350.0 | 23 |
| Total | 154 | | 249 |

(Adapted from Brott T, Thalinger K, Hertzberg V. Hypertension as a risk factor for spontaneous intracerebral hemorrhage. Stroke 1986;17:1078–1083.)

cinnati metropolitan area of 15 per 100,000.[7] For the entire period 1961 to 1983, ICH incidence was higher in men, 220 per 100,000, than in women, 70 per 100,000.[9] Overall, ICH accounted for 19.3% of all stroke events during a fifteen-year follow-up of 1621 Hisayama residents above age 40.[9]

The advent of the cranial CT scan in the 1970s has made it possible to diagnose small ICH. It has been estimated that 24% of strokes labeled as cerebral infarcts in prior decades were probably hemorrhages.[4]

Since the incidence of ICH increases with advancing age, and amyloid or congophilic angiopathy generally occurs after age 70, distinguishing "hypertensive or primary" hemorrhage from bleeding as a consequence of amyloid angiopathy is not easily accomplished.[12] Characteristics such as advanced age, absence of a history of hypertension, presence of Alzheimer disease, lobar location of the hemorrhage, and other features, such as multiple hemorrhages in different sites occurring simultaneously or serially, are thought to be characteristic of amyloid angiopathy.[12] However, in the recent Cincinnati data, the proportion of hemorrhages that were lobar in location did not increase with age.[13] Furthermore, hypertension was not substantially less frequent among patients sustaining lobar hemorrhage than in those whose bleeding was at sites commonly associated with hypertension, that is, deep in the basal ganglia or thalamus, cerebellum, and

**Table 2.4.** Incidence of Spontaneous Intracerebral Hemorrhage among Blacks and Whites, Men and Women Combined, Greater Cincinnati 1988

| Age in Years | Incidence/100,000* | | | Blacks/Whites Odds Ratio (95% CI) |
|---|---|---|---|---|
| | Blacks | Whites | Total | |
| 0–34 | 2 (2)[†] | 0.5 (3) | 0.7 (5) | 3.8 (0.7–20.1) |
| 35–54 | 27 (9) | 7 (17) | 10 (26) | 3.7 (1.8–8.0) |
| 55–74 | 58 (14) | 33 (59) | 36 (73) | 1.8 (1.0–3.2) |
| >75 | 36 (2) | 156 (80) | 144 (82) | 0.23 (0.1–0.8) |
| Total | 16 (27) | 15 (159) | 15 (159) | 1.4[‡] (0.9–2.1) |

* Crude unadjusted annual rates.
† Number of cases in parentheses.
‡ Adjusted for age and sex to the 1980 U.S. population.
Abbreviations: CI = Confidence interval.
(Adapted from Broderick JP, Brott T, Tomsick T, et al. The risk of subarachnoid and intracerebral hemorrhages in blacks as compared with whites. N Engl J Med 1992;326:733–736.)

pons.[13] In the absence of a pathognomonic or specific sign to diagnose hemorrhage due to amyloid angiopathy, epidemiological assessment of this entity will be problematical.

### Risk Factors

#### Hypertension

The importance of elevated blood pressure as a risk factor for non-aneurysmal spontaneous ICH is underscored by the name most commonly applied to the condition, "hypertensive" ICH. There seems little doubt that a substantial portion of ICH is attributable to hypertension, though probably not all. Based on an autopsy study of nontraumatic brain hemorrhage, McCormick and Rosenfield [14] concluded that in only about one-fourth could hypertension be considered to be responsible for the bleeding. In a report of the Rochester, Minnesota, ICH data, 89% of cases had prior hypertension as judged by documented blood pressures above 160/90 mm Hg, heart weight over 400 g, or both.[3] The authors noted a decline in the prevalence and severity of hypertension in hemorrhage cases over this thirty-two-year period.[3] In addition, the relationship of hypertension to ICH was not uniform across the age span.[4] In contrast to the rarity of normotension (17%) prior to hemorrhage in younger patients, that is, those ages 35 to 55, normotension was quite prevalent in those above age 75, occurring in 37% of elderly hemorrhage patients. Furthermore, younger patients had higher pressures; 28% of those ages 35 to 55 had mean pressures above 150 mm Hg, while no patient above age 75 had a mean blood pressure at this level.[4]

As noted, hypertension has not been uniformly found in systematic epidemiological studies of ICH. In the Cincinnati report, the proportion of the cases attributable to definite hypertension was 39%.[7] When other presumptive evidence of elevated blood pressure was included, the attributable risk increased to 49%. According to the authors,

eliminating hypertension from the Cincinnati population would result in elimination of ICH in only 49% of cases. One can take issue with inclusion of 27 of their patients, since they had hemorrhages secondary to primary and metastatic brain tumors, leukemia with bleeding diatheses, and other known causes of hemorrhage.[6] These represent 18% of the cases that would not properly be categorized as *primary* ICH. This misclassification and the retrospective determination of an asymptomatic condition, hypertension, in an urban metropolitan population is probably at least partially responsible for the low attributable risk.

#### Cigarette Smoking

Cigarette smoking has been clearly shown to increase the risk of thrombotic stroke and subarachnoid hemorrhage; the relationship to ICH is less well established. However, recent data from the Honolulu Heart Program firmly link cigarette smoking in Hawaiian men of Japanese ancestry to stroke, both "thromboembolic and hemorrhagic."[10] Risk of "hemorrhagic" stroke was 2.5 times greater in cigarette smokers than in nonsmokers and this excess risk of stroke was independent of other risk factors: age, diastolic blood pressure, serum cholesterol, alcohol consumption, hematocrit, and body mass index. It is likely that the majority of the hemorrhages were intracerebral. However, verification of hemorrhage type by imaging, autopsy, or angiography was often not available.[10]

#### Alcohol

Increased incidence of ICH has been related to alcohol consumption in the Honolulu Heart Program with a strong dose-response relationship.[15] However, alcohol consumption is also related to increasing levels of blood pressure, cigarette smoking, and to lower serum cholesterol levels, all of which are risk factors for ICH. Nevertheless, after taking these factors into account, alcohol consumption was independently related to

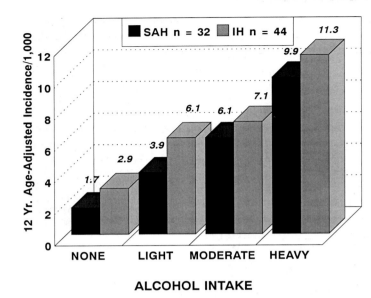

**Figure 2.1.** Alcohol use and hemorrhagic stroke, the Honolulu Heart Program. Age-adjusted twelve-year incidence of hemorrhagic stroke per 1000 population in relation to alcohol intake. (Data taken from Donahue RP, Abbott RD, Reed DM, et al. Alcohol and hemorrhagic stroke: The Honolulu Heart Program. JAMA 1986;255:2311–2314, with permission.)

incidence of intracranial hemorrhage, both subarachnoid and intracerebral; no such significant relationship was found between alcohol and thromboembolic stroke.[15] Age-adjusted estimated relative risk of ICH for light drinkers (1 to 14 oz per month) as compared with nondrinkers was 2.1, for moderate drinkers (15 to 39 oz per month) 2.4, and for heavy drinkers (over 40 oz per month) 4.0 (Figure 2.1). After adjustment was made for the other associated risk factors, ICH was still 2.0, 2.0 and 2.4 times as frequent, respectively, in these alcohol consumption categories. In a working population, heavy alcohol use (more than three drinks daily) was associated with higher rates (relative risk 3.64) of hospitalization for ICH.[16] Age, higher blood pressure, and black race (but not heavy alcohol consumption after these factors were taken into account), were independent predictors of ICH. The authors suggested that the effect of heavy alcohol consumption on "hemorrhagic" stroke was mediated by elevated blood pressure. A lower incidence of "occlusive" stroke hospitalizations was seen among heavy drinkers, but the reduced relative risk of 0.62 was not statistically significant (95% confidence interval 0.29 to 1.31).[16]

## Serum Cholesterol

A surprising but consistent finding has been the strong relationship between low total serum cholesterol and the increased incidence of ICH.[17,18] When initially noted in Japanese persons with very low serum cholesterol levels by Western standards (less than 160 mg per dl), no cause and effect relationship was seriously considered. However, an etiological link has been suggested by the recent confirmation of this relationship in other Asian populations, in Hawaiian persons of Japanese ancestry, and in 1989 in the white men in the United States who were Multiple Risk Factor Intervention Trial (MRFIT) screenees.[19]

Prospective epidemiological studies of Japanese men and women in Japan have shown this relationship, which has also been confirmed in Hawaiian-Japanese men.[20] Evidence that the low cholesterol, high ICH relationship is not restricted to Asians has recently emerged from follow-up in the United States of MRFIT screenees, 90% of whom were white.[21] Despite the large size of the study group of 350,977 men, ages 35 to 57 at screening, followed for six years for mortality, only 83 deaths from ICH and 55 deaths

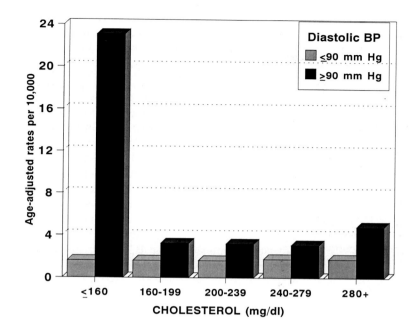

**Figure 2.2.** Serum cholesterol and hemorrhagic stroke, the Multiple Risk Factor Intervention Trial. Incidence of hemorrhagic stroke as a function of serum cholesterol level, in relation to diastolic blood pressure measurements. (Data taken from Iso H, Jacobs DR, Wentworth D. Serum cholesterol levels and six-year mortality from stroke in 350,977 men screened for the Multiple Risk Factor Intervention Trial. N Engl J Med 1989;320:904–910, with permission.)

from subarachnoid hemorrhage occurred. In the lowest serum cholesterol category (less than 160 per dl), the risk factor–adjusted relative risk of intracranial hemorrhage was considered to be 1.0; relative risk at all higher levels of serum cholesterol was lower at approximately 0.32. When deaths from intracranial hemorrhage were examined by entry blood pressure, the age-adjusted rates were significant only in those screenees with low cholesterol whose diastolic pressure was greater than 90 mm Hg[20] (Figure 2.2). Death rates per 10,000 were 23.07 in the lowest serum cholesterol category (less than 160 mg per dl), and ranged from 3.09 to 4.83 per 10,000 in the four highest categories. The interaction of high diastolic blood pressure and low serum cholesterol in promoting ICH suggested to some investigators "that very low serum cholesterol levels weaken the endothelium of intracerebral arteries, resulting in hemorrhagic stroke in the presence of hypertension."[21] It has been suggested that other factors were also operating to increase hemorrhage risk, including heavy alcohol consumption, dietary protein deficiency, and a higher intake of polyunsaturated fatty acids,

both linoleic acid derived from vegetable oils and eicosapentanoic acid from fish oil, acting to reduce platelet aggregability.[22]

*Aspirin for Primary Prevention of Coronary Heart Disease*

The report of a 44% reduction in myocardial infarction incidence in half of the 22,071 male physicians randomly assigned to aspirin (the other half received a placebo) and followed for 60.2 months also included a "warning" of a substantial increase in the incidence of "hemorrhagic" stroke in the aspirin group.[23] Relative risk of hemorrhagic stroke was of borderline statistical significance (relative risk 2.14, 95% confidence interval 0.93 to 4.77, P = 0.06), based on 10 mild hemorrhages in the aspirin group and 6 in the placebo group (relative risk 1.67; 95% confidence interval 0.61 to 4.57; P = 0.32) and 13 moderate, severe or fatal hemorrhagic strokes in the aspirin group and 6 in the placebo group (relative risk 2.19; 95% confidence interval 0.84 to 5.69; P = 0.11).[23] The finding of increased "hemorrhagic stroke" had not been reported in the aspirin trials for transient ischemic attacks or to prevent stroke recurrence[24] that were published at the time of the Physician's Health Study report. Was this finding real or merely an artifact of diagnostic coding or death certification? How many of these "hemorrhagic" strokes were subarachnoid hemorrhages from aneurysm and how many were spontaneous intraparenchymatous hemorrhages?

Since then, the SALT (Swedish Aspirin Low-dose Trial) Collaborative Group,[25a] a secondary stroke prevention trial that compared 75 mg of daily aspirin with placebo, reported a significant increase in the frequency of intracerebral hemorrhage in the aspirin group (8 events) as compared with placebo (3 events). All five instances of fatal "hemorrhagic stroke" (intracerebral and subarachnoid) occurred in the aspirin group. This issue clearly needs further study. It is curious that the increased rate of intracranial hemorrhage occurred with low doses of aspirin in the Physicians' Health Study[23] and in the SALT trial,[25a] but not with the use of 1300 mg daily in the Canadian aspirin trial and 990 mg daily in the AICLA study.[24]

*Other Causes*

A variety of situations in which ICH followed everyday circumstances such as migraine, exposure to cold weather, and severe dental pain have been described.[25] Other less common causes of hemorrhage, including drug abuse, carotid endarterectomy, surgery for trigeminal neuralgia, correction of congenital heart disease in children, and "spät" apoplexy, have been discussed in an editorial.[25] The unifying hypothesis offered was to relate these events to "acute augmentation of cerebral blood flow, most often by abrupt increase in blood pressure in regions of either normal or injured blood vessels."[25]

## Declining Mortality and Incidence

Hypertensive ICH and hypertensive encephalopathy were not rare diseases during the first half of the twentieth century. In the past forty years, however, these conditions, both a consequence of severe uncontrolled hypertension, have become quite uncommon. It is of interest that S. A. Kinnier Wilson, in the 1940 edition of his textbook, *Neurology* noted, "It is my impression that the proportion of haemorrhagic forms among cerebral vascular disease in general has been diminishing steadily during the last 30 years, mainly owing to improved social and personal habits, but I have no means of confirming it."[26] To verify an impression of an apparent decline in the frequency of ICH during the prior decade, a systematic study was conducted in Göteborg, Sweden.[27] In fact, the number of hospital admissions for ICH had declined, particularly in persons below age 55. They found that most patients presenting with ICH in that period were untreated hypertensives with markedly elevated blood pressures. Based on cases confirmed at autopsy (autopsies had been performed on nearly 100% of all hospital deaths), analysis disclosed cerebral hemorrhage rates to be lower among persons below age 65 during the period under study than in prior decades.[27] In Göteborg, ICH occurred, on average, in older persons in 1961 than in 1948, representing a ten-year "delay" in the onset of hemorrhage. The authors concluded that this delay resulted from control of severe hypertension in the latter time period.

Since the Göteborg report, a decline in the incidence of ICH has been documented in several populations.[3,9,28] In the United States, reduction has been related to better detection and more effective treatment of hypertension.[4] In Japan, including rural areas, substantial changes in the diet have occurred in the past twenty years.[18,28] These include an increase in the percentages of animal fat and animal protein and a reduction in the amount of sodium chloride in the diet.[28] In addition, the prevalence of hypertension in Japan fell and, coincident with it, the incidence of brain hemorrhage. The authors found that the incidence of massive ganglionic hemorrhages declined between 1961 and 1983 in the two cohorts studied in Hisayama, Japan.[9]

A stroke registry in Shibata, Japan, for three years, 1976 through 1978, disclosed the average annual incidence of stroke in those above age 20 to be 261 per 100,000; 61 per 100,000 was the incidence of ICH.[8] These data from Japan represent the composite incidence of three five-year periods, 1961 to 1966, 1967 to 1971, and 1972 to 1976. Age-adjusted incidence of ICH fell from 13.4 to 11.9 to 7.3 per 100,000 over these serial quinquennia.[8]

It seems ironic that the explosion of precursor data is appearing as the disease itself is decreasing in incidence and severity. Continued detection and control of hypertension, particularly in blacks, should help to continue to reduce the incidence rates of ICH. However, as life expectancy continues to increase there will be growing numbers of the elderly surviving into the ninth and tenth decades of life. These age groups are most susceptible to ICH secondary to amyloid or congophilic angiopathy. Whether the incidence of this condition is of sufficient magnitude to increase the overall incidence of ICH is uncertain. Concern has been expressed that the recent impetus to reduce serum cholesterol levels in Western populations by means of dietary and pharmacological measures may also increase the incidence of ICH.[19] In time, the impact of increasingly routine use of aspirin for cardiovascular disease prevention on the incidence of intracranial hemorrhage should also become clearer.

# References

1. Sacco RL, Wolf PA, Bharucha NE, et al. Subarachnoid and intracerebral hemorrhage: natural history, prognosis, and precursive factors in the Framingham Study. Neurology 1984;34:847–854.
2. Wolf PA, Cobb JL, D'Agostino. Epidemiology of stroke. In Barnett HJM, et al., eds. Stroke: pathophysiology, diagnosis, and management. Second edition. New York: Churchill Livingstone, 1992;6.
3. Furlan AJ, Whisnant JP, Elveback LR. The decreasing incidence of primary intracerebral hemorrhage: a population study. Ann Neurol 1979;5:367–373.
4. Drury I, Whisnant JP, Garraway WM. Primary intracerebral hemorrhage: impact of CT on incidence. Neurology 1984;34:653–657.
5. Gross CR, Kase CS, Mohr JP, et al. Stroke in south Alabama: incidence and diagnostic features - a population based study. Stroke 1984;15:249–255.
6. Brott T, Thalinger K., Hertzberg V. Hypertension as a risk factor for spontaneous intracerebral hemorrhage. Stroke 1986;17:1078–1083.
7. Broderick JP, Brott T, Tomsick T, et al. The risk of subarachnoid and intracerebral hemorrhages in blacks as compared with whites. N Engl J Med 1992;326:733–736.
8. Tanaka H, Ueda Y, Date C, et al. Incidence of stroke in Shibata, Japan: 1976–1978. Stroke 1981;12:460–466.
9. Ueda K, Hasuo Y, Kiyohara Y, et al. Intracerebral hemorrhage in a Japanese community, Hisayama: incidence, changing pattern during long-term follow-up, and related factors. Stroke 1988;19:48–52.
10. Abbott RD, Yin Y, Reed DM, et al. Risk of stroke in male cigarette smokers. N Engl J Med 1986;315:717–720.
11. Yano K, Reed DM, MacLean CJ. Serum cholesterol and hemorrhagic stroke in the Honolulu Heart Program. Stroke 1989;20:1460–1465.
12. Vinters HV. Cerebral amyloid angiopathy: a critical review. Stroke 1987;18:311–324.
13. Broderick J, Brott T, Tomsick T, et al. Lobar hemorrhage in the elderly: The undiminishing importance of hypertension. Stroke 1993;24:49–51.
14. McCormick WF, Rosenfield DB. Massive brain hemorrhage: a review of 144 cases and an examination of their causes. Stroke 1973;4:946–954.
15. Donahue RP, Abbott RD, Reed DM, et al. Alcohol and hemorrhagic stroke: The Honolulu Heart Program. JAMA 1986;255:2311–2314.
16. Klatsky AL, Armstrong MA, Friedman GD. Alcohol use and subsequent cerebrovascular disease hospitalizations. Stroke 1989;20:741–746.
17. Ueshima H, Iida M, Shimamoto T, et al. Multivariate analysis of risk factor for stroke: eight year follow-up study of farming villages in Akita, Japan. Prev Med 1980;9:722–740.
18. Tanaka H, Ueda Y, Hayashi M, et al. Risk factors for cerebral hemorrhage and cerebral in-

farction in a Japanese rural community. Stroke 1982;13:62–73.

19. Jacobs D, Blackburn H, Higgins M, et al. Report of the conference on low blood cholesterol: mortality associations. Circulation 1992; 86:1046–1060.

20. Kagan A, Popper JS, Rhoads GG. Factors related to stroke incidence in Hawaii Japanese men: The Honolulu Heart Study. Stroke 1980;11:14–21.

21. Iso H, Jacobs DR, Wentworth D, et al. Serum cholesterol levels and six-year mortality from stroke in 350,977 men screened for the Multiple Risk Factor Intervention Trial. N Engl J Med 1989;320:904–910.

22. Goodnight SH, Harris WS, Connor WE, et al. Polyunsaturated fatty acids, hyperlipidemia and thrombosis. Arteriosclerosis 1982;2: 87–113.

23. Steering committee of the Physicians' Health Study Research Group. Final report on the aspirin component of the ongoing Physicians' Health Study. N Engl J Med 1989;321:129–135.

24. Taylor DW, Barnett HJM. Physicians' Health Study: aspirin and primary prevention of coronary heart disease. N Engl J Med 1989; 321:1827 (letter).

25. Caplan L. Intracerebral hemorrhage revisited. Neurology 1988;38:624–627.

25a. The SALT Collaborative Group. Swedish Aspirin Low-dose Trial (SALT) of 75 mg aspirin as secondary prophylaxis after cerebrovascular ischaemic events. Lancet 1991;338:1345–1349.

26. Wilson SAK. Neurology. Volume II. London: Butterworth, 1940;1064. (Reprinted by Hafner Publishing, London, 1970.)

27. Aurell M, Hood B. Cerebral hemorrhage in a population after a decade of active antihypertensive treatment. Acta Med Scand 1964;176:377–383.

28. Shimamoto T, Komachi Y, Inada H, et al. Trends for coronary heart disease and stroke and their risk factors in Japan. Circulation 1989;79:503–515.

# Chapter 3
# General Symptoms and Signs

## Louis R. Caplan

Symptoms and signs in patients with intracerebral hemorrhage can be broadly separated into *general* and *focal* categories. By general symptoms, we refer to such things as headache, vomiting, and so forth that occur in patients with intracerebral hemorrhage irrespective of cause and location. Although the frequency of the general findings may vary with hemorrhages due to different causes and in different places, the findings are common to all hematomas. Focal findings, in contrast, relate almost entirely to the site of intracerebral hemorrhage and other factors depending on the particular anatomy and pathology of the lesion. Focal symptoms and signs are discussed in individual chapters in Part Three of this book. In this chapter, general symptomatology is discussed.

Most articles, texts, and reviews of intracerebral hemorrhage in the pre–computed tomography era emphasized (1) sudden catastrophic onset of symptoms, often with physical activity; (2) nearly invariable presence of headache and reduced alertness; and (3) importance of blood in the cerebrospinal fluid (CSF) as a diagnostic clue. Although Fisher began to raise doubts about these generally accepted rules,[1] not until computed tomography (CT) provided an accurate means of antemortem diagnosis of intracerebral hemorrhage could the validity of these dicta be formally studied.

## Onset and Early Course

The earliest symptoms are most often focal neurological symptoms. The nature of the symptoms, of course, depends entirely on the region of the brain where the hemorrhage begins. Usually the location is in the deeper brain structures, such as the basal ganglia, middle of the pons, white matter of cerebral lobes, or the cerebellum. When bleeding occurs very near pial or ependymal surfaces and blood quickly dissects into the ventricles or the CSF near the surface of the brain, then headache or vomiting may precede or overshadow focal symptoms. The bleeding in intracerebral hemorrhage is usually from small intraparenchymatous arteries. Bleeding is under less pressure and is less brisk than in aneurysmal subarachnoid hemorrhage in which blood is jetted into the CSF under arterial pressure. Brain parenchyma does not contain pain-responsive nerve endings so that blood within the brain should not cause pain or headache unless pain-sensitive fibers in the meninges or along superficial or basal blood vessels are distorted. For these reasons, the initial symptoms reflect loss of neurological function due to destruction of neurons or interruption of white matter pathways within the brain. In putaminal or capsular hematomas, the earliest symptoms might be numbness or weakness of a contralateral limb or of the contralateral face, arm, and leg; in cerebellar hemorrhage, ataxia or disturbed equilibrium or balance; in left temporal lobar hematomas, abnormal language function. In the Stroke Data Bank, 93% of patients with putaminal hemorrhage, 90% of patients with thalamic hemorrhage, and 90% of patients with pontine hematomas had focal deficits at onset.[2]

Once the neurological symptoms begin, most often they evolve and progress gradually during a period usually of minutes. Table 3.1 includes data from the Harvard and Michael Reese Stroke Registries on the early course of patients with intracerebral hemorrhage contrasted with the course in other stroke syndromes.[3] The two most common evolutions were gradual and maximal at onset deficits. Similarly, in the Lausanne Stroke Registry, among 109 patients with intracerebral hemorrhage, 44 were "immediately complete," 52 were "progressive," and 4 fluctuated.[4] Maximal at outset or "immediately complete" are descriptive designations assigned to the clinical course when the patient is as bad as he or she will get and can give no account of prior worsening. Some of these patients can not, of course, give a history because of decreased consciousness, aphasia, or lack of awareness of the deficit (anosognosia). If they do not worsen under further observation, the course is designated as maximal at outset. In all of these series, very few patients had stepwise or stuttering accumulation of their deficits or fluctuated from abnormal to normal, or improved

quickly. The smooth, gradual progression of symptoms in intracerebral hemorrhage is an important diagnostic point that helps to separate intracerebral hemorrhage from other stroke syndromes. Most often, the gradual progression occurs during a few minutes (10 to 30) but rarely progression continues for hours and occasionally during a few days.

Patient descriptions may illustrate the progression of symptoms and signs. One of the first patients with intracerebral hemorrhage seen by LR Caplan was in 1962. A previously healthy Chinese man came to the emergency ward of the Boston City Hospital because of numbness of the right arm and leg. Blood pressure was 210/125. In the emergency area he was alert and could use his right limbs, but they were slightly weak and hyperreflexic. The right plantar response was extensor, the left flexor. Language was normal. As he was being wheeled on a stretcher through the tunnel beneath the hospital, he said that his right limbs were weaker and in fact he could not now lift his arm or leg or move his fingers. Moments later, his speech deteriorated and was very thick and slurred. By the time he reached the elevator to the Medical Building, he was mute, sleepy, and had a severe right hemiplegia. His head and eyes were deviated to the left but his pupils were normal. When he reached the seventh floor and was placed in bed, he had no voluntary or reflex horizontal gaze, the left pupil was dilated and poorly reactive, and the left plantar response had become extensor. Thirty minutes later, he was bilaterally decerebrate

**Table 3.1.** Course of Development of Symptoms and Signs in Subtypes of Stroke

|  | Thrombosis | | Lacune | | Embolus | | ICH | | SAH | |
|---|---|---|---|---|---|---|---|---|---|---|
|  | HSR | MRSR | HSR | MRSR | HSR | MRSR | HSR | MRSR | HSR | MRSR |
| Maximal at onset | 40% | 45% | 38% | 40% | 79% | 89% | 34% | 38% | 80% | 64% |
| Stuttering or stepwise | 34% | 30% | 32% | 28% | 11% | 10% | 3% | 9% | 3% | 14% |
| Gradual or smooth | 13% | 14% | 20% | 24% | 5% | 1% | 63% | 51% | 14% | 18% |
| Fluctuant | 13% | 11% | 10% | 8% | 5% | 0% | 0% | 2% | 3% | 4% |

Note: ICH = intracerebral hemorrhage, SAH = subarachnoid hemorrhage, HSR = Harvard Stroke Registry, MRSR = Michael Reese Stroke Registry.
(From Caplan LR, Stein RW. Stroke: a clinical approach. Stoneham, MA: Butterworths, 1986, p. 13. With permission of the publisher.)

and had no eye movements. One hour after presentation, he was dead. Needless to say, it was very frustrating and humbling to see his brain function decline during the trip through the bowels of the hospital.

Another illustrative case was a middle-aged surgeon whose stroke began while he was arguing with a merchant who sold fruit and vegetables in Boston's North End. He first noted that his left hand was numb. A minute or so later, his hand was weak and he stumbled and tripped when he walked. He hailed a cab and on the way to the Massachusetts General Hospital, very close by, his left limbs became weaker. By the time he arrived at the Hospital, he could not support his weight and was obviously hemiplegic.

A 70-year-old minister came to the Hospital complaining of weakness and numbness of his right limb. He and his wife reported that he had awakened with the deficit. Each day for the first three days he worsened, first becoming more paretic on the right, then aphasic, then drowsy. Blood pressure was 165/100. Two lumbar punctures revealed slightly increased pressure but no blood (he was studied in 1969 before the advent of CT). Because of the "progressing stroke" he was given heparin and continued to worsen. Angiography showed no occlusion, but a large lateral ganglionic avascular zone. Now the wife told us that she had given erroneous information on admission. Actually he noted the right limb symptoms after rather vigorous coition. At necropsy there was a very large putaminal hematoma with considerable mass effect and brainstem compression but no communication with the ventricular system and no drainage on the surface of the brain.

Fisher's studies of the pathology of intracerebral hemorrhage yield important insights into the explanation of the gradual onset of symptoms. Fisher analyzed several specimens of intracerebral hemorrhage by serial section.[5] In the center of the hematomas was a mass of blood; cellular features and blood vessels could not be distinguished. However, along the periphery of the lesion were many small "fibrin globes" which were masses of agglutinated platelets encircled by thin layers of fibrin. These globular fibrin-platelet masses capped capillaries that had ruptured because of the pressure of the expanding hematoma. In trying to recapitulate the events, Fisher assumed that the initial rupture occurred in the center of the mass of blood. The initial hemorrhage caused pressure on adjacent capillaries and arterioles causing them to break. As they ruptured, blood was added at the circumference of the lesion, gradually expanding the hematoma. The process could be likened to a snowball rolling downhill with snow accruing along the circumference enlarging the snowball as it rolled. As the hematoma grew, local and later general intracranial pressure rose and the surrounding pressure acted to stop the bleeding. Dissection of blood into the ventricular system or at the surface acted to decompress the growing local mass effect. The alternative to CSF or ventricular bleeding was further hemorrhage into brain tissue. Figure 3.1 is from Fisher's neuropathological study illustrating the fi-

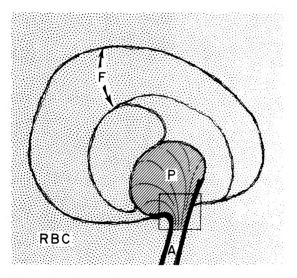

**Figure 3.1.** Fibrin globe. A = ruptured artery; P = platelet mass; F = fibrin, RBC = red blood cells. (From Fisher CM. Pathological observations in hypertensive cerebral hemorrhage. J Neuropathol Exp Neurol 1971; 30:536–550, with permission.)

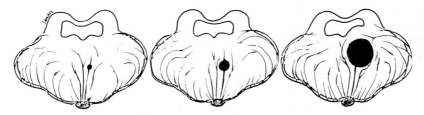

**Figure 3.2.** Artist's conception of development of pontine hematoma. (From Caplan LR, Stein RW. Stroke: a clinical approach. Stoneham, MA: Butterworths, 1986, p. 47, with permission.)

brin globes he found.[5] In Chapter 1, Figure 1.5 shows the location of the bleeding points in relation to the pontine hematoma. Figure 3.2 is an artist's reconstruction of the evolution of the bleeding.

Two recent studies have documented progression of bleeding in patients with intracerebral hemorrhage. Kelley and colleagues reported four patients with spontaneous intracerebral hemorrhages that clearly increased in size in the few minutes between plain and contrast enhanced CT scans.[6] Each patient worsened clinically while being studied. In one patient, a CT six hours after onset of symptoms and three and one-half hours after the first CT scan showed continued bleeding. More recently, another CT study documented continued bleeding in eight patients with intracerebral hemorrhage, six of which were thalamic.[7] The interval between CT scans ranged from two hours to nearly nine days. Clinical deterioration occurred within the first six hours in three patients (three, five, and six hours); in three others the clinical deterioration occurred between twelve and twenty-four hours (twelve, twelve, and twenty-two hours), and in two patients, deterioration occurred five and seven days after onset.[7] A prior study by Herbstein and Schaumberg involved radionuclide studies of patients with large hypertensive hematomas.[8] Red blood cells were labeled with $Cr^{51}$ and injected into the patients before death. Labeled erythrocytes were not found within the hematoma but

were found within the Duret hemorrhages in the brainstem. At least preterminally, the primary hematomas did not continue to bleed. The studies cited do not define whether the bleeding was gradual or occurred in starts and stops. Probably, most hematomas initially enlarge gradually. The vast majority then stop bleeding and do not enlarge further. Some continue to bleed, possibly sporadically during the first days after onset. In a recent study, Broderick et al.[9] performed CT evaluation in eight patients with intracerebral hemorrhages within two and one-half hours from onset of symptoms, and then repeated the CT several hours later. The second CT documented a mean increase of 107% in the volume of the hemorrhage. The largest increases in hematoma volume occurred in patients with putaminal (Figure 3.3) and thalamic (Figure 3.4) hemorrhages. The authors pointed out that these unique data obtained by "ultra-early" CT evaluation of intracerebral hemorrhage indicate that enlargement of the hematoma in the initial hours after onset is common, and is a likely mechanism of early clinical deterioration. The factors that lead to progressive bleeding have not been clarified. A review of anticoagulant-related hemorrhages showed that clinical evolution in patients treated with anticoagulants was over a longer period than in patients with hypertensive hematomas.[10] After the initial bleeding, edema develops in the regions around the hematoma during the first twenty-four to forty-eight hours after

## First CT-35 Minutes From Onset

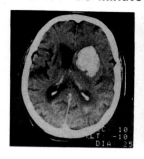 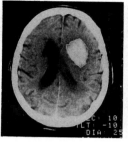 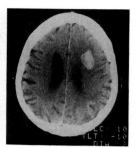

## Second CT-105 Minutes From Onset

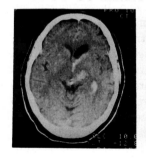 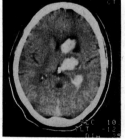 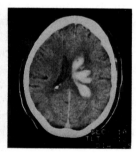

**Figure 3.3.** Enlargement of left putaminal hemorrhage, from an initial volume of 25 cm$^3$ on CT performed thirty-five minutes after onset (top row), to 44 cm$^3$ on CT done 105 minutes after onset (bottom row). (From Broderick JP et al. Ultra-early evaluation of intracerebral hemorrhage. J Neurosurg 1990; 72:195–199, with permission.)

## First CT-50 Minutes From Onset

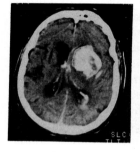 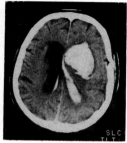 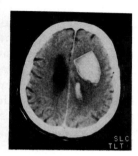

## Second CT-210 Minutes From Onset

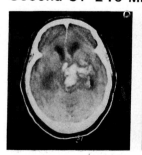 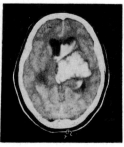 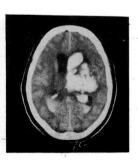

**Figure 3.4.** Enlargement of left thalamic hemorrhage, from an initial volume of 8 cm$^3$ on CT performed fifty minutes after onset (top row), to 35 cm$^3$ on CT done 210 minutes after onset (bottom row). (From Broderick JP et al. Ultra-early evaluation of intracerebral hemorrhage. J Neurosurg 1990; 72:195–199, with permission.)

onset. Edema and increased mass effect as well as continued leakage can lead to worsening of clinical symptoms and signs.

## Activity at Onset

Wilson commented that "conventional excitants" such as "straining at stool, lifting weights, coughing, sneezing, vomiting, laughing, running, during coition, and emotional experience" could trigger intracerebral hemorrhage.[11] Most neurologists, we believe, still feel that onset during "stress" is very common in patients with intracerebral hemorrhage. Before collecting data in the Harvard Stroke Registry, our bias was also that activity at onset was probably a feature that helped separate infarction from hemorrhage. However, the data from large series and registries have proved disappointing in this regard. In the Michael Reese Stroke Registry[12] (Table 3.2) most hemorrhages (64%) occurred during activities of daily living and only 10% occurred during physical activity or emotional duress. However, when compared with other stroke subtypes, fewer patients with intracerebral hemorrhage had stroke onset upon awakening. Similarly, in both the Harvard Stroke Registry (HSR)[13] and the Stroke Data Bank (SDB)[14] relatively few patients had onset of intracerebral hemorrhage noted upon awakening (15% in the SDB). We conclude that most often intracerebral hemorrhage begins during ordinary activities: sitting, standing, watching TV, and so forth. Onset during physical exertion favors intracerebral hemorrhage or subarachnoid bleeding but is not very common. Onset discovered on awakening is unusual in intracerebral hemorrhage and favors other stroke mechanisms.

## Headache

In descriptions of the clinical features of intracerebral hemorrhage written in the pre-CT era, headache was emphasized as a very prominent feature. These same series included mostly patients with large hematomas who subsequently died, allowing necropsy confirmation of the diagnosis of intracerebral hemorrhage. Most non-neurologists still hold to the rule that most intracerebral hemorrhage patients have headache. In the Harvard Stroke Registry, among patients with CT confirmation of the diagnosis of intracerebral hemorrhage, less than half had headache.[13] In a subgroup of 60 patients with putaminal hemorrhage analyzed separately, headache was present at onset in 17 (28%) and developed only later in an additional 7 patients (12%).[15] In 12 stuporous or comatose patients, headache history was unobtainable; 24 patients (40%) had no headache at any time during the hospitalization for acute stroke.[15] Similarly, severe headache at onset was present in only 41% of 237 patients with hematomas in the Stroke Data Bank[14] and headache at onset was noted in 40% of 109 intracerebral hemorrhage patients in the Lausanne Stroke Registry.[4]

**Table 3.2.** Activity at Onset in Subtypes of Stroke (From Michael Reese Stroke Registry)

| Activity at Onset | Thrombosis | Lacune | Infarct (U) | Embolus | ICH | SAH |
|---|---|---|---|---|---|---|
| On arising | 40% | 50% | 31% | 17% | 13% | 15% |
| Stress | 1% | 1% | 5% | 5% | 10% | 15% |
| ADL | 54% | 47% | 50% | 68% | 64% | 64% |
| Unknown | 5% | 2% | 14% | 10% | 13% | 6% |

Note: Infarct (U) = cause of infarct undetermined, ICH = intracerebral hemorrhage, SAH = subarachnoid hemorrhage, Stress = increased activity: exertion, coition, cough, sneeze, etc., ADL = activities of daily living.
(From Caplan LR, Stein RW. Stroke: a clinical approach. Stoneham, MA: Butterworths, 1986; p. 11. With permission of the publisher.)

Headache in intracerebral hemorrhage is explained by one of three mechanisms: (1) increase in pressure locally with distortion and traction effects on the overlying meninges and pial vessels, (2) generalized increase in intracranial pressure, or (3) release of blood into the ventricle or CSF on the surface of the brain. Pain fibers are concentrated within the meninges and the basal and pial vessels. Small hematomas that remain entirely intraparenchymal usually do not cause headache. Older patients often have brain atrophy so that despite mass effect there may be little increase in CSF pressure. Figure 3.5 shows a CT (first generation) of an older person with a very large intracerebral hemorrhage with ventricular spread, who had no headache during her hospitalization.

Hematomas that are near the surface are more likely to be associated with headache than those that are deep seated. In the Stroke Data Bank, headache was most frequent in patients with cerebellar hemorrhage, and lobar hematomas had the second highest frequency of headache.[2] When bleeding is from aneurysms (meningocerebral hemorrhage) headache is an invariable feature when the patient is alert enough to give an accurate account. Similarly, arteriovenous malformations that are near the sur-

face and leak into the CSF have a high frequency of associated headache.

## Level of Alertness—Loss of Consciousness

A decrease in the level of alertness was considered a common feature of intracerebral hemorrhage by authors in the pre-CT era (Osler, Gowers, Wilson, Aring and Merritt). Among the 60 patients with intracerebral hemorrhage in the Harvard Stroke Registry, 30 (50%) were fully alert on admission, 14 (23%) were lethargic, and 16 (27%) were stuporous or frankly comatose.[13] The prognosis was very poor for those who were stuporous or comatose on admission since all died. In the Stroke Data Bank, a higher percentage had a decrease in level of consciousness (57%) and coma (21%).[14] In the Lausanne Stroke Registry, 50% of intracerebral hemorrhage patients had some reduction in level of consciousness (28% somnolent, 22% comatose).[4] In the Stroke Data Bank, coma was most common in patients with pontine hemorrhage, followed in frequency by caudate and putaminal loci.[2]

Reduced alertness in patients with intracerebral hemorrhage is due to either a generalized increase in intracranial pressure, or to compromise of both hemispheres or the reticular activating system bilaterally in the brainstem tegmentum. Supratentorial hemorrhages (putaminal, caudate, lobar) cause coma by increasing intracranial pressure or by compressing the contralateral cerebral hemisphere or the upper brainstem. Ropper and Gress showed significant shift of midline structures in stuporous patients with cerebral lesions.[16] Patients with very large supratentorial hemorrhages often are stuporous or comatose by the time they arrive at the hospital. Among 17 patients with supratentorial hematomas larger than 55 cm$^3$, 14 were comatose on admission, 2 were stuporous, and 1 was drowsy.[17] Pontine and cerebellar hematomas cause coma when the brainstem tegmentum is involved directly by the he-

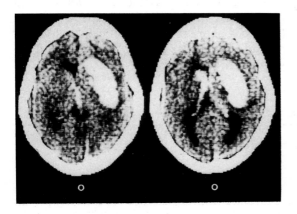

**Figure 3.5.** CT (early generation scanner) showing large right putaminal hemorrhage with extensive ventricular spread. The patient had no headache.

matoma or is compressed. In cerebellar hemorrhage, the patient may be alert on admission, but becomes unconscious when the fourth ventricle is compressed from above.[13] In thalamic hemorrhage, involvement of the rostral reticular activating system in the diencephalon or midbrain is responsible for stupor or hypersomnolence. Only in the case of thalamic hemorrhage does the state of alertness not correlate well with outcome. Stuporous patients with thalamic hemorrhage may recover well after the blood is reabsorbed. In caudate and primary intraventricular hemorrhage, reduced alertness is due to leakage of blood into the ventricles and accompanying increase in intracranial pressure. Patients may also recover well from hemorrhage at these sites despite early stupor. However, in patients with putaminal, lobar, pontine, or cerebellar hemorrhages, stupor or coma is a very ominous prognostic sign.

## Vomiting

Vomiting is a very important and diagnostic symptom in patients with intracerebral hemorrhage especially if the hematoma lies within the supratentorial compartment. In the Harvard Stroke Registry, we analyzed for the presence of vomiting in relation to the subtype of stroke and its location.[13] In patients with lacunar infarction, vomiting was quite rare irrespective of location. When the stroke involved the posterior circulation, whether the cause was embolic, "thrombotic," or intracerebral hemorrhage, vomiting was quite common. In posterior circulation strokes, 29% of ischemic stroke (embolism and thrombosis) patients vomited, while 2 out of 3 of the small number of patients with hemorrhages within this circulation vomited. Though there is a difference in the incidence of vomiting in vertebrobasilar ischemia and posterior fossa intracerebral hemorrhage, vomiting is still a common finding irrespective of stroke mechanism. However, in stroke patients with lesions in the anterior circula-

tion, vomiting proved a key symptom in separating hemorrhage and ischemia. Only 2% of patients with ischemia within the carotid territory vomited, while 48.5% of patients with hematomas in the supratentorial region vomited. This difference—2 in 100 versus nearly 1 of 2—is very impressive. The data regarding vomiting in the Harvard Stroke Registry are shown in Table 3.3. The Stroke Data Bank found a lower incidence of vomiting (29%) in patients with intracerebral hemorrhage.[14] However, within the Stroke Data Bank, intracerebral hemorrhage was the second most common stroke mechanism that caused vomiting, exceeded only by subarachnoid hemorrhage (45%). Vomiting was most frequent among patients with caudate, pontine, and cerebellar hemorrhages.

There are probably different mechanisms of vomiting among stroke patients. Any lesion that affects the vestibular nuclei and the so-called vomiting center in the floor of the fourth ventricle can cause vomiting.[18] This happens frequently in vertebrobasilar occlusive disease that involves the medulla and cerebellum, and in pontine and cerebellar hemorrhages that distort these structures. In the anterior circulation there are no structures that directly relate to vomiting. Vomiting in anterior circulation lesions relates to increased intracranial pressure which sec-

**Table 3.3.** Vomiting and Location and Type of Stroke (From Harvard Stroke Registry[13])

| ICH | | |
|---|---|---|
| Anterior circulation | 19/29 | 48.5% |
| Posterior circulation | 8/12 | 67% |
| Thrombosis | | |
| Anterior circulation | 3/141 | 2% |
| Posterior circulation | 24/83 | 29% |
| Embolus | | |
| Anterior circulation | 4/198 | 2% |
| Posterior circulation | 6/21 | 29% |

(From Caplan LR, Stein RW. Stroke: a clinical approach. Stoneham, Butterworth-Heinemann, 1986, p. 15. With permission of the publisher.)

**Table 3.4.** Seizures in Patients with Various Stroke Mechanisms

| | Thrombosis (Arteriosclerosis) | Lacune | Embolism | All Infarcts | ICH | SAH |
|---|---|---|---|---|---|---|
| Harvard Stroke Registry[13] | 0.4% | 0% | 4% | 1.7% | 6% | 7% |
| Lausanne Stroke Registry[4] | 1% | — | 0% | <1% | 7% | not included |
| Stroke Data Bank*[14] | 3% | <1% | 3% | 2% | 9% | 7% |
| Melbourne Hospital Study[19] | 10% | — | 5% | 5.6% | 14% | 8% |

*In the Stroke Data Bank data considered only seizures at onset.

ondarily stimulates the vomiting centers in the hindbrain. Caudate intracerebral hemorrhage probably produces vomiting because of sudden release of blood into the ventricular system and CSF, causing rapid change in intracranial pressure. Other supratentorial hematomas cause vomiting if they acutely distort structures and increase intracranial pressure, or if they drain sufficiently into the CSF pathways.

## Seizures

Seizures may develop during the course of any acute brain lesion. In the Harvard Stroke Registry, seizures occurred in 6% of patients with hematomas, a figure surpassed only by subarachnoid hemorrhage patients (7%).[13] Among patients with embolic stroke in the Harvard Stroke Registry, 4% had seizures, but only 0.4% of patients with large artery occlusions had seizures during the acute stroke.[13] Other stroke registry data confirm that seizures are more common in patients with intracerebral hemorrhage than in ischemic stroke of any cause. In the Lausanne Registry, 7% of intracerebral hemorrhage patients had convulsions compared with less than 1% with ischemic strokes.[4] In the Stroke Data Bank, intracerebral hemorrhage was the most frequent stroke mechanism that caused seizures, 9% being the frequency.[14] In a recent study from the Royal Melbourne Hospital, 15.4% of patients with intracerebral hemorrhage had seizures compared with 6.5% of patients with "cortical infarction."[19] The

composite figures for seizures in these studies are listed in Table 3.4.

The vast majority of patients with intracerebral hemorrhage and seizures had hematomas within the supratentorial compartment. In the Harvard Stroke Registry[13] and the Royal Melbourne Hospital Studies,[19] all the seizure producing lesions were within the anterior circulation, while a few patients with pontine hemorrhage in the Stroke Data Bank were reported to have seizures at onset.[2] Patients with pontine and cerebellar hemorrhages often have a variety of movements, such as decerebrate spasms, shivering, dystonic postures, and opisthotonus, that can easily be confused with convulsions. Lobar hematomas were the location most often associated with seizures, but caudate nucleus and putaminal hemorrhage patients also had seizures. Thalamic hematoma patients rarely had seizures unless the lesion spread to the adjacent subcortical regions.

In the Stroke Data Bank, 16.3% of the 65 patients with lobar hematomas had seizures compared with deep (caudate-putaminal-thalamic) hemorrhages in which 8.3% of 107 patients had seizures.[20] In a very large study of CT-documented patients with intracerebral hemorrhages, the differences in seizure incidence between superficial lobar hemorrhages and deep hematomas was even more striking.[21] In that study, 29 of 98 patients (29.5%) with lobar hemorrhages had seizures at some time after intracerebral hemorrhage while only 4 of the 110 patients (3.6%) with deep (caudate-putamen-thalamic) hematomas had seizures.[21] Most seizures occurred at or near onset (23 of 33; 70%). Among patients with lobar hemorrhages, 23 seizures were immediate, 2 delayed by one to three days and 4 were delayed longer than three days.[21]

Partial seizures were more common than tonic-clonic generalized convulsions.[19] The partial seizures could be motor or partial complex seizures and could remain focal or become generalized. Clearly, the type of partial seizure depends on the subcortical region involved. Most often seizures were single events and repeated convulsions were rare. The timing of the seizures varied. In the Royal Melbourne study, among all strokes, 43 of 44 first seizures occurred within 48 hours, and 26 occurred at or shortly after stroke onset.[19]

Two studies analyzed the chronology of seizures in more detail.[22,23] Berger et al. reported that 19 of 112 patients (17%) with spontaneous supratentorial hemorrhages had seizures.[22] All occurred at stroke onset. Patients who did not have seizures at onset did not convulse later. Faught et al. followed 123 patients with spontaneous intracerebral hemorrhages and found that 31 (25%) had seizures during the five years after their strokes.[23] Most often, seizures occurred early. Thirteen occurred while being evaluated in emergency wards after onset, four more during the first twenty-four hours, and another four during the second day.[23] Thus, two-thirds of seizures occurred within the first forty-eight hours. Between thirty days and two years, the prevalence rate for seizures was 13% and between two and five years, 6.5%.[23] All seizures in this series had motor manifestations, either at onset or after spread. In this large series, no patient with thalamic hemorrhage had seizures, and lobar hematomas were the location most often associated with convulsions.

Most studies do not subclassify the spontaneous hematomas by cause. Arteriovenous malformations, trauma, and drug-related hematomas are the most likely lesions associated with seizures. Hematomas in these disorders are most often lobar, cortical, or subcortical, and each of these disorders has an increased frequency of seizures even when intracerebral hemorrhage is not present. Intracerebral hemorrhage–related seizures are probably explained by undercutting of the cortex by the hematoma and partial injury to tissue at the edge of the hematomas. Seizures do not correlate well with hematoma size, but small linear subcortical hemorrhages and very large hemispherical hematomas are particularly likely to be complicated by seizures. In our experience, presentation of stroke with repeated partial seizures is often associated with subcortical hemorrhages and is rarely due to other stroke mechanisms.

## Other Features

### Stiff Neck

Stiff neck was commented upon by early authors as suggesting the diagnosis of either subarachnoid or intracerebral hemorrhage. In the Harvard Stroke Registry, 17% of intracerebral hemorrhage patients had a stiff neck.[13] In the Stroke Data Bank, neck stiffness was most often found in patients with caudate hemorrhage, probably because of the very high frequency of ventricular and subarachnoid blood.[2] Putaminal, thalamic, and cerebellar hemorrhage patients had a significant, but lower, frequency of stiff neck, and pontine and lobar locations had the least frequency.[2]

### Fever

Fever had been noted by Aring and Merritt[24] and early authors to be common in intracerebral hemorrhage patients during the acute phase of the illness. Most often, the temperature elevation is due to intercurrent infection, especially pneumonia or urinary tract infection. Some patients with pontine or other brainstem locations of intracerebral hemorrhage do have hyperthermia, possibly of central origin. The presence of fever in a patient with intracerebral hemorrhage should trigger a search for infection or pulmonary embolism. Fever should not be automatically attributed to the hematoma.

Few studies have reported systemic complications in patients with intracerebral hemorrhage. In the Stroke Data Bank, 15% of intracerebral hemorrhage patients developed pneumonia and 15% had urinary infections.[2] Gastrointestinal bleeding (5%), pulmonary embolism (1%), and arrythmia (8%) occurred less often.[2]

### Cardiac Changes

Cardiac changes are now known to frequently complicate acute brain lesions of any cause. In the 1940s, cardiologists became aware that prominent changes in the T waves of electrocardiograms could be due to subarachnoid hemorrhage.[25] Burch et al. in 1954 described seventeen patients, fourteen with intracranial, mostly subarachnoid, hemorrhage with an electrocardiographic pattern of: prolonged Q-T interval; wide, increased-amplitude T waves, either upright or inverted; and U waves.[26] These changes were considered diagnostic of brain disease. Subsequent studies have revealed an unexpectedly high incidence of T wave and S-T interval changes, elevated cardiac enzymes, and various arrhythmias in patients with acute stroke who have had continuous electrocardiographic monitoring.[27–30] The electrocardiographic changes reported most often include prolonged Q-T intervals, depressed S-T segments, flat or inverted T waves, and U waves.[29,30] Less often, tall, peaked T waves and elevated S-T segments have been described. Elevated enzymes, presumed to be of myocardial origin, were present in 30% of acute strokes in one series of one hundred consecutive stroke patients.[28] Enzyme elevations often accompanied electrocardiographic changes and were found in both hemorrhagic and ischemic strokes.[29,31] Ar-

rhythmias, especially sinus bradycardia and tachycardia, and premature contractions, are commonly found in acute stroke of any cause.[27,31] Stober et al. monitored fifty-four patients with intracerebral hemorrhage by continuous electrocardiographic recording during a period of five days.[32] Sinus tachycardia and bradycardia, and premature supraventricular contractions were maximal on the first day. Other arrhythmias, ventricular bigeminy, atrioventricular dissociation and block, ventricular tachycardia, atrial fibrillation, and bundle branch blocks were seen but much less often.[32] This study found no relationship between hematoma site and arrhythmias, but there were few posterior fossa hematomas.[32] All arrhythmias were more common when brainstem compression occurred. Especially frequent among the 21 patients with transtentorial herniation were sinus arrhythmias, frequent supraventricular beats, multifocal premature ventricular contractions, and ventricular tachycardias.[32]

Except for the few reports already cited, there are few detailed studies of the effect of acute stroke on the heart. The frequency and significance of the cardiac findings are still unclear. Examination of the hearts of patients dying of stroke, especially subarachnoid hemorrhage, have often found two prevalent pathologies, subendocardial hemorrhages and myocytolysis.[29,30,33] Some hearts show necrosis of cardiac muscle fibers, fibrillary degeneration of fibers with deposition of lipofuscin, and histiocytic infiltration into the necrotic regions.[29,30,33] Cardiac fibers become necrotic in a hypercontracted state. Often the focal lesions are calcified. These pathological findings presumably explain the T wave and S-T interval changes, and the elevation of cardiac enzymes. Increased sympathetic activity and stimulation of the hypothalamus can cause the same myocardial lesions as can increased blood catecholamine levels.[31,33,34] Catecholamine levels are often elevated in patients with subarachnoid hemorrhage but have been seldom measured systematically in patients with intracerebral hemorrhage. The cardiac lesions are probably due to excitotoxin toxicity. Catecholamines cause cardiac muscle hypercontraction that leads to cell death and early calcium entry.

There are a number of cortical, subcortical, and brainstem centers that help regulate cardiac rhythm. Especially prominent are the limbic portions of the temporal lobes, frontal agranular cortex, the insular cortex, hypothalamus, the nucleus of the tractus solitarius, and the ventrolateral medullary reticular formation.[31] Clearly, more cardiac studies are needed in patients with intracerebral hemorrhage.

### Pulmonary Edema

Pulmonary edema has been noted after subarachnoid hemorrhage and other conditions that suddenly increase intracranial pressure. Changes in intracranial pressure somehow disrupt normal ventilation-perfusion balances and lead to fluid accumulation in the lungs. We could find no reports of pulmonary congestion or edema after intracerebral hemorrhage but, undoubtedly, it must occasionally occur.

## Summary

Hematomas begin gradually. The earliest symptoms are focal neurological dysfunctions related to the area of parenchymal bleeding. Less often, when bleeding is near the ependymal or pial surface, onset is with headache and vomiting. As deep hematomas enlarge, focal signs gradually worsen. In supratentorial lesions, if the hematomas remain relatively small (less than 2 cm in greatest diameter) patients usually do not have headache, vomiting, or prominent changes in level of consciousness. In larger lesions, these symptoms develop when the hematoma becomes big enough to distort the meninges, compress the contralateral hemisphere or brainstem, or when the hematoma drains into the CSF. In infratentorial lesions, vomiting, loss of consciousness, and head-

ache are common, even in smaller hematomas. Loss of consciousness is an ominous prognostic sign in patients with lobar, posterior fossa, and putaminal hematomas. Seizures, especially focal or generalized with focal onset, are common in lobar intracerebral hemorrhage in contrast to other stroke syndromes. Some patients with intracerebral hemorrhage have arrhythmias and electrocardiographic changes consistent with myocardial injury or ischemia.

## References

1. Fisher CM. Clinical syndromes in cerebral hemorrhage. In Fields WS, ed. Pathogenesis and treatment of cerebrovascular disease. Springfield: Charles C Thomas, 1961;318–342.
2. Hier DB, Babcock DJ, Foulkes MA, et al. Influence of site on course of intracerebral hemorrhage. J Stroke Cerebrovasc Dis 1993;3:65–74.
3. Caplan LR, Stein RW. Stroke: a clinical approach. Boston: Butterworth, 1986; 11, 13.
4. Bogousslavsky J, Van Melle G, Regli F. The Lausanne Stroke Registry: analysis of 1,000 consecutive patients with first stroke. Stroke 1988; 19:1083–1092.
5. Fisher CM. Pathological observations in hypertensive cerebral hemorrhage. J Neuropathol Exp Neurol 1971;30:536–550.
6. Kelley RE, Berger JR, Scheinberg P, et al. Active bleeding in hypertensive intracerebral hemorrhage: computed tomography. Neurology 1982;32:852–856.
7. Chen ST, Chen SD, Hsu CY, et al. Progression of hypertensive intracerebral hemorrhage. Neurology 1989;39:1509–1514.
8. Herbstein DJ, Schaumburg HH. Hypertensive intracerebral hematoma: an investigation of the initial hemorrhage and rebleeding using chromium $Cr^{51}$-labeled erythrocytes. Arch Neurol 1974;30:412–414.
9. Broderick JP, Brott TG, Tomsick T, et al. Ultraearly evaluation of intracerebral hemorrhage. J Neurosurg 1990;72:195–199.
10. Kase CS, Robinson RK, Stein RW, et al. Anticoagulant-related intracerebral hemorrhage. Neurology 1985;35:943–948.
11. Wilson SAK, Bruce AN. Neurology Second Edition. London: Butterworth, 1955;1371.

12. Caplan LR, Hier DB, D'Cruz I. Cerebral embolism in the Michael Reese Stroke Registry. Stroke 1983;14:530–536.

13. Mohr JP, Caplan LR, Melski JW, et al. The Harvard Cooperative Stroke Registry: a prospective registry. Neurology 1978;28:754–762.

14. Foulkes MA, Wolf PA, Price TR, et al. The Stroke Data Bank: design, methods and baseline characteristics. Stroke 1988;19:547–554.

15. Caplan LR, Mohr JP. Intracerebral hemorrhage: an update. Geriatrics 1978;33:42–52.

16. Ropper AH, Gress DR. Anatomical causes of coma in large cerebral hemorrhage. Ann Neurol 1989;26:161 (abstract).

17. Ropper AH, Gress DR. Computerized tomography and clinical features of large cerebral hemorrhages. Cerebrovasc Dis 1991; 1:38–42.

18. Borison HL, Wang SC. Physiology and pharmacology of vomiting. Pharmacol Rev 1953; 5:193–230.

19. Kilpatrick CJ, Davis SM, Tress BM, et al. Epileptic seizures in acute stroke. Arch Neurol 1990;47:157–160.

20. Massaro AR, Sacco RL, Mohr JP, et al. Clinical discriminators of lobar and deep hemorrhages: the Stroke Data Bank. Neurology 1991; 41:1881–1885.

21. Weisberg LA, Shamsnia M, Elliott D. Seizures caused by nontraumatic parenchymal brain hemorrhages. Neurology 1991;41:1197–1199.

22. Berger AR, Lipton RB, Lesser ML, et al. Early seizures following intracerebral hemorrhage: implications for therapy. Neurology 1988; 38:1363–1365.

23. Faught E, Peters D, Bartolucci A, et al. Seizures after primary intracerebral hemorrhage. Neurology 1989;39:1089–1093.

24. Aring CD, Merritt HH. Differential diagnosis between cerebral hemorrhage and cerebral thrombosis: a clinical and pathologic study of 245 cases. Arch Int Med 1935;56:435–456.

25. Byer E, Ashman R, Toth LA. Electrocardiograms with large, upright T waves and Q-T intervals. Am Heart J 1947;33:796–806.

26. Burch GE, Meyers R, Abildskov JA. A new electrocardiograph pattern observed in cerebrovascular accidents. Circulation 1954; 9:719–723.

27. Lavy S, Yaar I, Melamed E, et al. The effect of acute stroke on cardiac functions as observed in an intensive stroke care unit. Stroke 1974; 5:775–780.

28. Dimant J, Grob D. Electrocardiographic changes and myocardial damage in patients with acute cerebrovascular accidents. Stroke 1977;8:448–455.

29. Talman WT. Cardiovascular regulation and lesions of the central nervous system. Ann Neurol 1985;18:1–12.

30. Rolak LA, Rokey R. Electrocardiographic features. In Rolak LA, Rokey R, eds. Coronary and cerebral vascular diseases. Mt. Kisco: Futura, 1990;139–197.

31. Goldstein DS. The electrocardiogram in stroke: relationship to pathophysiological type and comparison with prior tracings. Stroke 1979;10:253–259.

32. Stober T, Sen S, Anstätt T, et al. Correlation of cardiac arrythmias with brainstem compression in patients with intracerebral hemorrhage. Stroke 1988;19:688–692.

33. Norris JW, Hachinski VC. Cardiac dysfunction following stroke. In Furlan AJ, ed. The heart and stroke. London: Springer-Verlag, 1987;171–183.

34. Levine SR, Patel VM, Welch KMA, et al. Are heart attacks really brain attacks? In Furlan AJ, ed. The heart and stroke. London: Springer-Verlag, 1987;185–216.

# Chapter 4

# Intracerebral Hemorrhage: Pathology of Selected Topics

Julio H. García, Khang-Loon Ho,
and Darío V. Caccamo*

Intracranial bleeding has various causes depending on the primary location of the hemorrhage. Epidural (extradural) hemorrhages are frequently the consequence of head trauma accompanied by fractures of the temporal bone and injury to branches of the middle meningeal artery.[1] Subdural (intradural) hemorrhages are, in most cases, the consequence of tears or rents in the bridging veins; frequently, these tears are also the result of traumatic events.[1]

Bleeding confined to the subarachnoid space frequently reflects the rupture of branches of the internal carotid artery. Injury to these vessels also may be traumatic in origin; however, spontaneous rupture may occur at the site of an aneurysm or as a result of bacterial or fungal infections localized to the arterial wall.[2]

Spontaneous bleeding into the brain parenchyma, or intracerebral hemorrhage (ICH), is associated in most adults with structural abnormalities of the penetrating arterial vessels, for example, hypertensive arteriopathy.[3] Selected diseases of the circulating cells, such as the leukemias, can also be complicated by spontaneous intracerebral bleeding; however, even in these cases, abnormalities such as thrombocytopenia are assumed to alter either the function or structure of the endothelial lining and allow the escape of red blood cells.[4] In this sense, even this type of hemorrhage could be considered secondary to a vascular abnormality.

The structural abnormalities characteristic of most angiopathies associated with ICH are discussed elsewhere in this book. Three selected topics are covered in this chapter:

1. Time-dependent structural changes affecting the blood clot and the surrounding brain tissues in cases of non-traumatic ICH.
2. Hemorrhage into an evolving brain infarct, that is, hemorrhagic brain infarct.
3. Hemorrhage into the brain parenchyma and subarachnoid space secondary to thrombosis of intracranial veins and sinuses.

## Definitions

*Hematoma* is a large localized collection of blood in an organ (brain), space (subarach-

*The authors are grateful to Drs. Suresh Patel and Bharat Mehta (Division of Neuroradiology, Henry Ford Hospital, Detroit, Michigan) for their contributions on the neuroimaging aspects of intracerebral hemorrhage, and to Ms. Barbara Caracciolo, Ms. Lisa Pietrantoni, and Ms. Harriet Stone for their help in the preparation of the manuscript.

45

noid), or membrane (intradural). *Hemorrhage* describes the escape of blood from arterial or venous blood vessels. The implied difference between these two words refers to the fact that a hematoma, due to its large volume, exerts a "mass effect" or displaces anatomical structures surrounding it. A hemorrhage may or may not have the same effect.

*Petechia* is a pinpoint, non-raised, localized hemorrhage. *Purpura* describes a condition in which many petechiae occur simultaneously at the same site. Brain purpura, or generalized petechiae confined to the white matter of the brain, has been observed in, among others, cases of cerebral malaria,[5] and fat embolism.[6]

## Time-Dependent Changes in Intracerebral Hemorrhages

This description of the sequential changes in ICH is based on the evolution of basal ganglionic hemorrhages occurring in association with hypertension; these are the prototypes of ICH. Hemorrhages at other sites and caused by other mechanisms probably follow a similar pattern of changes, but these have not been described in detail. The gross and microscopic features of the conditions responsible for the hemorrhage (miliary aneurysms, arteriovenous malformations, amyloid angiopathy, and others) are described in detail elsewhere in this book. The following is a description of the evolutionary changes in the hematoma; where appropriate, correlation between morphological changes and neuroimaging studies is indicated.

Since the early 1930s[7] several authors have distinguished cerebral hemorrhage (a diffuse extravasation of blood infiltrating and destroying the cerebral tissue) from cerebral hematoma (a well-circumscribed area of bleeding, compressing and displacing, but not destroying, the cerebral tissue). Russell[8] chose a minimal diameter of 3 cm to define a symptomatic hemispheric ICH; for lesions

in the brainstem she suggested a minimal diameter of 1.5 cm. In this section, the terms hemorrhage and hematoma are employed interchangeably and regardless of size.

The sequential changes affecting the brain after spontaneous intraparenchymal hemorrhage have interested pathologists for the past 150 years.[9] Observations on the sequential changes occurring in ICH include those of Neumann,[10] who recognized two pigmented layers within the hemorrhage: an inner one negative for the traditional stains for iron-containing pigments (bilirubin or hematoidin), and a peripheral one positive for iron (hemosiderin). Later, Böhne[11] described *Gitterzellen* (macrophages) in the wall of the ICH, and Spatz[12] outlined three stages in the evolution of intracerebral hematomas. The first stage, lasting approximately four days, includes deformation, edema, and necrosis of the surrounding tissues; the second stage involves absorption of the hematoma and typically lasts five to fifteen days; in the final stage, there is conversion of the hematoma into either a scar or a cavity.[12] This "staging system" of ICH is still employed by some pathologists, and although many of these classical descriptions are accurate, the information provided is fragmentary; also, in many instances a precise correlation between the clinical events and the histological changes is poorly documented.

The macroscopic changes in the brain vary according to the site involved by the ICH, but the general appearance is similar. In the acute stages, the ICH consists of a liquid or semiliquid mass of blood displacing the surrounding brain tissue. Small fragments of necrotic brain tissue may be identified in the center of the hematoma. However, the ICH is primarily a collection of pure red blood cells that in most instances is easily distinguished macroscopically from a hemorrhagic infarct. After washing away the contents, sometimes it is possible to recognize small torn vessels at the periphery of the ICH; this is especially true in large hemorrhages of the basal ganglia. Edema develops at the periphery of the hemorrhage after a few days; edema is particularly prominent in ICH located in the white matter. This rim of brain around the ICH often contains small petechiae that give a "flea-bitten" appearance to the brain; these are referred to as Staemller's marginal hemorrhages.[13] After a few days, the hematoma increases in consistency and adopts a brown color, while edema in the surrounding parenchyma begins to recede. The edge of the hematoma often develops a golden-green tinge, attributable to the formation of hemoglobin-derived pigments in the macrophages; these cells begin to invade the marginal zone of the hematoma sometime after forty-eight to seventy-two hours. After several months or years, depending on the size, the hematoma becomes a cavity lined by cells (mostly astroglial) containing brown or rusty pigment, the "apoplectic cyst." At this stage, the cavity may be considerably smaller than the original ICH. There are, however, notable differences of opinion concerning the evolution of ICH. According to some authors, an ICH becomes a solid clot a few hours after the original bleeding, undergoing partial liquefaction twelve to fifteen hours later.[14] Others report that clotting in ICH occurs only after the first day.[15] Lamination of the clot has been interpreted as evidence of recurring hemorrhages at the same site.[16] Most authors believe that an ICH becomes at least partially liquefied by the end of the first week, but solid clots may persist for several weeks.[14,17]

Small ICH can be reabsorbed almost completely, leaving behind a small linear scar (Figure 4.1). Microscopic confirmation of hemosiderin presence is necessary to establish that these glial scars developed as the result of previous bleeding. In contrast, large ICH become "encapsulated" by a fibroglial membrane that has been compared to the capsule of chronic subdural hematomas. This "membrane," according to some authors, becomes established five to six weeks after the original bleeding.[18] The earliest tissue reactions include edema of adjacent tissues and neutrophilic exudate; macrophages appear later and begin a slow process of digestion. The re-

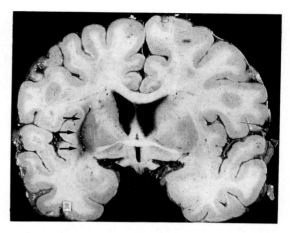

**Figure 4.1.** Old right putaminal hemorrhage reduced to a "slit" with brown edges (arrows), resulting from the presence of hemosiderin pigment.

sulting cavity becomes encapsulated after a period of several weeks and is finally surrounded by collagen fibers.[19] The older literature contains several reports of calcifications of the hematoma's "capsule,"[20] but this event is, in our opinion, very rare.

The microscopic changes in ICH are also essentially similar regardless of the site of the bleeding. In the early stages, the ICH consists of extravasated blood cells whose shape and structure are relatively preserved, and the interphase with the adjacent brain is well defined (Figure 4.2). The edge of the hematoma is in contact with disrupted and necrotic parenchyma; no inflammatory infiltrates are yet present. After several hours or days, depending on the size and site of the hemorrhage, extracellular brain edema may become evident in the parenchyma adjacent to the hematoma.[13] The hemispheric white matter appears expanded and microscopically displays pale-staining and swollen, vacuolated myelin sheaths. Physical changes also affect the red blood cells in the ICH, but these changes may be difficult to identify in tissue sections. After approximately four to ten days, depending on the size of the ICH, the red blood cells begin to lyse; this is thought to reflect depletion of the intracellular energy reserves.

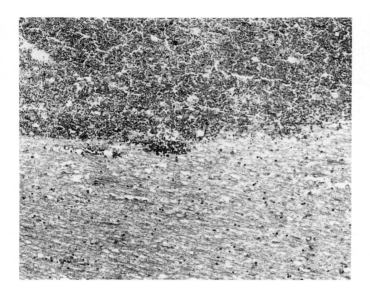

**Figure 4.2.** Acute stage (less than 48 hr) of intracerebral hemorrhage. The hematoma (top) is demarcated from the surrounding, slightly compressed brain parenchyma (bottom) (H&E, ×33).

Individual erythrocytes are more difficult to identify and their shape and outline become blurred or swollen and eventually their plasma membranes rupture and erythrocytes become an amorphous mass of methemoglobin. Once the metabolic reserves are depleted, erythrocytes rapidly accumulate deoxygenated hemoglobin and methemoglobin (oxidized deoxyhemoglobin).

Cellular infiltrates begin to appear at the periphery of the hemorrhage within a few days. One of the earliest events is the appearance of polymorphonuclear leukocytes (PMN) and activated microglial cells or *Gitterzellen*. Studies detailing the chronology of the arrival of PMN in human brain hemorrhages are not available, but experimental studies suggest that PMN appear at the margin of the ICH after two days and that their numbers peak at four days.[21] The appearance of macrophages or "gitter cells" (*gitter* means "lattice" in German) is better documented in human hematomas than is the appearance of PMN. Macrophages display a round shape, few processes, foamy or granular cytoplasm, and round nuclei located close to the plasma membrane (Figure 4.3); macrophages have strong acid phosphatase activity, can be immunostained by antibodies

to macrophages such as KP-1 or Mac 387, and also with biotynilated lectins, such as *Ricinus communis* agglutinin.[22] Immunophenotipically, gitter cells also express major histocompatibility (MHC) antigens class II, suggesting that they can act as antigen-presenting cells.[22] In many cases, transitional forms between activated and resting microglial cells are visible; the resting cells have elongated, rod-shaped nuclei in hematoxylin-eosin sections and thin short processes stainable in frozen sections by the Davenport method. However, it is still unsettled whether resting microglia are the main source of lipid-containing phagocytes or whether these cells derive from circulating mononuclear cells.[22]

The time-dependent appearance of hemoglobin-derived products in the ICH is of interest, especially because the interpretation of neuroimaging studies is based on the presence of these products of blood breakdown. The two major hemoglobin-derived pigments identifiable in tissue sections are hemosiderin and hematoidin. Hemosiderin represents aggregates of ferritin micelles within phagosomes (lysosomes of phagocytic cells); hemosiderin is a coarse, golden brown, granular intracytoplasmic pigment

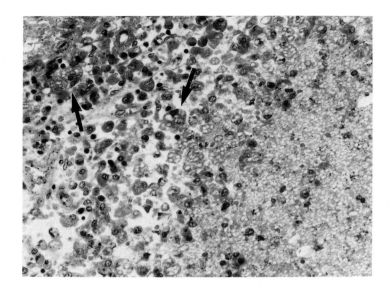

**Figure 4.3.** Organizing intracerebral hematoma (about two to three weeks old), showing lysed red blood cells (right lower corner), and abundant macrophages, some of which contain fragments of red blood cells (arrows) (H&E, ×100).

(Figure 4.4). The ferritin micelles contain ferric ions and this makes hemosiderin demonstrable with histochemical methods, such as the Prussian blue reaction of Perls. In this reaction, colorless potassium ferrocyanide reacts with the ferric ions to create insoluble ferric ferrocyanide that gives a deep blue color. Hematoidin, in contrast, is chemically identical to bilirubin, a pigment that forms locally as a result of hemoglobin breakdown;

this process is favored by reduced oxygen tension. Hematoidin appears as more coarse and globular deposits than hemosiderin, and is frequently extracellular. The main difference between the two pigments is that hematoidin does not contain iron and, therefore, is Prussian blue negative.[10,23]

In experimental ICH in mice, hemosiderin becomes visible first at forty-eight hours and is prominent after seventy-two hours; hema-

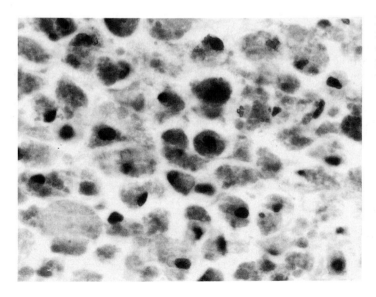

**Figure 4.4.** Hemosiderin-laden macrophages, showing ''plump'' bodies, coarse granular cytoplasm, and peripherally-displaced nuclei (H&E, ×200).

toidin is demonstrable at eleven days.[23] In human ICH, hemosiderin appears first at six days and remains visible for a long time; hematoidin becomes visible ten days after the hemorrhage, and its appearance is always more delayed than that of hemosiderin. Most hemorrhages contain two layers of histiocytes: an inner one, where the oxygen tension may be lowest, and which contains hematoidin, and an outer one rich in hemosiderin.

One of the final events in the microscopic changes of cerebral hematomas involves the astrocytes. These cells proliferate at the periphery of the hemorrhage in a manner similar to what is observed after other types of focal cerebral injury. The precise sequence of astrocytic reactions after ICH is not known, but experimental studies suggest that astrocytic reactivity may take place as early as two to three days after the hemorrhage.[21] The increase in size and number of astrocytes is best seen at the periphery of the hematoma, where these cells become enlarged and rounded and exhibit a homogeneously eosinophilic cytoplasm (gemistocytic astrocytes) (Figure 4.5). With time, reactive astrocytes around a hematoma become less evident and are replaced by abundant glial fibrils. In many cases, hemosiderin granules

are readily demonstrable in the astrocytic cytoplasm.[22] The presence of hemosiderin in astrocytes is a reflection of their phagocytic activity, which has been clearly demonstrated after experimental neuronal damage.[24] The source of hemosiderin in astrocytes is not known, but it seems likely that hemosiderin is transferred from macrophages or that hemosiderin is completely metabolized from hemoglobin within the astrocytic cytoplasm.[25]

ICH in newborn, especially premature, infants evolve in a manner similar to that observed in adults; however, there are some important qualitative differences. Darrow et al.[25] divided the evolution of ICH in premature infants, from occurrence to reabsorption, into seven stages. A major difference between the adult and neonatal brain is that the hemosiderin is completely cleared from the premature brains, while the pigment remains for years in the adult brain. This appears to be related to the transfer of hemosiderin from macrophages to astrocytes, an event that rarely happens in infants but is common in the adult. Brain cavitation after an ICH is much more rapid in the premature infant, probably because of the much smaller size of the hematoma as compared with that in the adult.[25]

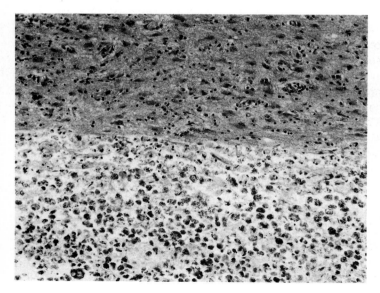

**Figure 4.5.** Organized intracerebral hematoma (older than four weeks); there is marked astroglial reaction (upper half of the field). The hematoma is being replaced by a fluid-filled cavity which at this stage still contains numerous hemosiderin-laden macrophages (lower half of the field). (H&E, ×40).

There are several studies of experimental ICH, but few of these detail the sequence of pathological changes. Most experiments are based on either the intracerebral injection of coagulated venous blood or the insertion of intracerebral balloons; neither of these reproduce the arterial bleeding of human ICH. Enzmann et al.[26] and Takasugi et al.[27] report good correlation between their observations on canine hemorrhages and the stages described in human ICH by Spatz.[12] In experimental hemorrhages in the rat, the ICH was induced at arterial pressure with an aliquot of liquid blood.[21] These authors also reported a sequence of histological changes that agrees with the timetable suggested by Spatz.[12] The extent of brain edema in these rats was greater than the original size of the ICH, suggesting that, in these animals, brain edema may be more harmful than the initial bleeding. PMN appeared at forty-eight hours and their numbers peaked at four days. Hemosiderin-laden macrophages appeared between four and fourteen days, and astroglial proliferation began at eight days and was well established by fourteen days. This resulted in the formation of a membrane (glia limitans) that clearly separated the residual hematoma from the adjacent neuropil.[21]

## Hemorrhagic Brain Infarct

An infarct is an area of coagulation necrosis caused by the occlusion of a vessel, usually an artery. Coagulation necrosis in the brain can also be the consequence of hemodynamic crises, venous occlusions, and viral infections, among others.[28] The brain lesions observed among patients who suffer hemodynamic crises (e.g., severe hypotensive attacks or cardiac arrest) may not be, in the strict sense of the word, infarcts. This is because the traditional definition of infarct (from the Latin *infarcere* meaning "to stuff") implies that an infarct is the lesion that results from the occlusion or "stuffing" of a vessel.[29] However, instead of defining a lesion by its cause, it is more appropriate to define brain infarcts as areas of coagulation necrosis that probably have an ischemic origin. The ischemic mechanism may be either occlusive or hemodynamic in origin.[30]

Most brain infarcts associated with arterial occlusions are classified as white, pale, bland, or anemic.[29] These adjectives describe the gross features of the infarct as being non-hemorrhagic, that is, the color and consistency of the area injured by ischemia are, in the initial stages, not too different from those of the surrounding brain. The bland, non-hemorrhagic characteristics of fresh (less than 24 hours) brain infarcts make the early identification of the lesion difficult either by neuroimaging methods or by direct examination of the brain.[28] In fixed specimens, brain infarcts cannot be identified unless forty-eight to seventy-two hours have elapsed since the time of the arterial occlusion.[31] Experimental brain infarcts in Wistar rats, induced by the permanent occlusion of an intracranial artery, become clearly outlined in histological preparations as areas of pallor and pannecrosis only when a minimum of seventy-two hours has elapsed after the arterial occlusion.[30]

In an autopsy survey of the causative mechanisms of brain infarcts, Fisher and Adams[32,33] identified a group of specimens in which the areas of ischemic necrosis contained petechiae throughout selected parts of the lesion; this type of ischemic injury is known as hemorrhagic brain infarct (HBI) (Figure 4.6). The analysis was limited to brain specimens in which the gross appearance of the lesion suggested an arterial occlusion as the cause of the infarct. Arterial HBI were characterized by Fisher and Adams[32] as localized areas of softening (secondary to an arterial occlusion) that contain multiple petechiae scattered throughout the gray matter of the injured brain; the extravasated red blood cells remain either visible as individual petechia or adopt a confluent purpuric pattern (Figures 4.7 and 4.8). In large brain infarcts containing both anemic and hemorrhagic areas, the hemorrhagic zone tends to involve the proximal areas of the infarct. Based on

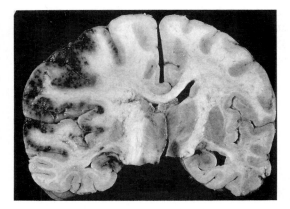

**Figure 4.6** Hemorrhagic brain infarct in the territory of the left middle cerebral artery in a patient with nonbacterial vegetations in the mitral valve. Several distal branches of the artery were occluded by thromboemboli.

these observations, Fisher and Adams[32] suggested that hemorrhagic transformation occurs in arterial infarcts when fragments of an embolus migrate downstream, thereby opening previously occluded vessels and reperfusing ischemic brain with abnormally permeable capillary endothelium under conditions of increased pressure.

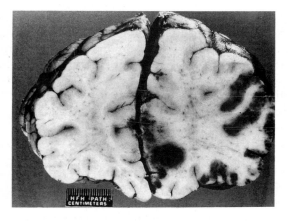

**Figure 4.7.** Hemorrhagic brain infarct in the territory of the anterior and middle cerebral arteries in a patient with myocardial infarct and mural thrombus in the left ventricle.

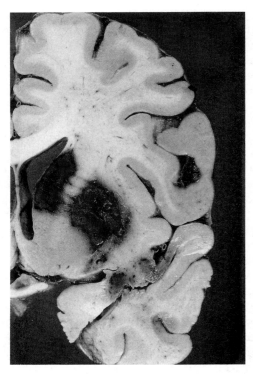

**Figure 4.8.** Hemorrhagic brain infarct in a patient with middle cerebral artery occlusion (proximal segment). The confluent hemorrhages are limited to the deep gray matter, mainly the putamen and caudate nuclei.

The diagnosis of HBI was once based solely on autopsy confirmation; but now computed tomography (CT) and, especially, magnetic resonance imaging (MRI) permit the clinical identification of HBI.[34–37] Improved neuroimaging has made possible the early recognition of these lesions and has identified increasing numbers of patients with HBI. These diagnostic advances and their corresponding therapeutic implications have renewed the interest in exploring the causes of secondary hemorrhage in brain infarcts.

Secondary bleeding in areas of ischemic brain may take the form of either petechiae or intra-infarct hematoma. The difference between these two conditions is of degree rather than of kind;[34,38] each represents an event associated with abnormalities in vascu-

**Table 4.1.** Hematoma and Hemorrhagic Infarction: Distinguishing Features

| Feature | Intracerebral Hematoma | Hemorrhagic Brain Infarct |
|---|---|---|
| Clinical | | |
| Deficit | Sudden → progression | Maximal from onset |
| ICP | Prominent increase | Normal |
| Embolic source | No | Yes |
| CT scan | | |
| High attenuation | Dense, homogenous | Spotted, mottled |
| "Mass effect" | Prominent | Absent or minimal |
| Location | Subcortical | Cortex > subcortical white matter |
| Distribution | Beyond arterial territories | Along branch distribution |
| Late enhancement | "Ring" | "Gyral" |
| Ventricular blood | Yes | No |
| Angiogram | "Mass effect" (avascular) | Branch occlusion |

Abbreviations: ICP = intracranial pressure; CT = computed tomography
(Adapted from Kase CS, Mohr JP, Caplan LR. Intracerebral hemorrhage. In: Barnett HJM, Mohr JP, Stein BM, et al. (eds): Stroke: pathophysiology, diagnosis, and management, 2nd ed. New York: Churchill Livingstone, 1992, pp. 561–616.

lar permeability and is perhaps the result of transiently increased pressure that may lead to secondary hemorrhage.

Kase et al.[39] have outlined clinical and imaging differences between ICH and HBI (Table 4.1). These differences apply to the timing of the hemorrhage with respect to the beginning of symptoms, and to the distribution of the hemorrhages within the ischemic lesion. Once the focal neurological deficit (or "stroke") occurs, an ICH can be demonstrated by CT within minutes;[40] in contrast, the petechiae of HBI appear either hours or days after the development of symptoms. Furthermore, the development of ICH at the site of a nascent brain infarct is accompanied by worsening of the patient's symptoms, whereas the appearance of petechiae at the site of a brain infarct is seldom reflected in further deterioration of neurological function.[39] Large hemorrhages at the site of a brain infarct have been associated with therapy aimed at preventing normal coagulation; petechial bleeding at the site of an ischemic infarct has not been described as a complication of anticoagulant therapy.[41,42] Rather, petechial bleeding is part of the natural evolution of some types of brain infarct.

The diagnosis of hematoma at the site of an evolving brain infarct is usually based on an initial CT evaluation suggesting an ischemic lesion; a subsequent CT scan, several hours later, shows a hematoma at the presumed site of the original infarct.[43] At autopsy, the infarcted brain is completely replaced by hematoma, rendering the identification of the infarct extremely difficult; in some large infarcts, ischemic brain tissue may be recognizable at the margin of the hematoma. In contrast to the features of a HBI in which necrotic brain tissue is recognizable among the petechiae, most cerebral hematomas do not contain identifiable brain tissue.

## Morphological Features of Hemorrhagic Brain Infarcts

The diagnosis of HBI in the past was a postmortem observation that had minimal impact on the treatment of patients with brain infarcts. Modern neuroimaging methods now allow the early identification of hemorrhagic infarcts, although occasionally the distinction between ICH and HBI, on either CT or MRI images, can be blurred.[44]

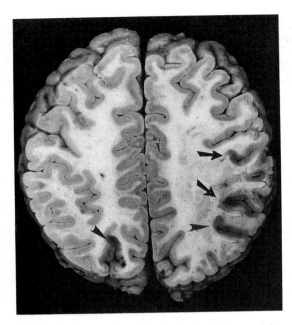

**Figure 4.9.** Hemorrhagic brain infarcts (arrows) in the "watershed" areas. The patient had suffered a cardiac arrest six days before death; the white matter lesions are nonhemorrhagic.

The distinction between pale and hemorrhagic infarcts may be slightly arbitrary; this is because most arterial brain infarcts contain occasional petechiae. However, a brain infarct is considered as being hemorrhagic only when the petechiae are grossly visible.[32,45]

In cases in which the cause of the brain infarct is either an arterial occlusion or a hemodynamic crisis, the hemorrhagic component preferentially involves cerebral or cerebellar cortices and deep gray matter structures, such as the basal ganglia and thalamic nuclei. Hemorrhages in HBI rarely involve the white matter, except when the infarct is caused by thrombosis of a venous sinus or vein.[33,46,47] In the cerebral cortex, the softening of HBI involves the full thickness of this structure and spreads along adjacent cortical gyri. The hemorrhages often are most marked in the depths of the sulci; the dusky-discolored cortex contrasts sharply with the adjacent white matter, rendering the HBI an easily identifiable lesion on gross examination (Figure 4.9).

An exception to the clear location of the hemorrhagic component to the cortex occurs when arterial infarcts are the result of infected thromboembolic material, for example, in aspergillosis; in such instances, the hemorrhagic component may involve both cortex and white matter, and the architectural landmarks of the brain may be blurred. Also, the margins of the lesion may not fit exactly the boundaries of an arterial territory.[48]

Under the microscope, many features of HBI are similar to those of anemic infarcts. Depending on the site of the infarct, there may be a combination of neuronal necrosis, sponginess of the neuropil, and astrocytic nuclear swelling, which are readily visible in standard histological preparations. Multiple, small collections of red blood cells around venules and capillaries are visible over variable extensions of the infarct (Figure 4.10). The petechiae are mainly located along small venules and capillaries, which are often distended; histological changes consistent with necrosis of the vessel walls are frequently seen but many vascular walls remain intact. HBI are easily identified under the microscope when they are less than one week old, although determining the exact age of the hemorrhage on the basis of microscopic features is often difficult. In

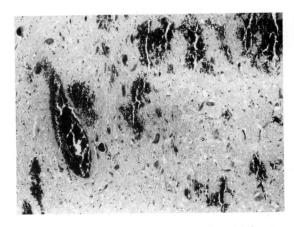

**Figure 4.10.** Coagulation necrosis and multiple hemorrhages in the cortex from the case shown in Figure 4.2 (H&E, ×40).

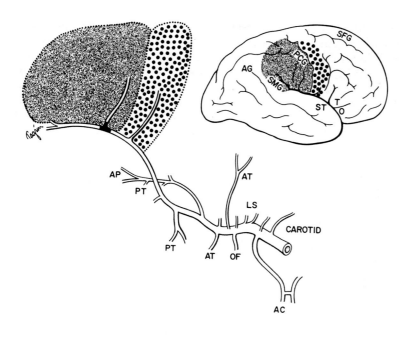

**Figure 4.11.** Mechanism of hemorrhagic infarction as a result of distal migration of occluding embolic material. The hemorrhagic portion (large dots) has been reperfused after distal migration of the embolus, which is occluding branches to the pale portion (small dots) of the infarct. Abbreviations: AC = anterior cerebral, LS = lenticulostriate, OF = orbitofrontal, AT = anterior temporal, PT = posterior temporal, AP = anterior parietal, SFG = superior frontal gyrus, PCG = postcentral gyrus, ST = superior temporal, SMG = supramarginal gyrus, AG = angular gyrus. (From Fisher CM, Adams RD: Observations on brain embolism with special reference to hemorrhagic infarction. In Furlan AJ, ed. The heart and stroke. Berlin: Springer-Verlag, 1987;17–36. With permission.)

some cases, collections of hemosiderin-laden macrophages and intact red blood cells coexist at the same site; this suggests that the bleeding may have occurred at two separate intervals. Old cavitary lesions in which the glial cells in the surrounding rim contain abundant hemosiderin are interpreted as representing the eventual outcome of either a hemorrhagic infarct or an intracerebral hematoma.

## Pathophysiology of Hemorrhagic Brain Infarct

One of the mechanisms involved in the induction of a hemorrhagic infarct assumes the existence of the phenomenon called "migratory embolus."[33] Most anemic brain infarcts in the study of Fisher and Adams[32,33] coexisted with thromboembolic arterial occlusions. Thromboembolic occlusion of the proximal artery was absent from specimens with hemorrhagic infarcts; instead, multiple "fragmented thrombi" were visible in several peripheral branches of the corresponding artery. This observation suggested embolus fragmentation and subsequent migration of the smaller components (Figure 4.11). Such interpretation is supported by what is now known about natural thrombolytic phenomena[49,50] and by sequential angiographic observations conducted in patients with intracranial arterial occlusions. According to several authors, up to 90% of intracranial arterial occlusions among patients with known embolism spontaneously reopen over a period of a few days.[51–53]

The mechanisms by which embolized vessels become recanalized are not fully understood; the embolic material is subject to the hydrostatic forces that compact, mold, and fragment its components. The embolus is also under the influence of endogenous thrombolytic factors that cause its breakdown and make possible its distal migration.[50] Restoring blood flow to the ischemic brain tissue at an appropriate time could allow escape of red blood cells through ischemic or disrupted capillary or venule walls, and this could lead to the development of a hemorrhagic infarction. This effect has been reproduced in selected instances of experimental brain infarcts. Cats with surgically-clipped intracranial arteries had the arteries opened (by removal of the clips) six hours later and the period of reperfusion lasted twenty-four hours. These animals developed multiple petechiae in the gray matter of the ischemic brain tissue, following a pattern essentially identical to that of HBI in humans.[54]

Additional support for the hypothesis of the migratory embolus has been obtained from other sources. In combined autopsy series, the frequency of hemorrhagic infarcts among patients with evidence of embolism approached 71%; in contrast, only 2% to 21% of brain infarcts were grossly hemorrhagic in cases in which the cause of the arterial occlusion was classified as being thrombotic.[33,45,55]

Postmortem evaluation of brains with hemorrhagic infarcts has shown in many cases a patent artery, suggesting that the occlusion was transient; however, petechiae also appear in brain infarcts in which the parent artery remains occluded.[56,57] This emphasizes the importance of the collateral circulation in the hemorrhagic transformation of some brain infarcts. The role of arterial reperfusion via the leptomeningeal collateral connections that exist among cerebral arteries has been well documented in experimental models of brain infarct[58-60] and is supported by clinical observations (Figure 4.12). Hemorrhagic transformation of brain infarcts in cases in which the proximal artery remains occluded may be the result of a surge in arterial blood pressure to the hypertensive range.[61] The resulting increased perfusion of the ischemic tissue, through the leptomeningeal collaterals, may be sufficient to

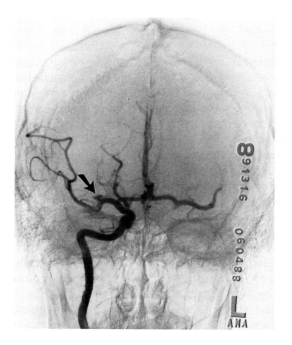

A

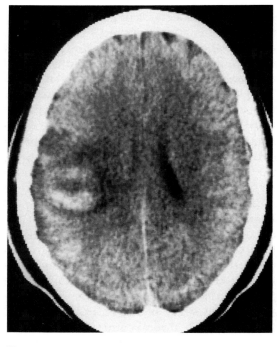

B

**Figure 4.12.** (A) Embolic occlusion of the upper division of the MCA (arrow), which did not reopen after treatment with tPA. (B) Hemorrhagic infarct involving the distal territory of the MCA in the same patient.

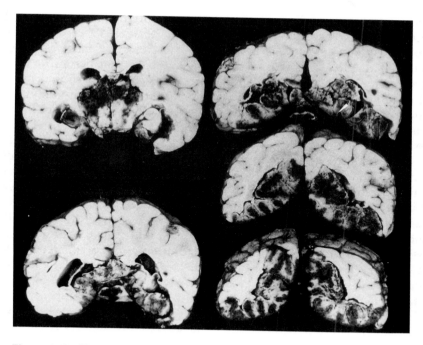

**Figure 4.13.** Hemorrhagic infarctions in a patient with bacterial endocarditis and embolism to the distal basilar artery.

cause hemorrhagic transformation of a previously anemic brain infarct.[57,60]

Among patients with infective endocarditis, the hemorrhagic transformation of infarcts secondary to septic embolism is the most common mechanism leading to the development of ICH (Figure 4.13). Rupture of an artery at a site of mural inflammation is thought to be the mechanism responsible for such hemorrhagic transformation.[62,63]

Most brain infarcts complicated by large hemorrhages are probably associated with cardiogenic embolism.[36,38,55] Analysis of combined autopsy data from Fisher and Adams,[33] Adams and van der Eecken,[64] and Jörgensen and Torvik[45] suggest that 50% of all embolic brain infarcts are hemorrhagic and that 88% of all HBI have a cardiac embolic source. In a recent autopsy series, 63% of cases with HBI had cardiac sources of embolism.[55] It is unclear why cardiogenic embolism is so frequently associated with hemorrhagic infarct.[44,55,61] In an analysis

of thirty patients with cardiogenic embolism, the frequency of HBI was not influenced by age.[65] However, a few reports have shown a possible association between aging and frequency of HBI.[36] Age alone may be an independent factor for the development of HBI; this is because elderly patients tend to have large brain infarcts as a result of the impaired collateral circulation that accompanies aging.[36]

The risk of secondary hemorrhage is significantly increased in patients who have large brain infarcts and severe neurological deficits. Neuroimaging studies and autopsy observations suggest that hemorrhagic transformation is closely related to the size of a brain infarct.[34,55,65-68] In a recent autopsy study, petechiae were much more frequent among brain infarcts large enough to produce uncinate herniation compared with patients with brain infarcts who died of extracerebral causes; the study emphasized that secondary bleeding relates more to the size than to the cause of the infarct.[55] The reason for the increased hemorrhagic transformation of large brain infarcts may relate to the extent of brain edema, compression of the small blood vessels, and the stasis of blood flow. After the edema subsides, reperfusion of the previously squeezed vessels could result in escape of erythrocytes through disrupted endothelium.[34,69,70]

Although some experimental studies suggest a correlation between hemorrhagic infarct and the level of blood pressure,[58,59] analysis of clinical data show no close correlation between acute or chronic hypertension and frequency of hemorrhagic infarcts.[66,71]

HBI in the territory of the posterior cerebral artery, which are frequent in cases of ipsilateral hemispheric mass effect and uncinate herniation, may develop through a different mechanism from that of embolic lesions (Figures 4.14, 4.15). The hemorrhagic component of the infarct is attributed in such cases to the extrinsic compression that the posterior cerebral artery undergoes as the initial segment of this vessel is pinched between the herniated uncus and the sharp edge of the tentorial incisura. HBI occurs because the extrinsic arterial compression results in incomplete occlusion of the lumen. In this situation, the residual blood flow may be inadequate to prevent tissue necrosis but

is sufficient to allow bleeding into the ischemic territory.[48]

Vasospasm may be involved in the secondary bleeding that occurs in some brain infarcts. Vasospasm, as a response to the embolic occlusion of an individual artery, remains a questionable issue, but arterial constriction is well documented by angiography among patients with aneurysmal subarachnoid hemorrhage; HBI develops in about one-third of patients with vasospasm secondary to the rupture of an aneurysm.[72,73] Hypertensive bursts during a presumed period of remission in the vasoconstriction may be one of the causes of hemorrhagic transformation observed in the brain lesions of some of these patients.[72,74]

After transient hemodynamic crises, ischemic lesions first appear in the brain at sites where the blood perfusion is lowest; these sites are the so-called arterial border (or boundary) zones, also referred to as "watersheds."[75] In the cerebrum, the most commonly involved sites are the boundary zones between the anterior and middle cerebral arteries. The lesions at these sites have many of the microscopic features of anemic or pale infarcts. The hemorrhagic components visible in some of these specimens are generally attributed to the effect of reperfusion,[48] which is a mechanism comparable

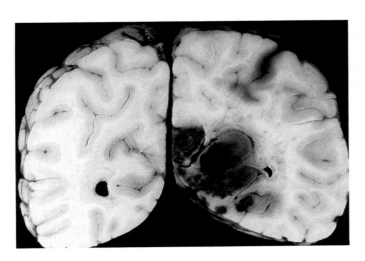

**Figure 4.14.** Hemorrhagic infarct in the territory of the posterior cerebral artery in a patient with an ipsilateral subdural hemorrhage and secondary uncinate herniation.

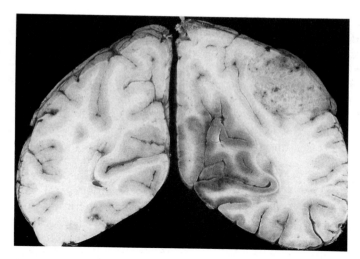

A

**Figure 4.15.** (A) Hemorrhagic infarct in the territory of the posterior cerebral artery in a patient with ipsilateral uncinate herniation. (B) A large glioblastoma multiforme was the cause of the herniation. The extension of the tumor to the posterior parietal lobe is shown in A.

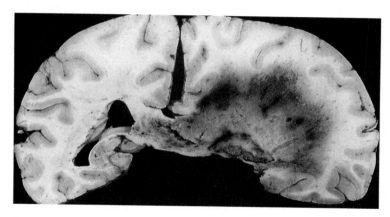

B

to what is believed to operate in cases of "migrating emboli."

The true incidence of hematoma formation at the site of a brain infarct is not known. Cerebral hematomas developing at the site of an infarct may be underdiagnosed, and bleeding at the site of an evolving infarct should be a diagnostic consideration in appropriately selected patients.[43,76]

The microenvironment of infarcted brain tissue may influence both the development and severity of secondary hemorrhage. Brain tissue is one of the richest sources of thromboplastin, or tissue factor, a known inhibitor

of the anticoagulant activity of heparin.[77] The activity of tissue thromboplastin in gray and white matter is similar; however, other factors, such as capillary density, may determine the tendency for hemorrhages to occur in the gray matter following an arterial occlusion.[78]

## Venous and Sinus Thrombosis as a Cause of Intracerebral Hemorrhage

Symptomatic thrombosis of intracranial sinuses and veins has been observed mainly in two groups of patients:

1. Those with bacterial and fungal infections, either systemic or localized to the cranium, as is frequently the case in patients with cavernous sinus thrombosis.[79] Infections have become a less frequent cause of venous thrombosis since the introduction of antibiotics in the early 1950s.[79]

2. Those with noninfectious miscellaneous and seemingly unrelated conditions, such as dehydration, puerperium, ulcerative colitis, hemoglobinopathies, protein C deficiency, and Behçet's syndrome, among others. In a substantial proportion of patients (about 25%) with angiographically confirmed intracranial sinus venous thrombosis (SVT), there was no identifiable risk factor.[80,81]

A predisposition to develop intravascular thrombi is often termed a "hypercoagulable" state. A preferred designation might be a "prethrombotic state," or one involving one or more of the following: activated blood coagulation, increased platelet reactivity, or impaired fibrinolysis.[82] Bousser and Barnett[81] have compiled a long list of the conditions identified in patients with SVT; among the least frequent causes are compression of sinuses by neighboring tumors (Figure 4.16).

Neuroimaging techniques allow early diagnosis of SVT, a condition that appears to be more common, less severe, and more diverse in its clinical presentations than previously thought. SVT should be considered in the differential diagnosis of patients with symptoms of pseudotumor cerebri. The symptoms recorded among patients with confirmed diagnosis of SVT also mimic those of arterial occlusions, brain abscesses, brain tumors, and subarachnoid hemorrhage. The CT scan is of major importance in ruling out these diagnoses, but either angiography or MRI is needed to verify a diagnosis of SVT, and to determine the nature and extent of the parenchymal abnormalities.[83]

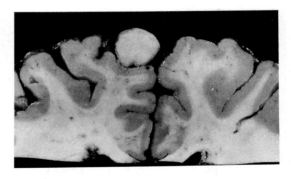

A

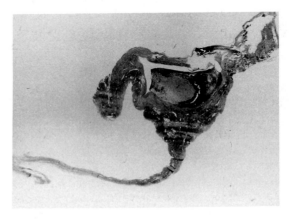

B

**Figure 4.16.** (A) Small parasagittal meningioma in a 72-year-old patient with a two-year history of headaches. (B) Thrombosis of the superior sagittal sinus in the same patient as shown in A.

### Pathological Anatomy of Sinus Venous Thrombosis

The abnormalities described in autopsy evaluations of brains with SVT are extremely variable. This is explained partly by the wide heterogeneity in the caliber of the occluded vessel; thrombosis may involve the superior sagittal sinus, a cortical vein, the cavernous sinus, or any of the tributaries of the great vein of Galen. In each case, the brain parenchymal lesions may be sufficiently different to result in widely variable circulatory changes. Baló[84] and Capra and Kapp[85] have reviewed the anatomical features of intracranial veins and sinuses.

Subarachnoid hemorrhage is a frequent consequence of intracranial SVT. In contrast with the subarachnoid hemorrhage of arterial origin, the hemorrhage in patients with SVT is located either on the lateral surface or over the convexity of the cerebral hemispheres. Hemorrhage in the brain parenchyma in patients with SVT is slightly less frequent than subarachnoid bleeding; in one clinical series, up to 28% of patients with confirmed diagnosis of SVT had evidence of ICH[86] (Figure 4.17). This percentage is probably higher among autopsy cases compared with clinical series, in part because large ICH may increase the lethality of SVT and also because hemorrhages less than 2 cm in diameter may not be readily detectable by standard CT.

In contrast to the predominantly cortical petechiae that develop in arterial infarcts, hemorrhages in venous infarcts may remain confined to the subcortical white matter or may spread into both gray and white matter structures. The distribution of the hemorrhages does not conform to the topography of an arterial territory and in cases in which the SVT involves midline channels, such as the sagittal sinuses or the great vein of Galen, the hemorrhagic softening involves structures located on both sides of the midline (Figures 4.18, 4.19).

Brain edema, expressed partly in the form of increased brain weight (10% to 15% above normal), is a prominent finding in cases of superior sagittal sinus thrombosis. This edema is especially pronounced in the white matter of the cerebral hemispheres and may be sufficiently marked as to result in a noticeable change in the consistency of the brain parenchyma. The supratentorial ventricular system may dilate in the initial stages of SVT, but in most patients the lateral ventricles are compressed by the swollen periventricullar white matter.[87] Dilatation of the ventricular system has been thought to be one of the

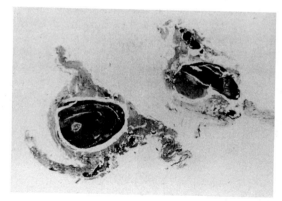

A

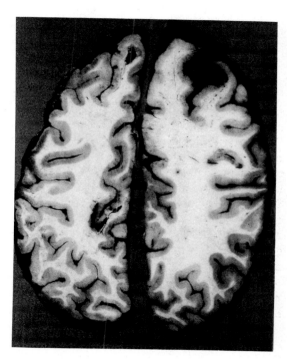

B

**Figure 4.17.** (A) Thrombosis of the superior sagittal sinus in a young patient with sickle cell disease. (B) Subarachnoid and minimal intracerebral hemorrhages with marked white matter edema in the same patient.

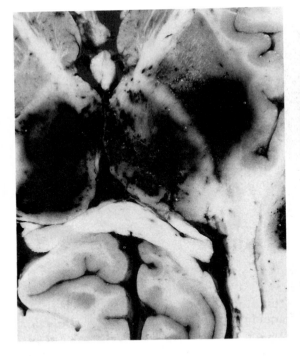

A

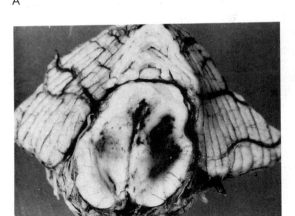

B

**Figure 4.18.** (A) Hemorrhagic infarct in the territory of the great vein of Galen involving both thalami and the right putamen. (B) Hemorrhagic midbrain infarct in the territory drained by the vein of Rosenthal in the same patient.

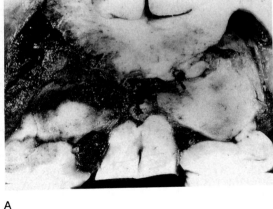

A

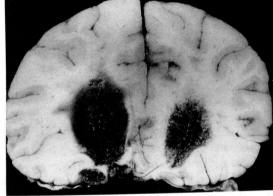

B

**Figure 4.19.** (A) Widespread thrombosis of deep cerebral veins in a patient with a large venous malformation. (B) Bilateral periventricular hemorrhages in the same patient.

complications developing after occlusion of the great vein of Galen, and a form of hydrocephalus called "otitic" was attributed by Symonds to the thrombosis of a transverse sinus.[88] This sinus is either unilateral or markedly asymmetric in many patients.[85]

Thrombosed cortical veins may be seen as stiff cords on the brain surface (Figure 4.20). The vessel caliber is enlarged compared with that of the neighboring veins or sinuses, and the lumen is filled with grayish white

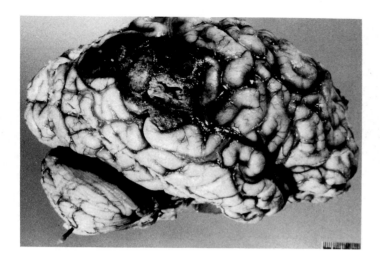

**Figure 4.20.** Hemorrhagic infarct secondary to thrombosis of a large cortical vein.

material that remains attached to the endothelial surface after opening the vessel.

Several microscopic features help distinguish the brain lesions accompanying SVT from those observed in ischemic lesions secondary to either arterial occlusions or hemodynamic crises. Coagulation necrosis (a common feature of arterial infarcts) is rare in venous infarcts, regardless of the age of the lesion; therefore, the identification of either eosinophilic or ghost neurons in these lesions is extremely rare.[46,47] In many foci of venous infarcts, the neuronal perikarya may appear almost entirely normal. The leukocytic infiltrates in cases of SVT are far more widespread and abundant, when compared with the infiltrates typical of arterial infarcts. Instead of focal coagulative necrosis, venous infarcts display large areas of neuropil sponginess and huge "plasma lakes" in the white matter. These lakes correspond to sites where extravasation of plasma (i.e., protein-rich fluid) can be readily identified in the form of accumulation of pale, eosinophilic, glassy material. Frequently, there are numerous hemorrhages of diverse sizes, most of which retain an angiocentric pattern; however, instead of a discrete petechial distribution, typical of the hemorrhagic arterial infarcts, the hemorrhages of venous infarcts spread diffusely into both gray and white

matter. Many of the venules and capillaries within the territory of the venous infarct are frequently distended and filled with pale, pink material that represents thrombi probably made of fibrin; this issue has not been clearly addressed in any of the autopsy studies published thus far.[46,47]

In experiments based on the induction of thrombi in the external jugular veins of laboratory dogs, histological examination revealed an organizing thrombus occupying between 20% and 90% of the lumen. Various stages of organization, ranging from extensive fibrosis and granulation tissue to relatively unorganized thrombus, were noted at various levels along the length of the thrombi. The extent of the vessel occlusion, the organization of the thrombus, and the extent of recanalization varied from thrombus to thrombus as well as within the same specimen. Venous thrombi in this study were made of fibrin, platelets, granulation tissue, and erythrocytes.[89] Based on these experimental studies, Erdman et al.[89] concluded that MRI at .35T does not allow establishment of the age of a venous thrombus, but that MRI may be helpful in following the thrombus resolution after three weeks.

The pattern of infiltration by PMN in venous infarcts is different from that seen in arterial infarcts; venous infarcts are infil-

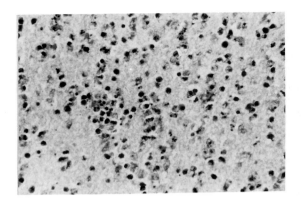

**Figure 4.21.** Abundant infiltrates by PMN in a cortical venous infarct. Symptoms had started three to four days before death (H&E, ×40).

trated early by large numbers of PMN that diffusely spread in sheets over most of the lesion (Figure 4.21). For this reason, the initial histological evaluation of these tissues may suggest infectious cerebritis. This profuse leukocytic infiltrate, much more abundant than that seen in arterial infarcts, is attributed to the preserved patency of the arterial and arteriolar tree; this probably facilitates the entry of these circulating cells into the area of infarct.[46,47]

Information concerning the long-term evolution of intracranial venous infarcts is scarce. This is partly attributable to the fact that, after many months, the morphological features of ICH, arterial hemorrhagic infarcts, and venous infarcts merge into a common pattern of a cavitary brain lesion in which the residual hemosiderin pigment deposited in the walls of the cavity suggests a hemorrhagic component. However, the histological features at this late stage lack specificity with respect to the cause of the lesion.

Schmiedek et al.[90] reported slight decreases in cerebral blood flow (CBF) values among patients with confirmed SVT; also, there was no correlation between the degree of ischemia and the severity of the neurological deficit. Similarly, Kristensen et al.[91] observed modest increases in intracranial pressure in ten patients in whom CSF hydro-

dynamics were recorded over a period of up to fifteen years; none of these patients developed hydrocephalus.

Detailed data based on the effects that SVT may have on intracranial pressure, CSF circulation, or CBF changes are scarce. This is because the number of experimental models of sinus venous thrombosis is very limited.[92,93]

Histological evaluation of feline brains with experimental occlusion of the superior sagittal sinus showed no visible changes at three to six hours. In cats with total sinus and venous occlusion, focal spongy changes in the absence of neuronal ischemic changes developed in the parasagittal white matter after one hour. After three hours, perivascular hemorrhages developed in the parasagittal cerebral cortex while the surrounding subcortical white matter became markedly spongy. Focal "ischemic neuronal changes" were noted in the cortex, but most neurons appeared normal. Animals with total sinus occlusion developed, at six hours, large hemorrhages in the parasagittal gray and white matter.[92]

Pronounced histological brain changes were observed in eleven of fourteen rats with experimental thrombosis of the superior sagittal sinus. Changes consisted of subarachnoid and intracerebral hemorrhages together with marked cortical edema. The most prominent finding was the development of sharply demarcated necrotic brain areas involving all layers of the parasagittal cortex. The areas containing necrotic neurons were only those topographically related to the thrombosed sinuses.[93]

### Spectrum of Neurological Symptoms Associated with Sinus Venous Thrombosis

The diagnosis of SVT was infrequently made before the 1970s. One of the first descriptions of SVT is attributed to Ribes who reported in 1825 the case of a 45-year-old patient who died six months after experiencing a syndrome of headache, epilepsy, and delirium; autopsy disclosed thrombosis of both the superior sagittal and transverse sinuses.[94] Additional patients have been sporadically reported, and only three publications have appeared within the last thirty years in which the collective experience of several groups has been recorded in individual volumes.[95–97]

The clinical manifestations of intracranial SVT vary according to the location and the size of the occluded vessel. Thrombosis of the cavernous sinus (in the absence of trauma) is associated in most instances with an infectious process (e.g., facial mucormycosis) that becomes manifest in an acute, precipitous manner, and includes unilateral exophthalmus, monocular blindness, and severe retroorbital pain.[98]

Clinical symptoms of SVT that involve the superior sagittal sinus, the transverse sinus, and the large intracranial veins differ from those observed in patients with cavernous sinus thrombosis. Bousser et al.,[80,83] Jacewicz and Plum,[99] Einhäupl et al.,[86] and Bousser and Barnett[81] each described several syndromes associated with angiographically proven intracranial SVT as follows:

1. The most frequent syndrome was one of subacute or progressive onset of intracranial hypertension; the overriding symptom was persisting, dull, generalized, noncrippling headache. Two additional findings among these patients should suggest a diagnosis of SVT: small ventricles as seen on CT, and bilateral papilledema. The syndrome tends to persist for long periods.[83]
2. A second pattern included the sudden onset of *focal* neurological deficits with a clinical syndrome very similar to that produced by an intracranial arterial occlusion; however, seizures and the absence of a neurological deficit that could be related to a specific arterial territory should suggest a diagnosis of SVT.[83]
3. A third type of presentation included the subacute onset of multiple deficits, with or without signs of increased intracranial pressure. Among these patients, an incorrect initial diagnosis of brain abscess or encephalitis was common, especially if there were fever, elevated sedimentation rate, and CSF pleocytosis, all of which have been recorded among patients with confirmed diagnoses of SVT. Several additional syndromes were observed in other patients.[81] Regardless of the type of syndrome, headache is the most common symptom (79%) and papilledema the most common sign (50%) observed in patients with confirmed SVT (Table 4.2).[81,86]

### Risk Factors or Conditions Associated with Sinus Venous Thrombosis

In the original cases of SVT reported in autopsy series between the 1880s and the 1960s, emphasis was placed on the association between intracranial SVT and two conditions: infections and purperium. Both of these are also identified in more recent series, but their proportional contribution to SVT seems to have decreased in Western countries.[81,86]

Close evaluations of several patients seen in the decades after the 1970s have uncovered a large number of seemingly unrelated hematological and systemic abnormalities among patients with confirmed SVT. Significantly, despite the assiduous investigations performed by several groups of investigators, up to 25% of patients with confirmed SVT do not have a clearly identifiable mechanism of intravascular thrombosis. Among the recently identified abnormalities detected in some patients with SVT are protein C deficiency, protein S deficiencies, circulating serum antiphospholipid antibodies, and Behçet's disease.[81,83,86]

A hereditary deficiency in protein C carries a high risk of venous thrombosis and embolism.[100] Most reports describe heterozygotes with a history of superficial thrombophlebitis, deep venous thrombosis, pulmonary embolism, or a combination of these. The clinical events in protein C deficiency are probably related to the role of this protein in

**Table 4.2.** Main Neurological Signs and Symptoms in 76 Patients with Cerebral Venous Thrombosis

|  | No. Patients | (%) |
|---|---|---|
| Headache | 61 | (80%) |
| Papilledema | 38 | (50%) |
| Motor or sensory deficits | 27 | (35%) |
| Seizures | 22 | (29%) |
| Drowsiness, mental changes, confusion, or coma | 18 | (27%) |
| Dysphasia | 5 | (6%) |
| Multiple cranial nerve palsies | 3 | (4%) |
| Cerebellar incoordination | 2 | (3%) |
| Nystagmus | 2 | (3%) |
| Hearing loss | 2 | (3%) |
| Bilateral or alternating deficits | 3 | (4%) |

Adapted from Bousser M-G, Barnett HJM. Cerebral venous thrombosis. In Barnett HJM, Mohr JP, Stein BM, et al. (eds): Stroke: pathophysiology, diagnosis, and management. New York: Churchill Livingstone, 1992, pp. 517–538.

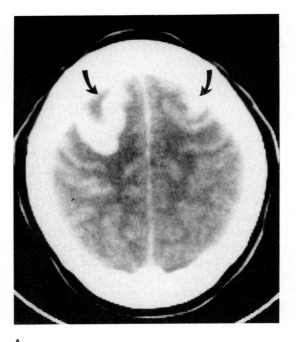

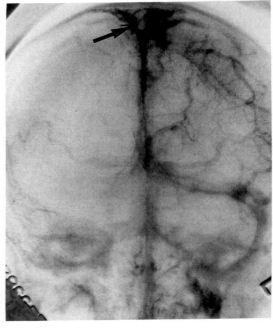

A

B

**Figure 4.22** (A) Noncontrast CT scan showing densely hemorrhagic infarcts bilaterally in the frontal lobes (arrows), secondary to thrombosis of the superior sagittal sinus. (B) Venous phase angiogram with filling defect (clot) in the superior sagittal sinus (arrow).

the formation and degradation of fibrin. Protein C is a vitamin K–dependent coagulation factor that inactivates cofactors V and VIII, thus stimulating fibrinolysis.[101] Among fifty-three patients with hereditary protein C deficiency belonging to twenty different families, each of three women, ages 27, 34, and 38, had cerebral hemorrhagic infarcts probably on the basis of SVT. All three also had venous thrombosis of the legs and pulmonary embolism either before or after the intracranial event.[102]

Diabetes mellitus does not appear in lists of risk factors for SVT. However, it is of interest that three of the patients with intracranial SVT reported by Snyder and Sachdev[103] and Goldberg et al.[104] were young, diabetic women who did not have other risk factors for SVT.

### Neuroimaging Diagnosis of Sinus Venous Thrombosis

Indirect signs of intracranial SVT on CT are less specific than the direct ones but, taken collectively, the following should suggest cerebral venous thromboses: low density areas suggestive of early brain infarct, parenchymal petechiae, post-contrast "gyral" enhancement, and small ventricles.[104] The areas of hypodensity visible in CT scans of patients with SVT have a poorly defined, rounded configuration as compared with the sharply marginated edge and either wedge or rectangular shape of most arterial infarcts. Venous infarcts are not confined to the territories of a single artery or to a watershed zone. The parenchymal hemorrhages associated with venous infarcts are often ill defined and have inhomogeneous densities. Multiple separate regions of hemorrhage, primarily involving the white matter, may be visible[105] (Figure 4.22). An additional feature of SVT is intense tentorial enhancement, which is attributed to enlargement of dural venous collaterals and increased capillary pressure leading to leakage of contrast material into the dura. Punctate or streak-like hyperdensi-

ties in the white matter may also be seen; this apparently is the consequence of the dilatation of medullary veins that serve as collateral channels between the cortical and deep venous systems.[106] Buonanno et al.[107] analyzed some of the CT features of dural sinus thrombosis in a group of eleven patients. They described the pathognomonic "empty delta sign," which corresponds to lack of contrast filling of the superior sagittal sinus posteriorly in axial cuts. The thrombosed sinus appears as a triangular structure with contrast at its periphery but without contrast centrally, on account of the presence of clot that is filling it.

The CT features of *deep* cerebral venous thromboses include high-density thrombi within the vein of Galen and straight sinus on noncontrast scans (Figure 4.23) and linear filling defects within a contrast-filled straight sinus. Nonspecific low-density areas of venous infarcts in the thalamic and basal ganglia regions have also been described.[108] A

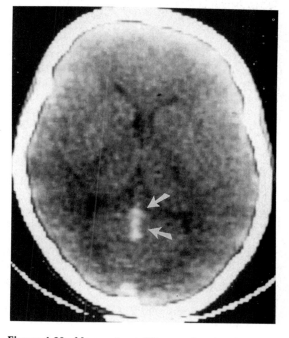

**Figure 4.23.** Noncontrast CT scan showing hyperdense clot in the vein of Galen and straight sinus (arrows).

thrombus within the thalamostriate veins was visualized on noncontrast scans as a V-shaped, high-density structure around the foramen of Monro.[109] The internal cerebral veins, the vein of Galen, and the straight sinus have been visualized on noncontrast CT as high-density structures in at least two instances.[109] Indirect signs of deep venous thrombosis include low-density areas in the thalamic and basal ganglia regions either unilaterally or bilaterally. These areas of low density change in size and shape on scans obtained at intervals of several days. Such changing patterns in the shape and density of venous infarcts may help differentiate these lesions from neoplasms.[109] Extension of a thalamic lesion across the midline serves to distinguish venous from arterial infarcts. None of the cases reviewed by Goldberg et al.[104] demonstrated ventricular dilatation; instead, some had compression of the adjacent lateral and third ventricles. Venous infarcts generally have greater "mass effect" than arterial infarcts of comparable size.[109]

# References

1. McCormick WF. Pathology of closed head injury. In: Wilkins RH, Rengachary SS, eds. Neurosurgery. New York: McGraw-Hill, 1985; 1544–1570.

2. Weir B. Intracranial aneurysms and subarachnoid hemorrhage: an overview. In: Wilkins RH, Rengachary SS, eds. Neurosurgery. New York: McGraw-Hill, 1985;1308–1329.

3. García JH, Ho KL. Pathology of hypertensive arteriopathy. Neurosurg Clin NA 1992; 3:497–507.

4. Weisberg LA, Stazio A, Shamsnia A, et al. Nontraumatic parenchymal brain hemorrhages. Medicine 1990;69:227–295.

5. White NJ, Looareesuwans. Cerebral malaria. In: Kennedy PGE, Johnson RT, eds. Infections of the nervous system. London: Butterworth, 1987;118–144.

6. Kamenar E, Burger PC. Cerebral fat embolism: a neuropathological study of a microembolic state. Stroke 1980;11:477–480.

7. Bagley C. Spontaneous cerebral hemorrhage: discussion of four types with surgical consideration. Arch Neurol Psychiat 1932;27: 1133–1174.

8. Russell DS. The pathology of spontaneous intracranial haemorrhage. Proc Roy Soc Med 1954;47:689–693.

9. Virchow R. Die patologischen Pigmente. Arch Pathol Anat Physiol Klin Med 1847;1:379–404, 407–486.

10. Neumann E. Nochmals die Pigmentfrage. Virchows Arch [Pathol Anat] 1904;177:401–426.

11. Böhne C. Kimpakte apoplektisch Hirnblutung und Hämorrhagische Hirnerweichung (Klinik, Pathologie, Pathogenese). Z klin Med 1931;117:30–54.

12. Spatz H. Patologische Anatomie der Kreislaufstorungen des Gehirns. Zeitschfrit für Neurologie 1939;167:301–351.

13. Zülch KH. Hemorrhage, thrombosis, embolism. In: Minckler J, ed. Pathology of the nervous system. New York: McGraw-Hill, 1971; 1499–1535.

14. Luyendijk W. Intracerebral haematoma. In: Vinken PJ, Bruyn GW, eds. Handbook of Clinical Neurology. Amsterdam: North-Holland, 1972;670–719.

15. Browder EJ, Turney F. Intracerebral hemorrhage of traumatic origin: its surgical treatment. NY State J Med 1942;42:2230.

16. Adson AW, McCraug WM. Spontaneous intracerebral hemorrhage: etiology and surgical treatment with a report of nine cases. Arch Neurol Psychiat 1936;35:701–720.

17. Weller RO. Spontaneous intracranial hemorrhage. In Adams J, Duchen L, eds. Greenfield's Neuropathology. New York: Oxford University Press, 1992;269–301.

18. Arseni C, Ionescu S, Maretsis M. Primary intraparenchymatous hematomas. J Neurosurg 1967;27:207–215.

19. Jellinger K. Pathology and aetiology of ICH. In: Pia HW, et al., eds. Spontaneous intracerebral hematomas: Advances in diagnosis and therapy. Berlin: Springer-Verlag, 1980; 131–135.

20. Lusignan FE. Calcified intracerebral hematoma: case report and review of the literature. Ann Surg 1950;132:268–272.

21. Jenkins A, Maxwell W, Graham D. Experimental intracerebral hematoma in the rat: sequential light microscopic changes. Neuropathol Appl Neurobiol 1989;15:477–486.

22. Duchen LW. General pathology of neurons and neuroglia. In: Adams JH, Duchen LW,

eds. Greenfield's Neuropathology. 5th edition. New York: Oxford University Press, 1992;1–68.

23. Strassmann G. Formation of hemosiderin and hematoidin after traumatic and spontaneous cerebral hemorrhages. Arch Pathol 1949;47: 205–210.

24. Nolan C, Brown A. Reversible neuronal damage in hippocampal pyramidal cells with triethyl lead: the role of astrocytes. Neuropathol Appl Neurobiol 1989;15:441–457.

25. Darrow V, Alvord E, Mack L, et al. Histologic evolution of the reactions to hemorrhage in the premature human infant's brain. Am J Pathol 1988;130:44–58.

26. Enzmann DR, Britt RH, Lyons BE, et al. Natural history of experimental intracranial haemorrhage: sonography, computed tomography and neuropathology. Am J Neuroradiol 1981;2:517–526.

27. Takasugi S, Ueda S, Matsumoto K. Chronological changes in spontaneous intracerebral hematoma: an experimental and clinical study. Stroke 1985;16:651–658.

28. García JH. The evolution of brain infarcts: a review. J Neuropathol Exp Neurol 1992;51: 387–393.

29. Fisher CM. The history of cerebral embolism and hemorrhagic infarction. In: Furlan AJ, ed. The heart and stroke. Berlin: Springer-Verlag, 1987;3–16.

30. García JH, Yoshida Y, Chen H, et al. Progression from ischemic injury to infarct following middle cerebral artery occlusion in the rat. Am J Pathol 1993;142:623–635.

31. Moossy J. Pathology of ischemic cerebrovascular disease. In: Wilkins RH, Rengachary SS, eds. Neurosurgery. New York: McGraw-Hill, 1985;1193–1198.

32. Fisher CM, Adams RD. Observations on brain embolism with special reference to the mechanism of hemorrhagic infarction. J Neuropathol Exp Neurol 1951;10:92–94.

33. Fisher CM, Adams RD: Observations on brain embolism with special reference to hemorrhagic infarction. In: Furlan AJ, ed. The heart and stroke. Berlin: Springer-Verlag, 1987; 17–36.

34. Hornig CR, Dorndorf W, Agnoli AL. Hemorrhagic cerebral infarction: a prospective study. Stroke 1986;17:179–185.

35. Laureno R, Shields RW, Narayan T. The diagnosis and management of cerebral embolism and hemorrhagic infarction with sequential computerized cranial tomography. Brain 1987;110:93–105.

36. Okada Y, Yamaguchi T, Minematsu K, et al. Hemorrhagic transformation in cerebral embolism. Stroke 1989;20:598–603.

37. Weisberg LA. Nonseptic cardiogenic cerebral embolic stroke: clinical—CT correlations. Neurology 1985;35:876–898.

38. Hart RG, Easton JD. Hemorrhagic infarcts. Stroke 1986;17:586–589.

39. Kase CS, Mohr JP, Caplan LR. Intracerebral Hemorrhage. In Barnett HJM, et al., eds. Stroke: pathophysiology, diagnosis and management. Second edition. New York: Churchill Livingstone, 1992;561–616.

40. Broderick JP, Brott TG, Tomsick T, et al. Ultraearly evaluation of intracerebral hemorrhage. J Neurosurg 1990;75:195–199.

41. Bogousslavsky J, Regli F. Anticoagulant-induced intracerebral bleeding in brain ischemia: evaluation in 200 patients with TIAs, emboli from the heart, and progressive stroke. Acta Neurol Scand 1985;71:464–471.

42. Shields RW, Laureno R, Lachman T, et al. Anticoagulant-related hemorrhagic stroke in acute cerebral embolism. Stroke 1984;15: 428–437.

43. Bogousslavsky J, Regli F, Uské A, et al. Early spontaneous hematoma in cerebral infarct: is primary cerebral hemorrhage overdiagnosed? Neurology 1991;41:837–840.

44. Bogousslavsky J, Cachin C, Regli F, et al. Cardiac sources of embolism and cerebral infarction—clinical consequences and vascular concomitants: the Lausanne Stroke Registry. Neurology 1991;41:855–859.

45. Jörgensen L, Torvik A. Ischemic cerebrovascular diseases in an autopsy series: II. Prevalence, location, pathogenesis, and clinical course of cerebral infarcts. J Neurol Sci 1969;9:285–320.

46. García JH. Thrombosis of cranial veins and sinuses: brain parenchymal effects. In: Einhäupl K, et al., eds. Cerebral sinus thrombosis: experimental and clinical aspects. New York: Plenum Press, 1990;27–38.

47. García JH. Trombosis venosa intracranial. In: Matías-Guiu J, et al., eds. Isquemia Cerebral. Barcelona: Editorial MRC, 1990;203–215.

48. García JH, Anderson ML. Circulatory disorders and their effect on the brain. In: Davis RL, Robertson DM, eds. Textbook of neuropathology. Baltimore: Williams & Wilkins, 1991; 621–718.

49. del Zoppo GJ, Zeumer H, Harker LA. Thrombolytic therapy in stroke: possibilities and hazards. Stroke 1986;17:595–607.

50. Sloan MA. Thrombolysis and stroke, past and future. Arch Neurol 1987;44:748–768.

51. Dalal PM, Shah PM, Sheth SC, Deshpande CK. Cerebral embolism: angiographic observations on spontaneous clot lysis. Lancet 1965;1:61–64.

52. Seki H, Yoshimoto T, Ogawa A, Suzuki J. Hemodynamics in hemorrhagic infarction: an experimental study. Stroke 1985;16:647–651.

53. Yamaguchi T, Minematsu K, Choki J-I, et al. Clinical and neuroradiological analysis of thrombotic and embolic cerebral infarction. Jpn Circ J 1984;48:50–58.

54. Kamijyo Y, García JH, Cooper J. Temporary regional cerebral ischemia in the cat: a model of hemorrhagic and subcortical infarction. J Neuropathol Exp Neurol 1977;36:338–350.

55. Lodder J, Krijne-Kubat B, Broekman J. Cerebral hemorrhagic infarction at autopsy: cardiac embolic cause and relationship to the cause of death. Stroke 1986;17:626–629.

56. Mohr JP, Duterte DI, Oliveira VR, et al. Recanalization of acute middle cerebral artery occlusion. Neurology 1988;38 (Suppl 1):215 (abstract).

57. Ogata J, Yutani C, Imakita M, et al. Hemorrhagic infarct of the brain without reopening the occluded arteries in cardioembolic stroke. Stroke 1989;20:876–883.

58. Faris AA, Hardin CA, Poser CM. Pathogenesis of hemorrhagic infarction of the brain: I. Experimental investigations on the role of hypertension and of collateral circulation. Arch Neurol 1963;9:36–40.

59. Laurent JP, Molinari GF, Oakley JC. Primate model of cerebral hematoma. J Neuropathol Exp Neurol 1976;35:560–568.

60. Saku Y, Choki J, Waki R, et al. Hemorrhagic infarct induced by arterial hypertension in cat brain following middle cerebral artery occlusion. Stroke 1990;21:589–595.

61. Beghi E, Boglium G, Cavaletti G, et al. Hemorrhagic infarction: risk factors, clinical and tomographic features and outcome. A case-control study. Acta Neurol Scand 1989;80: 220–231.

62. Masuda J, Yutani C, Waki R, et al. Histopathological analysis of the mechanisms of intracranial hemorrhage complicating infective endocarditis. Stroke 1992;23:843–850.

63. Salgado AV, Furlan AJ, Keys TF, et al. Neurologic complications of endocarditis: a 12-year experience. Neurology 1989;39:173–178.

64. Adams RD, van der Eecken HM. Vascular diseases of the brain. Ann Rev Med 1953;4: 213–252.

65. Cerebral Embolism Study Group. Immediate anticoagulation of embolic stroke: brain hemorrhage and management options. Stroke 1984;15:779–789.

66. Cerebral Embolism Study Group. Immediate anticoagulation of embolic stroke: a randomized trial. Stroke 1983;14:668–676.

67. Lodder J. CT-detected hemorrhagic infarction: relation with the size of the infarct, and the presence of midline shift. Acta Neurol Scand 1984;70:329–335.

68. Matías-Guiu J, Alvarez J, Dávalos A, Codina A. Heparin therapy for stroke. Neurology 1984;34:1619–1620 (letter).

69. Denny-Brown D, Meyer JS. The cerebral collateral circulation: 2. Production of cerebral infarction by ischemic anoxia and its reversibility in early stages. Neurology 1957;7:567–579.

70. García JH, Lowry SL, Briggs L, et al. Brain capillaries expand and rupture in areas of ischemia and reperfusion. In: Reivich M, Hurtig HI, eds. Cerebrovascular diseases: thirteenth research (Princeton) conference. New York: Raven Press, 1983;169–179.

71. Seto H, Nonaka N, Kuratsu I, et al. Clinical features of hemorrhagic infarction. Neurol Med Chir 1986;24:706–711.

72. Terada T, Komai N, Hayashi S, et al. Hemorrhagic infarction after vasospasm due to ruptured cerebral aneurysm. Neurosurgery 1986; 18:415–418.

73. Ohta H, Yasui N, Suzuki A, et al. Hemorrhagic infarction following vasospasm due to ruptured intracranial aneurysm. Neurol Med Chir 1982;22:716–724.

74. Uemura Y, Nagasawa S, Yonekawa Y, et al. Hemorrhagic infarction following cerebral vasospasm in relation to induced hypertension therapy. In: Iwabuchi T, ed. Proceedings of 11th conference of surgical treatment of stroke. Tokyo: Neuron, 1982;285–290.

75. Howard R, Trend P, Ross-Russell RW. Clinical features of ischemia in cerebral arterial borderzones after periods of reduced cerebral blood flow. Arch Neurol 1987;44:934–940.

76. Caplan L. Intracerebral hemorrhage revisited. Neurology 1988;38:624–627 (editorial).

77. Björklid E, Storm-Mathisen J, Storm E, et al. Localization of tissue thromboplastin in the human brain. Thromb Haemost 1977;37: 91–97.

78. Friede RL. Capillarization. In Topographic brain chemistry. New York: Academic Press, 1966;1–16.

79. Southwick FS, Richardson EP, Swartz MN. Septic thrombosis of the dural venous sinuses. Medicine 1986;5:82–106.

80. Bousser M-G, Chiras J, Bories J, et al. Cerebral venous thrombosis: a review of 38 cases. Stroke 1985;2:199–213.

81. Bousser M-G, Barnett HJM. Cerebral venous thrombosis. In: Barnett HJM, et al., eds. Stroke: pathophysiology, diagnosis, and management. Second edition. New York: Churchill Livingstone, 1992;517–538.

82. Bauer KA, Rosenberg RD. The pathophysiology of prethrombotic state in humans: insights gained from studies using markers of hemostatic activation. Blood 1987;70:343–350.

83. Bousser M-G, Goujon C, Ribeiro V, et al. Diagnostic strategies in cerebral sinus vein thrombosis. In: Einhäupl KM, et al., eds. Cerebral sinus thrombosis: experimental and clinical aspects. New York: Plenum Press, 1990;187–200.

84. Baló J. The dural venous sinuses. Anat Rec 1950;106:319–325.

85. Capra NF, Kapp JP. Anatomic and physiologic aspects of the venous system. In: Wood JH, ed. Cerebral blood flow. New York: McGraw-Hill, 1987;37–58.

86. Einhäupl KM, Villringer A, Haberl RL, et al. Clinical spectrum of sinus venous thrombosis. In: Einhäupl KM, et al., eds. Cerebral sinus thrombosis: experimental and clinical aspects. New York: Plenum Press, 1990;149–156.

87. Cervós-Navarro J, Kannuki S. Neuropathological findings in the thrombosis of cerebral veins and sinuses: vascular aspects. In: Einhäupl K, et al., eds. Cerebral sinus thrombosis: experimental and clinical aspects. New York: Plenum Press, 1990;15–26.

88. Symonds CP. Hydrocephalic and focal cerebral symptoms in relation to thrombophlebitis of the dural sinuses and cerebral veins. Brain 1937;60:531–550.

89. Erdman WA, Weinreb JC, Cohen JM, et al. Venous thrombosis: clinical and experimental MR imaging. Radiology 1986; 161:233–238.

90. Schmiedek P, Einhäupl K, Moser E, et al. Cerebral blood flow in patients with sinus vein

thrombosis. In: Einhäupl K, et al., eds. Cerebral sinus thrombosis: experimental and clinical aspects. New York: Plenum Press, 1990; 75–84.

91. Kristensen B, Malm J, Markgren P, et al. CSF hydrodynamics in superior sagittal sinus thrombosis. J Neurol Neurosurg Psychiat 1992;55:287–293.

92. Kannuki S, Cervós-Navarro J, Matsumoto K, et al. Experimental model in the cat for cerebral sino-venous occlusion. In: Einhäupl K, et al., eds. Cerebral sinus thrombosis: experimental and clinical aspects. New York: Plenum Press, 1990;43–62.

93. Deckert M, Frerichs K, Mehraein P, et al. A new experimental model of sinus vein thrombosis. In: Einhäupl K, et al., eds. Cerebral sinus thrombosis: experimental and clinical aspects. New York: Plenum Press, 1990;39–42.

94. Ribes MF. Des recherches faites sur la phlébite. Revue Médicale Francaise et Etrangère et Journal de clinique de l'Hôtel-Dieu et de la Charité de Paris, 1825;3:5.

95. Kalbag RM, Woolf AL. Cerebral venous thrombosis with special reference to primary aseptic thrombosis. New York: Oxford University Press, 1967.

96. Kapp JP, Schmidek HH. The cerebral venous system and its disorders. Orlando: Grune and Stratton, 1984.

97. Einhäupl KM, Kempski O, Baethmann A. Cerebral sinus thrombosis: experimental and clinical aspects. New York: Plenum, 1990.

98. Johnson EV, Kline LB, Julian BA, et al. Bilateral cavernous sinus thrombosis due to mucormycosis. Arch Ophthalmol 1988;106: 1089–1092.

99. Jacewicz M, Plum F. Aseptic cerebral venous thrombosis. In: Einhäupl K, et al., eds. Cerebral sinus thrombosis: experimental and clinical aspects. New York: Plenum Press, 1990; 157–170.

100. Broekmans AW, Veltkamp JJ, Bertina RM. Congenital protein C deficiency and venous thrombo-embolism: a study of three Dutch families. N Engl J Med 1983;309: 340–344.

101. Marlar RA, Kleiss AJ, Griffin JH. Mechanisms of action of human activated protein C, a thrombin-dependent anticoagulant enzyme. Blood 1982;59:1067–1072.

102. Wintzen AR, Broekmans AW, Bertina RM, et al. Cerebral haemorrhagic infarction in young patients with hereditary protein C de-

ficiency: evidence for "spontaneous" cerebral venous thrombosis. Br Med J 1985;20:350–352.

103. Snyder TC, Sachdev HS. MR imaging of cerebral dural sinus thrombosis. J Comput Assist Tomogr 1986;10:889–891.

104. Goldberg AL, Rosenbaum AE, Wang H, et al. Computed tomography of dural sinus thrombosis. J Comput Assist Tomogr 1986;10:16–20.

105. Beal MF, Wechsler LR, Davis KR. Cerebral vein thrombosis and multiple intracranial hemorrhages by computed tomography. Arch Neurol 1982;39:437–438.

106. Banna M, Groves JT. Deep vascular congestion in dural venous thrombosis on computed tomography. J Comput Assist Tomogr 1979;3:539–541.

107. Buonanno FS, Moody DM, Ball MR, et al. Computed cranial tomographic findings in cerebral sinovenous occlusion. J Comput Assist Tomogr 1978;2:281–290.

108. Solomon GE, Engel M, Hecht HL, et al. Progressive dyskinesia due to internal cerebral vein thrombosis. Neurology 1982;32:769–772.

109. Kim KS, Walczak TS. Computed tomography of deep cerebral venous thrombosis. J Comput Assist Tomogr 1986;10:386–390.

# Chapter 5

# CT and MR Imaging of Intracerebral Hemorrhage

Kevin Dul and Burton P. Drayer

Hemorrhage within the central nervous system (CNS) occurs in a variety of pathological processes, and its presence has important therapeutic implications. Any imaging modality used for diagnosing CNS disorders should, therefore, detect or exclude hemorrhage with a high degree of accuracy. Historically, cerebral angiography was the primary imaging tool available for this purpose. The advent of computed tomography (CT) revolutionized management of the patient with an acute neurological deficit by its ability to diagnose or exclude acute intracerebral hemorrhage (ICH) accurately and noninvasively. Unfortunately, the CT diagnosis of ICH becomes less accurate in the subacute and chronic stages of hemorrhage. This problem for the most part has been solved by the addition of magnetic resonance imaging (MRI) to the diagnostic armamentarium. High field strength magnets and gradient-echo techniques render MRI quite sensitive to the detection of hemorrhagic foci.

This chapter reviews the CT and MRI findings of hemorrhage within the brain parenchyma during all stages of evolution, discusses the physiological and pathological mechanisms thought to be responsible for these findings, and, when possible, emphasizes features suggestive of specific causes of ICH. Pitfalls of CT and MRI imaging of hemorrhage are also discussed.

## Pathophysiology

ICH is most commonly of arterial origin with resultant extravasation of approximately 95% to 98% oxygen-saturated oxyhemoglobin into the tissues.[1,2] Cerebral angiography has demonstrated that ICH usually originates from a single artery or arterialized vein. Serial histological sections of intracerebral hematomas demonstrate that hemorrhage occurs not only at the primary angiographically detected arterial site but also from torn arterioles at the margin of the expanding hematoma.[3] These are secondary bleeding sites and are created as blood dissects along the path of least resistance, the white matter fiber tracts. Angiographically, these secondary bleeding sites have been identified at the periphery of intracerebral hematomas as late as twenty days after clinical onset.[4] Thus intracerebral hematomas are typically heterogeneous, slowly expanding collections of blood.

Following the extravasation of blood, clot formation occurs with progressive extrusion of serum and clot retraction. Hemoconcentration occurs and oxygen is released from oxyhemoglobin, thereby increasing the relative concentration of deoxyhemoglobin. Local phenomena associated with decreases in pH and $Po_2$ hasten this conversion.[5-7]

As the subacute phase of hematoma evolution begins, the oxidative denaturation of hemoglobin continues with deoxyhemoglobin converting to methemoglobin. Methemoglobin is initially present within intact red blood cells (RBC), but over time the lysis of RBC membranes results in extracellular methemoglobin. Both methemoglobin formation and RBC lysis begin in the periphery of the hematoma and progress centrally, concurrent with the ingrowth of macrophages and neovascularity at the periphery of the hematoma.[8] White-matter edema surrounding the hematoma reaches its peak in the early subacute phase and subsequently diminishes over time in the absence of an underlying lesion, such as neoplasm, where vasogenic edema would persist and even increase over time.

Chronic hematomas are characterized pathologically by cystic cavities with orange-yellow borders. Occasionally, fibrotic plaques entirely obliterate the cavity.[9] The orange-yellow margin consists of macrophages laden with hemosiderin, an end product of hemoglobin degradation. Central cavities often have high protein concentrations from the non-iron-containing heme pigment, hematoidin.[10,11] Marginal edema is now absent and is replaced by gliosis in the adjacent parenchyma.

## Computed Tomography

Despite the advances made with MRI, CT remains the modality of choice for evaluation of acute ICH. As shown by Zimmerman et al.,[12] the MRI signal from acute intraparenchymal hemorrhage may be indistinguishable from that of the surrounding brain within the first twenty-four hours following presentation. However, these patients were studied on a midfield MRI system and without the benefit of gradient-echo sequences. Subarachnoid hemorrhage may be difficult to detect by MRI at any time.[13]

While the diagnosis of acute hemorrhage on CT is relatively straightforward, the subacute and chronic stages have a more non-specific appearance. This occurs because the attenuation coefficient of the hematoma approximates that of brain as the clot is resorbed. An understanding of the various CT imaging characteristics of subacute and chronic hemorrhage as well as of acute hemorrhage, is nonetheless critical because hemorrhage may not be suspected clinically in a patient who presents with a more subacute or chronic clinical picture.

### Technical Considerations

A computed tomographic image is a display of the anatomy of a thin slice of the body obtained from a mathematical reconstruction of multiple x-ray absorption measurements made around the body's periphery. The ability of CT to differentiate between various tissues of the body is based primarily upon the differential attenuation of the x-ray beam by these tissues. This, in turn, is dependent on the atomic number and density of that tissue and also on the energy spectrum of the x-ray beam.[14]

In CT, a numbering system has been developed which relates a given CT number to the linear attenuation coefficients of x-rays. Tissues of water density will have a CT number of zero while tissues that attenuate the x-ray beam to a greater or lesser degree than water will have positive or negative CT numbers, respectively. Soft tissue structures, such as the brain parenchyma, will have CT attenuation values ranging from 25 to 34 Hounsfield units (HU) for normal white matter to 30 to 40 HU for normal gray matter.[15] The attenuation unit is named in honor of the inventor of CT, Godfrey Hounsfield.

### Computed Tomography of Intracerebral Hemorrhage

The CT imaging appearance of ICH can be divided into four stages: hyperacute (0 to 4

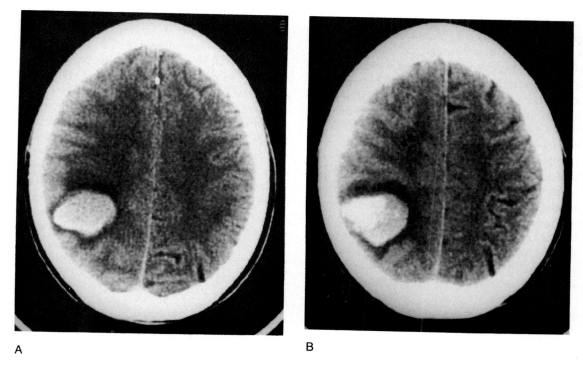

A            B

**Figure 5.1.** Hyperacute hematoma on CT. (A) The hematoma is hyperdense relative to gray matter. (B) Variable attenuation within the hematoma may be due to early clot formation or repeated hemorrhage in patients predisposed.

hours), acute (5 to 72 hours), subacute (4 to 21 days), and chronic (more than 22 days).[16]

In the *hyperacute stage*, blood has extravasated but not yet clotted. Several studies have been performed to delineate the imaging characteristics of extravasated blood on CT.[17–19] A direct linear relationship between the CT attenuation value and the hemoglobin concentration of the blood was determined. The increased attenuation of whole blood is based primarily on the protein concentration (globin portion) of the blood. Whole blood was determined to have an attenuation value of 56 HU, while the attenuation value of a cerebral hematoma will increase up to the range of 85 HU over the next twenty-four to forty-eight hours as clot retraction progresses. A hyperacute hematoma will thus appear as a hyperdense parenchymal lesion on unenhanced CT, often with variable attenuation

within the lesion (Figure 5.1). This variable attenuation may be due to early multifocal clot formation or repeated bouts of hemorrhage in predisposed patients (i.e., with bleeding diathesis, underlying arteriovenous malformation [AVM] or neoplasm).[20] Fluid/blood levels have been described that may or may not be associated with hemorrhage into a pre-existing cavity.[21,22] A caveat to consider is hemorrhage in the anemic patient, whereupon extravasated blood may be isodense to brain parenchyma and thus indistinguishable by attenuation criteria alone because of the lower hemoglobin concentration.[23]

In the *acute stage*, a cerebral hematoma becomes progressively dense as a result of clot formation and serum extrusion, with subsequent increase in relative hemoglobin concentration. A small surrounding region of hypodensity is usually present and is caused by the extruded serum (Figure 5.2). The circumferential hypodensity increases and reaches a maximum at approximately five to seven days because of associated vasogenic edema. The extent of the mass effect correlates with hematoma size so that mass effect much greater than apparent hematoma size should raise suspicion for an underlying neoplasm.

As the *subacute stage* begins, the surrounding white matter edema reaches its peak and then begins to recede. The density of the hematoma decreases, first at the periphery of the hematoma and subsequently in the center. The process evolves through a stage of isodensity with brain parenchyma (Figure 5.3). Smaller hematomas reach the isodense phase sooner than larger hematomas, which may remain hyperdense for up to four weeks.[24]

While an unenhanced CT examination performed at the isodense phase may appear nearly normal (with only mild mass effect evident),[25] the administration of intravenous contrast will produce ring enhancement at the periphery of the hematoma[26,27] (see Figure 5.3). Mechanisms postulated to account for this finding include (1) hypervascularity of the granulation tissue surrounding the hematoma, (2) loss of autoregulation with luxury perfusion, and (3) extravasation of contrast material due to localized blood-brain-barrier (BBB) breakdown.[27] This appearance is quite nonspecific; ring-enhancing isodense lesions may also be seen with cerebral abscess, neoplasm, infarct, and multiple sclerosis.

As ICH enters the *chronic stage*, it progresses from isodense to hypodense relative to brain parenchyma (Figure 5.4). Mass effect resolves and focal atrophy becomes apparent. Interestingly, a late (approximately one to two months postictus) nonenhanced CT scan may sometimes reveal a high-density rim. This rim represents hemosiderin-laden macrophages detectable by CT.[28] The chronic, resolved hematoma is seen as a cystic, encephalomalacic low-density region. There is rarely contrast enhancement beyond six weeks following the initial event.[27]

## Magnetic Resonance Imaging

MRI has dramatically improved our ability to evaluate the patient with ICH. Not only can hemorrhagic foci be identified with great sensitivity but often the hemorrhagic event can be dated, having important clinical and therapeutic ramifications. The literature is replete with articles describing the appearance and evolution of intracerebral hematoma with MRI, often with conflicting results.[5,8,12,29–35] The reason for such controversy is the extreme complexity of the MRI aspects of ICH. There are multiple factors, both physiological and operator-dependent,

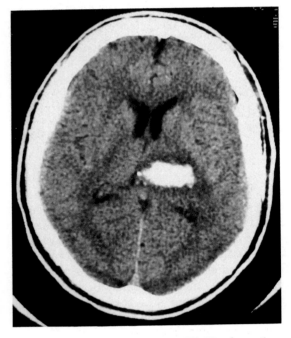

**Figure 5.2.** Acute hematoma on CT. Clot formation and relative increase in hemoglobin concentration account for marked hyperdensity of the hematoma. Surrounding rim of hypodensity is caused by extruded serum/edema. Mass effect is present with minimal left-to-right midline shift at the level of the third ventricle.

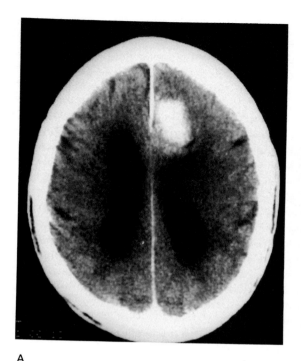

A

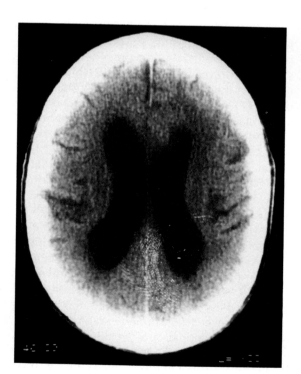

B

**Figure 5.3.** Subacute hematoma on CT. (A) Unenhanced CT at presentation demonstrates acute hematoma in the left frontal lobe adjacent to the lateral ventricle. (B) Unenhanced CT four weeks later shows the hematoma to be isodense to brain parenchyma. (C) Enhanced CT demonstrates ring enhancement of the isodense hematoma.

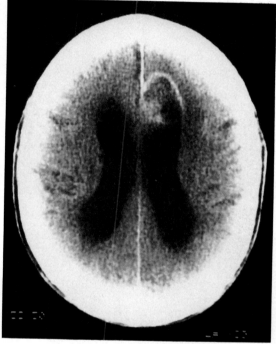

C

that potentially influence the signal intensity patterns of hemorrhage. The factors critical to an understanding of the appearance of ICH on MRI are reviewed here. For the interested reader, several excellent, detailed reviews are referenced.[36-38]

*Technical Considerations*

MRI utilizes the phenomenon of nuclear magnetic resonance to obtain signal in the form of alternating current from the body's tissues. This signal, through the process of Fourier transformation, is converted into the

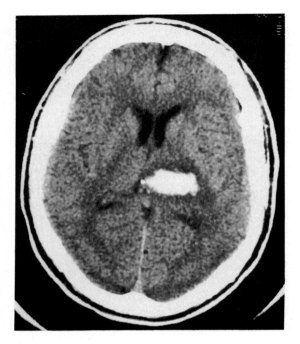

A

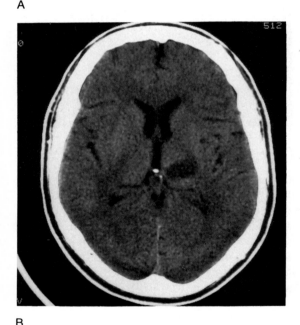

B

**Figure 5.4.** Chronic hematoma on CT. (A) Unenhanced CT at presentation demonstrates acute hematoma within the left thalamus. (B) Unenhanced CT six weeks later shows residual low density within the left thalamus. Mass effect has resolved leaving the pineal gland calcification in the midline.

digitized images used clinically. Signal generation is achieved by placing the patient within a strong magnetic field and then inducing tissue resonance by the addition of energy in the form of radio frequency (RF) waves. The particular RF wave chosen is that equal to the precessional frequency of $^1$H nuclei (protons) because hydrogen is abundant biologically and because protons possess strong magnetic moments, thus allowing maximum signal detection. From the above discussion, one can see how, in general, tissues with high proton content (free-water) will produce more signal than those with low proton content (cortical bone). To understand the MRI appearance of hemorrhage, however, review of additional technical factors is necessary. These include the concepts of T1, T2, paramagnetic properties, and field strength.

The RF pulse sequences used in standard spin-echo MRI can be varied to produce images with different tissue contrast. T1 and T2 are time constants that describe the rate of "relaxation" of protons back to equilibrium from the resonant state produced by the RF pulse. T1 time is related to magnetization in the longitudinal plane while T2 time is related to magnetization in the transverse plane. Different tissues of the body have variable relaxation times, thus providing outstanding tissue contrast. In general, tissues with a short T1 time will produce more MRI signal on a T1-weighted image (e.g., fat), while tissues with a long T2 time will produce more MRI signal on a T2-weighted image (e.g., CSF).

Tissues placed within a magnetic field generate their own magnetic field, which may enhance or reduce the effect of the externally applied field. This property, known as magnetic susceptibility, can be classified by the response of the tissue. Paramagnetic tissues enhance the applied magnetic field while diamagnetic tissues weakly oppose the magnetic field. Research has shown that the MRI appearance of hemorrhage is dominated by the paramagnetic properties of the various stages of hemoglobin degradation.[36–38] Oxyhemoglobin, deoxyhemoglobin, methemoglobin, and hemosiderin have different magnetic properties; each influences an image as it occurs in the evolution of an intracerebral hematoma.

The two main mechanisms by which paramagnetic tissues affect MRI signal include dipole-dipole interactions and magnetic susceptibility effects. Dipole-dipole interactions occur when water protons closely approach a paramagnetic region ($\approx 3$Å) causing an intermolecular proton-electron/dipole-dipole interaction and subsequent proton relaxation enhancement in both the longitudinal and transverse plane. Such action causes shortening of both the T1 and T2 times, respectively, and is responsible for the T1 shortening of methemoglobin in subacute hematoma and the resultant high signal intensity on T1-weighted images. While deoxyhemoglobin and hemosiderin are paramagnetic, the conformation of these molecules shields the water protons from access to the paramagnetic component (unpaired electrons) and there is no T1 shortening.

Paramagnetic tissues also produce local variations in the magnetic field, causing protons to experience a changing magnetic field as they diffuse over time. This results in spin dephasing and loss of transverse coherence with subsequent T2 shortening. There is no effect on T1. This magnetic susceptibility effect is responsible for the characteristic low signal intensity of an acute hematoma on the T2-weighted images when deoxyhemoglobin is present. It is also responsible for the low signal intensity seen on T2-weighted spin-echo images in patients with chronic or remote hemorrhage when hemosiderin- or ferritin-laden macrophages, or both, are present. Gradient-echo pulse sequences are even more sensitive to the presence of deoxyhemoglobin and hemosiderin.

Conflicting reports in the literature regarding the MRI appearance of hemorrhage may exist because different studies were performed with magnets of different field strengths.[39] While an increase in field strength causes a prolongation of the T1 relaxation time, it has no significant effect on the appearance or detection of a hematoma on T1-weighted images.[40] T2-weighted images, however, can show dramatic variation at different field strengths; the effect of T2-shortening associated with magnetic susceptibility increases with increasing field strength. The magnitude of this effect is proportional to the square of the field strength. Thus, the T2 shortening associated with magnetic susceptibility at 1.5 Tesla (high field) is one hundred times that at 0.15 Tesla (low field), and nine times that at 0.5 Tesla (mid-field).[37]

## Magnetic Resonance Imaging Appearance of Intracerebral Hemorrhage

Using the concepts discussed above, it is possible to gain an appreciation of the MRI appearance of hemorrhage. While there is some overlap, hematoma evolution can be divided into distinct stages: (1) hyperacute, (2) acute, (3) subacute, and (4) chronic. This discussion presents the appearance of these stages using high-field imaging systems.

### Hyperacute Hematoma

In the first several hours following hemorrhage, the RBC within the hematoma contain oxygenated hemoglobin. Other components of the blood are present but contribute little to the MRI image.[32,41] As oxyhemoglobin is diamagnetic, there can be no proton relaxation enhancement by dipole-dipole interactions and, thus, no shortening of T1 or T2. The hyperacute hematoma will, therefore, appear virtually identical to many brain lesions with high proton density—exhibiting slightly prolonged T1 and T2 relaxation times relative to brain parenchyma, demonstrating mild hypointensity to isointensity on T1-weighted images, and featuring high signal intensity on the T2-weighted images.[42] In clinical practice, hyperacute hematomas are rarely seen because in most instances at least several hours elapse between the onset of symptoms and scanning the patient. A clue that may possibly distinguish a hyperacute hematoma from other CNS lesions with high proton density would be a rim of marked hypointensity at the periphery of the lesion on T2-weighted images. The rim may represent initial conversion of oxyhemoglobin to deoxyhemoglobin with the hypointense signal representing T2 shortening caused by the magnetic susceptibility effect of paramagnetic deoxyhemoglobin[38] (Figure 5.5).

*Acute Hematoma*

As oxyhemoglobin is converted to deoxyhemoglobin, the acute stage of hematoma evolution begins. This process begins several hours following hemorrhage and lasts from a few days to as long as one week. Conversion initially occurs at the periphery of the hematoma and then progresses centrally. Deoxyhemoglobin is paramagnetic yet does not appear bright on T1-weighted images because its molecular geometry does not allow access of water protons to the paramagnetic component, its unpaired electrons. The mild hypointensity seen on the T1-weighted image is actually a reflection of T2-shortening, which "shines through," so to speak, onto the T1-weighted image. T2-weighted images demonstrate marked signal hypointensity representing magnetic susceptibility. At this early state of hematoma development, the surrounding edema and serum from clot retraction give a high-intensity perimeter on the T2-weighted images (Figure 5.6). As opposed to CT imaging, fibrin clot formation and retraction may not affect the appearance of the acute hematoma at 1.5 Tesla.[41]

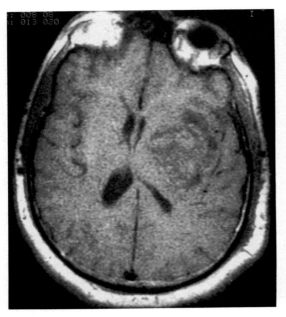
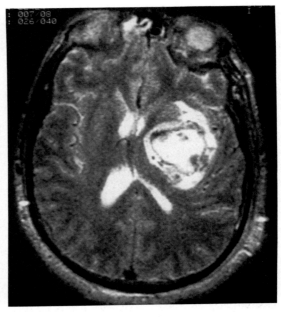

A    B

**Figure 5.5.** MRI of hyperacute hematoma. (A) Axial fast-spin-echo short TR/TE (866/14) MRI. (B) Axial fast-spin-echo long TR/TE (2900/80) MRI. Left basal ganglia hematoma demonstrates slight hypointensity on short TR/TE image (A) and high intensity on long TR/TE image (B), the usual features of a nonhemorrhagic mass, but in this case indicative of diamagnetic oxyhemoglobin. Thin rim of hypointense signal on long TR/TE image (B) separates the hematoma from adjacent serum/edema and may help distinguish hyperacute hematoma from nonhemorrhagic mass lesions.

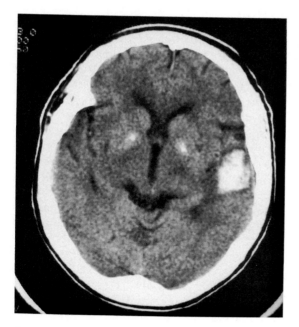

A

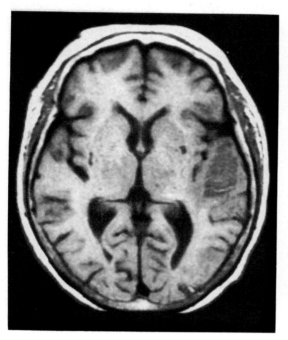

B

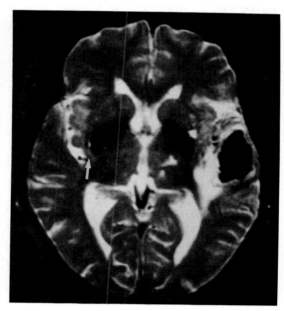

C

**Figure 5.6.** Acute hematoma on MRI. (A) Unenhanced CT at presentation demonstrates acute hematoma in the posterior left temporal lobe. Note symmetric physiological calcifications within the basal ganglia. (B) Short TR/TE (800/16) MRI. The lesion is slightly hypointense to gray matter on the T1-weighted image. (C) Long TR/TE (2500/90) MRI. The lesion is markedly hypointense on this T2-weighted image, while surrounding edema shows high signal intensity. Note that the basal ganglia calcifications seen on CT are not identified on MR in this case. Additional note is made of slit hemosiderin residua from prior right putaminal hemorrhage (arrow) and chronic small infarction in the left putamen and left thalamus.

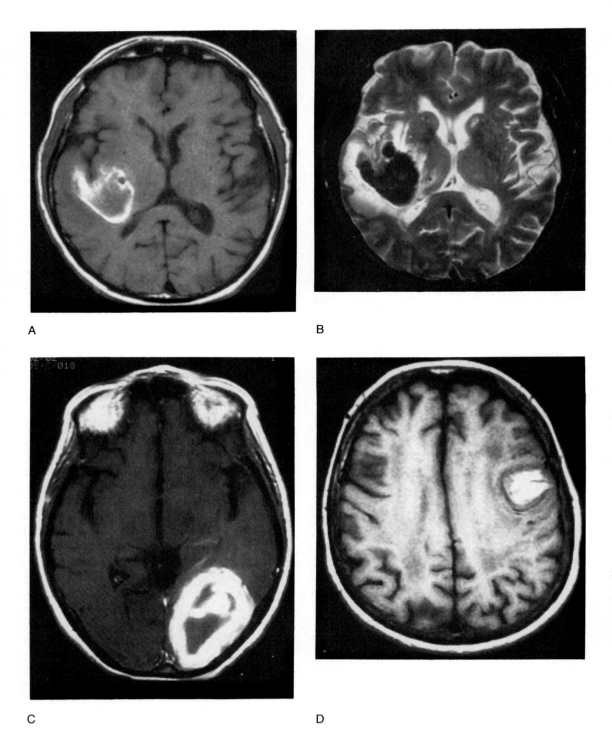

A

B

C

D

**Figure 5.7.** Progressive early subacute hematoma on MRI in three separate patients. Patient 1: (A) Short TR/TE (800/16) image shows early peripheral methemoglobin formation as high signal intensity. (B) Long TR/TE (2500/90) image shows diffuse hypointense signal within the hematoma and surrounding hyperintense edema. Patient 2: (C) Short TR/TE (800/16) image shows thick rim of hyperintense signal. Patient 3: (D) Short TR/TE (800/16) image shows uniform hyperintensity while long TR/TE (2500/90) image (E) demonstrates hypointense signal.

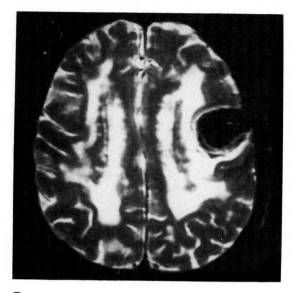

E

*Subacute Hematoma*

The initial subacute stage of hematoma evolution on MRI begins a few days postictus and lasts for a few weeks. Subacute hematomas are characterized by their high signal intensity on T1-weighted images. While both deoxyhemoglobin and methemoglobin are paramagnetic, the molecular configuration of methemoglobin allows close contact between its unpaired electrons and subjacent protons. The subsequent T1 shortening via dipole-dipole interactions results in the characteristic "bright" appearance of hematomas in the subacute stage on T1-weighted images. Once again the process begins peripherally and progresses toward the center (Figure 5.7).

Evaluation of the T2-weighted images allows further categorization of the subacute stage into "early" and "late" components. Early subacute hematomas remain dark on T2-weighted images, while late subacute hematomas become bright on T2-weighted images. The mechanism believed to be responsible is the location of the methemoglobin. When it is contained within intact red blood cells (intracellular), the magnetic sus-

ceptibility effect predominates and the early subacute hematoma will be dark on the T2-weighted images. This signal hypointensity is highlighted using gradient-echo pulse sequences. When RBC lysis occurs and methemoglobin is extracellular, the hematoma becomes bright on the T2-weighted image (Figure 5.8). Several factors probably contribute to this appearance. Rather than being due to a prolongation of T2-relaxation time, current theory stresses the importance of T1 shortening of a high-spin density solution.[43,44] The phenomenon serves to emphasize that although MRI sequences can be designed to "weight" T1 or T2 tissue characteristics, the signal obtained will always contain both a T1 and a T2 component. The late subacute phase of hematoma evolution on MRI is also characterized by a progressive decrease in the signal hyperintensity (edema) surrounding the hematoma related to the water concentration on the spin-echo T2-weighted images.

*Chronic Hematoma*

The chronic stage of hematoma evolution on MRI begins as methemoglobin is phagocytosed by macrophages and glial cells, and is converted to hemosiderin. Hemosiderin behaves like deoxyhemoglobin in the sense that it is paramagnetic yet exhibits no T1 shortening due to its molecular configuration. Magnetic susceptibility effects thus predominate, whereupon hemosiderin formation is identified as a thin peripheral rim of low signal intensity around the hematoma that becomes most marked on T2-weighted images. This signal hypointensity is differentiated from the acute and "early" subacute hematoma by the absence of edema in the chronic setting.

As the hematoma cavity is further resorbed over time, the rim of hemosiderin thickens slightly. Eventually the cavity may completely obliterate, leaving only a cleft of hypointensity. This finding persists throughout the patient's life and acts as a marker of any prior hemorrhagic event. Alternatively, a variable-sized central cavity may persist.

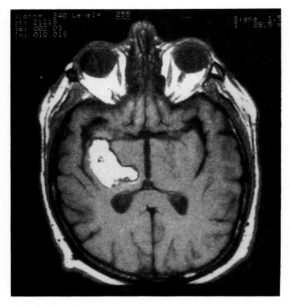

A

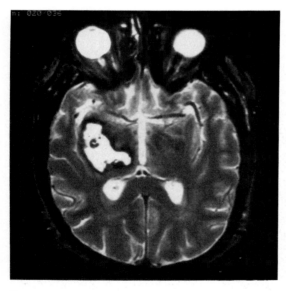

B

**Figure 5.8.** Late subacute hematoma on MRI. The hematoma demonstrates marked hyperintense signal on both the T1-weighted image (A) TR/TE (800/16) and the T2-weighted image (B) TR/TE (2500/90) caused by the presence of extracellular methemoglobin. Thin rim of hypointense signal at the hematoma margin results from hemosiderin and ferritin-laden macrophages.

This central cavity may have signal intensity either with methemoglobin or CSF characteristics[38] (Figure 5.9). The white matter edema which surrounded the subacute hematoma resolves and may be replaced by a variable amount of gliosis, seen as high signal on $T_2$-weighted images.

The MRI appearance of hemorrhage at its various stages is summarized in Table 5.1.

### Gradient-echo Magnetic Resonance Imaging of Hemorrhage

Gradient-echo pulse sequences play an important adjunctive role in the evaluation of hematoma. These partial-flip angle scans are considerably more sensitive than standard spin-echo images to susceptibility differences. Two particularly important applications of gradient-echo pulse sequences include evaluation of patients with traumatic brain injury and patients with suspected occult cerebrovascular malformations (OCVM), that is, cavernous angiomas. In both situations, small foci of hemosiderin deposition from prior episodes of hemorrhage may be detected as foci of hypointense signal on T2* (susceptibility)-weighted images, even when standard spin-echo sequences are normal. Multiple OCVM suggest that the condition is familial and may warrant MRI screening of family members (Figure 5.10).[45]

**Figure 5.9.** (opposite) Evolution of hematoma on MRI. (A) Short TR/TE (800/16) MRI thirty-six hours after presentation. (B) Long TR/TE (2500/90) MRI thirty-six hours after presentation. (C) Short TR/TE (800/16) MRI four months later. (D) Long TR/TE (2500/90) MRI four months later. In the early subacute phase the hematoma is hyperintense on short TR/TE (A) and diffusely hypointense on long TR/TE (B). Surrounding hyperintense signal on long TR/TE is due to edema (B). Four-month followup (C and D) demonstrates partial resolution of hematoma with central cavity having predominantly high signal intensity on short TR/TE (C) and high signal intensity on long TR/TE (D). Surrounding rim of hypointense signal on long TR/TE (D) represents hemosiderin deposition. Edema of the early subacute phase is replaced by gliosis or demyelination in the chronic phase.

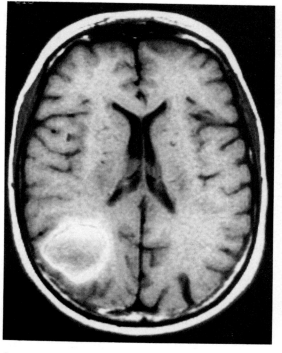

A

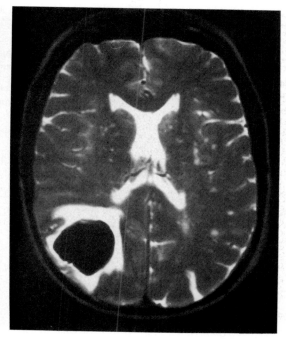

B

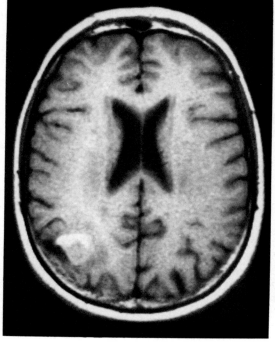

C

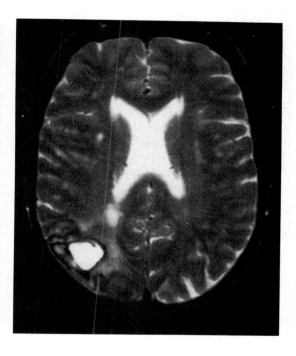

D

**Table 5.1.** Hemoglobin and MRI Evolution in Hematoma

| Stage | Time | Hemoglobin Form | Magnetic Property | Hematoma SI T1 | Hematoma SI T2 | Hemosiderin rim (SI* T2) | Edema (SI* T2) |
|---|---|---|---|---|---|---|---|
| Hyperacute | Hours | Oxyhemoglobin | Diamagnetic | $\approx$ or $\downarrow$ | $\uparrow$ | — | $\uparrow\uparrow$ |
| Acute | Days | Deoxyhemoglobin | Paramagnetic | $\approx$ or $\downarrow$ | $\downarrow\downarrow$ | — | $\uparrow\uparrow$ |
| Early subacute | Weeks | Methemoglobin (intracellular) | Paramagnetic | $\uparrow$ | $\downarrow$ | $\downarrow\downarrow$ | $\uparrow\uparrow$ |
| Late subacute | Weeks– months | Methemoglobin (extracellular) | Paramagnetic | $\uparrow\uparrow$ | $\uparrow\uparrow$ | $\downarrow\downarrow$ | — |
| Chronic | Months– years | Hemosiderin | Paramagnetic | $\approx$ or $\downarrow$ | $\downarrow\downarrow$ | $\downarrow\downarrow$ | — |

Abbreviations: SI = signal intensity relative to normal gray matter; $\approx$ = equal to brain, $\downarrow$ = hypointense to brain, $\downarrow\downarrow$ = markedly hypointense to brain, $\uparrow$ = hyperintense to brain, $\uparrow\uparrow$ = markedly hyperintense to brain.

### Magnetic Resonance Imaging Characteristics Distinguishing Primary Hemorrhage from That due to Intracranial Malignancy

Aside from the detection of brain hematoma, it is obviously very important to attempt to identify the cause of the hemorrhage. While conventional and MR angiography assist in the diagnosis of aneurysm or AVM, angiography is generally inconclusive in distinguishing primary from tumoral parenchymal hemorrhage. CT patterns of intratumoral hemorrhage are extremely variable.[46] Atypical location, multiplicity of lesions, and contrast enhancement of adjacent foci of acute hemorrhage may suggest malignancy as the cause of intracranial bleeding on CT.[47]

Whereas the imaging findings of ICH on angiography and CT are often inconclusive, the MRI signal intensity patterns of hemorrhagic intracranial malignancies are often distinct from the signal intensity patterns seen in primary hematomas.[48] As opposed to the stage-like progression of signal changes seen with primary hematomas, the sequence of changes in intratumoral hematoma are often atypical, demonstrating multiple concomitant stages of hemorrhage evolution within the lesion. Nonhemorrhagic neoplastic tissue within or adjacent to the hematoma confers additional heterogeneity to the lesion.[46–48] In addition, sequential MRI studies demonstrate delayed evolution of MRI signal patterns in neoplastic hematomas; for example, intracellular deoxyhemoglobin (seen as markedly hypointense to gray matter on T2-weighted images) is present only for several days in primary acute hematomas[8] but can persist for weeks in intratumoral hemorrhage.[48] The mechanism postulated to account for this delay in hemoglobin breakdown is intratumoral hypoxia.[48] Such hypoxia has been well documented in human tumors,[49] and it has long been known that methemoglobin formation is directly and intimately related to local oxygen tension,[50] further substantiating this hypothesis.

An additional consistent feature of hemorrhagic tumors is lack of well-defined, complete hemosiderin rim in the late subacute to chronic stage—seen as a hypointense signal rim on T2-weighted images in primary hematomas. While reestablishment of the BBB occurs after primary ICH, intracranial malignancies are known to have persistent BBB disruption. Current theory postulates that this persistent disruption allows for more efficient removal of hemosiderin-filled macrophages from the CNS, and thus the absent or incomplete hemosiderin ring seen on MRI.[48]

A final MRI finding that helps distinguish primary from intratumoral hemorrhage is the persistent and prominent perilesional

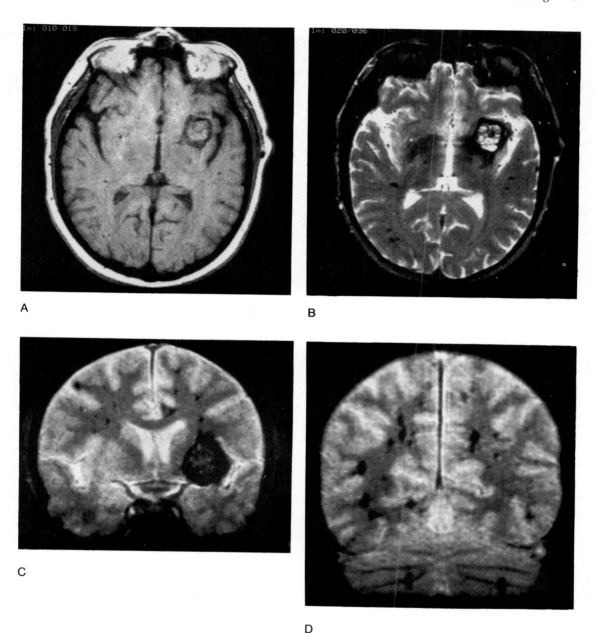

**Figure 5.10.** MRI of familial cavernous malformations. (A) Short TR/TE (800/16). Well-circumscribed left subinsular angioma with chronic hemorrhage. (B) Long TR/TE (2600/90). Typical reticulated core of cavernous angioma with chronicity affirmed by the thick surrounding hemosiderin/ferritin rim and absent edema. Multiple additional punctate angiomas evidenced as hypointense foci at gray/white junctions. (C and D) Gradient echo (550/15). The multiple cavernous angiomas are highlighted using gradient echo technique as it is more sensitive to the magnetic susceptibility effects of chronic hemosiderin accumulation.

**Table 5.2.** Primary versus Tumoral ICH: MRI

|  | Primary | Tumoral |
| --- | --- | --- |
| Signal | | |
| homogeneity | Yes | No |
| Associated mass | No | Yes |
| Evolution of hemo- | | |
| globin changes | Timely | Delayed |
| Peripheral | | |
| hypointense rim | Complete | Partial |
| Edema/mass effect | Resolution | Persistent |

high signal intensity on T2-weighted MRI images—even when the hemorrhage is in the chronic stage.[48] This may represent vasogenic edema, tumor infiltration, or a combination of the two. The MRI features distinguishing primary from intratumoral ICH are summarized in Table 5.2.

## Pitfalls in Computed Tomography and Magnetic Resonance Imaging Diagnosis of Hemorrhage

Unfortunately, all that is dense on CT or bright on T1-weighted MRI images is not hemorrhage. Multiple processes, both physiological and pathological, can mimic hemorrhage utilizing either modality. In most instances, however, these processes can be distinguished from hemorrhage with a high degree of certainty.

### Computed Tomography

Hyperdensity seen intracranially on an unenhanced CT scan falls into five categories: (1) high cellular density, (2) high protein content, (3) calcification or bone, (4) hemorrhage, or (5) prior contrast administration.[51] Examples of these nonhemorrhagic entities causing increased density include tumors, such as pineaoblastoma (high cellular density), and colloid cyst of the third ventricle (high protein content).[51] The location of the lesion and the presence of additional imaging and clinical findings may aid in proper diagnosis. With colloid cyst, for example, the additional finding of obstructive hydrocephalus at the level of the foramen of Monro and the clinical history of positional headache would be suggestive.

The most common cause of intracranial hyperdensity that must be distinguished from hematoma is calcification. Sites of physiological calcification include the pineal gland, habenula, choroid plexus, dura mater, falx, and basal ganglia (see Figure 5.6A). Note should be made that while basal ganglia calcifications may be physiological, they may also be associated with pathological states, including hypoparathyroidism and ischemic encephalopathy. Pathological calcifications may be seen in a variety of congenital, inflammatory, vascular, metabolic, and neoplastic conditions. In most instances, the distinction between hemorrhage and calcification can be made by measurement of the attenuation coefficient of the lesion. Calcification, depending on size and partial volume averaging, will have an attenuation from 70 to 200 HU.[51] As stated earlier, the attenuation value of whole blood corresponds to approximately 56 HU and that of the acute stage of a hematoma may reach a maximum of approximately 85 HU.

### Magnetic Resonance Imaging

Various nonhemorrhagic entities can be confused with hemorrhage on MRI. Calcifications may be confused with either subacute or chronic blood products because the appearance of calcium on MRI is variable. It may be (1) isointense to brain and thus not identified, (2) hypointense to brain on all pulse sequences and confused with hemosiderin, or (3) hyperintense to brain on T1-weighted images and confused with methemoglobin[52–54] (Figure 5.11).

Normal flow voids on T2-weighted spin-echo images may be confused with the hypointensity of hemosiderin and perhaps deoxyhemoglobin. A flow void will be hy-

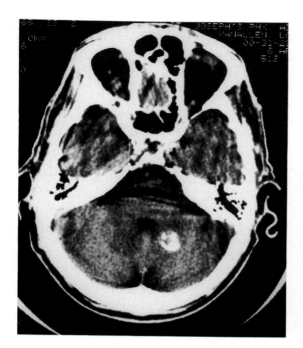

A

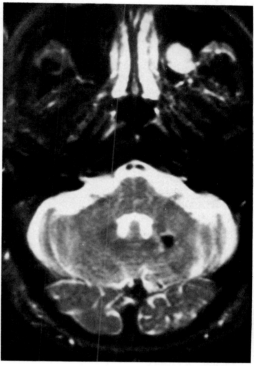

C

**Figure 5.11.** MRI of calcification mimicking hemorrhage. (A) Unenhanced CT showing dense chronic calcification of left dentate nucleus of cerebellum. (B) Short TR/TE (800/16) image shows paradoxical hyperintensity related to surface characteristics of the calcium. (C) Long TR/TE (2500/90) image demonstrates low signal within the left dentate calcification. A secondary finding, the absence of edema, favors calcification over early subacute hemorrhage.

B

pointense on a dual echo, spin-echo pulse sequence and become less prominent on the second echo (even-echo rephasing), while the hypointensity is more prominent on the second echo when blood product is present. A simple way to distinguish the hypointensity of hemosiderin from flow is to perform an imaging sequence with gradient-echo technique that emphasizes flow. While different variations of this technique exist, the end result is that blood vessels with flow can be seen as areas of high rather than low signal.

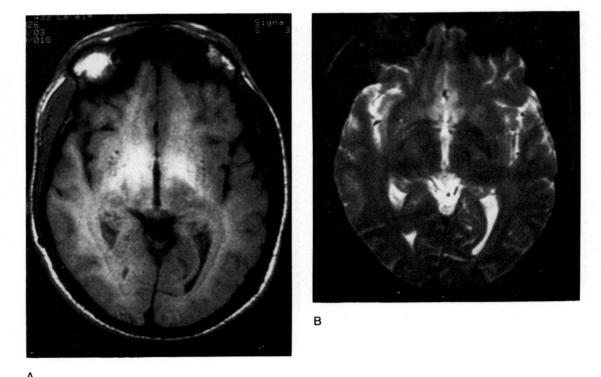

A

B

**Figure 5.12.** Brain MRI of hepatic failure. (A) Signal hyperintensity in globus pallidus on T1-weighted images (TR/TE, 800/16). (B) Normal low signal within the globus pallidus on the T2-weighted image (TR/TE, 2500/90).

Multiple compounds aside from methemoglobin cause T1 relaxation enhancement and high signal on T1-weighted images. Examples include lipid,[55] proteinaceous fluid,[56] mucin,[57] and the melanotic variant of melanoma.[58] Craniopharyngioma and colloid cyst are often of increased signal intensity on the T1 images. Recent work has shown nonheme T1 shortening may also be seen with laminar necrosis in cerebral infarction.[59] An additional potential cause of nonheme T1 shortening is paramagnetic cation deposition associated with chronic liver disease.[38] The responsible cation (possibly manganese) is deposited relatively symmetrically within the globus pallidus. Because coagulation abnormalities may be associated with ICH in patients with chronic liver disease, the finding of signal hyperintensity in the globus pallidus on T1-weighted images with hepatic en-

cephalopathy should not be confused with hemorrhage (Figure 5.12).

## Conclusions

With the use of CT and MRI, the clinical suspicion of brain hemorrhage can be readily confirmed or excluded noninvasively. An understanding not only of the appearances of hemorrhage but of the mechanisms responsible for these appearances is critical as the imaging findings may be complex. Additionally, different causes of bleeding can show important, but sometimes subtle, variations from the temporal patterns characteristic of primary hematomas. The ability of MRI to detect small foci of hemorrhage not discernible by CT and also to determine the age of the hemorrhagic event has had a significant effect upon patient diagnosis and management. Proper correlation of clinical history and imaging findings will often lead to correct identification of not only an ICH but also the underlying cause.

## References

1. Bradley WF. MRI of hemorrhage and iron in the brain. In: Stark DD, Bradley WG, eds. Magnetic resonance imaging. St. Louis: CV Mosby, 1988;359–374.
2. Nelson DA, Morris MW. Hematology and coagulation: basic methodology. In: Henry JB, ed. Clinical diagnosis and management by laboratory methods. Part IV. (17th ed). Philadelphia: WB Saunders, 1984;578–625.
3. Fischer CM. Pathological observations in hypertensive cerebral hemorrhage. J Neuropath Exp Neurol 1971;30:536–549.
4. Bergstrom K, Lodin H. An angiographic observation in intracerebral haematoma. Br J Radiol 1967;40:228–229.
5. Gomori JM, Grossman RI, Hackney DB, et al. Variable appearances of subacute intracranial hematomas on high-field spin-echo MR. Am J Neuroradiol 1987;8:1019–1026.
6. Grossman RI, Gomori JM, Goldberg HI, et al. MR imaging of hemorrhagic conditions of the head and neck. Radiographics 1988;8:441–454.
7. Wintrobe MM, Lee GR, Boggs DR, et al. Clinical Hematology. Eighth edition. Philadelphia: Lea and Febiger, 1981;88–102.
8. Gomori JM, Grossman RI, Hackney DB, et al. Intracranial hematomas: imaging by high-field MR. Radiology 1985;157:87–93.
9. Okayaka H. Hypertensive vascular disease of the CNS. In: Oayaki H, ed. Fundamentals of neuropathology. Tokyo: Igaku-Shoin, 1983; 59–62.
10. Bradley WG. Pathophysiologic correlates of signal alternations. In Brant-Zawadzki M, Norman D, eds. Magnetic resonance imaging of the central nervous system. New York: Raven Press, 1987;23–42.
11. Whisnant JP, Sayre GP, Millikan CH. Experimental intracerebral hematoma. Arch Neurol 1963;9:486–592.
12. Zimmerman RD, Heier LA, Snow RB, et al. Acute intracranial hemorrhage: intensity changes on sequential MR scans at 0.5T. Am J Neuroradiol 1988;9:47–57.
13. Bradley WG, Schmidt PG. Effect of methemoglobin formation on the MR appearance of subarachnoid hemorrhage. Radiology 1985; 156:99–103.
14. Christenson EE. X-ray attenuation. In: Christenson EE, et al., eds. An introduction to the physics of diagnostic radiology. Philadelphia: Lea and Febiger, 1978;59–76.
15. Weinstein MA, Duchesneau PM, MacIntyre WJ. White and gray matter of the brain differentiated by computed tomography. Radiology 1977;122:699–702.
16. Cohen WA, Hayman LA. Computed tomography of intracranial hemorrhage. Neuroimag Clin NA 1992;2:75–87.
17. Scott WR, New PFJ, Davis KR, et al. Computerized axial tomography of intracerebral and intraventricular hemorrhage. Radiology 1974;112:73–80.
18. New PFJ, Aronow S. Attenuation measurements of whole blood and blood fractions in computed tomography. Radiology 1976;121: 635–640.
19. Norman D, Price D, Boyd D, et al. Quantitative aspects of computed tomography of the blood and cerebrospinal fluid. Radiology 1977;123:335–338.
20. Greenberg J, Cohen WA, Cooper P. The "hyperacute" extra-axial intracranial hematoma: computed tomographic findings and clinical significance. Neurosurgery 1985;17:48–56.
21. Weisberg LA, Stazio A, Shamsnia M, et al. Nontraumatic parenchymal brain hemorrhage. Medicine 1990;69:277–295.
22. Zilkha A. Intraparenchymal fluid-blood level: a CT sign of recent intracerebral hemorrhage. J Comput Assist Tomogr 1987;7:301–305.
23. Smith WP, Batnitzky S, Rengachary SS. Acute isodense subdural hematomas: a problem in anemic patients. Am J Neuroradiol 1981;2: 37–40.
24. Dolinskas CA, Bilaniuk LT, Zimmerman RA, et al. Computed tomography of intracerebral hematomas. I. Transmission CT observations on hematoma resolution. Am J Radiol 1977; 129:681–688.
25. Zimmerman RA, Bilaniuk LT, Gennarelli T, et al. Cranial computed tomography in diagnosis and management of acute head trauma. Am J Radiol 1978;131:27–34.
26. Messina AV. Computed tomography: contrast enhancement in resolving intracerebral hemorrhage. Am J Radiol 1976;127:1050–1052.

27. Zimmerman RD, Leeds NE, Naidich TP. Ring blush associated with intracerebral hematoma. Radiology 1977;122:707–711.

28. Som PM, Patel S, Nakagawa N, et al. The iron rim sign. J Comput Assist Tomogr 1979;3:109–112.

29. Sipponen JT, Sepponen RE, Sivula A. Nuclear magnetic resonance (NMR) imaging of intracerebral hemorrhage in the acute and resolving phases. J Comput Assist Tomogr 1983;7:954–959.

30. DeLaPaz RL, New PFJ, Buonanno FS, et al. NMR imaging of intracranial hemorrhage. J Comput Assist Tomogr 1984;8:599–607.

31. Di Chiro G, Brooks RA, Girton ME, et al. Sequential MR studies of intracerebral hematomas in monkeys. Am J Neuroradiol 1986;7:193–199.

32. Cohen MD, McGuire W, Cory DA, et al. MR appearance of blood and blood products: an in vitro study. Am J Radiol 1986;146:1293–1297.

33. Dooms GC, Uske A, Brant-Zawadzki M, et al. Spin-echo MR imaging of intracranial hemorrhage. Neuroradiology 1986;28:132–138.

34. Hayman LA, Taber KH, Ford JJ, et al. Mechanisms of MR signal alteration by acute intracerebral blood: old concepts and new theories. Am J Neuroradiol 1991;12:899–907.

35. Zyed A, Hayman LA, Bryan RN. MR imaging of intracerebral blood: diversity in the temporal pattern at 0.5 and 1.0T. Am J Neuroradiol 1991;12:469–474.

36. Gomori JM, Grossman RI. Head and neck hemorrhage. In: Kressel HY, ed. Magnetic resonance annual 1987. New York: Raven Press, 1987;71–112.

37. Barkovich AJ, Atlas SW. Magnetic resonance imaging of intracranial hemorrhage. Radiol Clin NA 1988;26:801–820.

38. Thulborn KR, Atlas SW. Intracranial hemorrhage. In: Atlas SW, ed. Magnetic resonance imaging of the brain and spine. New York: Raven Press, 1991;175–222.

39. Chaney RK, Taber KH, Orrison WW, et al. Magnetic resonance imaging of intracerebral hemorrhage at different field strengths. Radiol Clin NA 1992;2:25–51.

40. Crooks LE, Arakawa M, Hoenninger J, et al. Magnetic resonance imaging: effects of field strength. Radiology 1984;151:127–133.

41. Clark RA, Watanabe AT, Bradley WG, et al. Acute hematomas: effects of deoxyhemoglobin hematocrit and fibrin-clot formation and retraction on T2 shortening. Radiology 1990;175:201–206.

42. Fullerton GD, Potter JL, Dornbluth NC. NMR relaxation of protons in tissues and other macromolecular water solutions. Magn Reson Imag 1982;1:209–228.

43. Brant-Zawadzki M, Kelly W, Kjos B, et al. Magnetic resonance imaging and characterization of normal and abnormal intracranial cerebrospinal fluid (CSF) spaces. Neuroradiology 1985;27:3–8.

44. Hackney DB, Atlas SW, Grossman RI, et al. Subacute intracranial hemorrhage: contribution of spin density to appearance on spin-echo MR images. Radiology 1987;165:199–202.

45. Rigamonti D, Hadley MN, Drayer BP, et al. Cerebral cavernous malformations: incidence and familial occurrence. N Engl J Med 1988;319:343–347.

46. Zimmerman RA, Bilaniuk LT. Computed tomography of acute intratumoral hemorrhage. Radiology 1980;135:355–359.

47. Gildersleeve N, Koo AH, McDonald CJ. Metastatic tumor presenting as intracerebral hemorrhage. Radiology 1977;124:109–112.

48. Atlas SW, Grossman RI, Gomori JM, et al. Hemorrhagic intracranial malignant neoplasms: spin-echo MR imaging. Radiology 1987;164:71–77.

49. Gatenby RA, Coia LR, Richter MP, et al. Oxygen tension in human tumors: in vivo mapping using CT-guided probes. Radiology 1985;156:211–214.

50. Pauling L, Coryell CD. The magnetic properties and structures of hemoglobin, oxyhemoglobin and carbonmonoxyhemoglobin. Proc Natl Acad Sci 1936;22:210–216.

51. Ross JS. Intracranial calcification. In Haaga JR, Alfidi RJ, eds. Computed tomography of the whole body. St. Louis: CV Mosby, 1988;334–354.

52. Oot RF, New PF, Pile-Spellman J, et al. The detection of intracranial calcifications by MR. Am J Neuroradiol 1986;7:801–809.

53. Atlas SW, Grossman RI, Hackney DB, et al. Calcified intracranial lesions: detection with gradient-echo acquisition rapid MR imaging. Am J Neuroradiol 1988;9:253–259.

54. Henkelman RM, Watts JF, Kucharczyk W. High signal intensity in MR images of calcified brain tissue. Radiology 1991;179:199–206.

55. Horowitz BL, Chari MV, Reese J, et al. MR of intracranial epidermoid tumors: correlation of

in vivo imaging with in vitro 13c spectroscopy. Am J Neuroradiol 1990;11:299–302.

56. Som PM, Dillon WP, Fullerton GD, et al. Chronically obstructed sinonasal secretion: observations on T1 and T2 shortening. Radiology 1989;172:515–520.

57. Maeder PP, Holtas SL, Basibuyuk LN, et al. Colloid cyst of the third ventricle: correlation of MR and CT findings with histology and chemical analysis. Am J Neuroradiol 1990;11:575–581.

58. Atlas SW, Grossman RI, Gomori JM, et al. MR imaging of intracranial metastatic melanoma. J Comput Assist Tomogr 1987;11:577–582.

59. Boyko OB, Burger PC, Shelburne JD, et al. Non-heme mechanisms for T1 shortening: pathologic, CT and MR elucidation. Am J Neuroradiol 1992;13:1439–1445.

# PART TWO

# Mechanisms of Intracerebral Hemorrhage

The causes of intracerebral hemorrhages (ICH) are multiple, and include *systemic illnesses* such as hypertension, bleeding disorders, and malignancies, *vascular abnormalities*, such as amyloid angiopathy, vascular malformations and vasculitis, and *exogenous factors*, such as sympathomimetic drug use and head trauma (Table II.1). The relative frequency of each of these factors varies among series, and reflects biases of geographic location, age, patterns of referral, and clinical versus autopsy origin of the series of patients studied. However, despite this variability, there is a degree of consistency in the relative frequency of these causal factors in series of patients with ICH[1-6] (Table II.2).

The different mechanisms of ICH in clinical series are represented with different frequencies, depending to some extent on the *age* of the population under study. Among young patients (under age 45), the most common mechanism is ruptured vascular malformations,[7] while in the elderly (over age 70), the dominant mechanism is cerebral amyloid angiopathy;[8] the intermediate age groups have the highest proportion of patients with hypertension as the mechanism[9] (Figure II.1). Other causes, such as trauma and bleeding disorders, have similar distributions across age groups, since some (trauma, leukemia) affect young patients as much as old patients, while others (ICH due to anticoagulants, fibrinolytic agents) occur as a function of the age group of patients affected by the disorders for which these treatments are prescribed (myocardial infarction, deep vein thrombosis). An increasingly frequent cause of intracranial hemorrhage, both ICH and subarachnoid hemorrhage, is the illicit use of sympathomimetic agents, in particular cocaine, by the young populations of urban communities.[10]

The mechanisms of ICH determine, to some extent, the *locations* in the brain. Although there is variability, hypertensive ICH favors the deep portions of the hemispheres (basal ganglia, internal capsule, thalamus), where the arterial lesions leading to rupture predominate,[11] whereas most other mechanisms tend to produce predominantly lobar hemorrhages.[12] The latter is partially accounted for by the more superficial location of the causative vascular lesions,

**Table II.1.** Mechanisms of Intracerebral Hemorrhage

| |
|---|
| Hypertension |
| Vascular malformations (aneurysms, AVM, CA) |
| Cerebral amyloid angiopathy |
| Intracranial tumors |
| Bleeding disorders (coagulopathies, anticoagulants, fibrinolytics) |
| Vasculitis |
| Sympathomimetic agents |
| Trauma |

Abbreviations: AVM = arteriovenous malformation; CA = cavernous angioma.

**Table II.2.** Mechanisms of Intracerebral Hemorrhage in Large Series from the Literature

| | Russell[1]<br>No. (%) | Mutlu et al.[2]<br>No. (%) | McCormick and<br>Rosenfield[3]<br>No. (%) | Schütz[4]<br>No. (%) | Jellinger[5]<br>No. (%) | Weisberg[6]<br>No. (%) |
|---|---|---|---|---|---|---|
| Hypertension | 232 (50) | 135 (60) | 37 (26) | 140 (56) | 80 (47) | 197 (66) |
| Vasc. malf. | 117 (25) | 50 (22) | 35 (24) | 30 (12) | 53 (31) | 28 (9) |
| Blood dyscr. | 36 (8) | 30 (13) | 28 (20) | 21 (8) | 5 (3) | 14 (5) |
| Brain tumor | 9 (2) | 2 (1) | 13 (9) | 8 (3) | 12 (7) | 5 (2) |
| Arteritis | 13 (3) | 2 (1) | 5 (3) | 2 (1) | 2 (1) | — |
| Other | 38 (8) | 6 (3) | 14 (10) | — | 13 (8) | 2 (1) |
| Unknown | 16 (4) | — | 12 (8) | 49 (20) | 5 (3) | 50 (17) |
| Total | 461 | 225 | 144 | 250 | 170 | 296 |

Abbreviations: Vasc. malf. = vascular malformations, dyscr. = dyscrasia.

such as amyloid angiopathy or vascular malformations, which predominate in the cortical-subcortical portions of the cerebral hemispheres.[8,13] A predominantly lobar location of ICH has been documented in patients with cerebral amyloid angiopathy,[8] vascular malformations,[13] granulomatous angiitis of the nervous system,[14] use of fibrinolytic agents[15] and anticoagulants,[16] and use of sympathomimetic agents, including cocaine[10] and phenylpropanolamine.[17] This predominance of lobar locations in instances of ICH due to nonhypertensive mechanisms results in the lowest frequency of the hypertensive cause in the group of patients with lobar ICH, in comparison with all other sites of ICH (Figure II.2).

These etiological and topographical patterns of ICH have undergone changes in recent decades. On one hand, the hypertensive

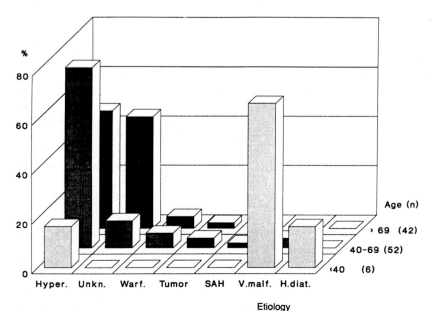

**Figure II.1.** Age-related mechanism of intracerebral hemorrhage in 100 consecutive patients. *Abbreviations:* Hyper. = hypertension; Unk. = unknown; Warf. = warfarin; SAH = subarachnoid hemorrhage; V. malf. = vascular malformation; H. diath. = hemorrhagic diathesis. (From Schütz H, Bödecker R-H, Damian M, et al. Age-related spontaneous intracerebral hematoma in a German community. Stroke 1990;21:1412–1418, reprinted with permission.)

## INTRACEREBRAL HEMORRHAGE

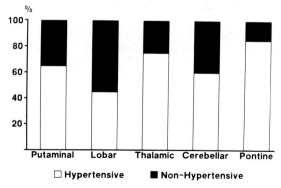

□ Hypertensive   ■ Non-Hypertensive

**Figure II.2.** Relative frequency of hypertensive and nonhypertensive mechanisms of intracerebral hemorrhage by location.

mechanism of ICH has been declining in frequency due to improvements in the treatment of hypertension and to increased awareness of the public and the medical community about the serious consequences of neglecting the control of hypertension. On the other hand, the nonhypertensive varieties of ICH have increased in frequency, due to a variety of reasons: an increase in the size of elderly populations in industrialized countries (presumably resulting in an increase in the number of patients with ICH due to cerebral amyloid angiopathy), the widespread use of anticoagulants and fibrinolytic agents for the treatment of coronary artery disease in the middle-aged and the elderly, and the alarming escalation in the use of illicit sympathomimetic drugs (especially cocaine) by urban young individuals. These patterns of ICH occurrence should promote further efforts at its prevention through monitoring and treatment of hypertension, judicious use of anticoagulants and fibrinolytics (i.e., proper selection of patients, with exclusion of the very elderly and hypertensive, and of those in need of other medications with potential additive effects in inducing bleeding), medical monitoring of the use of over-the-counter sympathomimetics with potential for causing ICH (such as phenylpropanolamine),

and increased education of the public on the dangers of cocaine use.[18]

## References

1. Russell DS. The pathology of spontaneous intracranial haemorrhages. Proc R Soc Med 1954;47:689–693.
2. Mutlu N, Berry RG, Alpers BJ. Massive cerebral hemorrhage: clinical and pathological correlations. Arch Neurol 1963;8:74–91.
3. McCormick WF, Rosenfield DB. Massive brain hemorrhage: a review of 144 cases and an examination of their causes. Stroke 1973;4:946–954.
4. Schütz H. Spontane intrazerebrale Hämatome: Pathophysiologie, Klinik, und Therapie. Heidelberg: Springer-Verlag, 1988.
5. Jellinger K. Zur Ätiologie und Pathogenese der spontanen intrazerebralen Blutung. Therapiewoche 1972;22:1440–1450.
6. Weisberg LA. Computerized tomography in intracranial hemorrhage. Arch Neurol 1979;36:422–426.
7. Gras P, Arveux P, Giroud M, et al. Les hémorragies intracérébrales spontanées du sujet jeune: étude de 33 cas. Rev Neurol 1991;147:653–657.
8. Vinters HV. Cerebral amyloid angiopathy: a critical review. Stroke 1987;18:311–324.
9. Schütz H, Bödeker R-H, Damian M, et al. Age-related spontaneous intracerebral hematoma in a German community. Stroke 1990;21:1412–1418.
10. Levine SR, Brust JCM, Futrell N, et al. Cerebrovascular complications of the use of the "crack" form of alkaloidal cocaine. N Engl J Med 1990;323:699–704.
11. Cole FM, Yates PO. The occurrence and significance of intracerebral micro-aneurysms. J Path Bact 1967;93:393–411.
12. Kase CS. Intracerebral hemorrhage: nonhypertensive causes. Stroke 1986;17:590–595.
13. Becker DH, Townsend JJ, Kramer RA, et al. Occult cerebrovascular malformations: a series of 18 histologically verified cases with negative angiography. Brain 1979;70:530–535.
14. Clifford-Jones RE, Love S, Gurusinghe N. Granulomatous angiitis of the central nervous

system: a case with recurrent intracerebral haemorrhage. J Neurol Neurosurg Psychiat 1985;48:1054–1056.

15. Kase CS, Pessin MS, Zivin JA, et al. Intracranial hemorrhage after coronary thrombolysis with tissue plasminogen activator. Am J Med 1992;92:384–390.

16. Rådberg JA, Olsson JE, Rådberg CT. Prognostic parameters in spontaneous intracerebral hematomas with special reference to anticoagulant treatment. Stroke 1991;22:571–576.

17. Kase CS, Foster TE, Reed JE, et al. Intracerebral hemorrhage and phenylpropanolamine use. Neurology 1987;37:399–404.

18. Kase CS. Differential diagnosis of intracerebral hemorrhage. In Adams HP, ed. Handbook of cerebrovascular diseases. New York: Marcel Dekker, 1993;287–314.

# Chapter 6
# Hypertensive Intracerebral Hemorrhage

## Louis R. Caplan

Utterance of the words "brain hemorrhage" evokes in the minds of most physicians and laypersons a single word response—hypertension. Hypertension and hemorrhage (involving the head or nose) are inseparably entwined in the common conceptualization of the pathogenesis of stroke. Yet hypertension, as we now understand it, is a relatively newly discovered disease, recognized and investigated in the twentieth century and little known before that. Clinicians in the nineteenth century knew that increased arterial pressure did exist but they had no method of measuring blood pressure during life. Richard Bright, writing in 1836, was aware of the large, heavy hearts of hypertensive patients with kidney disease.[1] During the nineteenth century, somehow, the idea evolved that certain personal characteristics predicted hypertension. Ruddy face, nervousness, lability of affect, hyperexcitability, and tenseness all indicated that the sufferer probably had high blood pressure, although there was no epidemiological or experimental evidence to support the idea and blood pressure was not measured. In the minds of many even today, equating hypertension with a low boiling point and a high-strung nature persists. Clinicians of the nineteenth century also knew that increased blood pressure somehow related to heart, kidney, and brain disease. Mahomed wrote in the latter part of the nineteenth century,

"My first contention is that high pressure is a constant condition in the circulation of some individuals and that this condition is a symptom of a certain constitution or diathesis. . . . These persons appear to pass on through life probably much as others do and generally do not suffer from their high blood pressure except in their petty ailments. . . . As age advances the enemy (hypertension) gains accession of strength . . . the individual has now passed forty years, perhaps fifty years of age . . . headache, vertigo, epistaxis, a passing paralysis, a more severe apoplectic seizure, and then the final blow."[2]

Osler, writing in 1903, was aware of some physiological aspects of increased blood pressure.[3] He wrote that hypertrophy of the heart could be caused by "all states of increased arterial tension induced by the contraction of the smaller arteries under the influence of certain toxic substances." Osler quoted Bright's idea that diseases of the "minute capillary circulation render greater action necessary to send the blood through the distant subdivisions of the vascular system."[3]

Important technological advances near the turn of the century led for the first time to the capability of measuring blood pressure in vivo. The initial method was introduced by Riva-Rocci[4] in 1896 and was later modified by Von Recklinghausen in the early years of the twentieth century. The technique involved the use of a cuff around the arm and a mercury manometer; the pulse was palpated as the cuff was inflated and deflated.[5] Later, following the work of Korotkoff, the auscultatory method we use today was introduced in 1905, allowing estimation of both systolic and diastolic blood pressures.[5,6] By the end of the first quarter of the twentieth century, sphygmomanometers were in common use and detection and quantification of blood pressure was widespread and relatively simple. Physicians then were able to turn their attention to the causes of hypertension and the effects of the elevated blood pressure on the blood vessels, heart, kidneys, and brain.

During the twentieth century, much interest and information has accrued about the effects of hypertension on systemic and brain vessels. Hypertension clearly leads to an accentuation of the development of both arteriosclerosis (literally vascular hardening and calcification) and atherosclerosis (the deposition of lipid-laden matter within the vascular wall). However, these changes are not specific for hypertension and occur in a qualitatively identical fashion in persons who have always had normal blood pressure. However, there are three vascular lesions that proponents have claimed are relatively specific and diagnostic of hypertension: fibrinoid necrosis, miliary (Charcot-Bouchard) aneurysms, and lipohyalinosis.

Fibrinoid necrosis was described and investigated mostly by Byrom and his colleagues.[5,7] The predominant abnormality is the appearance of a fibrinoid substance in the media with disappearance of muscle elements in smaller arteries in the kidneys, brain, and viscera. There are four major pathological features: necrosis of muscle fibers, infiltration of the media and intima with plasma proteins and often with erythrocytes, inflammatory reaction within and occasionally around the artery, and invasion of the infiltrated tissue by connective tissue cells.

Fisher popularized the designation lipohyalinosis as a descriptive term for chronic vascular changes seen in the small penetrating arteries in hypertensive patients.[8–11] Fisher defined lipohyalinosis as "a hypertensive cerebral vasculopathy in which the lumen of an artery, usually less than 200 micra in diameter, is occluded, the wall of the artery is thinned and reduced to connective tissue threads, hemosiderin-filled macrophages lie scattered in the vicinity, and the wall stains bright red with oil-red-o".[11] Deposition of lipid material and hyalinization and fibrinoid changes in the vessel wall were emphasized. The pathology especially affected the arteries penetrating into the putamen, thalamus, and the basis pontis. To describe the degenerative changes, Fisher also used the term "segmental arterial disorganization" emphasizing the striking loss of the usual arterial architecture. "Whorls, tangles, or wisps of more or less fine connective tissue entirely replaced the vessel and obliterated the normal vascular coats. Muscular and elastic elements were often not recognizable."[8] Fatty macrophages and foam cells often were seen within the vessel wall, and focal enlargements, hemorrhagic extravasations, and microaneurysms often affected the same arteries. At times, subintimal foam cell accumulations obliterated the lumen of arteries and homogeneous hyaline pink material replaced the vessel wall.[8] Fisher thought that these underlying changes were due to hypertension and caused both ischemic small infarcts (lacunes) and deep hypertensive intracerebral hemorrhage (ICH).

Although miliary aneurysms had been noted previously, Ross-Russell rediscovered their presence during the middle of the century and related the changes to hypertension.[12] Bouchard, working in Charcot's laboratory, had in 1872 reviewed his own work and that of prior observations by Gendrin, Heschl, and others regarding the so-called miliary (or Charcot-Bouchard) type aneurysms.[13] Pickering, in the second edition of his classic work *High Blood Pressure*, commented on advances since publication of the first edition in 1956, "the most important event in this field is Ross-Russell's rediscovery of Charcot and Bouchard's miliary aneurysms of the cerebral vessels and their relation to cerebral haemorrhage."[5] Others have more recently confirmed the presence of these microaneurysms in patients with ICH and in laboratory animals rendered hypertensive. Although Bouchard had claimed that all hypertensive ICH was explained by these aneurysms, further pathological study has raised doubts about this claim.

Even after one hundred or more years of study, many questions remain about the cause of hypertensive brain hemorrhage. Are all cases of so-called spontaneous "hypertensive" ICH due to chronic degenerative vascular damage caused by hypertension? If so, are the causative lesions Charcot-Bouchard aneurysmal ruptures, or are there other lesions that bleed? Can acute changes in the brain circulation cause bleeding despite the absence of prior or chronic hypertensive vascular changes? If some cases of ICH are due to chronic degenerative changes, and some due to acute circulatory perturbations, do these two different pathogenic situations produce hemorrhages that are different clinically?[14] Does hematoma size, location, course, or outcome differ in acute or chronic disease? The remainder of this chapter reviews the data on miliary aneurysms and other degenerative hypertensive vascular lesions, cites observations that raise questions about their importance in causing the majority of cases of ICH, and then reviews situations in which acute circulatory changes have been related to brain hemorrhage.

## Charcot-Bouchard Aneurysms and Other Chronic Hypertensive Vasculopathies Causing Intracerebral Hemorrhages

In 1862, Charles Bouchard came to the hospitals of Paris as an extern of the hospitals and two years later he joined the medical service of Jean Martin Charcot at the Salpetrière Hospital. In 1866, when Bouchard was 29 years old, he began, at Charcot's suggestion, to study the pathogenesis of cerebral hemorrhage.[15] His work under Charcot's tutelage was the subject of Bouchard's doctoral thesis and papers written with Charcot in 1868.[16] Four years later, Bouchard wrote a book on his studies of the pathology of cerebral hemorrhage.[13]

Bouchard cited the work of prior authors. Gendrin, in a doctoral thesis, had described a method for finding small ruptured aneurysms. The aneurysms were said to arise from fourth or fifth degree branches.

> In a great many cases the rupture can be detected by very carefully washing away the coagulated blood, by means of a very fine stream of water, from the walls of the cavity to which it adheres. The arterioles may thus be traced from their origin onwards into the clot, by the detritus of which their extremities are surrounded. Their sudden termination in the middle of these pieces of extravasated blood and the presence of fibrinous striae which seem to prolong the extremities of the vessels in the clot, leave no doubt as to the connection between the clot resulting from the extravasation and the blood which traversed these arterioles. This arrangement is rarely found in only one arteriole; it is generally common to all the ramifications of many of these small vessels springing from the same vascular branch.[13]

Bouchard also gave credit to Cruveilher and Heschl who had also described these small vascular lesions but, according to Bouchard, had not recognized their connection with cerebral hemorrhage. In fact, Bouchard chose the name "miliary aneurysms" from Cruveilher's term, miliary cavities, which sprung from the resemblance to millet seed.[13] Bouchard quoted Heschl's observations that these miliary aneurysms were more common with increasing age. Among 394 autopsies in patients over age 40, Heschl found the aneurysms 15 times (4%), but among 800 autopsies in persons under age 40, they occurred but once (0.1%).[13]

Bouchard described the vascular abnormalities he found as follows:

> All these aneurysms are visible to the naked eye; they look like little globular particles, varying in diameter from 2/10th of a millimetre to 1

millimetre, and even more, attached to a vessel which is likewise visible to the naked eye—a simple lens, at least suffices to make them quite distinct. The diameter of the vessel may vary from a third of a tenth of a millimetre to one-fourth of a millimetre and even more. The colour of these aneurysms varies according to the state of the blood which they contain and the conditions of the walls. When the wall is thin, as it usually is, the aneurysm is a purplish colour . . . if the blood, long coagulated, has already been transformed into haematoidin, the aneurysm is reddish-brown or ochrey, or even blackish, and the surrounding cerebral tissue generally presents in a less degree a similar coloration.[13]

The lesions were within the brain and different from the "ampillary dilatation" of the vessels in the pia mater described by Virchow. Bouchard found "my aneurysms have never been awanting in 12 cases of cerebral hemorrhage which I have collected since I became aware of their existence."[13] He believed they were *the* cause of cerebral hemorrhage. Bouchard rapidly rose to become full professor in the chair of General Pathology in the hospitals of Paris but later broke with his mentor Charcot, and the two ultimately became rivals and antagonists.[15] The aneurysms are shown in Figure 1.3 in the first chapter of this book.

In the ensuing years, pathologists were unable to corroborate the findings of Bouchard, and cast doubts as to whether these lesions existed or were small dissections or fragments of adherent blood clot.[17] Green, in 1930, wrote "the prevalent view seems to be that miliary aneurysms of the intracerebral arteries are a rarity, and some authors have expressed doubt as to whether they actually occur."[17] Green studied the brains of ten hypertensive patients whose blood pressures all exceeded 200/100 mm Hg during life. Three of the patients died of ICH. Green largely relied on "naked eye" methods to identify the aneurysms but used hematoxylin-and-eosin-stained frozen sections to analyze the lesions found. In all, he found three aneurysms, two in one patient dying of ICH and the other in an artery supplying a pontine infarct in another patient. The fatal ICH was a fourth ventricle hemorrhage; in this patient there were also small pea-sized hemorrhages in the left frontal region and the pons, and aneurysms were clearly seen in relation to these two small hematomas. The parent artery containing the pontine aneurysm was severely damaged. The subendothelial portion of the intima and the full thickness of the media were completely "necrotic" and consisted only of fatty and hyaline material. No intact muscle fibers or elastica were seen. The vessel fit the description later given by Fisher of a lipohyalinotic artery. The aneurysm arising from this vessel was saccular and "apparently resulted from a stretching and bursting of the diseased tunica media in a portion of its circumference."[17] Figure 6.1, from Green's article, shows a section from the aneurysm and parent artery. The other two miliary aneurysms also arose from lipohyalinotic arteries and, in fact, in one, the aneurysm was thrombosed and the artery led to a small pontine infarct. Charcot and Bouchard had not described disease of the parent artery and, in fact, had speculated about an arteritis

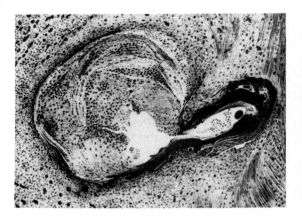

**Figure 6.1.** Section of a pontine aneurysm stained with H&E and Sudan III. The sac is partially occluded by organizing blood clot. There is recent hemorrhage around the aneurysm. (From Green FHK. Miliary aneurysms in the brain. J Pathol Bacteriol 1930;33:71–77. With permission of the publisher.)

or periarteritis of the parent artery as a cause of the bulges.[13,17]

After Green's observations, the issue of the presence and significance of miliary aneurysms lay relatively dormant until the observations of Ross-Russell in 1963.[12] Ross-Russell, a British neurologist, made his observations during a seven-month period when he worked at the Boston City Hospital, Harvard Neurological Unit, under the tutelage of Dr. Derek Denny-Brown. Ross-Russell studied the brains of 54 patients (38 normotensive and 16 known hypertensives). The mean blood pressure of the hypertensive group was 205/113 mm Hg. Among the hypertensive group, there were five recent massive brain hemorrhages and four small, old hemorrhages. There were no hypertensive patients under age 50 and only two were under 60. Some patients in the normotensive group had old putaminal hemorrhages and each had a large heart at autopsy, probably indicating past hypertension. Ross-Russell studied the brains after injecting a radiopaque barium sulfate mixture and then taking x-rays on special films.[12] This technique allowed satisfactory filling of arteries down to small arterioles 30 microns in diameter. Ross-Russell described the appearance of normal arteries and those affected by hypertension. In hypertensives, the walls of both penetrating and cortical arteries were thickened. Stenosis of the basal arteries was also more extensive in hypertensive subjects. Aneurysms were very frequently found. "A striking and unexpected finding in all but one of the brains in the hypertensive group and in ten of the brains in the normotensive group was the presence of saccular dilatations on the small intracerebral vessels."[12] The number of aneurysms varied from one to twenty, but all patients with more than ten aneurysms had been hypertensive. (One was normotensive at the time of death, but had old slit hemorrhages and a large heart.) The aneurysms were most often found in the putamen, globus pallidus, and thalamus, but also occurred in the caudate nucleus, internal capsule, white matter, and cortical gray matter.[12] The aneurysms were found on small arteries 100 to 300 microns in diameter. The diameter of the aneurysms varied from 300 to 900 microns. They most often arose at branch points and were often multiple. Figure 6.2 from Ross-Russell illustrates his findings. The muscular tissue of the parent vessel ended abruptly at the point of origin of the aneurysms and elastica was visible only for a short distance into the aneurysm before disappearing. The wall of the aneurysm was composed mostly of connective tissue with hyaline material being prominent. Red blood cells and hemosiderin-containing macrophages were seen around the aneurysms some of which were thrombosed.

Ross-Russell did not identify a ruptured aneurysm leading to any of the macroscopic sites of hemorrhage. The pathogenesis of the aneurysms was discussed. "It seems likely that once the two main causative factors, increased intraluminal pressure and weakness of the arterial wall, are present, the critical event is rupture of the elastic lamina allowing aneurysmal bulging of the wall composed only of connective tissue and the remnants of muscular elements."[12] Later, further stretching of the aneurysm occurs. Like Green, Ross-Russell was also impressed with the association of degenerative atherosclerotic changes in patients with the aneurysms.

Several years later, Cole and Yates[18] were able to corroborate the findings of Ross-Russell. They studied one hundred normotensive and one hundred hypertensive subjects. The criteria for inclusion in the hypertensive group was diastolic blood pressure of 110 mm Hg or higher and heart weight of over 400 g in men or 350 g in women. Like Ross-Russell, they also used injection of opaque material and x-ray filming. Aneurysms correlated highly with hypertension and age. Forty-six percent of hypertensive patients had miliary aneurysms while they were present in only 7% of normotensives. No brain that contained aneurysms had fewer than nine, and the usual range was fifteen to twenty-five per patient.[18] The

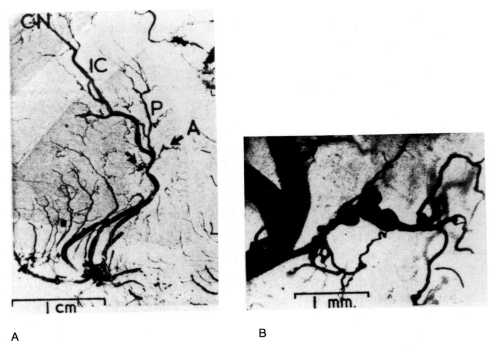

A                                          B

**Figure 6.2.** (A) x-Ray of striate arteries after injection of radiopaque material. Note irregularity of the main trunks, attenuation of small arteries and number of small aneurysms (arrows). CN = caudate nucleus; IC = internal capsule; P = putamen; A = aneurysm (B) Enlarged view of the same area. (From Ross-Russell RW. Observations on intracerebral aneurysms. Brain 1963;86:425–442. With permission.)

most frequent sites were the basal ganglia and thalamus, but many aneurysms were also found at the gray-white junctions and in the pons and cerebellum. Nearly a third of the hypertensive patients with aneurysms also had hematomas, but no hematomas were found in the normotensive group. All of the patients with hematomas had aneurysms, but Cole and Yates comment that "it is difficult to be quite certain that a particular hemorrhage has arisen from a specific aneurysm. This is possibly due to the fact that an aneurysmal sac may be so torn by even a small hemorrhage that few remnants of it can be identified."[18] Small cystic infarcts (lacunes) were also common especially, but not exclusively, in hypertensives. The evidence supporting an etiological relation between aneurysms and hemorrhage was substantial but indirect: (1) both hemato-

mas and aneurysms occurred predominantly in hypertensives, (2) aneurysms were present in each patient with hemorrhage, and (3) hematomas and aneurysms involved the same brain sites.[17,18]

The next important observations were those of Fisher. In 1971, he reported the results of exhaustive serial sections of two patients with hypertensive ICH.[10] The first patient had a large pontine hemorrhage. The center of the lesion was a sea of blood which had essentially obliterated the parenchyma. Around the border of the hematoma were many "fibrin globe" sites from which bleeding had occurred (see Figure 1.5, Chapter 1). Fibrin globes refer to large masses of platelets which are partially encircled by thin, concentric layers of fibrin; the fibrin-platelet conglomerate caps torn vessels to provide hemostasis (see Figure 3.1, Chapter 3). The arterial defects at the bleeding sites took varied forms. "In 19 instances, the artery appeared to have completely parted while in 5, the break involved only a segment of the arterial circumference."[10] In only four could the distal part of the artery be identified; the walls of the interrupted arteries were often attenuated and frayed at their ends. The arterial segment adjacent to the break was usually hyalinized with poor staining and definition of muscular and elastic elements. Neither aneurysms nor dissections were observed. Fisher interpreted the rupture of the arteries as a peripheral avalanche effect of pressure building in the center. These were then "secondary" ruptures, an effect of the bleeding in the center and not the primary cause of the initial bleeding.[10]

Fisher's second patient had a recent large lobar hematoma and two small putaminal hemorrhages judged to be about six days old. There were also old slit lobar hemorrhages and an old cerebellar hematoma. Fisher examined blocks from the small putaminal hemorrhages. The arteries in the region had severe lipohyalinosis. The larger putaminal hemorrhage seemed to derive from one torn artery that was capped by a large fibrin globe. The wall of the parent artery was a thin hyaline structure without internal structure. The proximal and distal torn edges were filled with fibrin. In the smaller putaminal hemorrhage, bleeding came from a torn artery with gaping edges whose parent artery was severely lipohyalinotic. No aneurysms were seen in the area of the hemorrhages, however in the pons there were three miliary aneurysms and two arterial "fibrous balls" at a distance from the hematoma. In the putaminal hemorrhage case, aneurysmal dilatations were found often and old ruptures of aneurysmal and nonaneurysmal segments of diseased arteries were common. Also many microinfarcts were found. Miliary aneurysms were formed in which arteries 80 microns in diameter enlarged segmentally to about 200 microns. The walls of these dilations were lined by a fibrin deposit, and a thick layer of red blood cells lay externally.

Fisher commented, "It is our impression that these structures are not an intermediate stage on the way to a major hemorrhage but represent the end stage of a limited extravasation."[10] Aneurysms and lipohyalinosis were consequences of hypertension, but Fisher did not find support for aneurysms as the cause of the hemorrhages. He noted, "The conclusion must be drawn that the same type of hypertensive vascular disease under some circumstances evokes ischemia and under others, tends to bleeding."[10]

Rosenblum also studied in serial section tissue from patients with ICH.[19] Only one of the patients was known to have been hypertensive during life. He found abundant examples of fibrinoid necrosis and miliary aneurysms. Some of the aneurysms were sclerosed, flask-shaped collections of collagen joined to a small artery by a narrow neck. Fibrous balls were believed to be sclerosed aneurysms. Fibrinoid changes occurred on surface arteries and were not always associated on the same artery with aneurysm development. Rosenblum emphasized that the presence of elastic tissue in the walls of the sclerosed aneurysms indicated that they were true aneurysms not merely organized extravasations of blood outside or adjacent to the vessels (so-called pseudoaneurysms). He did not see aneurysmal rupture at the site of the hemorrhages. Goto et al.[20] also found fibrinoid degeneration with and without aneurysmal dilatation and fibrous and fibrohyalinoid changes in both cerebral and retinal arteries in patients with cerebrovascular disease.

One group studied the relationship of aneurysm formation to cerebral hemorrhage by inducing hypertension in an experimental animal, the rabbit.[21] Iris aneurysms developed proportionately to the severity of the hypertension and highly correlated with the risk of ICH. Among the rabbits with iris aneurysms 42.5% had brain hemorrhages while only 11% without iris aneurysms had ICH. The iris vessels developed increasing thickness and tortuosity and aneurysm formation. The brain arteries of the hypertensive rabbits showed abundant miliary aneurysms and fibrinoid and lipohyalin changes very similar to those described in studies of human pathology. Clearly, hypertension could cause these changes in the brain and retina.

A recent study of surgical specimens of patients who had surgery for lobar ICH confirmed the presence of microaneurysms.[22] Of particular interest, some of the patients with microaneurysms had never been hypertensive. Takebayashi et al. have recently added important observations on the pathology of ICH and microaneurysms. In two separate studies, they examined by electron microscopy specimens from patients with fresh brain hemorrhages.[23,24] In the first study, the material came from twenty patients operated on within four hours of ICH and from sixteen necropsies of patients with recent hemorrhages.[23] Sixty-one rupture sites were identified. At all the rupture sites, there was breakage of the elastic lamina which otherwise showed no abnormality by electron microscopy. Medial degeneration characterized by atrophy and segmentation of medial smooth muscle cells and widening of the intracellular matrix with basement-membrane-like material and granular and vesicular cell debris was present in all ruptured arteries. In fifty-nine cases rupture was at or very near bifurcation points and in the other two ruptures, a microaneurysm was present at the break point. The medial degenerative changes emphasized the middle and distal portions of the penetrating arteries and were not found in the proximal portions of the arteries.

Takebayashi and colleagues studied carefully seven microaneurysms they found in their specimens, five of which were unruptured.[23] In the arterial wall connected to the aneurysm there was severe degeneration of smooth muscle cells and subendothelial deposition of fibrin and plasma materials. They believed the appearance of the microaneurysms indicated that they were cavities formed by reabsorption of minimal hemorrhages formed at rupture sites at vascular bifurcations. Lipohyalinosis was believed to be a separate process from microaneurysm formation. A later study of ten microaneurysms came to the same conclusion.[24] No vascular elements were seen in the walls of microaneurysms except for endothelial cells which "were easily regenerated." Some of the aneurysms were composed only of thin layers of fibrin and monocytes and macrophages. Ruptured arteries were 200 to 700 microns in diameter while the connecting artery to microaneurysms was always less than 200 microns. They made the following hypothesis regarding the cause of hypertensive ICH: "The medial degeneration which was the most important finding in ruptured arteries would cause the vascular wall to lose its elasticity and would induce dissection at the bifurcation which is a highly susceptible site to tensile forces. The various factors such as intravascular pressure, stress forces, and size of arteries determine whether complete or incomplete rupture occurs."[24]

To summarize the pathological data: (1) fibrinoid necrosis, medial degeneration, lipohyalinosis, and microaneurysm formation are abundantly found in the penetrating arteries in the brains of hypertensive patients especially those with ICH; (2) when rupture sites have been identified, the site does not usually show a microaneurysm; (3) microaneurysms (Charcot-Bouchard type) have never been clearly identified as the definitive cause of even a single hematoma despite very extensive study; (4) microaneurysms may well represent, at least in some instances, the effects of small vascular rupture rather than the cause; (5) ruptured arteries show changes in the elastic lamina and degeneration in the vascular media especially affecting smooth muscle elements; (6) rupture usually occurs in the middle or distal portions of penetrating arteries at or very near bifurcations.

## Evidence Against the Theory that Intracerebral Hemorrhage Is Always Caused by Chronic Vascular Degenerative Changes

Data from a variety of different sources raise serious doubts concerning the time-honored

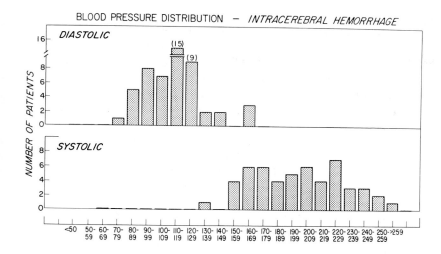

BLOOD PRESSURE DISTRIBUTION — *INTRACEREBRAL HEMORRHAGE*

**Figure 6.3.** Blood pressure distribution in patients with ICH from the Harvard Stroke Registry. (From Caplan LR, Mohr JP. Intracerebral hemorrhage: an update. Geriatrics 1978;33:42–52. With permission.)

concept that so-called hypertensive ICH is always caused by rupture of arteries chronically damaged by hypertension. In the preceding section, it was emphasized that there are no direct data that show that rupture of miliary aneurysms is a common cause of hypertensive ICH. In fact, in several of the reports, patients with hematomas had no history of being hypertensive in the past and were not hypertensive when examined after their hemorrhage.[19,22]

Epidemiological and stroke registry data show that many patients with deep hematomas in locations usually identified as loci for hypertensive ICH have no history of hypertension and have no other recognized cause of hematoma formation (e.g., trauma, aneurysm, arteriovenous malformations, bleeding diathesis, amyloid angiopathy, drugs). In the Harvard Stroke Registry, 41% of the patients with ICH had no past history of hypertension.[25,26] Their blood pressures on initial examination are charted in Figure 6.3; some had pressures within normal limits and in others, blood pressure elevation was modest. Brott et al. studied hypertension as a risk factor for spontaneous ICH in Cincinnati.[27] They reviewed all cases of ICH seen among sixteen hospitals in the Cincinnati metropolitan area during 1982. Patients with trauma, aneurysms, and hemorrhagic infarcts were excluded. Of 154 patients with spontaneous

ICH, only 69 (45%) had known hypertension, defined as blood pressure greater than 140/90 mm Hg prior to the hemorrhage. An additional 18 patients had cardiomegaly on chest x-ray or left ventricular hypertrophy on EKG but had no history of hypertension. In total, 67 patients (44%) with spontaneous ICH had neither a history of hypertension nor evidence of cardiomegaly or left ventricular hypertrophy.[27] Among those with no history of hypertension, 24 had blood pressure greater than 160 mm Hg systolic or greater than 90 diastolic on admission. Even in patients with deep hematomas, only 24 of 51 (47%) had a past history of hypertension. Brott and colleagues cited four other studies that were not epidemiologically based in which the incidence of hypertension in spontaneous ICH varied from 59% to 90%.[27] In the Stroke Data Bank, among 237 patients with ICH only 64% had a history of either treated or untreated hypertension.[28] Of interest, in the Cincinnati study, age did show an effect; there was a rising incidence of ICH with advancing years.[27]

Because historical data may be incomplete, evidence of left ventricular hypertrophy detected by electrocardiography, echocardiography, chest x-ray or CT, or at necropsy, may be a more reliable guide to the presence of chronic hypertension. With this in mind, Bahemuka studied the heart weights of patients coming to necropsy with ICH.[29] He searched the files of the Neuropathology Department of the Armed Forces Institute of Pathology for autopsies from 1965 through 1981. Only large hematomas were included, and patients with other causes of ventricular hypertrophy, for example, congenital or valvular heart disease, were also excluded. ICH occurred in 407 patients, and 218 were classified as primary intracerebral hemorrhage since they did not have aneurysms, arteriovenous malformations, reticuloendothelial cancers, hematological disorders, or brain tumors. Clinical evidence of past hypertension, that is, blood pressure of at least 160/95 mm Hg on several occasions, was present in only 57 patients (26.1%).[29] Nearly 40% of the patients with basal ganglionic hematomas were normotensive. Using heart weight as a criterion, only 94 patients (46%) had heart weights greater than or equal to the mean heart weight of autopsy controls matched for sex plus 1.5 standard deviations. The author noted, "patients who bled from primary ICH had been healthy all their lives with no evidence of cardiovascular or cerebrovascular disease, and the ICH was their first evidence of disease."[29]

## Is There Evidence that Acute Changes in Blood Pressure and Blood Flow Can Cause Intracerebral Hemorrhage in the Absence of Chronic Hypertension?

One of the authors (L.R.C.) recently examined an elderly retired college professor (H.F.) who was curious and perplexed by his diagnosis. It seemed that several years before he had developed a left hemiparesis, was hospitalized, and told he had a hypertensive intracerebral hematoma. He was puzzled because he had never had high blood pressure before the stroke nor were blood pressures elevated since. He had made a good recovery and was not disabled. The CT was requested and sure enough, it showed a typical right putaminal hemorrhage. His physicians were contacted and H.F.'s blood pressures had in-

deed always been quite normal. L.R.C. elicited the history of the events of that evening. It was a dreadful day, H.F. said. He was supposed to meet his wife in town for dinner and the symphony. He was detained and so began quite late; as he hurried, he knew his wife would be quite upset. After arriving at the restaurant, they had to wait to be seated and had a hurried, rather tasteless meal. They hurried to the symphony, arriving just as the last patrons were seated. Their seats were in the front of the hall. He collapsed in his seat next to his wife who was also harried, upset, and angry with him. He then, within moments, developed left limb weakness, slight headache, and had to be taken to the hospital. Blood pressure was slightly elevated on arrival but quickly normalized without treatment. H.F. asked, "Might the emotional and physical strain of events that evening cause enough circulatory stress to produce the hemorrhage?"

In many patients with ICH, although there is no history of past hypertension, the blood pressure is quite elevated on admission and remains high unless treated. In these patients, it has always been difficult to decide if the blood pressure elevation was caused by increased intracranial pressure related to the ICH, or if hypertension had developed recently and led to the ICH. In our experience in many of these cases, the hematoma size is insufficient to cause increased intracranial pressure. The subsequent sustained blood pressure elevation provides evidence that the patients indeed had recently developed their hypertension. ICH is often the initial symptom of clinical hypertensive disease. There is some evidence from other medical illnesses that elevated blood pressure and flow might make normal vessels break. In rheumatic mitral stenosis, hemoptysis is an early occurrence. The stenosed mitral valve causes an elevation of left atrial pressure which then leads to an increase in pressure in the pulmonary veins draining into the atrium. Pulmonary artery pressure rises in order to perfuse the pulmonary capillary bed. The lung arterioles and capillaries, when exposed to the higher pressure, break. Later, pulmonary arteries and arterioles become hypertrophied, thicken, and the smaller arterioles and capillaries are protected so that hemoptysis no longer occurs. Instead, right heart failure may develop because of the increased resistance in the pulmonary artery bed. Similarly, in acute hypertension, the systemic arteries and arterioles are unprotected. Brain hemorrhage, epistaxis, and hematuria might develop when these smaller vessels break under the increased pressure. With time, the systemic arteries and arterioles hypertrophy leading to protection of the smaller vessels, but left ventricular hypertrophy develops because of the increased resistance in the systemic vascular bed.

In recent years, there have been reports of ICH occurring under unusual circumstances. Review of these cases may shed light on the pathogenesis of so-called spontaneous or primary ICH.[14]

### Drug-related Intracerebral Hemorrhage

During recent years, there have been many reports of both subarachnoid and intracerebral bleeding in patients after taking drugs. This topic is reviewed fully in Chapter 10 and is mentioned only briefly here. The drugs involved have most often been sympathomimetic agents known to have effects on the pulse and blood pressure. Amphetamines (including dextroamphetamine and methamphetamine) and cocaine are the most commonly implicated agents. Other substances known to have autonomic effects, such as ephedrine, phencyclidine, mescaline, and lysergic acid diethylamide, have also been associated with intracranial hemorrhage. Some patients have had aneurysms or arteriovenous malformations but the majority of patients with drug-related ICH have no other causative lesions or abnormalities. In many, the blood pressure is elevated during the early hours after the bleeding. The pathogenesis of drug-related ICH is widely believed to be the sudden, dramatic increase in blood

pressure precipitated by the sympathomimetic effects of the agents used.

### Cold-related Intracerebral Hemorrhage

In 1984, Caplan et al. described three patients who developed ICH during a very severe winter freeze in Chicago when temperatures were below −10°F.[30] The first patient was an alcoholic man who was "shaky" from alcohol withdrawal; he went outside in −34°F weather without a warm coat in order to buy whiskey. On the way home, the bottle slipped from his left hand and he became hemiplegic. Initial blood pressure was 130/106 mm Hg but, later, normal pressures were obtained during hospitalization for his right putaminal hemorrhage. The second patient developed a thalamic hemorrhage after wiping snow manually from the windshield. He had a history of slight hypertension and the admitting blood pressure was 170/110 mm Hg. The blood pressure quickly returned to normal after hydrochlorothiazide. The third patient developed a cerebellar hemorrhage while waiting in a line (−25°F) to pay rent. He had a history of hypertension and blood pressure was 220/110 mm Hg on admission. After clonidine, the blood pressure fell to 140/80 mm Hg. The hematomas were attributed to sudden rises in blood pressure caused by a "cold pressor" response. Hines and Brown had observed, in 1933, that immersion of the hands in ice water for at least one minute could sometimes cause a significant elevation of blood pressure.[31] This cold pressor response has been well known since, but elevation of blood pressure during the test does not accurately predict subsequent clinical hypertension.[30] One of the most effective ways to elevate blood pressure is to immerse individuals in ice cold water. Takahashi et al. studied the effects of cold on blood pressure and brain hemorrhage.[32] They recorded higher blood pressures in winter than summer and a higher proportion of hypertensive patients lived in poorly heated compared to warm houses.

### Trigeminal Nerve Stimulation

The trigeminal nerves and their fibers play an important role in the innervation and control of cerebral blood vessels.[33] Pressor effects and alterations in pressure and flow follow trigeminal stimulation in animals and acute rises in blood pressure and tachycardia accompany pain in humans and follow stimulation of the trigeminal nerves.[34] Haines et al. in 1978, described five patients who developed post-craniotomy supratentorial hemorrhages in locations customary for hypertensive ICH.[35] All the posterior fossa operative procedures were near the trigeminal nerve and four of the five patients had elevated blood pressures, three transient and one more sustained. The hematomas were quite remote from the operative site and no other cause of ICH was identified.[35] Waga et al. also described four patients with ICH remote from their operative sites.[36] Sudden exacerbation of pre-existing hypertension or traction on the trigeminal nerve (suboccipital decompression of presumed Chiari malformation) were possible causes of the unexpected ICH complication. Similarly, intracerebral hemorrhages have been described after radiofrequency lesions for treatment of trigeminal neuralgia,[37] and dangerous rises in blood pressure are sometimes noted after heating of trigeminal rootlets[38] and during percutaneous trigeminal rhizoto-mies.[39] Neurosurgeons and neuroanesthetists advocate continuous blood pressure monitoring during surgery on the trigeminal nerve because of the lability of blood pressure during and after trigeminal stimulation.

In 1987, Barbas et al. reported the case of a woman who suddenly developed a fatal ICH while a dentist was treating her for toothache.[34] The 52-year-old woman had previously been well and had no history of hypertension. In preparation for a root canal procedure, the dentist washed her mouth (tooth) with sodium hypochlorite to clean away unwanted tissue near (in) the operative site. No anesthetic or epinephrine was given. She complained of severe mouth pain and then almost immediately clutched her head, slumped in the chair, and became comatose. Blood pressure was 170/92 mm Hg when she was evaluated in the emergency room a few minutes later. CT, and later necropsy, confirmed a large left cerebral hematoma involving the temporal and parietal lobes, the basal ganglia, and thalamus. There was no arteriovenous malformation or aneurysm and no microscopic evidence of hypertensive vascular changes in the brain or other organs. The heart was not enlarged.[34] One of the authors (L.R.C.) has recently reviewed the details of another patient who developed a spontaneous ICH during a dental procedure, again with no obvious cause. Dental pain or stimulation of trigeminal branches might have precipitated a sudden pressor response and ICH. Cawley et al. reported two other patients with hemorrhage during dental procedures, one with ICH and one with SAH.[40] The patient with a cerebellar hemorrhage had no pain during the dental procedure but copious irrigation that tasted bitter was used.

### Other Circumstances Causing Acute Hypertension

Intracerebral hemorrhage is a known and feared complication of carotid endarterectomy. ICH is particularly prone to occur in patients who have been previously hypertensive and nearly all reported cases have been hypertensive at the time of their brain hemorrhage. The hematoma most often occurs on the side of the surgery in common loci for hypertensive ICH.[41–43] It is now well known that hypertension can develop acutely in the postoperative period after endarterectomy. Usually this occurs within hours to days, but may be delayed as long as ten days after carotid surgery. Accelerated hypertension can be severe and cause a hypertensive encephalopathy-like syndrome of agitation, confusion and severe headache. The usual explanation for the hypertension is loss of the baroreceptor carotid sinus reflex.[44,45]

Lehv et al. first documented the frequent occurrence of increased blood pressure after carotid artery surgery.[44] These authors reported an elevation of systolic blood pressure of greater than 15 mm Hg over preoperative levels in fifteen of twenty-seven patients having unilateral carotid endarterectomy. In five of the fifteen the blood pressure was very high, in the 195–250/105–130 range.[44]

Piatt described a single patient with ICH that developed during cardiac catheterization shortly after a dose of ergonovine maleate.[46] At the beginning of the catheterization, the blood pressure was 125/85 mm Hg but it had been up to 160/85 mm Hg previously. Before the injection, the aortic blood pressure was 170/80 mm Hg. After two injections of ergonovine maleate of 0.05 mg, then 0.1 mg used to precipitate coronary vasospasm, the blood pressure rose to 200/95 mm Hg and the patient became unresponsive. CT showed a very large, left lobar hemorrhage that was evacuated surgically.

Another situation in which acute hypertension can develop is the so-called autonomic dysreflexia syndrome seen in paraplegic patients.[47] In this syndrome, various visceral or other usually painful stimuli cause sudden, often dramatic, elevations in blood pressure. In one patient given intrathecal prostigmine to induce penile erection and ejaculation, a sudden elevation in blood pressure was noted after the injection and he developed a fatal ICH.[47] Brain hemorrhage has also been noted after scorpion bites, another situation in which autonomic changes can occur.[48] One young person developed a lobar hematoma while break dancing, an activity requiring unusually vigorous movements.[49] Although hypertension was not documented, increased blood pressure is a possible explanation for the occurrence. One patient developed a lobar hemorrhage after treatment with electroconvulsive therapy for depression.[50] When electrically induced seizures occur, sympathomimetic activity increases with resulting increases in blood pressure and pulse rate.[50]

## Circumstances Causing Changes in Blood Flow to the Brain

In some patients with ICH, hemorrhage developed after acute or subacute changes in blood flow. In 1975, Humphreys et al. reported that sixteen children operated on by them to correct congenital cardiac lesions had intracranial hemorrhages.[51] The most common cardiac lesions were transposition of the great vessels and ventricular septal defects. Hemorrhages occurred intracerebrally or into the extradural or subdural spaces and developed intraoperatively or immediately during the postoperative period. The authors were puzzled and could not be certain of the cause but sudden change in intracranial blood flow, in retrospect, seems a likely cause. Intracerebral hemorrhage was also a complication in a recent series of patients who had cardiac transplantation.[52,53] At the Cleveland Clinic, 5% of early transplants had lobar ICH without a known vascular anomaly, chronic hypertension, or coagulopathy.[52,53] The patients with ICH were all young, had smaller body surface areas than other transplant patients, and the indication for transplantation in all was cardiomyopathy. All had relatively low mean arterial pressure before operation and higher mean arterial pressure and cardiac index after operation. Sila wrote that she believed the mechanism of ICH was probably relative cerebral hyperperfusion from abrupt increases in blood flow or blood pressure in the presence of abnormal autoregulation.[53]

Carotid endarterectomy is another situation in which there may be an abrupt increase in blood flow postoperatively. A hyperperfusion syndrome has been described characterized by headache, vomiting, and increased cerebral blood flow presumably due to disordered autoregulation and sudden increase in flow.[54] This could also contribute to ICH in some individuals.

Cerebral embolism, so-called spät apoplexy, and migraine are three other conditions in which alterations in blood flow to portions of the brain could contribute to bleeding. Unlike the situations described so far, they also share potential injury to brain tissue and blood vessels as an additional factor. Fisher and Adams commented, in 1951, that hemorrhagic infarction often indicated an embolic mechanism of ischemia.[55] Over three decades later they analyzed the mechanism of bleeding into infarcted tissue in more detail.[56] Emboli block previously normal arteries leading to ischemic damage to the brain parenchyma and small vessels supplied by that recipient artery. When the embolic plug moves distally, the previously ischemic territory may be suddenly flooded with blood. The damaged capillaries may bleed when the influx occurs. Fisher and Adams showed that reperfusion of previously ischemic tissue was the predominant mechanism of hemorrhagic infarction.[56] Reperfusion also occurs after cardiac arrest and systemic hypotension, situations also associated with hemorrhagic infarction. Most often, bleeding in patients with hemorrhagic infarction is made of petechiae by diapedesis of red blood cells into the infarcted tissue, but occasionally a frank hematoma may develop.

The topic of spät apoplexy is covered in detail in Chapter 11 on traumatic ICH. The term refers to a delayed onset stroke, usually ICH, in an area in which bleeding was not apparent immediately after the injury.[57,58] Recent studies indicate that tissue is injured, contused acutely and edema develops. The local tissue pressure and retraction and occlusion of blood vessels limits initial bleeding. When the edema subsides, perfusion increases. By that time fibrinolysis has developed and the injured blood vessels then bleed, producing a hematoma in the region of the initial pale contusion.[59]

Recently, Cole and Aubé described three patients with migrainous headaches who developed delayed hematomas.[60] In one patient, CT during the migraine was normal. In others, there were no focal signs. Carotid artery tenderness and angiographically demonstrated extracranial internal carotid

artery narrowing were prominent features. All three patients had the onset of focal signs and a CT demonstrated hematoma as their migraine cleared. Presumably, perfusion in focal regions fed by the carotid artery was decreased during the migraine phase. Tissue fed by the vasoconstricted arteries might have been ischemic. When vasoconstriction ceased, perfusion was increased and bleeding developed. None of the patients had aneurysms, arteriovenous malformations, or other known causes of ICH.[60]

In summary, in the unusual circumstances described, there are three common threads that seem to relate to the development of ICH:

1. *Acute elevation in blood pressure.* Elevation frequently occurs in persons who had slight or controlled hypertension, but it also could develop in persons previously normotensive.

2. *Acute increase in brain blood flow.* The change in blood flow could be regional, for example, after carotid endarterectomy and reperfusion or after an embolus passes, or more global, for example, after cardiac transplantation and correction of congenital heart lesions.

3. *Damage to local blood vessels and tissues preceding the influx of blood.* Intact blood vessels may be more resistant to breakage than those damaged. The examples given herein were cerebral embolic infarction, spät apoplexy, and migrainous ischemia. In some cases, particles of talc or microcrystalline cellulose contained in pills made for oral use but injected intravenously by addicts have caused vascular damage leading to ICH.[61] Also, perhaps more important is prior vascular injury due to slight, but chronic hypertension. Fibrinoid and lipohyalin deposition, and thinning and wearing away of muscular and elastic elements of penetrating arteries can make these vessels more susceptible to rupture when circulatory changes occur.

## A Hypothesis Based on the Data Discussed

The evidence presented leads us to conclude that there are probably two rather different important mechanisms of hypertensive ICH:

1. *Rupture of small penetrating arteries damaged by chronic hypertension and aging.* The evidence is overwhelming that both high blood pressure and aging cause degenerative changes in arteries that make them susceptible to both occlusion and rupture. The evidence, however, weighs against the theory that rupture is due to breakage of microaneurysms.
2. *Acute perturbations in blood pressure and blood flow lead to rupture of normal arterioles and capillaries unaccustomed and unprotected from these circulatory changes.* Of course, the more sudden and the more severe the change, the more likely is breakage. This theory also allows for the possibility and even likelihood of a third, or intermediate, group in which some damage to blood vessels, for example, incurred during protracted but slight hypertension, might make blood vessels more susceptible to breakage when circulatory changes occur.

We might again cite a discussion by Wilson in the first chapter of this book on the history of ICH.[62] Wilson noted the importance of transient fluctuations of blood pressure occurring during daily activities. He said, "Prolonged or severe muscular effort is a conventional excitant as in straining at stool, lifting weights, coughing, sneezing, vomiting, laughing, running, during coitus and so on . . . emotional experience, joy, anger, fear, or apprehension may disturb the action of the heart, trivial though the incident may be—an address at a public meeting, trouble with a cook, and so on."[62] Recently, Guyton, a distinguished physiologist, in an opinion piece called "Hypertension: A neural disease?" reviewed evidence that stimulation of the sympathetic nervous system

might underlie "all or almost all essential hypertension."[63] Guyton studied this theory in experimental animals and found that lesions or ischemia in vasomotor control centers or continuous stimulation of peripheral sympathetics commonly caused acute hypertension but that it was difficult to cause chronic hypertension in this way.[63] Others have shown that stress or emotional stimuli can cause catecholamine secretion and related circulatory changes.[64–68] Nestel gave young people with either normal blood pressure or labile hypertension mental puzzles to solve and found significant rises in epinephrine secretion, especially in those with labile hypertension.[65] Emotional state prior to gravitational stress also causes increase in epinephrine levels.[67] Varying the type of stimulation does help determine whether norepinephrine or epinephrine will be secreted.[66] Driving a racing car induces an increase in both norepinephrine and epinephrine.[68] Stoica and Enulescu studied patients who had either cerebral infarction or ICH as well as normotensive and hypertensive control subjects.[64] In normotensive controls and in those with infarction, most of whom were also normotensive, emotional stimuli caused a rise in norepinephrine secretion. In patients with ICH, most of them hypertensive and in hypertensive controls, the same emotional stimuli led to an increase in epinephrine secretion.[64] Emotional or physical stress can clearly cause circulatory changes mediated in part by catecholamine secretion. Can we answer the query posed by our Professor H. F. with the putaminal hemorrhage that developed while rushing to the symphony? Indeed, "Yes, the stress that night could have led to the ICH despite the absence of chronic hypertension."

If the theory we have proposed herein and previously[14] is correct, there should be two different subgroups of "hypertensive" ICH patients—those with a history of hypertension and possibly end organ changes in the heart, retina, and kidneys, indicative of the chronic pressure changes, and those with no history or evidence of prior sustained hypertension who bleed because of relatively recent changes in blood pressure and flow. Could the location, size, or outcome be different in these two groups? In a preliminary study, Estol et al. studied the effects of a history of hypertension and/or the presence of left ventricular hypertrophy as determined by chest x-ray or electrocardiography on the locale and size of hematomas.[69] Patients with no history of hypertension but documented left ventricular hypertrophy had the largest hematomas (52.6 cm$^3$) while those with a history of hypertension and left ventricular hypertrophy had the smallest (14.5 cm$^3$).[69] Location was not affected by the history of hypertension or the presence of ventricular hypertrophy. Weisberg[70] reviewed the clinical features and CT findings among 340 patients with spontaneous ICH, that is, no etiology other than hypertension. Smaller hematomas were present in normotensive or hypertensive patients with chronic vascular changes (evidence of left ventricular enlargement by chest x-ray, electrocardiogram or echocardiogram, and retinopathy). Larger hematomas developed in hypertensive patients without chronic vascular changes.[70] Chronic hypertension, by causing hypertrophy and increased peripheral resistance in large and medium-sized brain arteries, protects the smaller, more distal arteries from the centrally measured increased blood pressure. This could lead to smaller, more benign hematomas. Recall that patients with chronic hypertension often have several prior healed small slit hemorrhages at necropsy, but patients with massive hemorrhages seldom have old lesions. The data to date are not adequate to test this hypothesis. Clearly, there is still much to learn about so-called hypertensive ICH and about hypertension in general.

## References

1. Bright R. Cases and observations illustrative of renal disease accompanied with secretion of albuminous urine. Guy's Hosp Rep 1836; 1:339.

2. Mahomed FA. Some of the clinical aspects of chronic Bright's disease. Guy's Hosp Rep 1879;24:363–436.

3. Osler W. The principles and practice of medicine. Fifth edition. New York: Appleton, 1903;736.

4. Riva-Rocci S. Un nuovo sfigmomanometro. Gazz Med Torino 1896;47:981.

5. Pickering G. High blood pressure. Second Edition. London: J and A Churchill, 1968;2.

6. Korotkoff NS. A contribution to the problem of methods for the determination of the blood pressure. Rep Imper Milit Med Acad. 1905; 11:365. Translated and reprinted in Ruskin A. Classics in medical hypertension. Springfield: Charles C Thomas, 1956;126–133.

7. Byrom FB, Dodson LF. The causation of acute arterial necrosis in hypertensive disease. J Path Bact 1948;60:357–368.

8. Fisher CM. The arterial lesions underlying lacunes. Acta Neuropath 1969;12:1–15.

9. Fisher CM. Cerebral miliary aneurysms in hypertension. Am J Path 1972;66:313–330.

10. Fisher CM. Pathological observations in hypertensive cerebral hemorrhage. J Neuropathol Exp Neurol 1971;30:536–550.

11. Fisher CM. Lacunar strokes and infarcts: a review. Neurology 1982;32:871–876.

12. Ross-Russell RW. Observations on intracerebral aneurysms. Brain 1963;86:425–442.

13. Bouchard CH. A study of some points in the pathology of cerebral haemorrhage. Translated by TJ Maclagan. London: Simpkin, Marshall, 1872. (Reprinted in the Classics of Neurology and Neurosurgery library. Birmingham: Gryphon Editions, 1990).

14. Caplan LR. Intracerebral hemorrhage revisited. Neurology 1988;38:624–627.

15. Iragui VJ. The Charcot-Bouchard controversy. Arch Neurol 1986;43:290–295.

16. Charcot JM, Bouchard C. Nouvelles recherches sur la pathogénie de l'hémorrhagie cérébrale. Arch Physiol Norm Path 1868;1:110–127, 643–665, 725–734.

17. Green FHK. Miliary aneurysms in the brain. J Pathol Bacteriol 1930;33:71–77.

18. Cole FM, Yates P. Intracerebral microaneurysms and small cerebrovascular lesions. Brain 1967;90:759–767.

19. Rosenblum WI. Miliary aneurysms and "fibrinoid" degeneration of cerebral blood vessels. Human Pathol 1977;8:133–139.

20. Goto I, Kimoto K, Katsuki S, et al. Pathological studies on the intracerebral and retinal arter-

ies in cerebrovascular and noncerebrovascular diseases. Stroke 1975;6:263–269.

21. Santos-Buch CA, Goodhue WW, Ewald BH. Concurrence of iris aneurysms and cerebral hemorrhage in hypertensive rabbits. Arch Neurol 1976;33:96–103.

22. Wakai S, Nagai M. Histological verification of microaneurysms as a cause of cerebral haemorrhage in surgical specimens. J Neurol Neurosurg Psychiat 1989;52:595–599.

23. Takebayashi S, Kaneko M. Electron microscopic studies of ruptured arteries in hypertensive intracerebral hemorrhage. Stroke 1983; 14:28–36.

24. Takebayashi S, Sakata N, Kawamura K. Reevaluation of miliary aneurysm in hypertensive brain: recanalization of small hemorrhage? Stroke 1990; 21(suppl. I):I59–I60.

25. Caplan LR, Mohr JP. Intracerebral hemorrhage: an update. Geriatrics 1978;33:42–52.

26. Mohr JP, Caplan LR, Melski JW, et al. The Harvard Cooperative Stroke Registry: a prospective registry. Neurology. 1978;28:754–762.

27. Brott T, Thalinger K, Hertzberg V. Hypertension as a risk factor for spontaneous intracerebral hemorrhage. Stroke 1986;17:1078–1083.

28. Foulkes MA, Wolf PA, Price TR, et al. The Stroke Data Bank: design, methods, and baseline characteristics. Stroke 1988;19:547–554.

29. Bahemuka M. Primary intracerebral hemorrhage and heart weight: a clinicopathologic case-control review of 218 patients. Stroke 1987;18:531–536.

30. Caplan LR, Neely S, Gorelick P. Cold-related intracerebral hemorrhage. Arch Neurol 1984; 41:227.

31. Hines EA, Brown GE. A standard test for measuring the variability of blood pressure: its significance as an index of the prehypertensive state. Ann Intern Med 1933;7:209–217.

32. Takahashi E, Sasaki N, Takeda J, et al. The geographic distribution of cerebral hemorrhage and hypertension in Japan. Hum Biol 1957;29:139–166.

33. Moskowitz MA. The neurobiology of vascular head pain. Ann Neurol 1984;16:157–168.

34. Barbas N, Caplan LR, Baquis G, et al. Dental chair intracerebral hemorrhage. Neurology 1987;37:511–512.

35. Haines SJ, Maroon JC, Janetta PJ. Supratentorial intracerebral hemorrhage following posterior fossa surgery. J Neurosurg 1978; 49:881–886.

36. Waga S, Shimosaka S, Sakakura M. Intracerebral hemorrhage remote from the site of the initial neurosurgical procedure. Neurosurgery 1983;13:662–665.

37. Sweet WH, Poletti CE. Complications of current standard treatments for trigeminal neuralgia: need for mechanism for prompt reporting of complications. Abstract. Poster presentation #82 in program of the annual meeting of the American Association of Neurological Surgeons, Denver, Colorado, 243, 1986.

38. Sweet WH, Poletti CE, Roberts JT. 1985, Dangerous rises in blood pressure upon heating of trigeminal rootlets: increased bleeding times in patients with trigeminal neuralgia. Neurosurgery 1985;17:843–844.

39. Kehler CH, Brodsky JB, Samuels SI, et al. Blood pressure response during percutaneous rhizotomy for trigeminal neuralgia. Neurosurgery 1982;10:200–202.

40. Cawley CM, Rigamonti D, Trommer B. Dental chair apoplexy. South Med J 1991;84:907–909.

41. Caplan LR, Skillman J, Ojemann R, et al. Intracerebral hemorrhage following carotid endarterectomy: a hypertensive complication? Stroke 1978;9:457–460.

42. Wylie EJ, Hein MF, Adams JE. Intracerebral hemorrhage following surgical revascularization for treatment of acute strokes. J Neurosurg 1964;21:212–215.

43. Bruetman ME, Fields WS, Crawford ES, et al. Cerebral hemorrhage in carotid artery surgery. Arch Neurol 1963;9:458–467.

44. Lehv MS, Salzman EW, Silen W. Hypertension complicating carotid endarterectomy. Stroke 1970;1:307–313.

45. Holton P, Wood JB. The effects of bilateral removal of the carotid bodies and denervation of the carotid sinuses in two human subjects. J Physiol 1965;181:365–378.

46. Piatt JH. Massive intracerebral hemorrhage complicating cardiac catheterization with ergonovine administration. Stroke 1984;15: 904–907.

47. Ozer M. The management of persons with spinal cord injury. New York: Demos, 1988.

48. Rai M, Shukla RC, Varma DN, et al. Intracerebral hemorrhage following scorpion bite. Neurology 1990;40:1801.

49. Lee K-C, Clough C. Intracerebral hemorrhage after break dancing. N Engl J Med 1990;323: 615–616 (letter).

50. Weisberg LA, Elliott D, Mielke D. Intracerebral hemorrhage following electroconvulsive therapy. Neurology 1991;41:1849.

51. Humphreys RP, Hoffman HJ, Mustard WT, et al. Cerebral hemorrhage following heart surgery. J Neurosurg 1975;43:671–675.

52. Sila CA, Furlan AJ, Stewart RW. Intracerebral hemorrhage complicating cardiac transplantation: hyperperfusion breakthrough. Neurology 1989;39(suppl. 1):161.

53. Sila CA. Spectrum of neurologic events following cardiac transplantation. Stroke 1989;20:1586–1589.

54. Sundt TM, Sharbrough FW, Piepgras DG, et al. Correlation of cerebral blood flow and electroencephalographic changes during carotid endarterectomy: with results of surgery and hemodynamics of cerebral ischemia. Mayo Clin Proc 1981;56:533–543.

55. Fisher CM, Adams RD. Observations on brain embolism with special reference to the mechanism of hemorrhagic infarction. J Neuropathol Exp Neurol 1951;10:92–94.

56. Fisher CM, Adams RD. Observations on brain embolism with special reference to hemorrhagic infarction. In Furlan AJ (ed.) The heart and stroke. London: Springer-Verlag, 1987;17–36.

57. Bollinger G. Uber traumatische Spätapoplexie: ein Beitagzurlehre von der Hirnerschutterung. In Internationale Beitrage zur wissen Schaftlichen Medecin, Festschrift Rudolf Virchow. Vol. 2. Berlin: Hirschwald 1891;457–470.

58. DeJong RN. Delayed traumatic intracerebral hemorrhage. Arch Neurol Psychiat 1942;48:257–266.

59. Tanaka T, Sakai T, Uemura K, et al. MR imaging as predictor of delayed posttraumatic cerebral hemorrhage. J Neurosurg 1988;69:203–209.

60. Cole AJ, Aubé M. Migraine with vasospasm and delayed intracerebral hemorrhage. Arch Neurol 1990;47:53–56.

61. Caplan LR, Thomas C, Banks G. Central nervous system complications of addiction to "T's and blues". Neurology 1982;32:623–628.

62. Wilson SAK, Bruce AN. Neurology. Second edition. London: Butterworth, 1955;1367–1383.

63. Guyton AC. Hypertension: a neural disease? Arch Neurol 1988;45:178–179.

64. Stoica E, Enulescu O. Abnormal catecholamine urinary excretion after emotional stimulus in patients with cerebral hemorrhage. Stroke 1981;12:360–366.

65. Nestel PJ. Blood-pressure and catecholamine excretion after mental stress in labile hypertension. Lancet 1969;1:692–694.

66. Elmadjian F, Hope JM, Lamson ET. Excretion of epinephrine and norepinephrine in various emotional states. J Clin Endocr 1957;17:608–620.

67. Goodall MC. Sympathoadrenal response to gravitational stress. J Clin Invest 1962;41:197–202.

68. Taggart P, Carruthers M. Endogenous hyperlipidemia induced by emotional stress of racing driving. Lancet 1971;1:363–366.

69. Estol CJ, Caplan LR, Lee P, et al. Hypertensive intracerebral hemorrhage: does past hypertension or left ventricular hypertrophy predict size? Stroke 1990;21:175 (abstract).

70. Weisberg LA. The natural history of nontraumatic parenchymal brain hemorrhage. Ann Neurol 1990;28:257 (abstract).

# Chapter 7
# Bleeding Disorders

## Carlos S. Kase

Bleeding disorders are a relatively uncommon cause of intracerebral hemorrhage (ICH). However, in conditions such as hemophilia and acute leukemia associated with thrombocytopenia, massive intracranial hemorrhage is often the cause of death.[1-3] The intracranial hemorrhages in bleeding disorders can be subdural, intracerebral, or subarachnoid, at times occurring in combination. This chapter analyzes the mechanisms, clinical features, and pathogenesis of ICH in patients with disorders of coagulation and hemostasis.

The *frequency* of bleeding disorders as a cause of ICH varies slightly among series (Table 7.1).[2,4-7] Jellinger[5] reported bleeding disorders and anticogulant therapy as the cause of 6.4% of 1214 instances of ICH studied in autopsy material. In a literature review of postmortem series of ICH, he quoted figures between 2.1% and 13.3% of hemorrhages

due to bleeding disorders. The highest frequency reported in autopsy series is that of McCormick and Rosenfield.[2] They found 28 of 144 cases (19.4%) of massive nontraumatic ICH in association with leukemia (21 patients, the majority of whom had severe thrombocytopenia) and other disorders of coagulation. They noted that the hematomas were multiple in about one half of the patients with leukemia, whereas no examples of multiple ICH occurred among the thirty-seven cases attributed to hypertension.[2] The unusually high frequency of leukemia as the cause of ICH in this postmortem series probably reflects a biased referral pattern to the authors' institution.

The *classification* of bleeding disorders associated with ICH is shown in Table 7.2, following the recently published outline of del Zoppo and Mori.[8] In this abbreviated list of hematological conditions with bleeding po-

**Table 7.1.** ICH Secondary to Bleeding Disorders

| Author | Total patients with ICH | Cases due to bleeding disorders No. cases (%) | |
|---|---|---|---|
| | | Anticoagulants | Bleeding diathesis |
| Schütz[4] | 250 | 17 (6.8%) | 4 (1.6%) |
| Jellinger[5] | 170 | 1 (0.6%) | 4 (2.4%) |
| McCormick and Rosenfield[2] | 144 | 3 (2.1%) | 27 (18.8%) |
| Mutlu et al.[6] | 225 | — | 30 (13.3%) |
| Russell[7] | 461 | — | 36 (7.8%) |

**Table 7.2.** Bleeding Disorders as a Cause of ICH

| DISORDERS OF HEMOSTASIS |
| --- |
| Primary |
|     Hemophilia A and B |
|     von Willebrand factor deficiency |
|     Afibrinogenemia |
| Secondary |
|     Nonneoplastic |
|         Idiopathic thrombocytopenic purpura |
|         Disseminated intravascular coagulation |
|         Thrombotic thrombocytopenic purpura |
|         Drug-induced thrombocytopenia |
|     Neoplastic |
|         Leukemia |
|         Thrombocythemia and the myeloproliferative disorders |
|         Multiple myeloma |
| ANTITHROMBOTIC AGENTS |
|     Antiplatelet drugs |
|     Anticoagulants |
|     Fibrinolytic agents |

(From del Zoppo GJ, Mori E. Hematologic causes of intracerebral hemorrhage and their treatment. Neurosurg Clin NA 1992;3:637–658, with permission of the publisher.)

tential we have included, for the purpose of discussion, only those that are associated with a substantial risk of ICH, and that affect primarily adults. We have omitted the congenital coagulation factor deficiencies that cause hemorrhagic complications mostly in young children.

## Disorders of Hemostasis

These conditions are divided into *primary,* generally congenital, deficiencies of coagulation factors, and *secondary,* or acquired, disorders of coagulation, which are either idiopathic, immune, or neoplastic in character. The primary disorders of coagulation are rarely a cause of ICH in the adult,[8] most of the information being in the pediatric literature and in small clinical series in adults. The secondary coagulation disorders are responsible for the majority of examples of clinically

relevant ICH in adults with abnormal hemostatic function.

### *Primary Deficiency of Coagulation Factors*

#### *Hemophilia*

Congenital deficiency of factor VIII (hemophilia A) or factor IX (hemophilia B, Christmas disease) is responsible for widespread bleeding into internal organs, joints, subcutaneous/muscular tissues, and intracranial structures. Martinowitz et al.[9] reported an annual incidence of ICH in hemophilia patients of 0.27%, the rate of ICH being higher in patients with factor VIII inhibitor (0.86%) than in those without the circulating inhibitor (0.18%). Kerr[1] documented 19 episodes of intracranial hemorrhage in 15 hemophilia patients from a group of 109 patients with the disease, representing a frequency of intracranial bleeding of 13.8%. Fourteen of the nineteen intracranial bleeding events corresponded to ICH, and five of the fifteen patients (33%) died as a result of the hemorrhage. In the large series of Eyster et al.,[10] the incidence of CNS bleeding was 2.7% for factor VIII–deficient patients, and 3.6% for factor IX–deficient patients. Similar data were reported by Silverstein,[11] who found a frequency of intracranial bleeding of 6.3% among the hemophilia patients admitted to the Mount Sinai Hospital in New York. The mortality figure in that series, published in 1960, was 71%, and Silverstein accurately predicted that future refinements in treatment would appreciably reduce the overall mortality in hemophilia complicated by intracranial bleeding. This reduction in mortality, to 33% to 35%, occurred largely as a result of the introduction of cryoprecipitate treatments in the early 1960s.[9]

The sites of intracranial bleeding in hemophilia are about equally distributed between subdural hematomas (SDH) and ICH, isolated subarachnoid hemorrhage (SAH) being the least common.[1,10–12] Among the risk factors for bleeding, most reports agree that young age and history of head trauma are the most common.[1,9,10–12] *Young age* as a risk factor for intracranial bleeding was suggested by the observation of Silverstein[11] who found that 27 of a group of 31 (87%) hemophilia patients were under age 20 at the time of the stroke. More recently, Eyster et al.[10] reported 71 patients with CNS bleeding, 51 (72%) of whom were under age 18. A less clear predominance of intracranial hemorrhage in the young was found in the series of Kerr,[1] although a local bias toward older patients being preferentially included was recognized. An additional risk factor that is partially linked to age is *disease severity,* as measured by factor VIII activity levels, of less than 1% in severe, 1% to 3% in moderate, and 3% to 30% in mild hemophilia.[1] Kerr[1] found a mean age of 16 (range 1 to 47) for severe hemophilia patients at the time of intracranial hemorrhage, whereas mild hemophilia patients had a mean age of 46 (range 39 to 50), leading him to conclude that intracranial hemorrhage is a risk for severe hemophilia patients at all ages, whereas mild hemophilia patients are at maximal risk during the fourth and fifth decades. In regard to *head trauma* as a risk factor for intracranial hemorrhage, Kerr[1] documented head injury in five (26%) of the nineteen episodes of intracranial bleeding in his fifteen patients, Silverstein[11] quoted a figure of 45% (14 of 31 patients) from the literature, and Eyster et al.[10] found a history of trauma in 54% (38 of 71 patients) in their series; in the series of Martinowitz et al.[9] the figure was 50%, and Pettersson et al.[12] reported head injury in 64% (seven of eleven) of their patients. The onset of symptoms of intracranial hemorrhage after head trauma is variable. At times, symptoms begin immediately following the traumatic event (in five of twenty-four patients, or 21%, with adequate histories regarding stroke onset in the series of Eyster et al.[10]). In other patients, there is a long symptom-free interval. In nineteen of the twenty-four patients (79%) reported by Eyster et al.,[10] the mean delay between trauma and onset of symptoms was 4 ± 2.2 days, and Martinowitz et al.[9] found

symptom-free intervals ranging from six hours to ten days. These data emphasize the often slow and indolent character of intracranial hemorrhage in patients with bleeding disorders, at times following seemingly trivial trauma to the head, both features contributing to the risk of delaying diagnosis and proper management. Although the importance of head trauma as a cause of intracranial hemorrhage in hemophilia patients is unquestionable, bleeding sometimes follows only slight blows to the head (such as in pillow-fighting[1]). It is also noteworthy that there are a number of remarkable instances in which hemophilia patients have experienced serious head trauma without any consequence. Kerr[1] reported thirteen patients (nine with mild, two with moderate, and two with severe hemophilia) who sustained head trauma after street fighting, being tackled at rugby, falling off a horse, or boxing (up to eighty bouts, at times being knocked out), without the development of intracranial hemorrhage.

The mortality of intracranial hemorrhage in hemophilia patients is still substantial (Table 7.3) despite the availability of modern therapies. In the series of Eyster et al.,[10] the overall mortality for intracranial hemorrhage was 35%, but there were major differences in mortality in relation to the type of hemorrhage: SDH and SAH had mortalities of 10% and 18%, respectively, whereas the mortality for ICH was 67%. These data were commented on by Martinowitz et al.,[9] who pointed out that the reduction in mortality of intracranial hemorrhage in hemophilia pa-

**Table 7.3.** Mortality in Hemophilia Patients with Intracranial Hemorrhage

| Author | Patients with intracranial hemorrhage | Deaths, No. cases (%) |
|---|---|---|
| Kerr[1] | 15 | 5 (33%) |
| Martinowitz et al.[9] | 7 | 4 (57%) |
| Eyster et al.[10] | 65 | 23 (35%) |

tients in the last three decades probably only applies to those with SDH and SAH, while mortality for ICH has remained unchanged. They suggested that the *incidence* of ICH may have decreased in the last few decades by the introduction of active home and preventive therapies for hemophilia patients prior or subsequent to engaging in potentially traumatic activities.

### von Willebrand Factor Deficiency

The diagnosis of von Willebrand factor (vWF) deficiency, an autosomal dominant trait with a high frequency in the population, is less often made after spontaneous hemorrhage than in hemophilia, but is frequently discovered because of bleeding complications after surgery or trauma. The laboratory diagnosis rests on finding a prolonged bleeding time despite a normal platelet count, and decreased factor VIII coagulant activity.[13] The common heterozygous form of the disease is generally benign, but the rare autosomal recessive form of vWF deficiency can produce severe hemorrhage and behave in a manner similar to hemophilia.[13]

Intracranial hemorrhage in vWF deficiency is rare. Rice[14] reported in 1982 a single case of SDH secondary to moderate head trauma in a 26-year-old patient with vWF deficiency. Despite being responsive to pain only, with decerebrate posturing and having a right third nerve palsy on admission, he recovered without residual deficits after surgical drainage of the hematoma. He was treated perioperatively with cryoprecipitate and fresh frozen plasma for the coagulopathy. Mizoi et al.[15] reported a child with vWF deficiency who developed a hemorrhage in the head of the right caudate nucleus and anterior limb of the internal capsule, with ventricular extension, following head trauma. She did well after surgical aspiration of the intraventricular component of the hemorrhage. These authors suggested that many undetected cases of vWF deficiency are likely to be included among patients with intracra-

nial hemorrhage. This opinion was shared by Almaani and Awidi,[16] who found four patients with vWF deficiency among fifty patients admitted with intracranial hemorrhage. Three of their patients had an ICH, while the fourth had an intraventricular hemorrhage. Three of the four patients died, despite the performance of ventricular drainage in the patient with intraventricular bleeding. They stressed the value of routine testing of bleeding time in patients with intracranial hemorrhage as a screening test for the detection of vWF deficiency.

### Afibrinogenemia

Afibrinogenemia is a rare, recessive, autosomally inherited trait that leads to bleeding early in life, at times immediately after birth with hemorrhage from the umbilical cord.[13] It is one of the genetic disorders associated with hemorrhagic stroke,[17] and ICH has been reported as a cause of death,[13] but the condition is more likely to present with less serious bleeding, including ecchymoses, hemoptysis, gastrointestinal or genitourinary bleeding; hemathrosis is comparatively less common. A single case of SDH in a young woman with afibrinogenemia was reported by Almaani and Awidi.[18] She recovered after drainage of the SDH and correction of the afibrinogenemia. Montgomery and Natelson[19] described a unique case of a 12-year-old girl with afibrinogenemia who had a right parietal ICH. She recovered after surgical drainage of the hematoma, while the coagulopathy was treated with concentrates of human fibrinogen. The patient's brother, who was suspected of having a congenital coagulopathy because of bleeding from the umbilical stump at birth, had previously died at age 7 after he developed a right hemiparesis.

### Secondary Deficiency of Coagulation Factors

These conditions are here arbitrarily divided into *nonneoplastic,* to include those of either immune or unknown cause, and *neoplastic*, in which the leukemias and other myeloproliferative and lymphoproliferative disorders are included. We recognize that this separation is artificial, since some overlapping between the two categories exists (as in cases of disseminated intravascular coagulation secondary to a systemic malignancy); at times conditions from both groups can lead to hemorrhagic phenomena through a common mechanism (the most frequent being thrombocytopenia), and some entities listed as "nonneoplastic" may be the result of a neoplastic condition (such as examples of immune thrombocytopenic purpura that result from a lymphoproliferative disorder). However, we will adhere to this categorization of disorders for the purpose of this discussion of ICH in adults.

In an autopsy study of intracranial hemorrhage in fifty-eight patients with bleeding disorders, Silverstein[20] found that thrombocytopenia was the underlying mechanism in fifty-one (91%). The majority of the thrombocytopenic patients (48%) had leukemia, while the rest had aplastic anemia, myeloproliferative disorders, and various forms of idiopathic thrombocytopenia.

*Nonneoplastic Conditions*

The most common conditions leading to intracranial hemorrhage in this group are idiopathic thrombocytopenic purpura (ITP), disseminated intravascular coagulation (DIC), and thrombotic thrombocytopenic purpura (TTP).

**Idiopathic (or Immune) Thrombocytopenic Purpura.** ITP is characterized by persistent thrombocytopenia caused by a circulating antiplatelet antibody (PAIgG) that results in platelet destruction by the reticuloendothelial system.[21] Life-threatening bleeding is common, and ICH has been reported in 1% of patients with ITP.[22] This serious complication generally occurs in children with platelet counts below 10,000 per mm,[3][22] who develop

either SDH[23] or ICH.[22] In young adults, ITP is very rarely the cause of ICH. Only five patients with ITP and ICH have been reported during recent years.[22–24] They were all young adults in their 20s with chronic ITP, and ICH developed during periods of severe thrombocytopenia, with platelet counts between 2,000 and 55,000 per mm$^3$. The ICH locations varied, with hemorrhages in the basal ganglia, thalamus, lobar white matter, and cerebellum. Head trauma was not a factor in any of these cases, and thrombocytopenia had become resistant to steroids at the time of the ICH. Outcome was poor, as only one of the five patients survived the event.[24]

**Disseminated Intravascular Coagulation.** DIC is commonly a manifestation of a severe systemic disorder, including infections, malignancies, trauma or surgery, shock, or obstetric complications.[25,26] The laboratory diagnosis of DIC is made in the presence of thrombocytopenia, elevated prothrombin time (PT) and activated partial thromboplastin time (aPTT) values, low fibrinogen, and elevated fibrin degradation products (FDP). These changes reflect the combination of intravascular coagulation and activation of the fibrinolytic system.[25] Microvascular thrombi in the brain and systemically are a routine finding in autopsy series, along with frequent petechial hemorrhages in the brain.

Large intracranial hemorrhages, either SDH or ICH are occasionally the cause of death in severe DIC.[25] Schwartzman and Hill[27] reported six adult patients with large intracranial hemorrhages and DIC who had fatal nonhematologic malignancies (three patients), bacterial endocarditis (two patients), and sickle-cell anemia (one patient). The ICH were multiple in three patients, and two patients had SAH and intraventricular hemorrhage without ICH. The coagulopathy resulted in large-vessel cerebral infarction in two of the six patients. Other conditions related to symptomatic ICH in patients with DIC have included primary cerebral tumors, abdominal aortic aneursym, head trauma, and leukemia.[28-30] Kawakami et al.[28] reported fatal postoperative bleeding into a bifrontal glioblastoma multiforme complicated by DIC. They also documented fatal recurrent SDH in a patient with an unruptured thoracoabdominal aneurysm. The pathogenesis of DIC in the latter patient is unclear. Exposure of the subendothelial layer of the aortic wall and relative stasis of blood within the aneurysm are thought to stimulate platelet adhesion and fibrin deposition, with resultant intravascular coagulation and secondary fibrinolysis.[28]

Head trauma complicated by delayed or recurrent intracranial hemorrhages has been described by Kaufman et al.[29] They found eight patients with either new ICH or extension of a previous ICH detected between one and eight days after head trauma, with development of DIC. In two instances the hematomas occurred as a result of the placement of a ventriculostomy catheter. Four patients died as a result of the intracranial hemorrhages. The mechanism of DIC after head trauma is thought to be the release of thromboplastic substances from injured brain tissue into the circulation.[29] For this reason, DIC is more likely to follow severe head trauma with extensive cerebral tissue destruction.[31] The ultimate mechanism of delayed hemorrhage after head trauma and DIC may involve a sequence of vascular occlusion by microthrombi, cerebral infarction, lysis of thrombi, and reperfusion of vessels with abnormal endothelia, leading to rupture and ICH.[29] The hemorrhagic complications related to DIC in patients with leukemia are discussed in the section on leukemia.

**Thrombotic Thrombocytopenic Purpura.** TTP occurs predominatly in young, otherwise healthy women, and is characterized by the pentad of consumptive thrombocytopenia, microangiopathic hemolytic anemia, renal involvement, fever, and neurological abnormalities.[32] Although platelet microthrombi and thrombocytopenia are characteristic of TTP, the disorder differs from DIC in that there is no associated systemic illness

or evidence of activation of the fibrinolytic system, with normal fibrinogen levels and no evidence of fibrinogen consumption.[32]

**Drug-induced Thrombocytopenia.** The list of drugs known to be potentially associated with thrombocytopenia is extensive (Table 7.4).[33] A few among them have been associated with ICH. *Heparin*, a parenteral anticoagulant widely used in the management of coronary artery disease, stroke, and venous thrombosis, can be associated with severe thrombocytopenia. Heparin-induced thrombocytopenia occurs in about 5% to 10% of patients treated. Among them, less than 10% will develop hemorrhagic complications.[34] Heparin-induced thrombocytopenia has two forms: (1) Type I, which is benign (rarely associated with thromboembolism), appearing one to five days after treatment onset, with platelet counts generally above 50,000 per mm$^3$, and with normalization of platelet counts despite continued heparin therapy; its mechanism is direct heparin-induced platelet aggregation; (2) Type II, a more severe thrombocytopenia with platelet counts below 10,000 per mm$^3$ and of later onset (during the second week of treatment), frequently associated with thromboembolic complications, and requiring discontinuation

**Table 7.4.** Agents Implicated in Drug-induced Thrombocytopenia

| | |
|---|---|
| Cytotoxic drugs | Digoxin |
| Estrogens | Nitroglycerin |
| Thiazides | Phenytoin |
| Furosemide | Carbamazepine |
| Chloramphenicol | Phenothiazines |
| Phenylbutazone | Desipramine |
| Antibiotics | Tolbutamide |
| Alpha-methyldopa | Chlorpropamide |
| Aspirin | Quinine |
| Acetaminophen | Heparin |
| Chloroquine | Propylthiouracil |
| Quinidine | Gold salts |

(From Burstein SA, Harker LA. Quantitative platelet disorders. In Bloom AL, Thomas DP, eds. Haemostasis and thrombosis. New York, Churchill Livingstone, 1981; 279–300, with permission of the publisher.)

of heparin in order to obtain gradual recovery of normal platelet counts; it is thought to result from immune-mediated platelet aggregation.[35] Heparin-induced thrombocytopenia occurs more commonly with heparin derived from bovine lung than with that from porcine gut.[36] *Quinidine* is well recognized for its association with immune thrombocytopenia, and it has been described as a possible cause of ICH in two patients reported by Glass et al.[37] Their Patient 1 developed a left basal ganglionic ICH while on treatment with warfarin (for deep vein thrombosis) for seven months and quinidine (for ventricular tachyarrhythmias) for two months. This patient had cutaneous and mucosal bleeding as well, and her PT was 15.7 seconds, with platelet count of 10,000 per mm$^3$ at presentation with the ICH. She did well after discontinuation of both medications and treatment with intravenous gamma globulin, with normalization of her platelet count within ten days from ICH onset. Patient 2 was on digoxin, verapamil, quinidine, and aspirin for coronary artery disease (and CABG one month previously), and developed epistaxis and a large left frontotemporal ICH. His platelet count on admission was 4000 per mm$^3$ and PT and aPTT were normal. Carotid angiography revealed no aneurysm, arteriovenous malformation (AVM), or tumor. He died despite drug discontinuation, steroids, platelet transfusions, immunoglobulins, and surgical drainage of the hematoma. These unique cases, in which drug-induced thrombocytopenia occurred in patients treated with warfarin and aspirin, respectively, raise concern about the simultaneous use of agents that can alter the coagulation system. They also stress the value of close monitoring of PT (when applicable) and platelet counts in those instances in which the condition under treatment requires such drug combinations.

### Neoplastic Conditions

**Leukemia.** Massive and fatal intracranial hemorrhage has long been recognized as a common complication in patients with leukemia, especially in the acute forms. Groch et al.,[38] in 1960, reported the findings in a necropsy series of ninety-three patients with leukemia managed at the Mayo Clinic. They found macroscopic ICH in forty-six (49%) instances. The ICH were described as "massive" (alone or with associated petechial hemorrhages) in fourteen, "small to moderate round zones of hemorrhage" in seventeen (with petechial hemorrhages in two, without them in fifteen), purely petechial hemorrhages in twelve, and "SAH alone" in three. The cases of ICH in patients with acute leukemia outnumbered those in chronic leukemia by a ratio of 10:1 (42:4 patients), and the predominant type leading to ICH was acute lymphocytic leukemia (ALL). The main site of location of ICH was the lobar white matter of the cerebral hemispheres, where thirty-six of forty-six (78%) hemorrhages occurred, favoring the temporal and frontal lobes. Deep hemorrhages also occurred frequently, with involvement of the corpus callosum (37%), basal ganglia (22%), thalamus (20%), and internal capsule (26%). Cerebellar and brainstem hemorrhages were equally common, being present in approximately 22% to 37% of the patients. As these various percentages indicate, it is apparent that multiple ICH of supra and infratentorial locations are often present in patients with leukemia who die from intracranial hemorrhage.[2,38] The series of Groch et al.[38] further documented a high frequency of systemic bleeding along with the occurrence of ICH: thirty-nine of forty-six (85%) patients with ICH had hemorrhages elsewhere, mainly mucocutaneous and gastrointestinal, whereas only twenty of forty-seven (43%) patients without ICH at autopsy had evidence of systemic bleeding. In every instance in which ICH was the direct cause of death (twenty-three patients), bleeding at other sites was found at postmortem examination. A correlation between ICH and low platelet counts was not clearly suggested by their data, as counts of 50,000 per mm$^3$ or less were almost equally as common in those patients with ICH (31 of

41, or 76%) and without ICH (24 of 38, or 63%). However, among twenty-three patients with fatal ICH, nineteen (83%) had platelet counts of 50,000 per mm$^3$ or less, all of whom had additional systemic sites of bleeding. In the autopsy series of twenty-one patients with leukemia and ICH of McCormick and Rosenfield[2] seventeen (81%) had platelet counts below 50,000 per mm$^3$. These authors also reported a marked predominance of the acute forms of leukemia (15 of 21, or 71%) in patients with ICH (Figure 7.1).

In addition to the potential role of thrombocytopenia, rising numbers of abnormal peripheral leukocytes ("blastic crisis") are recognized as a risk factor for ICH in patients with leukemia. Fritz et al.[39] studied eighty-one patients with acute leukemia who died, eighteen of them as a result of ICH. Among the eighty-one deceased patients, thirteen

had leukocyte counts above 300,000 per mm$^3$, and this group contributed nine (69%) to those who died of ICH. On the other hand, of the remaining sixty-eight patients with leukocyte counts below 300,000 per mm$^3$, only nine (13%) died of ICH. This was a highly significant difference (p <0.001) in the frequency of fatal ICH between patients with leukocyte counts above and below 300,000 per mm$^3$. Furthermore, in the group of patients with leukocyte counts above 300,000 per mm$^3$, eight of nine with ICH had greater than 90% circulating leukemic cells or "blasts." McCormick and Rosenfield[2] reported comparable data, as about one half of their twenty-one patients with leukemia and ICH had markedly elevated leukocyte counts, with up to 95% being circulating "blasts." In comparing platelet counts in patients with ICH and leukocyte counts above

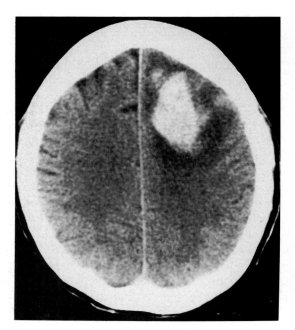 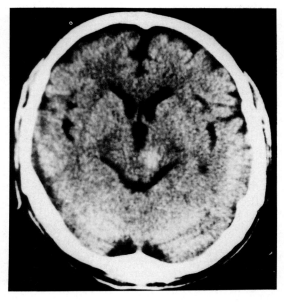

A                                    B

**Figure 7.1.** ICH in acute mylogenous leukemia with thrombocytopenia. (A) Left frontal lobar ICH in 51-year-old woman, with platelet count of 7,000/mm$^3$ (Courtesy of Mark T. D'Esposito, M.D., Braintree Hospital, Braintree, MA). (B) ICH on the left side of the midbrain in 66-year-old man with platelet count of less than 10,000 per mm$^3$ at the time of the hemorrhage.

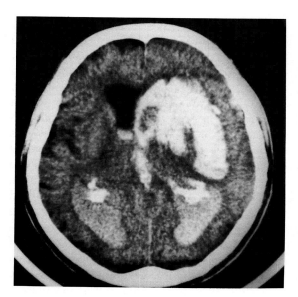

**Figure 7.2.** Massive left basal ganglionic ICH in 58-year-old man with acute myelogenous leukemia with leukocyte count of 316,000 per mm³, and 96% blasts; platelet count was 49,000 per mm³ (Courtesy of Michael S. Mega, M.D., Boston VA Medical Center, Boston, MA.)

and below 300,000 per mm³ (nine in each group), Fritz et al.[39] found significantly *higher* counts in those in "blastic crisis." These authors also reported a high frequency of intracerebral white matter hemorrhages (six of seven patients) at postmortem examination of patients in "blastic crisis," as opposed to exclusively extracerebral (SDH or SAH) hemorrhages in all five patients with neuropathological examination in the group with leukocyte counts below 300,000 per mm³. These data suggested a risk of ICH five times greater in patients reaching leukocyte counts above 300,000 per mm³, and the rise in counts to that level carried a 60% chance of having a fatal ICH within a few days.[39] In addition to the level of circulating leukocytosis, the rate of rise of the white cell count had an impact on ICH occurrence. In patients with rapidly rising leukocyte counts and myeloblastic leukemia, despite having the highest platelet counts, ICH followed four to five days after onset of the "blastic crisis." In contrast, in those with lymphoblastic leukemia with a more gradual rise in leukocyte counts, fatal ICH developed as late as two weeks or more after the onset of the "blastic crisis."[39] Among the risk factors for ICH, comparing patients with leukocyte counts above and below 300,000 per mm³, head injury, hypertension, and drug therapy were not significantly different. The differences in platelet counts between the two groups were indicative of a primary thrombocytopenic mechanism of bleeding in those patients who were not in "blastic crisis," whereas in the group with leukocyte counts above 300,000 per mm³ thrombocytopenia seemed less important, suggesting that intracerebral growth of leukemic cells causing blood vessel damage is the main factor responsible for the high frequency of ICH in this group (Figure 7.2).

In the last decades, since the description of acute promyelocytic leukemia (APL) as a distinct subcategory of acute myeloid leukemia,[40] it has become apparent that this form of leukemia has a marked propensity to produce severe hemorrhagic complications,

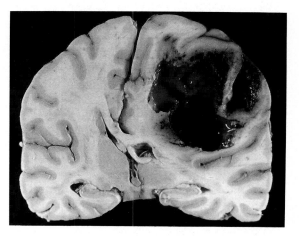

**Figure 7.3.** Massive right parietal lobar hemorrhage in 54-year-old man with acute promyelocytic leukemia. Platelet count on day of hemorrhage was 36,000 per mm³ (Courtesy of Michael S. Mega, M.D. and Flaviu C. A. Romanul, M.D., Boston VA Medical Center, Boston, MA.)

including ICH. This is the cause of death in more than 60% of patients with APL[30] (Figure 7.3). The coagulopathy that accompanies APL corresponds to DIC, which results from the release of a procoagulant factor from the promyelocyte granules.[25] In the series of Graus et al.,[30] acute myelogenous leukemia (AML), including APL, was responsible for thirty-three of forty-nine (67%) episodes of symptomatic ICH in patients with leukemia, while ALL only accounted for five episodes (10%). Other types of leukemia (acute monocytic and myelomonocytic, chronic lymphocytic, hairy cell, and erythroleukemia) resulted in eleven (23%) episodes of ICH. These authors[30] also confirmed the strong association between hyperleukocytosis and ICH in patients with acute leukemia,[39] thrombocytopenia being an adjuvant but not a major factor in the production of ICH.[30,39]

**Thrombocythemia and the Myeloproliferative Disorders.**    Thrombocythemia is characterized by recurrent hemorrhages, generally preceded or accompanied by venous thromboses, in patients with markedly elevated platelet counts, splenomegaly, leukocytosis, and anemia.[41] ICH is an uncommon manifestation of this syndrome,[8,42] which typically leads to chronic bleeding, mainly gastrointestinal, for periods of years.[41] Large hematomas after trivial trauma can occur. On occasion the thrombotic manifestations have been arterial in the CNS, leading to cerebral infarction,[43] but hemorrhage is more often its presentation. A case of lobar ICH in an 82-year-old man with thrombocythemia and platelet count of 1,000,000 per mm$^3$ was reported by Kase et al.[44] Korenman[45] reported five patients with neurologic complications of primary thrombocythemia, one of whom was on oral anticoagulants for thrombophlebitis, and had a probable SDH after head trauma. His platelet count was 1,700,000 per mm$^3$, and the PT was 20 seconds.

The diagnosis of thrombocythemia is suspected by the finding of high platelet counts, which were in the range of 900,000 to 14,000,000 per mm$^3$ (mean 3,200,000 per mm$^3$) in the series of Gunz.[41] The mechanism of hemorrhage despite abnormally high platelet counts is thought to relate to a dysfunctional state of these blood cells, at times in association with an abnormal morphology.[41]

A closely related myeloproliferative disorder, myelosclerosis with myeloid metaplasia of the spleen (MMM), is one of the hematological disorders that is consistently associated with marked thrombocythemia.[41] On occasion, ICH can occur, either spontaneously or, more commonly, after head trauma (Figure 7.4).

**Multiple Myeloma.**    Multiple myeloma rarely results in intracranial hemorrhage.[8] The malignant plasma cell proliferation with accumulation of a paraprotein frequently leads to disorders of hemostasis. These include (1) decrease in platelet survival: the half-life of platelets was decreased to a mean of 73 hours, as compared with 107 hours in normal controls, in thirty patients with multiple myeloma;[46] this occurred in the absence of thrombocytopenia or bleeding phenomena; (2) impaired platelet aggregation: a 62-year-old man with multiple myeloma presented with mucocutaneous petechial hemorrhages followed by a fatal gastrointestinal hemorrhage, despite an adequate platelet count (110,000 per mm$^3$) and normal PT, aPTT, fibrinogen, and FDP; he was found to have impaired platelet aggregation due to binding of the myeloma paraprotein to the glycoprotein IIIa portion of the platelet;[47] (3) fibrinolytic activity and thrombocytopenia: Niléhn and Nilsson[48] showed evidence of fibrinolysis and thrombocytopenia in one-half of sixty-three patients with multiple myeloma, but found no correlation between these abnormalities and bleeding phenomena; hemorrhages occurred in seventeen patients, and involved mucocutaneous tissues and the gastrointestinal tract, but not the CNS.

ICH in multiple myeloma is occasionally seen as a preterminal event in severely thrombocytopenic patients, the hemorrhages at times being an autopsy finding (Figure 7.5).

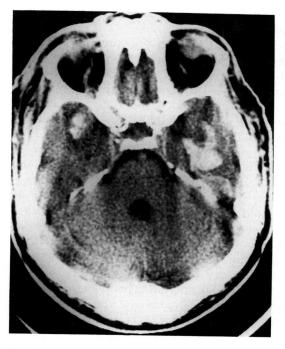 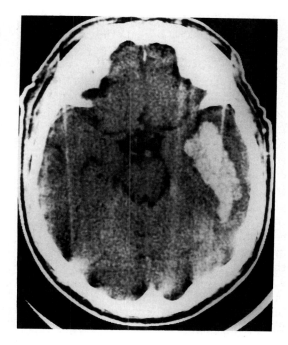

A                                    B

**Figure 7.4.** Bilateral temporal lobe hemorrhages (A), extensive on the left side (B), in a 69-year-old man with a myeloproliferative disorder (MMM), who sustained head trauma with loss of consciousness prior to the onset of the neurological symptoms (Courtesy of Judy S. Fine-Edelstein, M.D. and Karla B. Kanis, M.D., Boston VA Medical Center, Boston, MA.)

## Antithrombotic Agents

The use of antithrombotic agents is widespread for the prevention and treatment of coronary artery thrombosis, stroke and systemic embolism, and veno-occlusive disease. These substances include antiplatelet agents (aspirin, ticlopidine), anticoagulants (warfarin, heparin), and fibrinolytics (tissue plasminogen activator, streptokinase, urokinase).

### Antiplatelet Agents

These substances derive their therapeutic benefit from their ability to inhibit platelet aggregation by mechanisms that are specific for the various classes of drugs in this group.

### Aspirin

Aspirin (acetylsalicylic acid, ASA) has a marked inhibitory effect on platelet aggregation. This is mediated by the irreversible inactivation of the enzyme cyclooxygenase, which in turn results in a decrease in the production of the natural platelet aggregant thromboxane $A_2$.[49] At low doses, ASA does not interfere with the synthesis of the natural platelet antiaggregant prostacyclin produced by the vascular endothelium.[50] This combination of inhibition of the natural platelet aggregant thromboxane $A_2$, without disturbing the antiaggregant prostacyclin, makes ASA an excellent antiplatelet agent in the clinical setting. These theoretical advantages of ASA have been extensively confirmed in randomized clinical trials during the last two de-

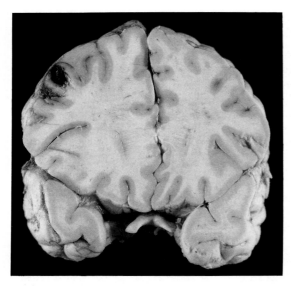

A

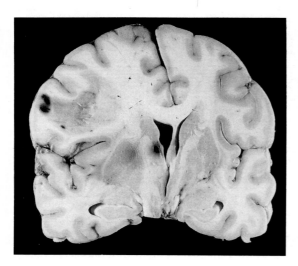

B

**Figure 7.5.** Multiple small incidental hemorrhages in patient with multiple myeloma associated with thrombocytopenia (platelet count: 20,000 per mm³). (A) Right frontal corticosubcortical hemorrhage. (B) Right subcortical parietal and capsular hemorrhages.

cades. At the same time, concern has been raised about a potential increase in hemorrhagic complications, besides those known to

occur in the upper gastrointestinal tract, including ICH.

Although there are no prospectively collected data on the specific issue of ICH occurrence in ASA users, a number of studies on the use of ASA for various purposes provide useful information in this regard (Table 7.5). Several of these studies[51,52,54–57,59,60] documented either the same frequency of ICH in patients on ASA and placebo, or a slight excess of hemorrhages in the ASA group, but without statistical significance for the difference in rates. The UK-TIA study group[59] reported thirteen intracranial hemorrhages among 1621 patients who received either 300 mg or 1200 mg of ASA, whereas three intracranial hemorrhages occurred in the 814 patients who received placebo, during a four-year follow-up period. This twofold increase in the risk of hemorrhage was however not statistically significant (p = 0.2). The Physicians' Health Study Research Group[60] reported twenty-three "hemorrhagic strokes" (encompassing ICH, SAH, and hemorrhagic infarction) among 11,037 subjects taking ASA, and twelve in the group of 11,034 subjects on placebo, a difference that was of borderline statistical significance (p = 0.06). Taylor and Barnett[61] argued that the evidence of an increased risk of hemorrhagic stroke in ASA-treated patients is less compelling than suggested by the Physicians' Health Study data. They contrasted the slight difference in hemorrhagic stroke events between the two groups with the lack of such association in secondary stroke prevention trials,[53,54] in which the precise separation of stroke subtypes was part of the design of the studies. However, the recently reported Swedish Aspirin Low-dose Trial (SALT)[62] also recorded an excess of intracranial hemorrhages in the group treated with ASA, as compared with those taking placebo: ten (1.5%) intracranial hemorrhages occurred among 676 patients on 75 mg of ASA per day, whereas three (0.4%) hemorrhages occurred in the 684 patients on placebo, during a mean follow-up period of thirty-two months. All five fatal intracranial hemorrhages were in the ASA-

**Table 7.5.** Randomized Trials of Aspirin Use: Incidence of ICH

| Study | Subject | Agent | Dose (mg) | Follow-up (yrs.) | N | ICH N | ICH %/yr |
|-------|---------|-------|-----------|------------------|---|-------|----------|
| AICLA[51] | TIA/st. | ASA/dip. | 990/225 | 3 | 202 | 1 | 0.16 |
| | | ASA | 990 | | 198 | 2 | 0.34 |
| | | Placebo | | | 204 | 2 | 0.33 |
| ACCSG[52] | TIA/st. | ASA/dip. | 1300/300 | 1.5 | 448 | 2 | 0.30 |
| | | ASA | 1300 | | 442 | 4 | 0.60 |
| UK-TIA[59] | TIA | ASA | 300/1200 | 4 | 1621 | 13* | 0.20 |
| | | Placebo | | | 814 | 3 | 0.09 |
| ESPS[53] | TIA/st. | ASA/dip. | 975/225 | 2 | 1250 | 3 | 0.12 |
| | | Placebo | | | 1250 | 3 | 0.12 |
| Swedish[54] | Stroke | ASA | 1500 | 2 | 253 | 3 | 0.59 |
| | | Placebo | | | 252 | 2 | 0.40 |
| Peto et al.[55] | Physician | ASA | 500 | 6 | 3429 | 14† | 0.07 |
| | | No Rx | | | 1710 | 6† | 0.06 |
| AFASAK[56] | AF | ASA | 75 | 2 | 336 | 0 | 0 |
| | | Placebo | | | 336 | 0 | 0 |
| PHS[60] | Physician | ASA | 163 | 5 | 11037 | 23† | 0.04 |
| | | Placebo | | | 11034 | 12† | 0.02 |
| SPAF[57] | AF | ASA | 325 | 1.13 | 517 | 1 | 0.20 |
| | | Placebo | | | 528 | 0 | 0 |
| Dutch[58] | TIA/st. | ASA | 30 | 2.6 | 1555 | 13 | 0.32 |
| | | ASA | 283 | | 1576 | 15 | 0.37 |
| SALT[62] | TIA/st. | ASA | 75 | 2.6 | 676 | 10 | 0.50 |
| | | Placebo | | | 684 | 3 | 0.16 |

Abbreviations: N = number of patients, dip. = dipyridamole, TIA = transient ischemic attack, st. = stroke, AF = atrial fibrillation, Rx = treatment.
*Difference not statistically significant
†Listed as "hemorrhagic stroke," not necessarily all ICH
(Modified from del Zoppo GJ, Mori E. Hematologic causes of intracerebral hemorrhage and their treatment. Neursurg Clin NA 1992; 3:637–658, with permission of the publisher.)

treated patients. The stroke subtype determination in the SALT trial was done by CT scan or autopsy in 98% of patients, a rate of confirmation of events similar to that of the Dutch trial,[58] but higher than in the UK-TIA trial[59] and the Physicians' Health Study.[60]

These data indicate a generally low risk of intracranial hemorrhage in the various trials of ASA for primary or secondary stroke prevention and primary prevention of myocardial infarction. In most studies the risk in the ASA group does not exceed that of the placebo group, whereas others[60,62] have shown a slight excess of intracranial hemorrhagic stroke in the ASA-treated patients. In view of these conflicting data, it is still unclear whether or not long-term ASA treatment increases the risk of intracranial hemorrhage.

### Ticlopidine

Ticlopidine hydrochloride is a platelet antiaggregant agent that acts by inhibiting the binding of fibrinogen to the platelet wall.[63] It has been tested in two separate trials in patients with TIA and strokes, against placebo[64] and against ASA.[65] In the former, the Canadian-American Ticlopidine Study (CATS),[64] two ICH (one of them fatal), occurred among 525 patients treated with 500 mg of ticlopidine for a median follow-up of about eighteen months. No ICH occurred in the 528 patients forming the placebo group, but two patients had a fatal SAH. When ticlopidine (500 mg per day) was tested against ASA (1300 mg per day) in patients with TIA or stroke in the Ticlopidine-Aspirin Stroke Study (TASS),[65] the same number of hemorrhages (seven) occurred in the ticlopidine group (N = 1,529) as in the ASA group (N = 1,540), after a mean follow-up period of 3.3 years.

These limited data on ticlopidine indicate that this drug does not have a significant association with intracranial hemorrhagic events. The frequency of this complication is clearly not higher with ticlopidine than with ASA, and both drugs have a marginally elevated, probably not statistically significant, rate of intracranial hemorrhage in comparison with placebo.

### Anticoagulants

The anticoagulant agents warfarin and heparin are used for the treatment of patients with ischemic cerebrovascular disease, ischemic heart disease, prosthetic heart valves, atrial fibrillation, and venous thromboembolism. Randomized clinical trials have documented the value of this therapy in virtually all these indications.[66] At the same time, they have emphasized the risk of hemorrhagic complications, at times leading to substantial morbidity and mortality.

### Warfarin

Warfarin, a 4-hydroxycoumarin compound, exerts its effect by interfering with the τ-carboxylation of the vitamin K–dependent coagulant proteins prothrombin and factors VII, IX and X, and the anticoagulant proteins C and S.[66] Long-term oral anticoagulation with warfarin carries a risk of hemorrhagic complications that is difficult to quantitate. This results from variations in patient populations, indications for anticoagulant treatment, and measurement of coagulation parameters in the different series. The lack of uniformity in the measuring and reporting of

anticoagulation parameters is particularly responsible for variations in intensity of anticoagulation in different series, as well as within a given institution.[67] This problem derives from the technique used to measure the PT as a way of monitoring anticoagulant treatment. The PT is sensitive to three of the four vitamin K–dependent clotting factors; the test is performed by the addition of thromboplastin to citrated plasma, followed by the addition of calcium, which results in clotting.[68] Due to variations in the sensitivity of thromboplastins of different origins used by coagulation laboratories, PT values are not equivalent when generated from different laboratories. This has even resulted in an unnoticed variation in the last decades within a given institution, because of unannounced changes in the sensitivity of the thromboplastins provided by the manufacturers. Thromboplastins used to perform PT can be prepared from either human brain, rabbit brain, a mixture of rabbit brain and lung, or placental tissues, and they all have different sensitivities.[67,68] Since laboratories in different countries use thromboplastins of different origins (human brain in the United Kingdom, rabbit brain or brain and lung in the United States, bovine brain in Scandinavia[67]), the World Health Organization (WHO) promoted a standardization effort. This resulted in the creation of the International Normalized Ratio (INR), which is derived by measuring the patient's PT and the control, to obtain a patient/control PT ratio, which in turn is elevated to the power of a value called the International Sensitivity Index (ISI). The ISI is the standardized value that results from adjusting the sensitivity of a given thromboplastin to that of the WHO standard. As a result, coagulation laboratories are now urged to report coagulation parameters for the purpose of monitoring anticoagulant treatment as the INR, also providing the measure of their thromboplastin sensitivity as the ISI value.[68] Current recommendations for monitoring anticoagulant treatment in North America are to use less intense levels of anticoagulation than in the past for the pre-

**Table 7.6.** Pooled Data on Incidence of Hemorrhage during Long-term
Anticoagulant Therapy

|  |  | Incidence of bleeding | | | |
| --- | --- | --- | --- | --- | --- |
| Indication | N | Total (%) | Minor (%) | Major (%) | Fatal (%) |
| Ischemic CVD | 588 | 169 (28.7) | 128 (21.8) | 41 (7.0) | 28 (4.8) |
| Prosthetic heart valves | 405 | 23  (5.7) | 13  (3.2) | 10 (2.4) | 7 (1.7) |
| AF | 302 | 46 (15.2) | 43 (14.2) | 3 (0.01) | 1 (0.003) |
| Ischemic heart disease | 1890 | 299 (19.1) | 199 (10.5) | 88 (4.7) | 19 (1.0) |
| Venous thrombosis | 159 | 36 (22.6) | 23 (14.4) | 13 (8.1) | 0 |

Abbreviations: N = number of patients, CVD = cerebrovascular disease, AF = atrial fibrillation.
(From Levine MN, Raskob G, Hirsh J. Risk of haemorrhage associated with long term anticoagulant therapy. Drugs
1985;30:444–460, with permission of the publisher.)

vention of thromboembolism, treatment of venous thrombosis and pulmonary embolism, and prevention of systemic embolism in patients with tissue heart valves, atrial fibrillation, acute anterior wall myocardial infarction, and valvular heart disease. The recommended monitoring parameters are an INR of 2.0 to 3.0, corresponding to PT of 1.3 to 1.5 times control, using an ISI of 2.4 for North American thromboplastin.[69] A more intense level of anticoagulation, INR of 3.0 to 4.5 (corresponding to PT ratios of 1.5 to 2.0, with North American thromboplastin of ISI of 2.4), is recommended for patients with prosthetic heart valves and in patients with recurrent systemic embolism.[69] Despite these specific recommendations, Bussey et al.[70] recently reported a disturbing lack of uniformity in reporting PT data in coagulation laboratories across the United States: among fifty-three laboratories surveyed, only eleven (21%) reported INR results, and sixteen (30%) could not provide ISI data for the thromboplastin used for the assay. Three manufacturers of thromboplastin marketed their products with ISI values from 1.2 to 2.8, but none had ISI values in the recommended range of 2.2 to 2.6.[70] This prompted a call for a change in the monitoring of warfarin anticoagulation in North America[71] to include: (1) the checking of ISI values for each new lot of thromboplastin by clinical laboratories, (2) reporting of PT results in INR values, (3) providing of thromboplastins with accurate ISI values of 2.2 to 2.4 by the manufacturers (ide-

ally made mandatory by the regulatory government agencies), and (4) the mandatory use of the INR standard in all manuscripts dealing with anticoagulant treatment published in medical journals.

In a literature review of hemorrhagic risk with long-term oral anticoagulation, Levine et al.[67] tabulated the incidence of bleeding for the various indications of oral anticoagulants (Table 7.6). They found the highest bleeding rates in patients with ischemic cerebrovascular disease, in whom the majority of hemorrhagic events were intracranial. They attributed this association to either the presence of cerebrovascular pathology or coexisting hypertension.[67] Petty et al.,[72] on the other hand, determined a cumulative risk of life-threatening and fatal hemorrhage of 2% at six months, 7% at one year, 12% at two years, and 14% at three years of oral anticoagulation. These authors did not document a difference in the frequency of hemorrhagic complications when they compared cerebrovascular with noncerebrovascular indications for anticoagulation. Other factors were found to increase the risk of bleeding on long-term oral anticoagulants in the literature review of Levine et al.[67] Hypertension increased the relative risk of bleeding more than twofold; risk factors such as cancer, recent surgery, and paraplegia markedly increased the bleeding rates in patients with venous thrombosis; and the addition of ASA (but not dipyridamole) to warfarin in patients with prosthetic heart valves was also associated with more frequent hemorrhagic complications. A relationship with the patient's age could not be established because of incomplete reporting of data in the literature. However, an increased risk of hemorrhage with increasing age has been found in some series[73,74] but not in others.[72,75,76]

Intracranial hemorrhage in patients treated with long-term warfarin anticoagulation has been extensively studied. The majority of these events take the form of SDH, but there is a substantial risk of ICH as well.[77] Since the early days of anticoagulant drug use, ICH was recognized as a major cause of fatal bleeding. In a literature review, Duff and Shull[78] found eight patients with ICH among twenty-three patients who died under dicumarol treatment, Russek and Zohman[79] reported 46 deaths from intracranial bleeding (24 ICH, 22 SAH) among 122 patients who died while on oral anticoagulants, and in the series of Riddick[80] six of eight deaths were due to ICH among 125 patients treated. Askey[81] reported twenty-two patients with anticoagulant-related ICH, nineteen (86%) of whom died.

The *frequency* of ICH in patients taking chronic oral anticoagulants is generally low. Coon and Willis[73] reported a frequency of 6.8% of bleeding complications (4.8% minor, 2.0% major) in 3862 courses of therapy. Among the total number of hemorrhagic events (N = 313), five (1.6%) were intracranial. Similarly, Forfar[76] reported a frequency of 8.2% of bleeding among 501 patients on anticoagulants followed for seven years; two of the fifty-one (4%) bleeding episodes were intracranial, one an ICH (2%), the other a SAH (2%). However, this low frequency of ICH is still significantly higher than that of comparable populations not receiving anticoagulants. ICH occurs eight to eleven times more frequently in patients on anticoagulants in comparison with those not receiving anticoagulants in population studies.[74,82] In a more recent study, Franke et al.[83] reported a 7.6 times higher relative risk of ICH in patients over age 50 who took anticoagulants

than in patients over age 50 who did not take anticoagulants.

The *clinical features* of anticoagulant-related ICH have been studied in detail. Barron and Fergusson[84] reported six patients with fatal ICH while on oral anticoagulants, and commented on the frequent occurrence of preceding embolic cerebral infarction in their patients. Such association was present in three of their six patients, and in four of twenty-two patients from the literature. Also, they found an excessively prolonged PT (from 35.4 to 45.4 seconds) around the time of the fatal ICH in five of their six patients. None of their patients had a vascular malformation at necropsy, and pathological evidence of recent embolic cerebral artery occlusions was present in only one patient. Head trauma was not a factor in any of the six patients, and hypertension was present in one. These authors[84] postulated that hypertension and, especially, recent (within a few weeks) cerebral infarction were risk factors for ICH in patients with excessive levels of oral anticoagulation. The presence of preexisting cerebral lesions as a risk factor for anticoagulant-related ICH is further emphasized by reported instances of ICH into tumors[85] and into a pineal cyst.[86]

In recent years, four large patient series[74,83,87,88] have analyzed the clinical aspects of ICH in anticoagulated patients. Findings in these studies varied concerning some aspects, while other features were rather consistent. Findings in common among these clinical series included (1) *Lack of correlation between ICH and preceding head trauma or cerebral infarction.*[87,88] Although ICH occasionally follows after an episode of cerebral infarction,[84] it does not necessarily occur at the site of the previous infarct.[87,88] Also, the long delays between the two events make their causal relationship doubtful, as ICH has occurred many days after the time when spontaneous hemorrhagic transformation of an embolic brain infarct was known to take place[89,90] (Figure 7.6). Finally, the occurrence of anticoagulant-related ICH in patients at

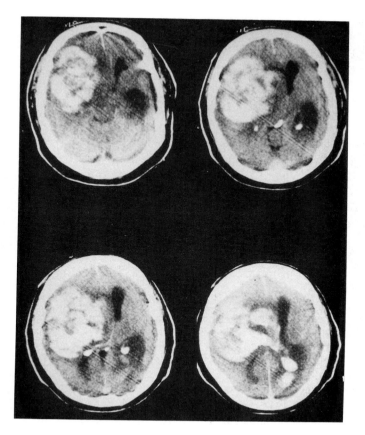

**Figure 7.6.** Massive right frontoparietal ICH with midline shift and hydrocephalus of the left lateral ventricle, eighteen days after onset of warfarin anticoagulation for right frontal nonhemorrhagic embolic infarct.

high risk of embolic phenomena, such as those with prosthetic heart valves,[91,92] raises the issue of embolic infarct rapidly becoming hemorrhagic and leading to massive ICH in the setting of pre-existing anticoagulation. Whether this phenomenon is operative or not is unclear, and in the event of its occurrence its frequency is probably very low, since patients with prosthetic valves are not significantly represented in any of the published series of anticoagulant-related ICH.[82–84,87,88] (2) *Lack of association of ICH with bleeding elsewhere in the body.*[87,88] ICH represents an isolated event rather than being just one more site in a generalized drug-induced bleeding disorder. (3) *Mean hematoma volumes substantially higher (close to double in size) in patients taking anticoagulants than in patients not taking anticoagulants.*[83,87,88] This has been

found to correlate occasionally with slow progression of the neurological deficits at onset, at times for periods as long as forty-eight to seventy-two hours (Figure 7.7), presumably reflecting a slow accumulation of blood in the brain substance. This, in turn, suggests the possibility of bleeding from different blood vessels, such as smaller arteries, in patients taking anticoagulants in comparison with those with hypertensive ICH, who usually have a more fulminant acute clinical course at onset.[87] (4) *Higher mortality figures, of 57% to 67%, in patients on anticoagulants as compared with patients not on anticoagulants (30% to 55%).*[83,87,88] This probably reflects the generally larger hematoma sizes, since this parameter is one of the main determinants of mortality in ICH in general.[93] Despite its generally poor prognosis, patients with

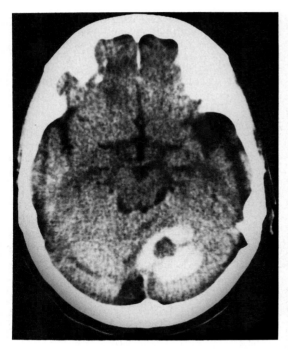 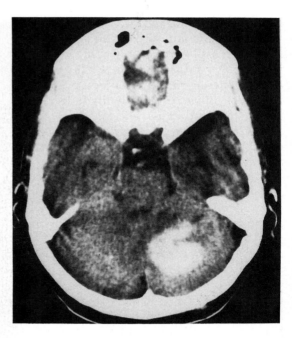

A                                          B

**Figure 7.7.** Left cerebellar hemorrhage in patient on chronic warfarin anticoagulation for prosthetic heart valve. (A) The admission CT shows a moderate hematoma in the area of the dentate nucleus, with slight mass effect on the quadrigeminal cistern. (B) Follow-up CT 24 hours later, coinciding with worsening lethargy and prominent vertigo, shows slight increase in size of the hematoma and more prominent effacement of the ipsilateral quadrigeminal cistern.

anticoagulant-related ICH can at times have satisfactory outcomes, often after surgical drainage of the hematoma.[94–97]

Other features of anticoagulant-related ICH have been discrepant in clinical series. These include (1) duration of anticoagulation before ICH onset: in some series[87,88] most of the hemorrhagic events (70%,[87] 54%[88]) occurred within the first year of treatment, while in others[74,82,83] the occurrence of ICH had no temporal predominance and spanned throughout periods of treatment duration between one and many years; (2) role of hypertension and increasing age as risk factors for ICH: a strong association between hypertension and ICH risk was found by Wintzen et al.[74] and a more than twofold increase in bleeding risk in general was reported by Levine et al.,[67] but others[82] failed to show a significantly higher frequency of hypertension in patients with anticoagulant-related ICH; increasing age was suggested as an association with ICH in patients on anticoagulants,[74,82] but other studies have failed to substantiate such correlation;[72,74,83] (3) relationship between intensity of anticoagulation and ICH risk: when considering hemorrhagic complications in general, there is clear evidence that increasing intensity of anticoagulation carries a higher risk of bleeding;[67,76] some studies of anticoagulant-related ICH[74,87] have also suggested an increased risk of hemorrhage with increasing intensity of anticoagulation; others[83,88,98] however have not found such an association, reporting the majority (71% to 87%) of ICH instances in patients with therapeutic or subtherapeutic anticoagulation[88,98] or showing only a slight excess of ICH in overtreated patients as compared with those treated in the therapeutic range;[83] (4) location of ICH: we reported an unusually high frequency (37.5%) of anticoagulant-related ICH located in the cerebellum,[87] where ICH in general occurs in only 5% to 10% of patients;[99] a similar, but less marked predilection for the cerebellum (14%) was reported by Rådberg et al.[88] among their twenty-eight patients with anticoagulant-related ICH, whereas that location accounted for 6% of their 172 patients with non-anticoagulant-related ICH; however, other authors[74,83] have found no differences in ICH location when comparing patients taking anticoagulants with patients not taking anticoagulants; (5) computed tomography (CT) aspects: some authors[100,101] have suggested that anticoagulant-related ICH (as well as ICH related to fibrinolytic therapy[101a]) have a propensity to show "fluid-blood levels" on CT scans done shortly after onset of symptoms of ICH; this has been interpreted as due to unequal clotting within the hematoma, some portions (usually the dependent ones) clotting, others remaining unclotted, thus resulting in two different absorption values within the hemorrhage;[101] although a similar CT aspect can be seen in acute ICH unrelated to the use of anticoagulants, a similar explanation of differential clotting within the hematoma has been given,[102] despite the lack of demonstration of two different portions of the hematoma at postmortem examination.[100]

The *mechanism* of anticoagulant-related ICH remains unclear. This is the result of the lack of adequate pathological studies of brains with anticoagulant-related ICH. These studies should be performed in order to determine the type of bleeding vessel and the eventual presence of local pathology, such as lipohyalinosis, microaneurysms, fibrinoid necrosis, or cerebral amyloid angiopathy (CAA), at bleeding sites. The suggestion that "elderly subjects (may) often have small ICHs without symptoms,"[83] resulting in

large symptomatic ICH in the event of being anticoagulated, is plausible but appears unlikely to us in view of the rarity of incidentally-found small ICH without specific local vascular pathology in routine autopsy material.

## Heparin

The parenteral anticoagulant heparin exerts its effect by binding to lysine sites of the plasma cofactor antithrombin III, which then becomes an inhibitor of thrombin and activated factors X, XII, XI, and IX.[36,103] Its anticoagulant effectiveness has been proven in the prevention and treatment of venous thrombosis and pulmonary embolism, in preventing mural thrombus formation after myocardial infarction (MI), in the treatment of patients with unstable angina and acute MI, and in preventing coronary reocclusion after thrombolytic treatment.[103]

Bleeding complications, in the form of major hemorrhage, in heparin-treated patients have been reported in 6.8% of those receiving the drug by continuous intravenous infusion.[103] Risk factors for this complication include the amount of heparin given, a concomitant serious concurrent illness, and chronic heavy alcohol use.[104–106]

ICH as a complication of heparin treatment is virtually limited to patients who have had preceding cerebral infarctions. For noncerebrovascular indications, such as in patients with acute MI, ICH has been reported in a minute fraction of patients (0.05%) receiving heparin treatment alone.[107–112] A similarly low frequency (0.08%) of "hemorrhagic stroke" was found in the heparin arm of a large multicenter trial of thrombolysis in MI.[113] When used for the treatment of transient ischemic attacks (TIA), in the absence of cerebral infarction, heparin has a negligible risk of ICH. Systemic bleeding complications occurred in 13% of 102 TIA patients treated with heparin in a recently reported trial,[114] but none had ICH. Similarly, no instances of ICH were recorded among 160 patients with TIA treated with heparin in another study.[115]

The only substantial risk of ICH after heparin use is in patients with acute brain infarcts.

Although it has not been proven beneficial in randomized clinical trials, heparin therapy after acute ischemic stroke is generally used for patients with brain embolism and progressing cerebral infarction.[116,117] For the former indication, anticoagulant treatment is felt to carry a particularly significant risk of ICH, since hemorrhagic transformation is part of the natural history of acute embolic brain infarction.[118] However, the importance of treatment with heparin in the pathogenesis of ICH after brain embolism is still controversial. Furlan et al.[119] found no examples of ICH after heparin treatment of fifty-four patients with acute nonseptic brain embolism of cardiac origin. Koller[120] reported similar results in a retrospective review of sixteen patients with embolic infarction who underwent heparin anticoagulation within forty-eight hours of onset, without having hemorrhagic complications. However, others have suggested a role for heparin in the development of ICH after anticoagulation of brain embolic infarcts. Drake and Shin[121] reported two patients who developed massive ICH at the site of a recent cardioembolic infarct, within twenty-four hours of onset of heparin treatment. Neither patient had CT evidence of hemorrhagic infarction prior to the onset of heparin therapy, and the degree of anticoagulation was not excessive in either patient at the time of onset of ICH symptoms. These authors suggested that massive ICH is a risk in patients acutely anticoagulated in the setting of an embolic stroke, even when the levels of anticoagulation are maintained within the recommended therapeutic range. However, it is unclear whether the frequency of this occurrence is high enough to justify restrictions in the use of this agent. Also, the risk factors for this complication of acute embolic stroke have not been fully elucidated.

Ramirez-Lassepas and Quinones[115] reported three instances of ICH among 269 patients (1.1%) with brain infarction treated with continuous intravenous heparin infu-sion. Two of the three patients with ICH died. In two patients, the ICH occurred within twelve hours of onset of heparin treatment, while the third patient bled on the sixth day of treatment. Potential factors associated with the occurrence of ICH in the three patients included the presence of severe initial neurological deficits secondary to cardiogenic embolism, history of hypertension, CT demonstration of cerebral infarction within twelve to twenty-four hours from onset of symptoms, and heparin loading doses greater than 100 U per kg. An excessive level of anticoagulation was not a significant risk factor for ICH in their series. These issues were systematically studied by the Cerebral Embolism Study Group (CESG).[122–124] Initial data on forty-five patients randomized to immediate heparin anticoagulation or no anticoagulation showed no instances of ICH among those receiving intravenous heparin.[122] These observations were further expanded in a second study,[123] which included thirty patients with cardiogenic embolism who developed hemorrhagic changes on follow-up CT, after an initial scan had not shown hemorrhage. From the analysis of those data, the authors identified large infarct size as a potential risk factor for the development of ICH after early heparin anticoagulation in patients with cardioembolic stroke. Also, a possible association with persistent hypertension above 180/100 mm Hg was detected. No consistent effect of excessive levels of anticoagulation on ICH risk was found by these authors.[124] These data were accepted as generally favoring the use of heparin anticoagulation in patients with nonmassive, acute cardioembolic strokes, based on the generally low risk of catastrophic ICH, along with a perceived protection against recurrent embolism.[125] These views were further tested by Rothrock et al.,[126] who randomized 121 patients with cardioembolic stroke to either heparin within ninety-six hours from onset or no anticoagulation for fourteen days after stroke onset. Their findings indicated a low frequency of hemorrhagic complications (2%) and recurrent embolism (2%) in *both* groups of pa-

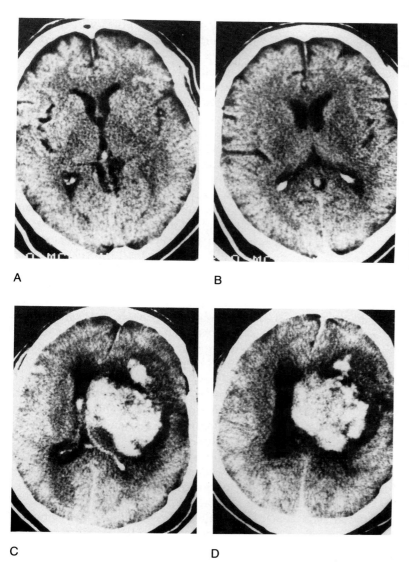

A    B

C    D

**Figure 7.8.** (A and B) CT of 70-year-old man with recent MI and atrial fibrillation, who developed a large left MCA infarct with right hemiplegia, global aphasia, and right homonymous hemianopia, with unremarkable CT on admission. After approximately twenty hours from initiation of heparin anticoagulation, he became lethargic and lapsed into coma with decerebrate rigidity of the limbs and bilaterally unreactive and dilated pupils. (C and D) CT showed massive left frontoparietal ICH, which was fatal.

tients. These data led the authors to conclude that the acute use of anticoagulants does not appear to increase the risk of ICH, but the value of such therapy for the prevention of recurrent embolism is still questionable.

The *clinical features* of ICH related to heparin use in acute stroke patients were reported by Babikian et al.[127] They studied ten patients of their own, and reviewed sixteen others from the literature. The main features that characterized these ICH included: (1) early onset of hemorrhage after initiation of heparin treatment, 80% of the cases developed symptoms of bleeding within twelve hours or less after onset of therapy (Figure 7.8), (2) generally large or medium-size infarcts, this complication not being described in patients with small brain infarcts, and (3) excessive levels of anticoagulation (aPTT more than twice that of control) in seven of their ten patients (70%) and in eleven of sixteen (69%) of those collected from the literature.

These data further confirmed the observation that infarct size appears to be a risk factor for ICH in acutely-anticoagulated patients with cardioembolic stroke, a complication that occurs early in the course of the stroke. The significance of the finding of excessively prolonged aPTT in about 70% of the patients with ICH is difficult to evaluate, without knowing the frequency of such prolongation of aPTT in similarly-treated patients who did not develop ICH in these authors' institutions.

### Fibrinolytic Agents

These substances produce dissolution of clots by activating the body's fibrinolytic system, through the conversion of plasminogen into plasmin, the natural fibrinolytic enzyme.[128] The lysis of fresh fibrin clots takes place at the clot itself by the binding of the fibrinolytic agent to fibrin, with generation of fibrin(ogen) degradation products. The degree of clot-specificity varies among the various fibrinolytic substances, some producing higher levels of activation of the circulating plasminogen than others, thus resulting in more significant systemic, rather than clot-specific, fibrinolysis.[129] The fibrinolytic agents that are currently used include the exogenous substances streptokinase (SK) and urokinase (UK), single-chain urokinase plasminogen activator (SCU-PA), anisoylated plasminogen-streptokinase activator complex (APSAC), and the endogenous recombinant tissue-type plasminogen activator (rt-PA). The agents that have been most widely used in the management of patients with thrombotic disorders are SK, UK, and rt-PA, and the discussion of hemorrhagic complications is limited to these three substances.

### Fibrinolytics in the Treatment of Myocardial Infarction

The main clinical use of fibrinolytic agents is in the treatment of acute MI. When administered early after onset of symptoms of MI, both SK and rt-PA produce recanalization of more than 70% of occluded coronary arteries.[130,131] This, in turn, results in improved ventricular function and survival in treated patients as compared with controls.[113,132,133] This proven beneficial effect of fibrinolysis is limited to some extent by its hemorrhagic complications, the most serious being ICH.

ICH has occurred in large clinical trials of patients with acute MI treated with fibrinolytic agents with a low frequency of about 0.18% for SK and 0.46% for rt-PA.[8] This frequency is slightly higher than that of the control groups (0.02%) of the same trials, suggesting that, albeit low, the frequency of ICH is increased by the use of fibrinolytic agents in patients with acute MI. Furthermore, data from one study[134] suggested a dose relationship between ICH and rt-PA (the single-chain agent alteplase) use, as an ICH frequency of 0.4% was recorded after a 100-mg dose of rt-PA, in contrast with 1.3% after a 150-mg dose. However, with the recent use of rt-PA or SK for acute MI in the community, outside multicenter controlled clinical trials, higher frequencies of ICH have been recorded, of 1.1%,[134a] 2.3%,[135] 2.8%,[136] and 5%,[137] despite use of the medications at the recommended doses. This raises a concern about a significantly higher rate of ICH in the routine clinical use of fibrinolytics for acute MI, the differences possibly being related to either looser adherence to parameters of patient selection in the community or under-reporting of ICH in clinical trials.[8] In some trials, no clear distinction between ischemic and hemorrhagic strokes was made, and the definition of cerebrovascular events was not rigorously applied across all study centers.[138,139]

A number of studies have reported the *clinical features* of ICH related to the use of SK or rt-PA in acute MI. With *SK*, Aldrich et al.[140] reported two patients among ninety-one treated (2.2%) who had ICH. Their Case 1, a 53-year-old woman with ischemia of digits of the left hand, was treated with an intravenous loading dose of 250,000 U of SK followed by a constant intravenous infusion of 100,000 U per hour. She developed symptoms of a right cerebellar hemorrhage within twenty-four hours from treatment onset, and recovered after surgical drainage of the ICH. She had not received anticoagulants along with the SK. Case 2, a 69-year-old woman with an acute inferior MI, was treated with 100,000 U of intracoronary SK and 5000 U of intravenous heparin, with lysis of a right coronary artery thrombus. She developed symptoms of a left ICH (lethargy, global aphasia, right hemiparesis, bilateral Babinski signs), with a possible additional SDH, approximately thirty-six hours after treatment onset. At that time, her coagulation parameters (PT, aPTT, platelet count) were normal, but she had previously received fresh-frozen plasma and antihemophilic factor for persistent bleeding at the angiography catheter entry site. She improved gradually over the following weeks, and was described as "nearly . . . normal" two months after the event. The authors[140] suggested that the frequency of ICH after SK use may be higher than the generally quoted figures of less than 1%.[141] Gorelick et al.[142] reported a 63-year-old hypertensive and diabetic woman who developed a fatal cerebellar hemorrhage after receiving 270,000 U of intracoronary SK followed by intravenous heparin for an acute anterior MI. This complication occurred in a patient with poorly controlled hypertension, excessive prolongation of the aPTT (more than 149 seconds), and hypofibrinogenemia. The onset of symptoms occurred "several hours" after the initiation of the thrombolytic-anticoagulant treatment. Ramsay et al.[143] described a 56-year-old man with an acute inferior MI who received 1.5 megaunits of intravenous SK during a one-hour period and subsequently became unresponsive eight hours after treatment onset. CT showed a large left SDH and multiple left ICH, with marked shift of the midline from left to right. He had prolonged aPTT (79 seconds) and thrombin clotting time, and died despite surgical evacuation of the left SDH. At autopsy, a left parieto-occipital lobar ICH

was present, and histological examination showed the typical features of CAA. Another example of multiple intracranial hemorrhages in a 75-year-old man treated with SK for acute MI was reported recently by Wijdicks and Jack.[101a] Following drainage of an occipital lobar ICH, histological examination of adjacent tissues disclosed CAA. These authors[101a,143] raised the issue of underlying vascular disease, other than atherosclerosis, being a possible risk factor for the occurrence of ICH in the setting of thrombolytic therapy. The finding of CAA in their patient, made Ramsay et al.[143] recommend caution in the use of thrombolytic agents in elderly patients or in those with dementia.

With the use of *rt-PA*, hemorrhagic complications occur in 15% to 33% of patients,[44,145] but mostly at vascular catherization sites. ICH is uncommon, occurring in 0.4% to 1.3% of the cases in controlled clinical trials,[146] and in 1.1% to 5% after the routine use of rt-PA in the community,[134a,135–137,147] These figures apply to the only FDA-approved rt-PA preparation available in the United States, the single-chain alteplase.

The clinical features of rt-PA-related ICH have been analyzed in a series of recent reports. Carlson et al.[148] reported two patients with ICH among 450 patients treated with rt-PA, for a frequency of ICH of 0.44%. The patients received 150 mg and 90 mg of alteplase, respectively, and they developed symptoms of intracranial bleeding within four hours from treatment onset. Both patients were treated with intravenous heparin, and one had a therapeutic aPTT (65 seconds), while the other had an excessively prolonged aPTT (100 seconds) at the onset of their subcortical (lobar) ICH. A systemic fibrinolytic state developed in both patients, with decreased fibrinogen levels and elevated fibrin degradation products. The authors postulated that the systemic fibrinolytic state was the likely cause of ICH in their patients. Following this report, a number of larger series of patients with rt-PA-related ICH have helped to clarify most features of this condition. O'Connor et al.[149] reported thirteen patients among 1696 (0.76%) treated with alteplase who developed intracranial hemorrhage, nine of whom had ICH, while the others had combinations of SDH and SAH. The mortality for the group was 61%. Ten of the thirteen patients had excessive prolongation of the aPTT (more than 100 seconds) at the time of the intracranial hemorrhage. The same group of authors[150] analyzed the risk factor profile of rt-PA-related ICH. They identified age greater than 65 years, history of hypertension, and ASA use as possible risk factors for ICH in patients treated with alteplase. Similarly, in the Thrombolysis in Myocardial Infarction (TIMI) study with alteplase, Gore et al.[134] reported an increased frequency of ICH with higher medication doses (150 mg vs. 100 mg), older patient age, history of hypertension, prior neurological history (including TIA and stroke), and use of calcium-channel blockers. However, in a study of 1700 patients treated with the double-chain preparation duteplase, Kase et al.[151] found no relationship between ICH occurrence and older age, sex, weight, hypertension (by history or on admission), history of previous stroke, and use of ASA, betablockers, or calcium-channel blockers. These conflicting data on two agents of different composition may reflect either biological differences between them, or risk factor profiles that are still not completely defined. Further experience with these relatively novel substances will hopefully increase our understanding of their risk profile, which should in turn improve our criteria for patient selection for therapy.

The rt-PA-related ICH generally occur relatively early after onset of treatment. In the series of Gore et al.,[134] in almost 40% of the patients the symptoms of ICH started during the infusion, and another 25% occurred within twenty-four hours after treatment onset. With the use of duteplase, ICH symptoms started between seven and ninety-six hours (median, twenty-one hours) after onset of treatment, and in 55% of the patients the symptoms developed within twenty-four hours from onset of therapy.[151] The location

of the ICH was lobar in 70% to 90% of the cases, and they were multiple in almost one-third of the patients, at times with an associated SDH[101a,134,137,151] (Figure 7.9). These hemorrhages generally carry a poor prognosis, with a mortality reported between 44% and 80% in different series.[101a,134,137,150,151] The following case illustrates the presentation of ICH after use of alteplase in a patient with an acute MI:

A 72-year-old man was admitted with an acute inferior MI, with persistent chest pain that did not respond to treatment with nitroglycerin. Because of hypotension, he received a bolus of 5000 U of intravenous heparin and was started on intravenous rt-PA (alteplase), receiving 100 mg between 3:30 and 6:30 P.M. At 8:45 P.M. he complained of headache. He later vomited once, and by 9 P.M. was obtunded. The aPTT was 63 seconds. Shortly afterwards he was comatose, with bilateral decerebrate posturing to painful stimulation, absent oculocephalic and corneal reflexes, dilated pupils without reactivity to light, and bilateral Babinski signs. A head CT showed a massive right hemispheric ICH, with an associated SDH, marked shift of the midline from right to left, and dilatation of the contralateral ventricular system (Figure 7.10). Despite treatment with intubation, hyperventilation, and intravenous mannitol, he expired 33 hours after onset of rt-PA treatment.

This case illustrates the generally early onset of symptoms of ICH after the infusion of rt-PA, its massive character on CT, and its dramatic course and frequently fatal outcome.

The mechanism of ICH after rt-PA use for acute MI is still unknown. In several studies,[137,150,151] a relationship between excessive heparin anticoagulation and ICH has been suggested by the finding of aPTT beyond 100 seconds in two-thirds of the patients with ICH. However, in the large TIMI II cohort, Gore et al.[134] found no differences in the proportion of patients with excessively prolonged aPTT among those with ICH, in comparison with those without ICH. A similar comparison in the duteplase-treated pa-

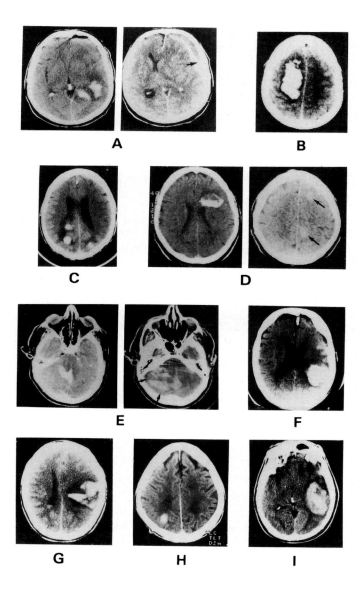

**Figure 7.9.** Sites of intracranial hemorrhage in nine patients treated with rt-PA for acute MI. (From Kase CS, Pessin MS, Zivin JA, et al. Intracranial hemorrhage after coronary thrombolysis with tissue plasminogen activator. Am J Med 1992;92:384-390, with permission of the publisher.) (A) Left temporal lobar hematoma (left panel), and chronic and acute SDH (arrow) (right panel). (B) Right parasagittal frontoparietal lobar ICH. (C) Bilateral multiple occipital lobar hematomas. (D) Left frontal and occipital hematomas (arrows). (E) Right cerebellar ICH (arrows) (right panel), with extension to the vermis and fourth ventricle (left panel). (F) Left posterior temporal lobar ICH. (G) Left frontoparietal lobar ICH with ventricular extension. (H) Small right posterior parietal parasagittal hematoma. (I) Left temporoparietal lobar hemorrhage.

tients reported by Kase et al.[151] showed significantly higher aPTT values in the ICH group only with measurements at four hours after treatment onset. Comparisons of aPTT values at all post-baseline times between the ICH and non-ICH groups was only marginally significant (p = 0.06). These apparently conflicting observations leave the role of excessively prolonged aPTT as a risk factor for rt-PA-related ICH still unresolved. However, the combined use of thrombolytic and antico-agulant agents appears to produce a slight increase in the frequency of ICH in comparison with the use of heparin alone. The latter was associated with ICH in 0.08% of 2493 patients forming the placebo-plus-heparin group of the ASSET study,[113] whereas a threefold increase to a frequency of 0.27% was found among the 2512 patients in the alteplase-plus-heparin arm of that study. Although this threefold increase in frequency was not statistically significant, it

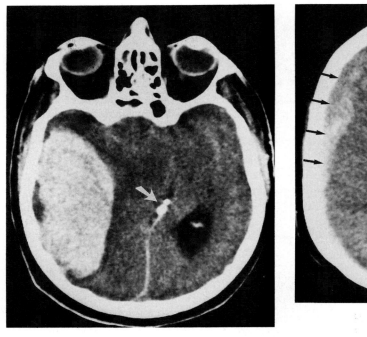

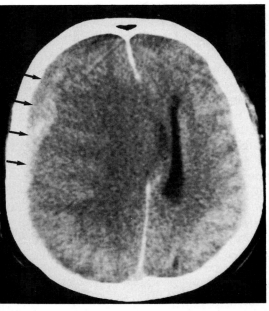

A                                    B

**Figure 7.10.** (A) Large right temporo-occipital ICH with effacement of basal cisterns and displacement of calcified pineal gland from right to left (arrow). (B) Upper cut with right frontal SDH (arrows), effacement of the right lateral ventricle, and shift of the midline to the left.

suggests a trend toward a higher risk of ICH by using the two agents together.

Other factors, such as local cerebrovascular lesions, may be important in the pathogenesis of rt-PA-related ICH. Preceding head trauma was a factor in two of the nine patients reported by Kase et al.,[151] but it was not mentioned in other reports.[101a,134,135,137,148–150] A preceding, "silent" embolic cerebral infarct is also a consideration, in view of the likelihood of this event in the setting of acute MI,[152] and the tendency of these infarcts to become hemorrhagic as part of their natural history.[118] However, this appears to be an unlikely explanation for most cases of rt-PA-related ICH. This complication has been reported in numerous instances in patients who have a low risk for brain embolism, in patients with inferior MI as often as in those with the high-embolic-risk anterior MI,[135,137,151] and in the absence of factors that are known to promote brain embolism after acute MI, such as atrial arrhythmias and congestive heart failure.[152] A more likely mechanism of ICH after rt-PA use for MI is the presence of concomitant angiopathies with bleeding potential, such as CAA. Its presence has been confirmed pathologically in patients with ICH after treatment with either rt-PA[153] or SK[101a,143] for acute MI. It is possible that this angiopathy, which is highly prevalent in the elderly and leads to superficial lobar ICH,[154,155] may be an important contributing factor in instances of rt-PA-related ICH in the elderly. This, in turn, calls for caution in the selection of this therapy for MI in elderly patients, especially those over age 70 who have dementia, as both conditions are associated with a high frequency of CAA.[154]

A systemic effect of rt-PA in the coagulation system also seems an unlikely explanation for the occurrence of ICH. The initial suggestion that a systemic fibrinolytic state contributes to the hemorrhagic complications of alteplase[148,156] has not been confirmed in subsequent studies.[134,137,145,151] Similarly, thrombocytopenia as a risk factor for ICH has not been documented.[134,135,137,151] An antiplatelet effect induced by rt-PA is supported by a delayed inhibition of platelet aggregation in vitro,[63] and prolongation of the bleeding time in rt-PA-treated patients.[157] Finally, the presence of elevated fibrin degradation products has been associated with an increased risk of ICH in two studies of alteplase[130,145] and one of duteplase[151] treatment of acute MI. These preliminary observations deserve further analysis in future trials of MI patients treated with fibrinolytic agents, in order to define an ICH risk profile, which in turn should result in improved patient selection and a decrease in the frequency of this complication of thrombolytic therapy.

*Fibrinolytics in the Treatment of Acute Ischemic Stroke*

The use of clot-dissolving agents is intuitively attractive for the treatment of acute thrombotic and embolic stroke, with the hope of producing early reperfusion of occluded cerebral arteries, thus salvaging brain tissue from irreversible ischemic infarction. Early attempts at treating patients with cerebral infarction with intravenous UK revealed no therapeutic benefit.[158] Furthermore, ICH occurred during the UK infusion or within twenty-four hours following it in four of the thirty-one patients treated, and it was fatal in three of them. Although unlikely, the possibility existed that those cases represented instances of ICH misdiagnosed as infarcts in that pre-CT study. However, autopsy examination of two of the ICH cases revealed ICH into areas of cerebral infarction caused by internal carotid artery occlusion,[159] suggesting that the initial clinical diagnosis of cerebral

infarction was correct. Based on its lack of therapeutic benefit and frequency of ICH, UK was abandoned as a treatment option in acute ischemic stroke. In recent years, a surge in new noninvasive methods of acute stroke diagnosis, thrombolytic administration techniques, and therapeutic agents has stimulated an interest in retesting these substances in patients with acute ischemic stroke.

In experimental stroke models of brain embolism, promising results have been obtained with rt-PA, resulting in clot lysis and reduction of neurological damage, without the occurrence of ICH.[160] This has led to the testing of UK, SK, and rt-PA in a number of pilot studies in acute stroke patients.[161] The intraarterial infusion of thrombolytic agents using superselective angiography catheters has shown adequate levels of arterial reperfusion, at times with concomitant clinical improvement and in the absence of an excessive risk of ICH. These studies have employed UK[162,163] or SK[163,164] in patients with vertebrobasilar occlusions, UK or SK in internal carotid artery occlusion,[165–167] and UK in middle cerebral artery (MCA) occlusion.[168] The rate of hemorrhagic complications has varied, with combined rates of hemorrhagic infarction and ICH between 9% and 25% of patients treated.[163,166–168] Analysis of the intracranial hemorrhagic complications in these trials shows that postfibrinolytic hemorrhagic transformation of the infarct (i.e., hemorrhagic infarction) is frequently asymptomatic and only detected by the routine performance of CT. ICH, on the other hand, is virtually always symptomatic and is often fatal. The frequency of hemorrhagic events, hemorrhagic infarction and ICH, was 14% (7% each) in a combined group of eighty-five patients treated with intraarterial thrombolytics for acute carotid and vertebrobasilar strokes from the literature.[161] The rate of reperfusion, partial or complete, of the occluded artery was 55% (47 of 85 patients), and clinical improvement correlated with reperfusion, but ICH did not.[161]

The recent increased interest in the use of the clot-specific rt-PA has resulted in two

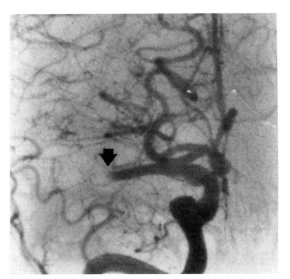

A

**Figure 7.11.** ICH after rt-PA treatment of acute right MCA occlusion (Courtesy of Michael S. Pessin, M.D., Tufts-New England Medical Center, Boston, MA). (A) Entry angiogram showing cut-off of the MCA stem by presumed acute embolic occlusion (arrow). Following a one-hour intravenous infusion of duteplase, the patient complained of headache during the post-rt-PA angiogram, which showed progressive extravasation of contrast medium from a lenticulostriate branch of the MCA (arrow), without significant recanalization of the MCA stem (B and C). Her condition rapidly deteriorated to coma with bilateral decerebrate rigidity of the limbs and dilated and unreactive pupils, and CT scan documented massive deep right ICH with ventricular extension (D and E).

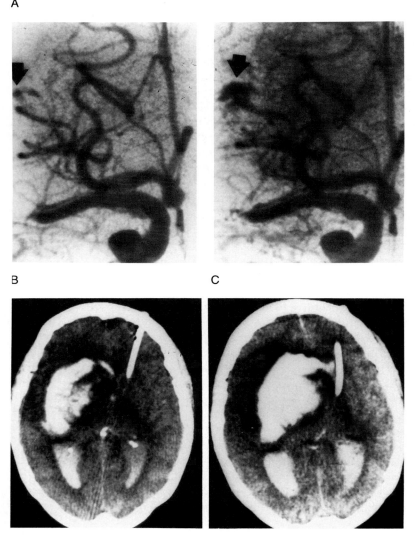

B    C

D    E

pilot studies of its intravenous administration in patients with acute ischemic stroke.[169,169a,170] Although their design varied in a number of probably significant ways, both studies enrolled a large number of patients (N = 74 in Brott et al.'s[169] study and N = 20 in Haley et al.'s study[169a], N = 93 in del Zoppo et al.'s[170] study) who were treated with intravenous rt-PA within ninety minutes[169] and between 91 and 180 minutes[169a] of stroke onset in one study, and within eight hours from stroke onset in the other.[170] The rate of reperfusion in the angiography-based study of del Zoppo et al.[170] was a disappointing 26.1% for MCA stem occlusions and 38.1% for MCA branch occlusions. Hemorrhagic events with clinical neurological deterioration occurred in 9.6% of the patients (Figure 7.11). In the nonangiographic study of Brott et al.[169] there was a 4% rate of ICH after rt-PA use within ninety minutes from stroke onset, and this complication was dose related, as all three patients who developed ICH had received a dose of 0.95 mg per kg, and no instances of ICH occurred in 48 patients treated with less than 0.95 mg per kg of rt-PA. Neurologic improvement was observed within two hours of treatment in 22 patients (30%), and 34 patients (46%) were improved 24 hours after treatment. Using a similar study design, but with onset of rt-PA treatment between 91 and 180 minutes from stroke onset, Haley et al.[169a] observed a low rate of 15% of clinical improvement after 24 hours of rt-PA treatment, with an alarming rate of 17% of ICH among 12 patients treated with the higher rt-PA doses (0.85 mg per kg and 0.95 mg per kg, six patients each). In a group of 32 patients with angiographically proven acute MCA occlusions, von Kummer and Hacke[169b] used intravenous rt-PA (alteplase) at the recommended dose for coronary thrombolysis (100 mg), in combination with intravenous heparin, the latter given to prevent arterial reocclusion. Patients were treated within six hours from stroke onset. The authors observed a rate of recanalization (assessed by either angiography or transcranial Doppler testing) of 34% (11 pa-

tients) immediately after the completion of rt-PA infusion, and 53% (17 patients) on assessment of MCA patency 12 to 24 hours after treatment. Fatal ICH occurred in three patients (9%).

The risk factors for ICH in acute ischemic stroke treated with rt-PA are still poorly understood. Preliminary observations suggest that delaying the onset of treatment beyond six hours from stroke onset may significantly increase the frequency of ICH.[171] It is possible that the safety of rt-PA in acute ischemic stroke closely depends on the timing of its use after stroke onset. This drug may be a feasible option only for patients presenting within a very short time after stroke onset. Other factors potentially related to the efficacy and safety of thrombolytic therapy include the dose of medication given, its route of administration (intravenous vs. intraarterial), the site of arterial occlusion (extracranial vs. intracranial, MCA stem vs. branch), and efficiency of collateral flow into the area of ischemia. The ultimate value and potential role of thrombolysis in acute stroke therapy will depend on its increased safety (i.e., lower rate of intracranial hemorrhagic complications), with better rates of arterial reperfusion and clinical improvement than those that have so far been observed in clinical trials.

## References

1. Kerr CB. Intracranial haemorrhage in haemophilia. J Neurol Neurosurg Psychiat 1964; 27:166–173.
2. McCormick WF, Rosenfield DB. Massive brain hemorrhage: a review of 144 cases and an examination of their causes. Stroke 1973;4: 946–954.
3. Omae T, Ueda K, Ogata J, et al. Parenchymatous hemorrhage: etiology, pathology and clinical aspects. In Vinken PJ, Bruyn GW, Klawans HL, eds. Handbook of clinical neurology. New York: Elsevier Science, 1989;287–331.
4. Schütz H. Spontane intrazerebrale Hämatome: pathophysiologie, klinik und therapie. Heidelberg: Springer-Verlag, 1988.

5. Jellinger K. Zur Ätiologie und Pathogenese der spontanen intrazerebralen Blutung. Therapiewoche 1972;22:1440–1450.

6. Mutlu N, Berry RG, Alpers BJ. Massive cerebral hemorrhage: clinical and pathological correlations. Arch Neurol 1963;8:644–661.

7. Russell DS. The pathology of spontaneous intracranial haemorrhage. Proc Roy Soc Med 1954;47:689–693.

8. del Zoppo GJ, Mori E. Hematologic causes of intracerebral hemorrhage and their treatment. Neurosurg Clin NA 1992;3:637–658.

9. Martinowitz U, Heim M, Tadmor R, et al. Intracranial hemorrhage in patients with hemophilia. Neurosurgery 1986;18:538–541.

10. Eyster ME, Gill FM, Blatt PM, et al. Central nervous system bleeding in hemophiliacs. Blood 1978;51:1179–1188.

11. Silverstein A. Intracranial bleeding in hemophilia. Arch Neurol 1960;3:141–157.

12. Pettersson H, McClure P, Fitz C. Intracranial hemorrhage in hemophilic children: CT follow-up. Acta Radiol (Diagn) 1984;25:161–164.

13. Bloom AL. Inherited disorders of blood coagulation. In Bloom AL, Thomas DP, eds. Haemostasis and thrombosis. New York: Churchill Livingstone, 1981;321–370.

14. Rice ML. Acute subdural haematoma associated with von Willebrand's disease: a case report. Aust NZ J Surg 1982;52:86–88.

15. Mizoi K, Onuma T, Mori K. Intracranial hemorrhage secondary to von Willebrand's disease and trauma. Surg Neurol 1984;22:495–498.

16. Almaani WS, Awidi AS. Spontaneous intracranial hemorrhage secondary to von Willebrand's disease. Surg Neurol 1986;26:457–460.

17. Natowicz M, Kelley RI. Mendelian etiologies of stroke. Ann Neurol 1987;22:175–192.

18. Almaani WS, Awidi AS. Spontaneous intracranial bleeding in hemorrhagic diathesis. Surg Neurol 1982;17:137–140.

19. Montgomery R, Natelson SE. Afibrinogenemia with intracerebral hematoma: report of a successfully treated case. Am J Dis Child 1977;131:555–556.

20. Silverstein A. Intracranial hemorrhage in patients with bleeding tendencies. Neurology 1961;11:310–317.

21. McMillan R. Chronic idiopathic thrombocytopenic purpura. N Engl J Med 1981;304:1135–1147.

22. Brenner B, Guilburd JN, Tatarsky I, et al. Spontaneous intracranial hemorrhage in immune thrombocytopenic purpura. Neurosurgery 1988;22:761–764.

23. Novak R, Wilimas J. Plasmapheresis in catastrophic complications of idiopathic thrombocytopenic purpura. J Pediatr 1978;92:434–436.

24. Awerbuch G, Sandyk R. Intracranial haemorrhage in a 26-year-old woman with idiopathic thrombocytopenic purpura. Postgrad Med J 1987;63:781–783.

25. Goodnight SH. Bleeding and intravascular clotting in malignancy: a review. Ann NY Acad Sci 1974;230:271–288.

26. Mant MJ, King EG. Severe, acute disseminated intravascular coagulation: a reappraisal of its pathophysiology, clinical significance and therapy based on 47 patients. Am J Med 1979;67:557–563.

27. Schwartzman RJ, Hill JB. Neurologic complications of disseminated intravascular coagulation. Neurology 1982;32:791–797.

28. Kawakami Y, Ueki K, Chikama M, et al. Intracranial hemorrhage associated with nontraumatic disseminated intravascular coagulation: report of four cases. Neurol Med Chir 1990;30:610–617.

29. Kaufman HH, Moake JL, Olson JD, et al. Delayed and recurrent intracranial hematomas related to disseminated intravascular clotting and fibrinolysis in head injury. Neurosurgery 1980;7:445–449.

30. Graus F, Rogers LR, Posner JB. Cerebrovascular complications in patients with cancer. Medicine 1985;64:16–35.

31. Jaap van der Sande J, Veltkamp JJ, Boekhout-Mussert RJ, et al. Head injury and coagulation disorders. J Neurosurg 1978;49:357–365.

32. Byrnes JJ. Thrombotic thrombocytopenic purpura. In Kassirer JP, ed. Current therapy in internal medicine. Philadelphia: B. C. Decker, 1991;891–893.

33. Burstein SA, Harker LA. Quantitative platelet disorders. In Bloom AL, Thomas DP eds. Haemostasis and thrombosis. New York: Churchill Livingstone, 1981;279–300.

34. Bell WR, Royall RM. Heparin-associated thrombocytopenia: a comparison of three heparin preparations. N Engl J Med 1980;303:902–907.

35. Becker PS, Miller VT. Heparin-induced thrombocytopenia. Stroke 1989;20:1449–1459.

36. King DJ, Kelton JG. Heparin-associated thrombocytopenia. Ann Intern Med 1984;100:535–540.

37. Glass JT, Williams JP, Mankad VN, et al. Intracranial hemorrhage associated with quinidine induced thrombocytopenia. Ala Med 1989;59:21–25.

38. Groch SN, Sayre GP, Heck FJ. Cerebral hemorrhage in leukemia. Arch Neurol 1960;2: 439–451.

39. Fritz RD, Forkner CE, Freireich EJ, et al. The association of fatal intracranial hemorrhage and "blastic crisis" in patients with acute leukemia. N Engl J Med 1959;261:59–64.

40. Hillestad LK. Acute promyelocytic leukemia. Acta Med Scand 1957;159:189–194.

41. Gunz FW. Hemorrhagic thrombocythemia: a critical review. Blood 1960;15:706–723.

42. Jabaily J, Iland HJ, Laszlo J, et al. Neurologic manifestations of essential thrombocythemia. Ann Intern Med 1983;99:513–518.

43. Delangre T, Mihout B, Borh J-Y, et al. Primary thrombocythemia in a patient with cerebellar infarction. Stroke 1985;16:524–526.

44. Kase CS, Williams JP, Wyatt DA, et al. Lobar intracerebral hematomas: clinical and CT analysis of 22 cases. Neurology 1982;32:1146–1150.

45. Korenman G. Neurologic syndromes associated with primary thrombocythemia. J Mt Sinai Hosp 1969;36:317–323.

46. Fritz E, Ludwig H, Scheithauer W, et al. Shortened platelet half-life in multiple myeloma. Blood 1986;68:514–520.

47. DiMinno G, Coraggio F, Cerbone AM, et al. A myeloma paraprotein with specificity for platelet glycoprotein IIIa in a patient with a fatal bleeding disorder. J Clin Invest 1986; 77:157–164.

48. Niléhn J-E, Nilsson IM. Coagulation studies in different types of myeloma. Acta Med Scand 1966;179(suppl 445):194–199.

49. Vane RJ. Inhibition of prostaglandin synthesis as a mechanism of action for aspirin-like drugs. Nature 1971:231:232–235.

50. Preston FE, Whipps S, Jackson CA, et al. Inhibition of prostacyclin and platelet thromboxane $A_2$ after low-dose aspirin. N Engl J Med 1981;304:76–79.

51. Bousser MG, Eschwege E, Haguenau M, et al. "AICLA" controlled trial of aspirin and dipyridamole in the secondary prevention of athero-thrombotic cerebral ischemia. Stroke 1983;14:5–14.

52. The American-Canadian Co-Operative Study Group. Persantine aspirin trial in cerebral ischemia. Part II: endpoint results. Stroke 1985;16:406–415.

53. The ESPS Group. The European Stroke Prevention Study (ESPS): principal end-points. Lancet 1987;2:1351–1354.

54. Swedish Cooperative Study. High-dose acetylsalicylic acid after cerebral infarction. Stroke 1987;18:325–334.

55. Peto R, Gray R, Collins R, et al. Randomised trial of prophylactic daily aspirin in British male doctors. Br Med J 1988;296:313–316.

56. Petersen P, Boysen G, Godtfredsen J, et al. Placebo-controlled, randomised trial of warfarin and aspirin for prevention of thromboembolic complications in chronic atrial fibrillation: the Copenhagen AFASAK study. Lancet 1989;1:175–179.

57. Stroke Prevention in Atrial Fibrillation Study Group Investigators. Preliminary report of the stroke prevention in atrial fibrillation study. N Engl J Med 1990;322:863–868.

58. The Dutch TIA Trial Study Group. A comparison of two doses of aspirin (30 mg vs. 283 mg a day) in patients after a transient ischemic attack or minor ischemic stroke. N Engl J Med 1991;325:1261–1266.

59. UK-TIA Study Group. United Kingdom transient ischaemic attack (UK-TIA) aspirin trial: interim results. Br Med J 1988;296:316–320.

60. Steering Committee of the Physicians' Health Study Research Group. Final report on the aspirin component of the ongoing Physicians' Health Study. N Engl J Med 1989;321:129–135.

61. Taylor DW, Barnett HJM. Letter to the editor. N Engl J Med 1989;321:1827.

62. The SALT Collaborative Group. Swedish Aspirin Low-dose Trial (SALT) of 75 mg aspirin as secondary prophylaxis after cerebrovascular ischaemic events. Lancet 1991;338:1345–1349.

63. Coller BS. Platelets and thrombolytic therapy. N Engl J Med 1990;322:33–42.

64. Gent M, Blakely JA, Easton JD, et al. The Canadian American Ticlopidine Study (CATS) in thromboembolic stroke. Lancet 1989;1:1215–1220.

65. Hass WK, Easton JD, Adams HP, et al. A randomized trial comparing ticlopidine hydrochloride with aspirin for the prevention of stroke in high-risk patients. N Engl J Med 1989;321:501–507.

66. Hirsh J. Oral anticoagulant drugs. N Engl J Med 1991;324:1865–1875.

67. Levine MN, Raskob G, Hirsh J. Risk of haemorrhage associated with long term anticoagulant therapy. Drugs 1985;30:444–460.

68. Hirsh J, Levine MN. The optimal intensity of oral anticoagulant therapy. JAMA 1987;258: 2723–2726.

69. Hirsh J, Poller L, Deykin D, et al. Optimal therapeutic range for oral anticoagulants. Chest 1989;95(Suppl):5S–11S.

70. Bussey HI, Force RW, Bianco TM, et al. Reliance on prothrombin time ratios causes significant errors in anticoagulation therapy. Arch Intern Med 1992;152:278–282.

71. Hirsh J. Substandard monitoring of warfarin in North America: time for change. Arch Intern Med 1992;152:257–258 (editorial).

72. Petty GW, Lennihan L, Mohr JP, et al. Complications of long-term anticoagulation. Ann Neurol 1988;23:570–574.

73. Coon WW, Willis PW. Hemorrhagic complications of anticoagulant therapy. Arch Intern Med 1974;133:386–392.

74. Wintzen AR, deJonge H, Loeliger EA, et al. The risk of intracerebral hemorrhage during oral anticoagulant treatment: a population study. Ann Neurol 1984;16:553–558.

75. Errichetti AM, Holden A, Ansell J. Management of oral anticoagulant therapy: experience with an anticoagulant clinic. Arch Intern Med 1984;144:1966–1968.

76. Forfar JC. A 7-year analysis of haemorrhage in patients on long-term anticoagulant treatment. Br Heart J 1979;42:128–132.

77. Silverstein A. Neurological complications of anticoagulation therapy; a neurologist's review. Arch Intern Med 1979;139:217–220.

78. Duff IF, Shull WH. Fatal hemorrhage in dicumarol poisoning: with report of necropsy. JAMA 1949;139:762–766.

79. Russek HI, Zohman BL. Anticoagulant therapy in acute myocardial infarction: a survey of specialists' opinions concerning indications, results and dangers. Am J Med Sci 1953; 225:8–13.

80. Riddick FA. Long-term anticoagulant therapy in an outpatient department: techniques and complications. J Chronic Dis 1960;12:622–638.

81. Askey JM. Hemorrhage during long-term anticoagulant drug therapy: Part 1: intracranial hemorrhage. Calif Med 1966;104:6–10.

82. Whisnant JP, Cartlidge NEF, Elveback LR. Carotid and vertebral-basilar transient ischemic attacks: effect of anticoagulants, hypertension, and cardiac disorders on survival and stroke occurrence—a population study. Ann Neurol 1978;3:107–115.

83. Franke CL, de Jonge J, van Swieten JC, et al. Intracerebral hematomas during anticoagulant treatment. Stroke 1990;21:726–730.

84. Barron KD, Fergusson G. Intracranial hemorrhage as a complication of anticoagulant therapy. Neurology 1959;9:447–455.

85. So W, Hugenholtz H, Richard MT. Complications of anticoagulant therapy in patients with known central nervous system lesions. Can J Surg 1983;26:181–183.

86. Apuzzo MLJ, Davey LM, Manuelidis EE. Pineal apoplexy associated with anticoagulant therapy: case report. J Neurosurg 1976;45: 223–225.

87. Kase CS, Robinson RK, Stein RW, et al. Anticoagulant-related intracerebral hemorrhage. Neurology 1985;35:943–948.

88. Rådberg JA, Olsson JE, Råådberg CT. Prognostic parameters in spontaneous intracerebral hematomas with special reference to anticoagulant treatment. Stroke 1991;22:571–576.

89. Lodder J, Krijne-Kubat B, van der Lugt PMJ. Timing of autopsy-confirmed hemorrhagic infarction with reference to cardioembolic stroke. Stroke 1988;19:1482–1484.

90. Okada Y, Yamaguchi T, Minematsu K, et al. Hemorrhagic transformation in cerebral embolism. Stroke 1989;20:598–603.

91. Lieberman A, Hass WK, Pinto R, et al. Intracranial hemorrhage and infarction in anticoagulated patients with prosthetic heart valves. Stroke 1978;9:18–24.

92. Nagano N, Tabata H, Hashimoto K. Anticoagulant-related intracerebral hemorrhage in patients with prosthetic heart valves: report of two cases. Neurol Med Chir 1991;31:743–745.

93. Tuhrim S, Dambrosia JM, Price TR, et al. Prediction of intracerebral hemorrhage survival. Ann Neurol 1988;24:258–263.

94. Dooley DM, Perlmutter I. Spontaneous intracranial hematomas in patients receiving anticoagulation therapy: surgical treatment. JAMA 1964;187:396–398.

95. Nassar SI, Khouri S, Afifi AK. Successfully treated acute intracerebellar hemorrhage secondary to anticoagulant therapy: case report. Leb Med J 1972;25:215–219.

96. Finney LA, Gholston D. Cerebral aneurysm rupture during anticoagulant therapy with survival. JAMA 1967;200:1127–1128.

97. Kanoff RB, Ruberg RL. Bilateral spontaneous intracerebral hematomas following anticoagu-

lation therapy: report of case with recovery following surgery. J Amer Osteopathic Assoc 1979;79:174–178.

98. Furlan AJ, Whisnant JP, Elveback LR. The decreasing incidence of primary intracerebral hemorrhage: a population study. Ann Neurol 1979;5:367–373.

99. Kase CS, Caplan LR. Hemorrhage affecting the brain stem and cerebellum. In Barnett HJM, et al., eds. Stroke: pathophysiology, diagnosis, and management. New York: Churchill-Livingstone, 1986;621–641.

100. Livoni JP, McGahan JP. Intracranial fluid-blood levels in the anticoagulated patient. Neuroradiology 1983;25:335–337.

101. Weisberg LA. Significance of the fluid-blood interface in intracranial hematomas in anticoagulated patients. Comput Radiol 1987;11:175–179.

101a. Wijdicks EFM, Jack CR. Intracerebral hemorrhage after fibrinolytic therapy for acute myocardial infarction. Stroke 1993;24:554–557.

102. Zilkha A. Intraparenchymal fluid-blood level: a CT sign of recent intracerebral hemorrhage. J Comp Assist Tomogr 1983;7:301–305.

103. Hirsh J. Heparin. N Engl J Med 1991;324:1565–1574.

104. Morabia A. Heparin doses and major bleedings. Lancet 1986;1:1278–1279 (letter).

105. Landefeld CS, Cook EF, Flatley M, et al. Identification and preliminary validation of predictors of major bleeding in hospitalized patients starting anticoagulant therapy. Am J Med 1987;82:703–713.

106. Walker AM, Jick H. Predictors of bleeding during heparin therapy. JAMA 1980;244:1209–1212.

107. Carleton RA, Sanders CA, Burack WR. Heparin administration after acute myocardial infarction. N Engl J Med 1960;263:1002–1005.

108. Wasserman AJ, Gutterman LA, Yoe KB, et al. Anticoagulants in acute myocardial infarction: the failure of anticoagulants to alter mortality in a randomized series. Am Heart J 1966;71:43–49.

109. The Working Party on Anticoagulant Therapy in Coronary Thrombosis. Assessment of short-term anticoagulant administration after cardiac infarction. Br Med J 1969;1:335–342.

110. Drapkin A, Merskey C. Anticoagulant therapy after acute myocardial infarction: relation of therapeutic benefit to patient's age, sex, and severity of infarction. JAMA 1972;222:541–548.

111. Handley AJ, Emerson PA, Fleming PR. Heparin in the prevention of deep vein thrombosis after myocardial infarction. Br Med J 1972;2:436–438.

112. Holzman D, Paraskos JA, Lyon AF, et al. Anticoagulants in acute myocardial infarction: results of a cooperative clinical trial. JAMA 1973;225:724–729.

113. Wilcox RG, von der Lippe G, Olsson CG, et al. Trial of tissue plasminogen activator for mortality reduction in acute myocardial infarction: Anglo-Scandinavian Study of Early Thrombolysis (ASSET). Lancet 1988;2:525–530.

114. Keith DS, Phillips SJ, Whisnant JP, et al. Heparin therapy for recent transient focal cerebral ischemia. Mayo Clin Proc 1987;62:1101–1106.

115. Ramirez-Lassepas M, Quinones MR. Heparin therapy for stroke: hemorrhagic complications and risk factors for intracerebral hemorrhage. Neurology 1984;34:114–117.

116. Jonas S. Anticoagulant therapy in cerebrovascular disease: review and meta-analysis. Stroke 1988;19:1043–1048.

117. Gordon DL, Linhardt R, Adams HP. Low-molecular-weight heparins and heparinoids and their use in acute or progressing ischemic stroke. Clin Neuropharmacol 1990;13:522–543.

118. Fisher M, Adams RD. Observations on brain embolism with special reference to the mechanism of hemorrhagic infarction. J Neuropathol Exp Neurol 1951;10:92–93.

119. Furlan AJ, Cavalier SJ, Hobbs RE, et al. Hemorrhage and anticoagulation after nonseptic embolic brain infarction. Neurology 1982;32:280–282.

120. Koller RL. Recurrent embolic cerebral infarction and anticoagulation. Neurology 1982;32:283–285.

121. Drake ME, Shin C. Conversion of ischemic to hemorrhagic infarction by anticoagulant administration: report of two cases with evidence from serial computed tomographic brain scans. Arch Neurol 1983;40:44–46.

122. Cerebral Embolism Study Group. Immediate anticoagulation of embolic stroke: a randomized trial. Stroke 1983;14:668–676.

123. Cerebral Embolism Study Group. Immediate anticoagulation of embolic stroke: brain hem-

orrhage and management options. Stroke 1984;15:779–789.

124. Cerebral Embolism Study Group. Cardioembolic stroke, early anticoagulation, and brain hemorrhage. Arch Intern Med 1987;147:626–640.

125. Yatsu FM, Hart RG, Mohr JP, et al. Anticoagulation of embolic strokes of cardiac origin: an update. Neurology 1988;38:314–316.

126. Rothrock JF, Dittrich HC, McAllen S, et al. Acute anticoagulation following cardioembolic stroke. Stroke 1989;20:730–734.

127. Babikian VL, Kase CS, Pessin MS, et al. Intracerebral hemorrhage in stroke patients anticoagulated with heparin. Stroke 1989;20:1500–1503.

128. Sharma GVRK, Cella G, Parisi AF, et al. Thrombolytic therapy. N Engl J Med 1982;306:1268–1276.

129. Verstraete M, Collen D. Thrombolytic therapy in the eighties. Blood 1986;67:1529–1541.

130. Mueller HS, Rao AK, Forman SA. Thrombolysis in myocardial infarction (TIMI): comparative studies of coronary reperfusion and systemic fibrinogenolysis with two forms of recombinant tissue-type plasminogen activator. J Am Coll Cardiol 1987;10:479–490.

131. Bates ER, Topol EJ. Thrombolytic therapy for acute myocardial infarction. Chest 1989 (supplement);95:257S–264S.

132. Guerci AD, Gerstenblith G, Brinker JA, et al. A randomized trial of intravenous tissue plasminogen activator for acute myocardial infarction with subsequent randomization to elective coronary angioplasty. N Engl J Med 1987;317:1613–1618.

133. O'Rourke M, Baron D, Keogh A, et al. Limitation of myocardial infarction by early infusion of recombinant tissue-type plasminogen activator. Circulation 1988;77:1311–1315.

134. Gore JM, Sloan M, Price TR, et al. Intracerebral hemorrhage, cerebral infarction, and subdural hematoma after acute myocardial infarction and thrombolytic therapy in the thrombolysis in myocardial infarction study: thrombolysis in myocardial infarction, phase II, pilot and clinical trial. Circulation 1991;83:448–459.

134a. Longstreth WT, Litwin PE, Weaver WD, and the MITI Project Group. Myocardial infarction, thrombolytic therapy, and stroke: a community-based study. Stroke 1993;24:587–590.

135. Blard JM, Vastene M, Labauge R, et al. Hémorragies du système nerveux central après fibrinolyse thérapeutique: 11 cas. Rev Neurol 1992;148:256–261.

136. Urban P, Reynard C, Meier B. Thrombolysis and risk of intracranial bleeding. Lancet 1992;339:817 (letter).

137. Kase CS, O'Neal AM, Fisher M, et al. Intracranial hemorrhage after use of tissue plasminogen activator for coronary thrombolysis. Ann Intern Med 1990;112:17–21.

138. Gruppo Italiano per lo Studio della Streptochinasi nell'Infarto Miocardico (GISSI). Effectiveness of intravenous thrombolytic treatment in acute myocardial infarction. Lancet 1986;1:397–402.

139. Loscalzo J, Braunwald E. Tissue plasminogen activator. N Engl J Med 1988;319:925–931.

140. Aldrich MS, Sherman SA, Greenberg HG. Cerebrovascular complications of streptokinase infusion. JAMA 1985;253:1777–1779.

141. Thrombolytic therapy in thrombosis: a National Institutes of Health Consensus Development Conference. Ann Intern Med 1980;93:141–144.

142. Gorelick PB, Parikh M, McDonald L. Intracoronary streptokinase and fatal cerebellar hemorrhage. Ill Med Journal 1987;171:28–30.

143. Ramsay DA, Penswich JL, Robertson DM. Fatal streptokinase-induced intracerebral haemorrhage in cerebral amyloid angiopathy. Can J Neurol Sci 1990;17:336–341.

144. Chesebro JH, Knatterud G, Roberts R, et al. Thrombolysis in Myocardial Infarction (TIMI) trial, phase I: a comparison between intravenous tissue plasminogen activator and intravenous streptokinase. Circulation 1987;76:142–154.

145. Rao AK, Pratt C, Berke A, et al. Thrombolysis in Myocardial Infarction (TIMI) trial, phase I: hemorrhagic manifestations and changes in plasma fibrinogen and the fibrinolytic system in patients treated with recombinant tissue plasminogen activator and streptokinase. J Am Coll Cardiol 1988;11:1–11.

146. The TIMI Study Group. Comparison of invasive and conservative strategies after treatment with intravenous tissue plasminogen activator in acute myocardial infarction: results of the Thrombolysis in Myocardial Infarction (TIMI) Phase II Trial. N Engl J Med 1989;320:618–627.

147. Linnik W, Tintinalli JE, Ramos R. Associated reactions during and immediately after rtPA infusion. Ann Emerg Med 1989;18:234–239.

148. Carlson SE, Aldrich MS, Greenberg HS, et al. Intracerebral hemorrhage complicating intravenous tissue plasminogen activator treatment. Arch Neurol 1988;45:1070–1073.

149. O'Connor CM, Aldrich H, Massey EW, et al. Intracranial hemorrhage after thrombolytic therapy for acute myocardial infarction: clinical characteristics and in-hospital outcome. J Am Coll Cardiol 1990;15:213A (abstract).

150. O'Connor CM, Aldrich H, Uglietta J, et al. Risk factor profile of patients with intracranial hemorrhage after thrombolytic therapy for acute myocardial infarction. Neurology 1990;40 (Suppl 1):192 (abstract).

151. Kase CS, Pessin MS, Zivin JA, et al. Intracranial hemorrhage after coronary thrombolysis with tissue plasminogen activator. Am J Med 1992;92:384–390.

152. Komrad MS, Coffey CE, Coffey KS, et al. Myocardial infarction and stroke. Neurology 1984;34:1403–1409.

153. Pendlebury WW, Iole ED, Tracy RP, et al. Intracerebral hemorrhage related to cerebral amyloid angiopathy and t-PA treatment. Ann Neruol 1991;29:210–213.

154. Vinters HV. Cerebral amyloid angiopathy: a critical review. Stroke 1987;18:311–324.

155. Kase CS. Intracerebral hemorrhage: non-hypertensive causes. Stroke 1986;17:590–595.

156. Marder VJ, Sherry S. Thrombolytic therapy: current status. N Engl J Med 1988;318:1512–1520, 1585–1595.

157. Gimple LW, Gold HK, Leinbach RC, et al. Correlation between template bleeding times and spontaneous bleeding during treatment of acute myocardial infarction with recombinant tissue-type plasminogen activator. Circulation 1989;80:581–588.

158. Fletcher AP, Alkjaersig N, Lewis M, et al. A pilot study of urokinase therapy in cerebral infarction. Stroke 1976;7:135–142.

159. Hanaway J, Torack R, Fletcher AP, et al. Intracranial bleeding associated with urokinase therapy for acute ischemic hemispheral stroke. Stroke 1976;7:143–146.

160. Zivin JA, Fisher M, DeGirolami U, et al. Tissue plasminogen activator reduces neurological damage after cerebral embolism. Science 1985;230:1289–1292.

161. Pessin MS, del Zoppo GJ, Estol CJ. Thrombolytic agents in the treatment of stroke. Clin Neuropharmacol 1990;13:271–289.

162. Zeumer H, Freitag H-J, Grzyska U, et al. Local intraarterial fibrinolysis in acute vertebrobasilar occlusion: technical developments and recent results. Neuroradiology 1989;31:336–340.

163. Hacke W, Zeumer H, Ferbert A, et al. Intra-arterial thrombolytic therapy improves outcome in patients with acute vertebrobasilar occlusive disease. Stroke 1988;19:1216–1222.

164. Zeumer H, Hacke W, Ringelstein EB. Local intraarterial thrombolysis in vertebrobasilar thromboembolic disease. Am J Neuroradiol 1983;4:401–404.

165. Zeumer H, Hündgen R, Ferbert A, et al. Local intraarterial fibrinolytic therapy in inaccessible internal carotid occlusion. Neuroradiology 1984;26:315–317.

166. Theron J, Courtheoux P, Casasco A, et al. Local intraarterial fibrinolysis in the carotid territory. Am J Neuroradiol 1989;10:753–765.

167. del Zoppo GJ, Ferbert A, Otis S, et al. Local intra-arterial fibrinolytic therapy in acute carotid territory stroke: a pilot study. Stroke 1988;19:307–313.

168. Mori E, Tabuchi M, Yoshida T, et al. Intracarotid urokinase with thromboembolic occlusion of the middle cerebral artery. Stroke 1988;19:802–812.

169. Brott TG, Haley EC, Levy DE, et al. Urgent therapy for stroke: Part I. Pilot study of tissue plasminogen activator administered within 90 minutes. Stroke 1992;23:632–640.

169a. Haley EC, Levy DE, Brott TG, et al. Urgent therapy for stroke: Part II. Pilot study of tissue plasminogen activator administered 91-180 minutes from onset. Stroke 1992;23:641–645.

169b. von Kummer R, Hacke W. Safety and efficacy of intravenous tissue plasminogen activator and heparin in acute middle cerebral artery stroke. Stroke 1992;23:646–652.

170. del Zoppo GJ, Poeck K, Pessin MS, et al. Recombinant tissue plasminogen activator in acute thrombotic and embolic stroke. Ann Neurol 1992;32:78–86.

171. Wolpert SM. Predictive factors for the effective treatment of acute stroke with intravenous thrombolytic agents. In Hacke W, et al., eds. Thrombolytic therapy in acute ischemic stroke. New York: Springer-Verlag, 1991;87–90.

# Chapter 8
# Aneurysms and Vascular Malformations

## Carlos S. Kase

Vascular malformations represent an important cause of intracerebral hemorrhage (ICH); in a series of 1214 autopsy cases of ICH from the reports reviewed by Jellinger,[1] 6.9% were caused by a ruptured aneurysm and 3.4% by a ruptured "angioma". In clinical series, among a total of 1145 cases of ICH collected from the literature, 22.1% were due to ruptured aneurysms and 18.6% to ruptured arteriovenous malformations (AVM).[1] On the other hand, such lesions (in particular, "angiomas") are relatively common incidental findings at autopsy: in a series of 4069 consecutive autopsies, Sarwar and McCormick[2] found angiomas in 165 brains (4%), which contained a total of 177 malformations. Their histological type and frequency are shown in Table 8.1.

## Classification of Vascular Malformations

Although there is still controversy about their origin, cerebral "saccular" or "berry" *aneurysms* are considered to be largely acquired lesions.[3] They are thought to originate in developmental gaps in the smooth muscle media at points of bifurcation.[4] Their tendency to usually become symptomatic by rupture in adulthood or as a result of slow and progressive increase in size with degen-

**Table 8.1.** Types of Angiomas Incidentally Found at Autopsy

| Type of Angioma | No. Cases (%) |
| --- | --- |
| Venous angioma | 105 (59%) |
| Telangiectasis | 28 (16%) |
| Arteriovenous malformation | 24 (14%) |
| Cavernous angioma | 16 (9%) |
| Varix | 4 (2%) |
| Total: | 177 |

(From Sarwar M, McCormick WF. Intracerebral venous angioma: case report and review. Arch Neurol 1978;35:323–325. With permission of the publisher.)

eration of their wall, makes these lesions truly acquired, at least in regard to their clinically relevant behavior. Vascular malformations or *angiomas*, which are the result of abnormal vascular embryogenesis, are congenital lesions that have the potential for becoming symptomatic through either rupture or progressive growth at a generally earlier age than cerebral aneurysms. These lesions are classified as AVM, cavernous angiomas, venous angiomas, or telangiectases, depending on their histological characters.[5] AVM are composed of a dense conglomerate of abnormal blood vessels, some of which have either arterial or venous histological features, while others correspond to abnormally dilated channels without a defined wall structure

(Figure 8.1). The latter connect the arterial and venous portions of the malformation, establishing abnormal, high-flow shunting of blood from arteries into dilated veins, without an intermediate capillary bed. This high-pressure, high-flow system promotes progressive enlargement of the abnormal vascular channels, as well as their tendency for sudden rupture causing acute hemorrhagic strokes. These lesions are most commonly located on the surface of the brain, in a subpial position ("pial" AVM), whereas less frequent varieties are located intradurally ("dural" AVM). Cavernous angiomas consist of masses of large sinusoidal vascular channels which do not have arterial or venous structure, but rather have thin, elementary walls that have a single layer of endothelial cells and contain connective tissue without muscular or elastic elements (Figure 8.2A). The vascular channels tend to become densely aggregated, thus leaving no cerebral parenchyma in between them, but rather being separated by loose, amorphous tissue which frequently contains remnants of local hemorrhage (hemosiderin-laden macrophages) (Fig. 8.2B). These bleeding sites frequently appear at various stages of evolution, reflecting the tendency to repeated episodes of hemorrhage that characterize this malformation. Other changes in these malformations include calcium and cholesterol deposition, and thrombosis of the abnormal vascular channels (see Figure 8.2A). Venous angiomas consist of aggregates of dilated venous channels in an area of the brain, generally adopting histologically the form of loosely arranged veins (with abundant normal brain parenchyma in between them) that drain into a larger venous channel that, in turn, is connected with one of the dural sinuses. This lesion is not associated with abnormal artery-to-vein shunting of blood, and it can coexist with one or several cavernous angiomas in its close vicinity. Telangiectases, also referred to as "capillary" telangiectases, are thought to represent abnormally dilated vessels of capillary structure, with connective tissue walls without muscular or elastic elements, and a single layer of endothelial cells. Telangiectases are separated by wide areas of normal brain parenchyma (Figure 8.3). Their site of predilection is the pons.[5] They are not generally associated with risk of ICH, unless they coexist with a cavernous angioma, when the latter, and not the telangiectases, has been the documented lesion responsible for bleeding.[6]

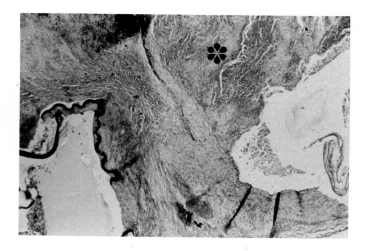

**Figure 8.1.** Microscopic section of cerebral AVM showing an arterial vessel with prominent internal elastic lamina (left lower corner) adjacent to a large vascular channel without defined histological character of its wall (right), next to an area of recent hemorrhage (asterisk) within the malformation. (Elastic-van Gieson, ×100.)

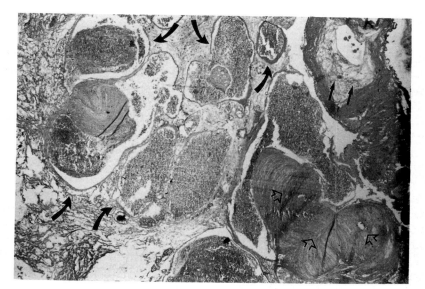

A

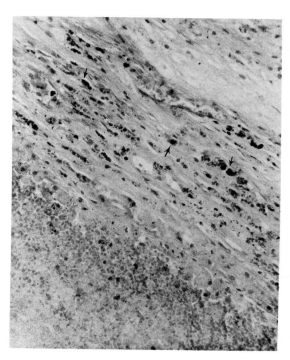

B

**Figure 8.2.** Cavernous angiomas. (A) Multiple thin-walled vascular channels (arrows) in a ''honey-comb'' pattern, without intervening brain parenchyma. Areas of thrombosis (open arrows) and old partially recanalized thrombus (double arrows) are shown. (H&E, × 25.) (B) Wall of pontine cavernous angioma with evidence of recent (left lower corner) and old (hemosiderin-laden macrophages, arrows) hemorrhage. (H&E, × 230.) Reprinted from Roberson GH, Kase CS, Wolpow ER. Telangiectases and cavernous angiomas of the brainstem: ''cryptic'' vascular malformations. Neuroradiology 1974;8:83–89. With permission.

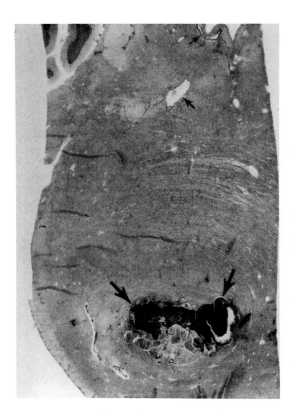

**Figure 8.3.** Capillary telangiectases in the tegmentum of the pons (small arrows), shown as widely separated vascular channels with thin walls, separated by normal intervening brain parenchyma. A cavernous angioma with surrounding hematoma is present in the basis pontis (large arrows). (PTAH, ×4.5.) (Reprinted from Roberson GH, Kase CS, Wolpow ER. Telangiectases and cavernous angiomas of the brainstem: "cryptic vascular malformations. Neuroradiology 1974;8:83–89. With permission.)

## Intracerebral Hemorrhage from Aneurysms and Vascular Malformations

### Aneurysms

The location of intracerebral aneurysms at sites of predilection in the intracranial circulation (Table 8.2)[7–9] results in a relatively predictable pattern of ICH location in the event of aneurysmal rupture into the adjacent brain substance. Due to the extracerebral position of the aneurysms, mostly at the base of the brain, their rupture leads virtually always to subarachnoid hemorrhage (SAH), less commonly to ICH. It is difficult to determine the true frequency of ICH after aneurysmal rupture, since most neurosurgical series that report this association have some degree of referral bias. Thus, the review of Wheelock et al.[10] cites figures from as low as 4% to as high as 25% from the world literature, and Benoit et al.[11] quote 30% to 40% in CT series and 30% to 70% from autopsy series. The sites of origin of ICH secondary to aneurysmal rupture are relatively consistent in autopsy[12–14] and clinical series.[9–11] In the former, a predominance of anterior cerebral artery aneurysms has been noted, whereas middle cerebral artery aneurysms have been the main source of ICH in clinical series (Table 8.3).

ICH secondary to aneurysmal rupture occurs in characteristic locations that depend on the site of the ruptured aneurysm. (1) *Anterior communicating artery:* These aneu-

**Table 8.2.** Location of Intracranial Aneurysms

| Aneurysm Site | Locksley[7] No. Cases (%) | Weir et al.[8] No. Cases (%) | Freger et al.[9] No. Cases (%) |
|---|---|---|---|
| Ant. commun. a. | 895 (33%)* | 19 (30%)* | 76 (38%) |
| Intracranial ICA | 1104 (41%) | 19 (30%) | 57 (28.5%) |
| MCA | 529 (20%) | 19 (30%) | 57 (28.5%) |
| Post. circulation | 144 (6%) | 6 (10%) | 7 (3.5%) |
| Other | — | — | 3 (1.5%) |

Abbreviations: ant. commun. a. = anterior communicating artery, ICA = internal carotid artery, MCA = middle cerebral artery.

*Includes all sites of ant. cerebral artery and ant. communicating artery.

**Table 8.3.** Site of Origin of ICH in Autopsy and Clinical Series of Ruptured Intracranial Aneurysms

| Site | Autopsy Series | | | Clinical Series | |
|---|---|---|---|---|---|
| | Robertson[12] No. Cases (%) | Crompton[13] No. Cases (%) | Reynolds and Shaw[14] No. Cases (%) | Benoit et al.[11] No. Cases (%) | Freger et al.[9] No. Cases (%) |
| ACA | 29 (45%) | 27 (44%) | 46 (46%) | 33 (25%) | 17 (30%) |
| Pericallosal a. | 6 (9%) | 6 (10%) | —* | 7 (5%) | 2 (3%) |
| MCA | 24 (37%) | 16 (26%) | 33 (33%) | 71 (54%) | 30 (53%) |
| ICA | 4 (6%) | 13 (21%) | 13 (13%) | 20 (15%) | 8 (14%) |
| Post. circulation | 2 (3%) | 0 | 8 (8%) | 1 (1%) | 0 |
| Total | 65 | 62 | 100 | 132 | 57 |

Abbreviations: ACA = anterior cerebral artery, MCA = middle cerebral artery, ICA = internal carotid artery.
*Pericallosal a. cases included with ACA group.

rysms most commonly bleed into one or both frontal lobes, frequently extending into the ventricular system via the frontal horn of the lateral ventricle. They can at times rupture directly into the third ventricle after the jet of blood pierces through the lamina terminalis, whereas more anterior lesions can rupture into the genu of the corpus callosum, with subsequent extension into the body of this structure (Figure 8.4). In some patients, the hematoma is limited to the septum pellucidum. In all these situations, the parenchymal component of the aneurysmal hemorrhage is located *above* the aneurysm, the rupture site being directed superiorly from the aneurysmal dome. An intracranial hematoma was

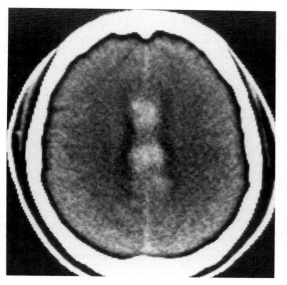

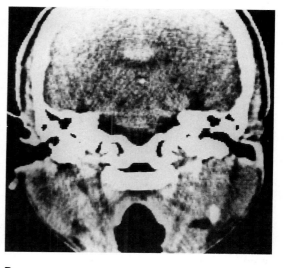

B

A

**Figure 8.4.** Noncontrast CT scan with hematoma of the corpus callosum secondary to ruptured anterior communicating artery aneurysm. (A) Axial view, with blood density in the corpus callosum, separating the bodies of the lateral ventricles. (B) Coronal view of the midline callosal hematoma.

documented in seventeen of seventy-six (22%) patients with ruptured anterior communicating artery aneurysms reported by Freger et al.[9] However, the hemorrhages reported by these authors were apparently not all intraparenchymal in location, since some of the computed tomography (CT) pictures in the paper depict hematomas that most likely corresponded to localized subarachnoid clots adjacent to a ruptured aneurysm. The most common location of the hematomas in their series was the medial frontal lobe (twelve cases), followed by the ventricular system (seven cases) and the septal-callosal area (two cases). (2) *Internal carotid artery (ICA):* In instances of bleeding from ICA aneurysms at the origin of the posterior communicating artery, the hemorrhage occurs laterally, into the medial temporal lobe, at times extending into the temporal horn of the lateral ventricle.[4] When the aneurysm is at the ICA bifurcation, it generally bleeds superiorly into the frontal lobe, at times producing a massive hematoma in the basal ganglia, which can be mistakenly interpreted as an example of "spontaneous," presumably hypertensive ICH (Figure 8.5). Intraparenchymal hematomas occurred in seven of fifteen

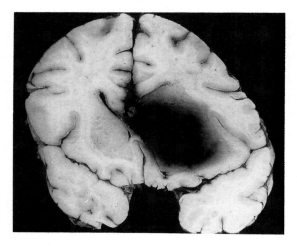

**Figure 8.5.** Large left ICH into the putamen, anterior limb of the internal capsule, and frontal horn of the lateral ventricle, secondary to ruptured aneurysm of the ICA bifurcation.

(47%) cases of ICA bifurcation aneurysms in the series of Freger et al.[9] (3) *Middle cerebral artery (MCA):* These aneurysms can rupture into the temporal or the frontal lobe, depending on the inferior or superior orientation of their dome, respectively; on occasion, both lobes can be the site of ICH after rupture of an MCA bifurcation aneurysm. At times, a localized hematoma of the Sylvian fissure, in a strictly subarachnoid, extracerebral location, can acquire such large size as to behave as an ICH, with prominent focal deficits and mass effect. ICH was reported in twenty-four of the forty-eight (50%) cases of MCA bifurcation aneurysms reported by Freger et al.,[9] this being the highest frequency of ICH among the various aneurysm sites in that series. The MCA site also accounted for the largest hematoma volumes in their series, a feature that correlated with a high mortality (67%) compared with mortalities of 53% for anterior communicating aneurysms and 29% for ICA bifurcation aneurysms.[9]

In analyzing the factors related to prognosis, Freger et al.[9] found that hematoma volumes of 50 ml or more were associated with a mortality rate of 76%, and the bulk of this poor prognosis was directly related to the presence of the ICH; with hematoma volumes below 50 ml, on the other hand, the mortality was 28%, and eight of the nine deaths resulted from the effects of delayed vasospasm, rather than from the ICH themselves. From the total analysis of their series, all hematoma sizes and locations considered, these authors concluded that about 10% of ruptured aneurysms will produce fatal ICH as a complication.[9] When aneurysm site was considered, hematomas determined the risk of fatal ICH in one of every four MCA aneurysms, whereas such complication only followed in one of every twenty-five cases of anterior communicating artery aneurysm, suggesting that surgery for unruptured, incidentally found aneurysms should be particularly considered for those located in the MCA system.[9] With regard to surgical therapy of symptomatic ICH for aneurysmal rupture, both Freger et al.[9] and Wheelock et al.[10]

stated that early surgical intervention with hematoma drainage and aneurysm clipping provide the best possibilities for good clinical outcome.

In a patient presenting with ICH, certain clinical and radiological features are suggestive of aneurysmal rupture as the mechanism. (1) Very abrupt and severe headache is a feature that characterizes 78%[15] to 86%[16] of cases of aneurysmal SAH, whereas primary ICH patients only report this symptom in about 33% of the cases.[15] (2) Subhyaloid hemorrhages on funduscopic examination occur in about 9% of cases of aneurysmal SAH,[16] but are exceptionally rare in primary ICH, thus their presence is virtually diagnostic of aneurysmal rupture in a patient presenting with ICH. (3) The CT documentation of diffuse SAH in association with an ICH is strong evidence of aneurysmal or AVM rupture, since primary ICH usually communicate with the CSF pathways through the ventricular system, not through the basal or convexity subarachnoid space.[4] In the rare situations when the latter occurs, as in cortical superficial ICH due to cerebral amyloid angiopathy (see Chapter 9, Figure 9.4), the subarachnoid component of the hemorrhage is limited to and occurs focally in the cerebral convexity, without extension to the basal subarachnoid space, where aneurysmal SAH characteristically occurs. (4) The CT or MRI finding of ICH in locations that are "atypical" for primary ICH and likely in aneurysmal ICH include the basal and medial frontal lobe, septal-callosal sites, medial temporal lobe, combined frontal and temporal lobe locations, and purely intraventricular hemorrhage into the lateral, third or, less commonly, fourth ventricle.

### Arteriovenous Malformations

AVM correspond to congenital malformations that result from an arrest in the developmental differentiation of blood vessels that occurs at about three weeks of gestation.[17] The result is a failure of the primitive capillary plexus to differentiate into afferent and efferent channels, which in turn produces an irregular array of multiple arterial feeders that drain directly into dilated, thin-walled veins, without a normal intervening capillary bed. The walls of these vascular channels, both arterial and venous, are irregular, frequently thicker than normal, with proliferation of fibromuscular tissue in the media, as well as with intimal thickening.[4] Thrombosis can occlude these vessels, and calcification is often present, whereas atherosclerotic changes are uncommon, and amyloid deposits are rarely documented.[18] Evidence of old or recent hemorrhage is often present within the malformation, as well as in the adjacent brain parenchyma. AVM are rarely multiple,[19] and occasionally occur on a familial basis in individuals affected by "hereditary hemorrhagic telangiectasia" (Rendu-Osler-Weber disease).[20] The vascular malformations found in this disorder usually display the characteristic angiographic features of AVM, with opacification of the malformation in the arterial phase of the angiogram, frequently associated with early draining veins.[21]

*Pial* AVM have a frequency that is between one-tenth and one-fifth of that of cerebral aneurysms, and they accounted for 7.7% of the cases entered into the Cooperative Study of Intracerebral Aneurysms and Subarachnoid Hemorrhage.[22] Their location is in the supratentorial compartment in over 90% of the cases. They are evenly distributed between the right and left hemispheres, and the parietal lobe is their most common site, that area accounting for up to one-third of the cases, whereas the frontal and temporal lobes contain about 20% of the AVM each.[22–24] The sites of pial AVM location from several series from the literature are shown in Table 8.4. Their clinical presentation can be with either seizures, headache, or hemorrhage, at times with a combination of them. These lesions have a tendency to become symptomatic at an earlier age than cerebral aneurysms: 20% of cases were younger than age 20 and an additional 44% were between ages 20 and 40

**Table 8.4.** Arteriovenous Malformation Locations in Series from the Literature

| | Authors | | |
|---|---|---|---|
| AVM Location | Perret and Nishioka[22] No. Cases (%) | Crawford et al.[23] No. Cases (%) | Graf et al.[24] No. Cases (%) |
| Frontal | 102 (23%) | 85 (21%) | 33 (25%) |
| Temporal | 92 (20%) | 41 (10%) | 25 (19%) |
| Parietal | 122 (27%) | 145 (36%) | 41 (30%) |
| Occipital | 23 (5%) | 69 (17%) | 7 (5%) |
| Brainstem | 11 (2%) | | 5 (4%) |
| Cerebellum | 21 (4%) | 36 (9%)[†] | 6 (4.5%) |
| Basal ganglia | | 27 (7%) | 14 (10%) |
| Other | 87 (19%)* | | 3 (2.5%) |
| Total | 458 | 403 | 134 |

*Basal ganglia locations not mentioned separately; this group probably includes that site (labeled as "paraventricular"), as well as intraventricular locations.
[†]Brainstem and cerebellar locations given together.

when entered into the Cooperative Study.[22] The hemorrhagic presentations (both SAH and ICH) account for over 70% of the cases, as opposed to seizures, which occur in less than 20% of the cases.[23] Among 126 patients with a documented site of hemorrhage from an AVM reported by Graf et al.,[24] eighty-two (65%) presented with ICH, whereas only forty-four (35%) had purely SAH (eight patients did not have the type of intracranial hemorrhage recorded). In addition to rupture of the AVM, intracranial hemorrhage in these cases can result from rupture of a coexisting aneurysm. In AVM cases, an associated aneurysm is reported in 6% to 8% of the cases.[22–24] Crawford et al.[23] found the aneurysms more commonly (75%) in an arterial feeder to the AVM than at a distance from it, but in the cases from the Cooperative Study, Perret and Nishioka[22] reported only 37% of them located on a feeding artery and 42% were anatomically unrelated to the AVM. In some instances of associated AVM and aneurysm with intracranial hemorrhage it is possible to determine the bleeding lesion (Figure 8.6), which was found to be the aneurysm in at least 50% of the patients with a combination of lesions reported by Graf et al.[24]

Infratentorial AVM can occur in the substance of the brainstem (generally the pons, and in relation to the floor of the fourth ventricle) or cerebellum, as well as in the cerebellopontine angle. Their presentation is with acute and dramatic posterior fossa hemorrhage more often than with progressive or fluctuating neurological deficits.[25] Progressive deficits are caused by repeated episodes of minor bleeding leading to the accumulation of neurological deficits. According to Abe et al.[25] it is possible that in rare occasions these progressive deficits result from "mechanical compression or ischemia" on adjacent brain tissue, "due to a slowly enlarging AVM." In regard to the potential for ischemia-related deficits in patients with AVM, the long-held notion that AVM can produce transient or permanent cerebral ischemia through a "steal" phenomenon (i.e., directing blood flow into the malformation, rendering adjacent or distal cerebral tissue ischemic), based on the abundant dilated and autoregulation-lacking vessels of the AVM, has received support from studies employing single-photon-emission computed tomography (SPECT). Homan et al.[26] studied eleven patients with proven AVM with SPECT, and documented decreased blood flow in areas

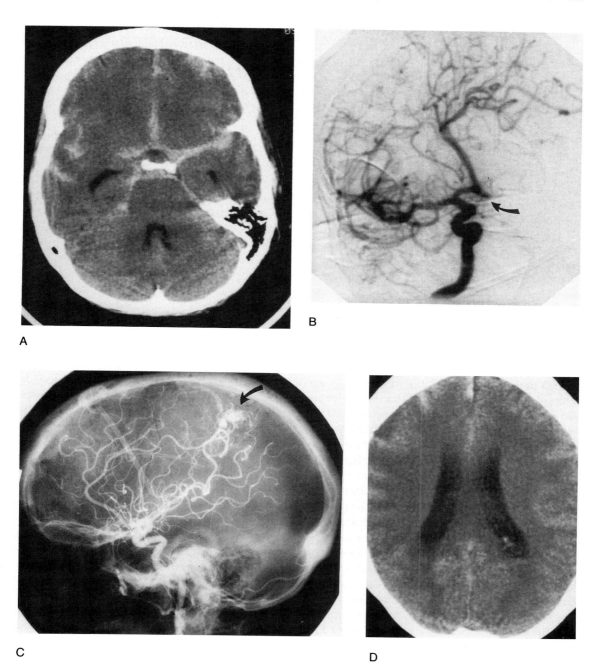

A

B

C

D

**Figure 8.6.** Diffuse basal SAH on admission CT (A) in a 58-year-old woman who was shown to have a ruptured anterior communicating artery aneurysm (B, arrow) and an incidental left parietal lobe AVM (C, arrow). The likely cause of the SAH was the aneurysm, since blood was heavily collected in the basal cisterns around it, whereas no blood density was present in the distant parietal convexity AVM on CT scan performed at onset of SAH (D). Signs of recent bleeding were also found around the aneurysm at the time of its surgical clipping (Courtesy of Joe I. Ordia, M.D., Department of Neurosurgery, Boston University Medical Center, Boston, MA.)

remote from the AVM, either ipsilaterally or contralaterally and affecting arterial territories different from the main arterial supply to the AVM, in eight of them; these focal perfusion abnormalities were generally correlated with either seizure foci or abnormalities in cognitive performance.

*Dural* AVM correspond to 5% to 20% of the intracranial vascular malformations.[27,28] They usually receive their arterial supply from meningeal branches of the external carotid, internal carotid, or vertebral arteries, and their venous drainage is via the dural venous sinuses or, less commonly, through pial veins.[28] They are located most commonly in the area of the transverse sinus, cavernous sinus, the anterior cranial fossa, and the incisura of the tentorium; less frequent sites are the middle cranial fossa and the convexity of the cerebral hemispheres.[27]

The *prognosis* of AVM-related intracranial bleeding has been extensively studied. The initial mortality from a bleeding AVM is approximately 10% to 12%, the majority of these patients (88%) presenting with ICH, which extends into the ventricular system in one-fourth of the cases.[24] Further mortality and morbidity result from the highly significant risk of rebleeding in unoperated AVM. Although the extensive literature data on rebleeding rates in AVM generally do not specify whether the hemorrhage is intracerebral or subarachnoid, ICH is likely to be the predominant event as judged by the information available on initial episodes of AVM-related hemorrhage. It is generally agreed that AVM that have bled once have a rebleeding rate of approximately 2% per year, with a cumulative rebleeding rate of 14% in five years, 31% in ten years, and 39% in twenty years.[24] Among the risk factors for rebleeding, AVM size was initially thought to be important as Graf et al.[24] found that small AVM (i.e., 3 cm or less) had a significantly higher bleeding rate (10% in the first year, 52% in five years) than that of larger lesions (0% at one year, 10% at five years, 34% at ten years, and 34% at twenty years). However, subsequent stud-

ies have failed to document a relationship between certain anatomical features of the AVM and frequency of rebleeding on long-term follow-up, including small versus large size, as well as superficial versus deep location of the AVM, except for a reduced risk of rebleeding in parietal AVM as compared with those at other sites,[23] and increasing rebleeding rates the older the patient at diagnosis.[23,24] Another feature related to rebleeding rates includes the form of initial presentation, hemorrhage carrying higher rebleeding rates (51%) than seizures (30%) after twenty years of follow-up; similar figures of 67% and 27%, respectively, were reported by Fults and Kelly[29] after fifteen years of follow-up. The rates of recurrent hemorrhage correlate with increasing mortality on long-term follow-up, having reached 18% at ten years and 29% at twenty years after diagnosis in the series of Crawford et al.[23]

In comparison with supratentorial AVM, those in the posterior fossa are, as expected, less prone to present with a seizure disorder, thus making hemorrhage or progressive neurological deficit the most common clinical manifestation. Their prognosis was felt to be generally poor in the series of Fults and Kelly,[29] with a high mortality (66.7%) from the initial hemorrhage, with frequent rebleeding episodes, most of which were fatal. However, other series have recorded a less dismal prognosis: Batjer and Samson[30] reviewed thirty-two cases, twenty-three (72%) of whom presented with intracranial hemorrhage, an event that had occurred previously in eleven (34%) of these twenty-three patients. The location of the AVM was in the cerebellar vermis (seventeen patients), cerebellar hemisphere (seven patients), brainstem (four patients), cerebellopontine angle and cerebellar tonsil (two patients each); an unusually high proportion of these patients (6 of 32 or 19%) had ten associated intracranial aneurysms, eight of which were located in branches of the vertebrobasilar system, and two of which presented with SAH. Among thirty patients who underwent operation, there were two deaths (7%) and four instances of surgery-related neurological morbidity (13%).

Dural AVM have less predictable behavior in regard to risk of bleeding in comparison with pial AVM. In some instances, they are fully asymptomatic and are unexpected angiographic findings,[31] in others, they are associated with cranial bruits or pulsatile tinnitus and headache.[32,33] Their potential for bleeding, causing SAH or ICH, is however considerable, occurring in approximately 15% of the cases,[28] and it depends to some extent on the anatomy and angiographic features of the malformation. The locations that carry a high risk of bleeding from dural AVM are the tentorial incisura and the anterior cranial fossa,[27,34–36] whereas those of the transverse-sigmoid sinus and cavernous sinus have a more benign prognosis.[27,35] There are, however, exceptions to the latter rule, since an added factor that increases their bleeding potential relates to the pattern of venous drainage. Dural AVM often (in 65% of the cases[28]) drain through the adjacent dural venous sinus alone, but on occasion they have in addition venous drainage through adjacent pial veins, a feature that confers them a substantially increased risk of bleeding.[27,34,35,37] The resulting venous hemorrhages occur after rupture of either the adjacent draining pial veins or an associated venous aneurysm or "varix," that frequently develops in the vicinities of dural AVM.[28,38] In the case of presenting with ICH, the venous origin of the hemorrhage usually results in a less violent clinical picture than that of ruptured intracranial aneurysm. Another difference between rupture of aneurysms and dural AVM is the rare tendency of the latter to rebleed and to become complicated by vasospasm.[28] The pattern of bleeding of dural AVM relates to the anatomical location of the malformation, tentorial AVM usually causing SAH, whereas those of the anterior fossa and cerebral convexity often cause ICH.[28] The treatment of dural AVM is limited to those that have pial venous drainage or an associated venous aneurysm, or both, and to those that have presented

with intracranial bleeding.[28] The treatment modalities available include resection of the AVM or embolization via endovascular techniques,[27,28,39] the latter at times being the definitive treatment, at others being done prior to its surgical resection.

The term "cryptic vascular malformations" was introduced by Crawford and Russell in 1956,[40] to refer to small malformations that had escaped detection by clinical diagnostic means (including angiography), and were found pathologically to have accounted for episodes of otherwise unexplained intracranial hemorrhage. They occurred generally in young subjects, as all twenty patients reported by these authors were age 40 or younger, and fifteen of them were under age 20 at the time of the ICH.[40] The common feature of these lesions is their small size, generally below 2 to 3 cm in diameter, and they generally correspond to small AVM, less commonly to cavernous angiomas, and rarely to venous malformations: among 159 cases from the literature and thirteen of their own (total, 172 cases), Wakai et al.[41] found ninety-nine (58%) labeled as AVM (apparently with inclusion of venous angiomas together with AVM), fifty-nine (34%) as cavernous angiomas, and fourteen (8%) as "unclassified angiomas." Their occurrence as incidental autopsy findings, in the absence of clinical evidence of rupture, lends further support to the notion that these "cryptic" lesions are to be considered when evaluating patients presenting with ICH.[42] This concept of "cryptic vascular malformations" rapidly gained acceptance in the neurological community, and further led to the frequent suggestion that in cases of unexplained ICH, such lesions may have been present,[43,44] but were said to have been "destroyed by the hemorrhage,"[42] thus even escaping postmortem detection.[45] This concept, which is "inherently difficult to substantiate,"[46] is often used when evaluating cases of ICH, and is at times considered, by default, to be the stated bleeding mechanism in a case of ICH that fails to show other documented cause.[45] In the autopsy series of forty-eight cases of "cryptic" vascular malformations reported by McCormick and Nofziger,[42] it was calculated that the "cryptic" lesions would be over nine times more frequent than the classic large malformations (forty-eight "cryptic," five "classic"). In ten of the forty-eight patients massive, fatal ICH resulted from rupture of the malformation, and two additional cases had evidence of minor hemorrhage. The ages of the patients varied across the full spectrum from newborn to elderly, with an average age of 49, and without differences in frequency by sex. The majority of the lesions were small AVM, but twelve telangiectases and one cavernous angioma were also reported. With regard to their location, contrary to the marked preponderance of large AVM supratentorially, these authors reported from their forty-eight cases and from another 260 from the literature, an almost equal distribution in the supratentorial and infratentorial compartments, the latter showing a predilection for the pons.[40,42]

In the clinical literature on ICH, these small malformations were frequently reported in the setting of nondiagnostic cerebral angiography,[47–50] presumably reflecting either a size of malformation below that of angiographic resolution, or the fact that an acute hematoma may compress a low-pressure malformation, precluding its visualization; such lesions were at times documented by angiography after the mass effect of the acute ICH had subsided[46] or, more commonly, were found on postsurgical biopsy specimens or at postmortem examination. This led to their being also labeled as "angiographically occult vascular malformations." The presurgical or premortem diagnosis of these small, angiographically occult lesions was slightly facilitated by the introduction of CT scan, with its ability to occasionally show calcium deposits adjacent to an area of ICH, and a tendency to show post-contrast enhancement in an area of fresh hemorrhage.[41,51] The latter, however, is not specific for a vascular malformation, since bleeding into a tumor may produce a similar CT picture.[52] The introduction of MRI has definitely changed the situation (and has made the terms "cryptic" and "occult" vascular malformations obsolete), as this technique is superior to any of the other radiological modalities in the demonstration of small vascular malformations, mainly due to its ability to detect small foci of hemorrhage, fresh or old, in the area of the malformation.[53,54] The value of MRI is particularly evident when using high-intensity magnetic field imaging at 1.0 to 1.5 Tesla. Gomori et al.[55] documented forty-six lesions (thirty-four supratentorial, twelve infratentorial) in nineteen patients with the use of a 1.5 Tesla unit, which depicted a characteristic picture for "occult" vascular malformations: circumscribed regions of hypointensity on T1-weighted sequences, with more prominent hypointensity on T2-weighted images (reflecting hemosiderin deposits), within which there would be areas with a different intensity pattern, either T1-isointensity plus T2-hypointensity, cyst-like T1- and T2-hyperintensity, or mild T1- and T2-hypointensity (Figure 8.7). These MRI changes suggest that the imaging features of small vascular malformations reflect the residual effects of multiple episodes of small hemorrhage around the central nidus of the malformation.[55] Most of the lesions these authors documented had characteristics suggestive of cavernous angiomas, and those located supratentorially favored the subcortical and periventricular areas of the cerebral hemispheres. Although the superior ability of CT to document calcium deposits is recognized, the MRI documentation of various stages of hemorrhage evolution around a central nidus is both more sensitive and more specific than CT in the diagnosis of small vascular malformations.[55] This greater sensitivity of MRI was reflected in that twenty-two of the forty-six lesions were missed by contrast-enhanced CT scan in the series of Gomori et al.[55] However, caution needs to be exercised in the diagnosis of vascular malformation by MRI, since at times the differential diagnosis with hemorrhage into a brain tumor may not be possible: Sze et al.[56] reviewed the cases of twenty-four pa-

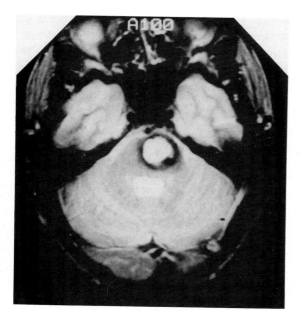

**Figure 8.7.** Midpontine cavernous angioma on T2-weighted (TR/TE = 3440/80) MRI sequence, characterized by a bright signal central nidus surrounded by a hypointense ring of hemosiderin deposition (Courtesy of J. P. Mohr, M.D., Neurological Institute, New York.)

tients who had high-field (1.5 Tesla) MRI features characteristic of "occult" vascular malformations, eighteen of whom had hemorrhagic tumors as the mechanism of the MRI changes. The difficulty in separating these lesions on MRI grounds alone derives from their having in common the presence of blood, generally along with peripheral hemosiderin deposits, adjacent to the vascular or tumoral lesion. Features helpful in distinguishing hemorrhagic tumor from vascular malformation include (1) the presence of prominent perilesional edema, which favors tumor, especially metastases, over vascular malformations, and (2) multiplicity of lesions, which also favors metastatic tumor,[56] despite the occasional occurrence of multiple vascular malformations.

Small, angiographically "occult" vascular malformations of the brainstem have been studied in detail, in part due to their ten-

dency to present with clinical syndromes uncharacteristic of brainstem hemorrhage. Although sudden, apoplectic onset of hemorrhage with devastating brainstem damage occurs, a common scenario is one of slow and gradual progression of brainstem signs over periods of several days, in the absence of headache,[25] at times taking a protracted course over months or years of recurrent or gradually progressive brainstem deficits that simulate the course of multiple sclerosis[57] or a slowly-growing glioma.[6,26] Although CT scan may be helpful in demonstrating acute hemorrhage or calcification with minimal or no mass effect,[25,58] the definitive diagnosis is made with MRI, which detects the typical hyperintense central nidus surrounded by a low-signal peripheral hemosiderin ring.[55] The natural history of these lesions has not been clearly established. It is apparent that the data on rebleeding rates, morbidity, and mortality of large, angiographically-documented, predominantly supratentorial AVM[24] cannot be extrapolated to small, angiographically occult vascular malformations. This may in part be due to the fact that the latter are a more heterogeneous group that includes AVM, cavernous angiomas, and venous angiomas, all of which have different rates of bleeding (maximal in AVM, minimal in venous angiomas, intermediate in cavernous angiomas). In addition, the patterns of bleeding may be different, the more benign gradual, progressive course of brainstem vascular malformations being distinctly uncommon for the large supratentorial AVM. However, the potential for major brainstem hemorrhage in angiographically occult vascular malformations is significant: Abe et al.[25] found that after an initial presentation with minor neurological deficits, 21% of their patients suffered a subsequent major episode of brainstem hemorrhage, whereas 45% of them remained with stable minor deficits. Based on their known tendency to produce either recurrent major hemorrhage or progressive brainstem deficits, small brainstem vascular malformations diagnosed by MRI are being increasingly treated surgically, with successful evacuation of the hematoma and the malformation, with relatively low morbidity and mortality rates.[41,59,60]

### Cavernous Angiomas

Cavernous angiomas are increasingly being recognized as an important cause of neurological morbidity, in great part due to their being reliably diagnosed since the advent of MRI. As a result, numerous series in the neurosurgical literature have analyzed the clinical and radiological features of these malformations, and recommendations on their preferred mode of treatment have followed.[61–69]

The frequency of cavernous angiomas has been estimated as 5% to 13% of the vascular malformations affecting the CNS.[2,42,68,70] They were found incidentally in 0.53% (131 cases) in an unselected series of 24,535 autopsies.[66] When comparing their incidence in relationship to the introduction of CT scanning, Yamasaki et al.[62] found a 2.6% frequency of cavernous angiomas among vascular malformations in the pre-CT era, whereas this figure increased to 23.2% after widespread use of CT became available. Since MRI is superior to CT as a means of diagnosing cavernous angiomas,[53–55,65,67] these frequency figures are expected to be even higher with the routine use of this diagnostic modality.

Cavernous angiomas are generally located supratentorially, where 60% to 75% of these lesions occur,[62,63,65] favoring the subcortical and cortical areas of the cerebral hemispheres, with a predilection for the temporal lobe, the frontal and parietal areas being intermediate in frequency, with a low frequency of lesions in the occipital lobes.[63–65,68] The infratentorial lesions favor the pons, followed by cerebellar locations, and rare examples of extra-axial lesions, mainly involving the cerebellopontine angle, have been described.[61–66] The sex distribution is roughly equal between males and females when all locations are considered together,[62–65] but a female predominance for the infratentorial

forms, especially pontine, has been detected in some series.[64,67] The age at diagnosis favors the younger age groups, and a peak has been noticed in the third and fourth decades.[61,63–69] A significant difference in age at presentation by sex was found in the series of forty-seven cases reported by Requena et al.,[65] as eleven of twenty-one (52.4%) men were diagnosed before age 30, whereas only three of twenty-six (11.5%) women presented clinically that early in life. Cavernous angiomas are generally single lesions, but multiplicity occurs in a substantial proportion of patients, in the order of 10% to 33% of the cases,[5,65,66,71,72] if those diagnosed by either MRI or autopsy are included (Figure 8.8). There appears to be a relationship between multiplicity of lesions and familial incidence of cavernous angiomas.[73,74] Rigamonti et al.[74] studied twenty-four patients with histologically verified cavernous angiomas, thirteen (54%) of whom had a positive family history; head MRI examination was performed in eleven first-degree and five other relatives of these individuals, showing cavernous angiomas in fourteen of them, the lesions being multiple in eleven of the fourteen subjects. In addition, four of the original thirteen patients with cavernous angiomas and a positive family history had multiple lesions on MRI examination, resulting in a 73% figure of multiple lesions within the familial group of cavernous angiomas. Study of the family pedigrees of these individuals suggested an autosomal dominant pattern of inheritance with variable expression and incomplete penetrance of the abnormal gene.[74] All individuals affected by this familial form of generally multiple cavernous angiomas were of Mexican-American descent, an association also suggested by other reports.[75] It is still unclear whether this ethnic predilection represents a regional bias or a true genetic association.

The *clinical presentation* of supratentorial cavernous angiomas is with seizures, hemorrhage, or progressive neurological deficits. Infratentorial malformations usually become symptomatic with either bleeding or progres-

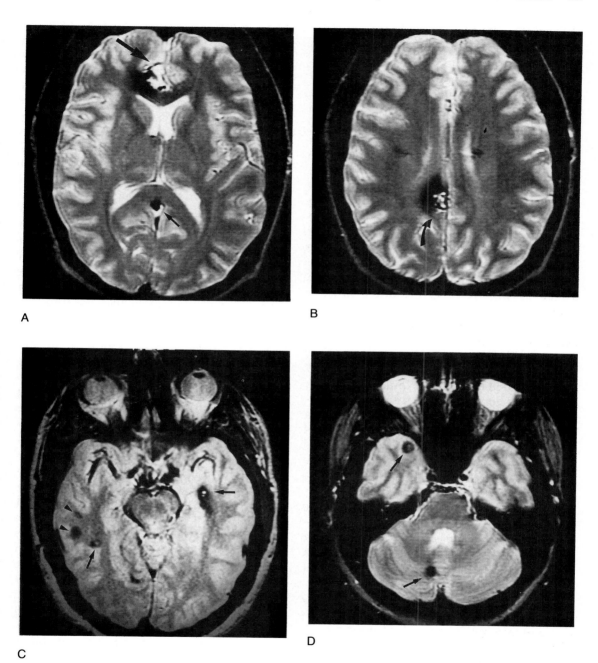

**Figure 8.8.** Multiple small cavernous angiomas on T2-weighted (TR/TE = 3243/80) MRI sequences in a 30-year-old woman with a long-standing seizure disorder. (A) Left medial frontal (large arrow) and callosal (splenium) (small arrow) cavernous angiomas with bright signal centrally and hemosiderin hypointensity peripherally. (B) Left medial frontal lesion (arrow) with mixed signal centrally and surrounding hemosiderin hypointense halo. (C) Bilateral temporal lesions, with either bright central signal surrounded by hypointensity (arrows) or diffuse hypointensity (arrowheads). (D) Left temporal and left cerebellar cavernous angiomas (arrows). (Courtesy of Philip A. Wolf, M.D., Department of Neurology, Boston University Medical Center, Boston, MA.)

sive signs of brainstem dysfunction.[61,63-65] Most of the reported series have documented *seizures* as the leading form of clinical presentation of cavernous angiomas, accounting for 27% to 70% of the cases.[61-65,68,69] Seizure types are about equally distributed between generalized tonic-clonic and simple or complex partial, and the most common age of onset is the third and fourth decades.[61,64] In a review of forty-nine cases from the literature, Simard et al.[61] noted that half of patients who consulted because of seizures exhibited neurological abnormalities at the time of diagnosis. The duration of the seizure disorder varied between the extremes of one month and twenty-three years in the series of Yamasaki et al.[62] The presentation of cavernous angiomas with *ICH* was a feature in forty (29%) of the 138 cases reviewed by Simard et al.[61] Eight of these forty patients had previously been evaluated for episodes of ICH or SAH. Similarly, ten of thirty patients (33%) had hemorrhage in the series of Yamasaki et al.,[62] half presenting with a sudden onset, the other half having an insidious course. ICH was the form of presentation in 31% of the thirteen patients reported by Tagle et al.,[63] in 10% of the nineteen supratentorial cases of Vaquero et al.,[69] and in 20% in the series of ten patients of Rigamonti et al.[72] The diagnostic suspicion of an underlying cavernous angioma in the setting of an acute ICH is facilitated by the rare history of preceding episodes of ICH at the same anatomic site.[61] In most cases, however, the ICH is an isolated event which is initially virtually indistinguishable from ICH from other mechanisms, as cerebral angiography invariably shows only the vascular mass effect secondary to the acute hematoma, without abnormal local vascular structures.[63-65] An underlying vascular malformation can at times be suggested by the CT demonstration of calcification near the ICH (shown in only 10% of the forty ICH cases reviewed by Simard et al.,[61] but found in 33% of those reported by Vaquero et al.[69]), and the presence of postcontrast enhancement.[61,62,69] In most instances, the diagnosis of cavernous angioma is only made after histological examination of surgical or autopsy tissue taken from the vicinities of the ICH. A syndrome of *progressive neurological deficits* is a well-known form of presentation of cavernous angiomas, in both the supratentorial and, especially, the infratentorial compartments. This frequently suggests other initial diagnoses such as multiple sclerosis[57] or primary brain tumor.[6,25,69] A progressive, tumor-like course was the form of presentation in forty-nine (35%) of the 138 patients reviewed by Simard et al.[61] The length of progression of symptoms varied between the extremes of five months and twenty-seven years. An apparently distinct group among these patients were those with extra-axial cavernous angiomas of the middle fossa, most of them being reported from Japan.[61] These frequently had imaging features suggestive of a preoperative diagnosis of meningioma, and they were difficult lesions to resect surgically, with high mortality and morbidity, mostly due to their tendency to bleed profusely intraoperatively.[61,62] Brainstem cavernous angiomas are particularly likely to present with a gradually progressive syndrome of brainstem and cerebellar dysfunction. Zimmerman et al.[67] analyzed twenty-four such lesions that were located in the midbrain tegmentum (five patients) or tectum (six patients), pons (nine patients), and medulla (four patients). A gradually progressive, at times stepwise course characterized at least one-third of this group. This protracted course of brainstem cavernous angiomas is thought to be due to recurrent small hemorrhages within or around the malformation, leading at times to actual increase in size of the lesion,[61,62] but without producing clinical or radiological evidence of acute, ictal brainstem hemorrhage. This point is illustrated by the following case:

A 54-year-old woman developed in 1968 "numbness" of the left arm, initially intermittently, later on becoming permanent, not extending to any other portions of that half of the body. Subsequently she developed gait imbalance, and evaluation in 1973 resulted in the diagnosis of probable multiple sclerosis. During the following years, she had progressive clumsiness of the left limbs, diplopia with deviation of OS inward, right facial palsy, and dysphagia. She was emphatic in that these deficits accumulated slowly, never with a sudden onset or with associated headache, nausea or vomiting.

On exam, mental status was intact. Speech was moderately dysarthric, with scanning character. Motor strength was intact and symmetric in all four limbs. The deep tendon reflexes were 2+ and symmetric, with flexor plantar reflexes. She had mild ataxia of the left limbs, in the arm more than in the leg. Her gait was with increased base, slow, with ataxia of the lower limbs, more prominent on the left than on the right side. Sensory testing was normal.

Cranial nerves showed bilateral 6th nerve palsies, left more severe than right; horizontal nystagmus; right facial palsy, predominantly inferiorly, with elements of hemifacial spasm, at times with rhythmic and synchronous movements of "palatal myoclonus." The tongue protruded in the midline, without atrophy or fasciculations, with normal strength bilaterally.

MRI showed a typical cavernous angioma of the midpons (Figure 8.9), which has remained stable on MRI follow-up for the last four years.

The radiological diagnosis of these lesions is favored by the documentation of calcification (found in 100% of the patients reported by Yamasaki et al.,[62] but in only 33% of those of Vaquero et al.[69]), and postcontrast enhancement on CT scan (reported in 83% of the sixty-four patients who had contrast studies in the series reviewed by Simard et al.[61]). Angiography generally only shows nonspecific avascular mass effect due to the presence of the slow-flow vascular malformation and adjacent hematoma.[61] On occasion, angiography can show contrast "blush" in the arterial phase and early draining veins[76] or, more commonly, an associated vascular anomaly, either capillary telangiectasia[6,64] or venous angioma,[64,67] the latter being a finding in 16% of the twenty-four patients with brainstem cavernous angiomas reported by Zimmerman et al.[67] This association is particularly important with regard to surgical treatment, since these two lesions appear to

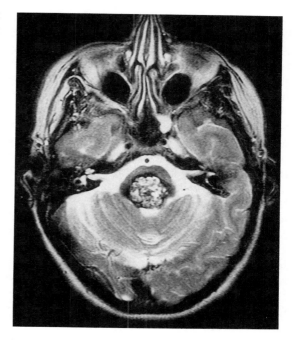

A

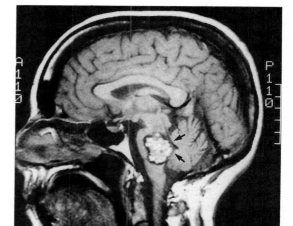

B

**Figure 8.9.** Large cavernous angioma of the midpons in axial (A, heavily T2-weighted, TR/TE = 4000/102 msec) and midsagittal (B, T1-weighted, TR/TE = 350/19 msec) MRI views, showing typical mixed-signal central nidus with peripheral hemosiderin ring. Marked replacement of the pontine tegmentum and basis by the malformation, with close apposition to the floor of the fourth ventricle dorsally (arrows) are also shown.

have radically different behavior in terms of bleeding potential. The mainstay in the radiological diagnosis of cavernous angiomas is MRI,[62,65,67,72] which shows, on T2-weighted sequences, a lesion of irregular, bright signal intensity mixed with mottled hypointensity in its central nidus, along with a typical hypointense peripheral ring corresponding to hemosiderin deposits. Smaller lesions only appear as round areas of decreased signal (hypointense) in the brain substance.[72]

The *treatment* of cavernous angiomas in the supratentorial space is frequently surgical in patients who present with ICH, seizures, or progressive neurological deficits.[62,68,69,71] The indication for surgery used to be most often the suspicion of a tumor as the mechanism of progressive neurological deficits or seizures,[63] but since the advent of MRI with increasingly accurate preoperative diagnosis of cavernous angiomas, surgery is performed in order to arrest or reverse neurological dysfunction and control seizures.[62] In both instances, the additional indication for surgery is the prevention of future bleeding episodes. In the setting of acute ICH from a cavernous angioma, surgery generally is performed for hematoma removal, frequently with the preoperative suspicion of cavernous angioma, since the visualization of the lesion is often possible with the use of MRI, even in the presence of an acute hematoma.[53,72]

The results of surgical treatment for supratentorial cavernous angiomas are encouraging: Yamasaki et al.[62] operated on twenty-two of their thirty patients, achieving complete removal of the lesion in seventeen, resulting in intact postoperative status in ten, residual neurological deficits in five, and persistent seizure disorder in two. The five patients who had partial resection of the lesion fared less well, since one died from massive intraoperative bleeding from a middle fossa cavernous angioma, and three were left with neurological deficits, only one patient being described as neurologically intact postoperatively.[62] Weber et al.[64] had one death (5.5%) among eighteen operated cases with cavernous angiomas. Their surgical results were

also generally favorable, reporting disappearance or decreased frequency of seizures in all ten patients who survived the procedure (the one death in their series was a patient who underwent surgery because of generalized seizures, with a cavernous angioma of the atrium of the right lateral ventricle). Among patients presenting with progressive neurological deficits (four patients) or hemorrhage (three patients), they reported excellent results in those with supratentorial lesions, whereas persistent neurological sequelae followed the removal of the malformation in all three patients with posterior fossa lesions.[64] Recent data, however, have indicated that surgical treatment of posterior fossa cavernous angiomas can be safely performed, and the results are encouraging, provided certain guidelines are followed.[67] Among twenty-four patients with posterior fossa cavernous angiomas, sixteen were deemed appropriate surgical candidates in the series of Zimmerman et al.,[67] based on previous history of symptomatic episodes of bleeding and surgical accessibility, the latter meaning a lesion located in close proximity to the pial surface of the brainstem. They reported no surgical mortality, but one patient died six months postoperatively because of shunt infection with sepsis; all four instances of new postoperative neurological deficits were transient. One patient who had partial resection of the cavernous angioma required reoperation thirty months later because of regrowth of the malformation. In their group of eight patients treated nonsurgically, with midbrain (five patients) or pontine (three patients) cavernous angiomas, follow-up revealed one fatal midbrain hemorrhage one year after diagnosis, while the rest remained minimally symptomatic or neurologically intact. Although there are no adequate data on the natural history of cavernous angiomas of the brainstem, the current recommendation is to consider surgical resection in those patients who are symptomatic (with either bleeding or progressive neurological deficits) from brainstem cavernous angiomas located near the pial surface.[62,67] In those with incidentally found or deeply located lesions, the logical approach is with clinical and MRI follow-up,[62,67] with plans for surgical treatment of the superficially located lesions in the event they become symptomatic. In the group of deep, surgically inaccessible malformations, the results of surgical treatment are poor,[69] and they are generally treated with radiation therapy,[62] following the reported beneficial results in the treatment of deep AVM,[77] although there are no adequate follow-up data to support its value in the treatment of cavernous angiomas.

### Venous Angiomas

Venous angiomas are often found on routine autopsy studies, and they occurred in 59% of the 165 brains with vascular malformations studied by Sarwar and McCormick[2] among 4069 consecutive autopsies. This contrasts with a relative paucity of reports of venous angiomas in clinical series, a feature that has been taken to underscore the frequently benign and asymptomatic character of these malformations.[78,79] Although they are generally considered to be benign lesions with a low potential for neurological morbidity as a result of hemorrhage and with a high frequency of presentation as incidental findings,[2,78,80,81] some authors have suggested that they have more serious implications, with a higher bleeding risk than generally estimated.[82] This, in turn, results in a controversy regarding their surgical management.

The majority of the venous angiomas reported in the literature have been supratentorial (about 70%), with a predilection for the frontal lobes (over two-thirds of the cases), while those in the posterior fossa (30% of the cases) favor the cerebellum, in a 4:1 ratio with the brainstem sites.[81] Their radiological diagnosis is made by CT scan, MRI, and cerebral angiography. *CT scan* commonly shows a hyperdense, round lesion on noncontrast studies,[79–81,83–85] felt to represent the in-

creased blood pool that results from the local aggregates of dilated venous channels, since these lesions are not characterized pathologically by the presence of calcification or surrounding acute extravasation of blood.[80,83] However, a substantial proportion of the cases (40% to 54%)[79,85] may show no abnormality in noncontrast CT scan.[80,83,84,86] Following contrast infusion, enhancement is seen in over 90% of the cases[79–81,85,86] in the form of either diffuse or, more commonly, linear enhancement, the latter representing the main draining vein of the malformation[80,81,84,86] (Figure 8.10A). *MRI* provides similar data, generally showing a linear "flow-void" in T1-weighted sequences in the area of the main draining vein, as well as its tributaries, the latter becoming particularly prominent after Gadolinium infusion[79] (Fig. 8.10B,C). At times, a central core of mixed increased and decreased signal intensity is detected in cases that show as round or globular enhancing lesions on CT scan.[79] The diagnostic sensitivity of MRI (94%)[81] approaches that of angiography in demonstrating the malformation. *Cerebral angiography* still represents the "gold standard" for the diagnosis of venous angiomas. It typically shows normal structures in arterial and capillary phases, and the venous phase shows the malformation composed of an array of small, generally parallel, deep medullary veins (the so-called "caput medusae") converging into one (or rarely two) large draining veins, which in turn drain into one of the dural sinuses or, less commonly, a superficial cortical vein or the deep venous system[2,78,79,83–87] (Figure 8.10D). This typical aspect is rarely subject to variations, but Wendling et al.[88] reported, with magnification angiography, the finding of enlarged arterial branches at the periphery of the malformation, as well as a capillary "blush" and early filling veins, in three cases of venous angiomas. These features, however, raise the suspicion about the diagnosis of AVM,[79] rather than venous angioma, as transitional forms between these two malformations are known to exist.[84,89] Angiographic distinction

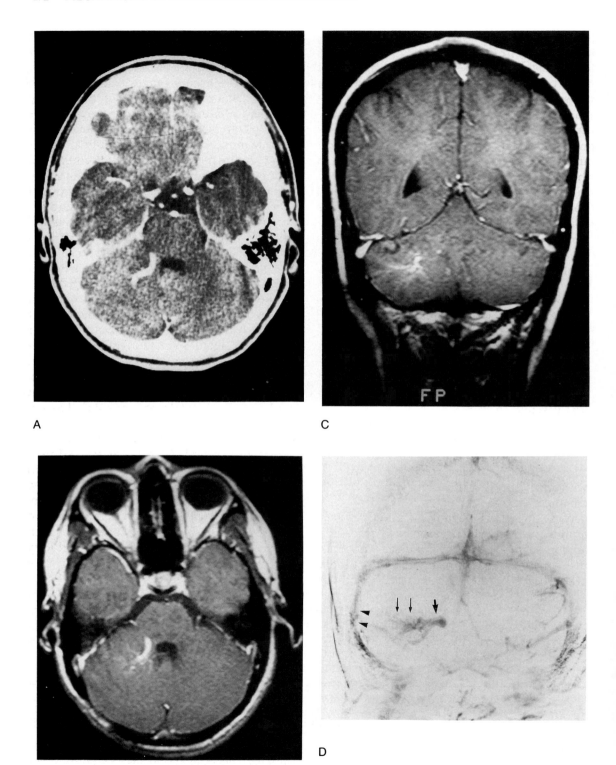

A

C

B

D

of the two may not be possible, requiring histological examination for a definite diagnosis.[90] This was the case in the patient reported by Wolf et al.[91] A 52-year-old man presented with a large ICH of the left temporal lobe, and cerebral angiography showed the mass effect related to the ICH, as well as a second lesion characterized by pathological arterial vessels and an early draining vein in the left parietal lobe. These findings were thought to represent cerebral metastases, but postmortem examination disclosed multiple bilateral hemispheric, cerebellar, and pontine venous angiomas, lesions that were also present near the left temporal ICH. Finally, another variant of the classic angiographic picture of the venous angioma is an isolated dilated vein without the prominent deep medullary veins of the "caput medusae,"[86] an aspect that has been interpreted as representing a different type of vascular anomaly, a so-called "varix,"[81] an entity that is not well characterized pathologically and is not included in most modern discussions of cerebral vascular malformations.

The association of venous angiomas with other vascular malformations, in particular cavernous angiomas, has been recently stressed in the literature,[79,92] in particular with regard to the bleeding potential of the combination, as opposed to that of pure venous angiomas. Rigamonti and Spetzler[92] found evidence of an associated cavernous angioma in 8% of their venous angioma cases, and in the rare instances (two patients) of cerebellar hemorrhage in association with a venous angioma, a cavernous angioma was detected at the hemorrhage site, with MRI in one and at the time of surgery in the other. These authors raise the concern that the rare cases of venous angioma with hemorrhage reported in the past, prior to the introduction of MRI, may have been erroneously attributed to that malformation, without the proper exclusion of a cavernous angioma by high-field MRI imaging.[79] Their view of the benign character of isolated venous angiomas, without associated cavernous angiomas, is further strengthened by the reported absence of bleeding episodes in their thirty patients over a mean follow-up period of forty-five months. However, other authors[81,82] have reported a substantially higher risk of hemorrhage in venous angiomas, in particular for those located in the cerebellum. Tannier et al.[81] reported four cases with hemorrhage (one SAH, three ICH) among twelve cases of venous angiomas, and nine (43%) of the twenty-one patients reported by Malik et al.[82] presented with hemorrhage. The latter authors collected a series of twenty-one patients with twenty-three venous angiomas, who presented with ICH (nine patients), intractable seizures (one patient), or as an incidental finding (eleven patients). The average age for the total group was 38, and that of the patients with ICH was 33. The ICH were frontal (two), parietal (three), pontine (three), and mesencephalic (one) in location. They were all treated surgically, with either complete (four) or partial (five) resection of the venous angioma, and no mortality resulted from the procedure, which was associated with significant morbidity (dysphagia, tongue paresis) in only one patient. On the basis of their experience, as well as that reported in the literature, Malik et al.[82] suggested that venous angiomas have a significant risk of bleeding and rebleeding, and recommended surgical treat-

**Figure 8.10.** Venous angioma of the cerebellum. (A) Postcontrast CT scan showing prominent vascular structure to the right of the fourth ventricle. B (axial) and C (coronal) are Gadolinium-enhanced MRI (TR/TE = 600/30 msec) views of the malformation which is made of a number of medullary veins draining into the single large vein adjacent to the fourth ventricle. (D) Vertebral angiogram of the venous phase, antero-posterior view, depicts the venous angioma as the "caput medusae" medullary veins (double small arrows) that drain into a large, medially placed vein (large arrow), which in turn drains into the transverse sinus (arrowheads).

ment as the preferred option. In addition, because of their observation of two patients who bled during pregnancy, they recommended surgical excision for asymptomatic venous angiomas in women of childbearing age. These opinions regarding the risk of hemorrhage and the treatment of venous angiomas were contested by Spetzler,[90] who argued that bleeding potential in venous angiomas is negligible in the absence of an associated cavernous angioma, and that considerable surgical morbidity and mortality can follow the surgical resection or obliteration of venous angiomas, especially those located in the posterior fossa. In support of the latter view, Senegor et al.[93] and Biller et al.[94] reported young patients who underwent resection of a midline cerebellar venous angioma with postoperative development of fatal posterior fossa venous hemorrhagic infarction. Similar instances of intraoperative or postoperative transient local brain swelling with reversible clinical deterioration were reported by Rigamonti and Spetzler[92] and by Inagawa et al.[95] following complete resection of a cerebellar and a parietal lobe venous angioma, respectively. Based on these instances of severe venous infarcts following resection of venous angiomas,[92,93–95] the notion (originally developed by Courville[96]) exists that these lesions are the result of a developmental defect in which there is either agenesis or occlusion of transcerebral veins during the embryogenesis of the venous system, between eight and twelve weeks of gestation.[81] This embryological defect leads to the development of a compensatory venous drainage system,[96] which constitutes the venous angioma, a developmentally anomalous structure that nevertheless performs the venous drainage of normal areas of brain. In the event of complete surgical resection or obliteration of this structure, at times extensive areas of the brain are deprived of venous drainage, resulting in venous hemorrhagic infarction. Using this same concept, Yamamoto et al.[97] postulated that thrombosis of a venous angioma resulted in ICH in their

patient, although they did not have pathological verification of the suspected thrombosis.

In view of the documented instances of severe morbidity from resection of venous angiomas, especially in the posterior fossa, current recommendations for the management of these lesions include (1) the routine performance of high-field MRI, in order to detect a possible associated cavernous angioma[79,90,92] (2) in the event of presentation with ICH, drainage of the hematoma and resection of an associated cavernous angioma are indicated, but without resection of the venous angioma, and (3) in asymptomatic patients with isolated venous angiomas a conservative approach is warranted, since resection/obliteration of the malformation is not indicated in these patients who have an extremely low risk of bleeding.

### Telangiectases

These lesions are considered to have the lowest bleeding potential among the cerebral vascular malformations, and they are usually incidental autopsy findings, occurring preferentially in the pons.[5,70] Among 164 posterior fossa malformations in the autopsy study of McCormick et al.,[70] thirty-eight (23%) were telangiectases, twenty-seven of which were pontine, six cerebellar, and five medullary. Fifty-one of the 164 malformations had bled, and only one of them was a telangiectasis; none of the twenty-seven pontine telangiectases bled. Well-documented examples of bleeding from these lesions are scanty in the literature. Teilmann[98] described two patients who died as a result of pontine hemorrhage, with postmortem diagnosis of telangiectases as the mechanism of the hemorrhage. A patient with a deep hemispheric hemorrhage, surgically drained, was reported by Girard et al.,[99] who subsequently documented multiple telangiectases of the cerebral hemispheres and brainstem at autopsy. Finally, McConnell and Leonard[100] reported one patient who had a massive, fatal hemorrhage described as "intraventricular," presumably originating in the medial aspect of the right caudate nucleus, where a "collection of distended vascular channels . . . with a single layer of lining endothelium . . . [and] walls made up of fibrous tissue, with small amounts of intermingled, disorganized smooth muscle and elastic fibers" were described histologically. Although the lesion was labeled a telangiectasis, its histological description is equivocal, possibly corresponding to a small AVM.

In rare instances, large aggregates of telangiectases in the brain substance have produced progressive neurological dysfunction in the absence of pathological evidence of hemorrhage.[101,102] In one patient,[101] extensive telangiectases of the basal ganglia, internal capsule, thalamus, and subthalamus were associated with hemiparesis and hemiparkinsonism. The remarkable patient of Farrell and Forno[102] developed progressive gait disturbance and bulbar palsy in the setting of virtual replacement of the medullary parenchyma by extensive telangiectases, without hemorrhage. Other rare cases of brainstem hemorrhage and telangiectases have corresponded to bleeding from an associated cavernous angioma,[6] rather than from the telangiectases. Since these two types of vascular malformation are known to frequently coexist,[6,99] the attribution of hemorrhage to telangiectases should only rest on convincing evidence of lack of an associated cavernous angioma on pathological examination.

## References

1. Jellinger K. Zur Ätiologie und Pathogenese der spontanen intrazerebralen Blutung. Therapiewoche 1972;22:1440–1450.
2. Sarwar M, McCormick WF. Intracerebral venous angioma: case report and review. Arch Neurol 1978;35:323–325.
3. Weller RO. Spontaneous intracranial haemorrhage. In Adams JH, et al., eds. Greenfield's neuropathology, 4th ed. New York: Wiley, 1984;223–224.
4. Stehbens WE. Intracranial arterial aneurysms. In Pathology of the cerebral blood vessels. St. Louis: CV Mosby, 1972;351–470.
5. Russell DS, Rubinstein LJ. Tumours and hamartomas of the blood-vessels. In Pathology of tumours of the nervous system, 4th ed. Baltimore: Williams & Wilkins, 1977; 116–145.
6. Roberson GH, Kase CS, Wolpow ER. Telangiectases and cavernous angiomas of the brainstem: "cryptic" vascular malformations. Neuroradiology 1974;8:83–89.
7. Locksley HB. Report on the cooperative study of intracranial aneurysms and subarachnoid hemorrhage. Section V, Part 1: natural history of subarachnoid hemorrhage, intracranial aneurysms and arteriovenous malformations. J Neurosurg 1966;25:219–239.
8. Weir B, Miller J, Russell D. Intracranial aneurysms: a clinical, angiographic and computerized tomographic study. Can J Neurol Sci 1977;4:99–105.
9. Freger P, Creissard P, Sevrain L, et al. Les hématomes intracraniens des anévrysmes rompus: a propos de 57 cas. Neurochirurgie 1987;33:1–11.
10. Wheelock B, Weir B, Watts R, et al. Timing for surgery for intracerebral hematomas due to aneurysm rupture. J Neurosurg 1983;58: 476–481.
11. Benoit BG, Cochrane DD, Durity F, et al. Clinical-radiological correlates in intracerebral hematomas due to aneurysmal rupture. Can J Neurol Sci 1982;9:409–414.
12. Robertson EG. Cerebral lesions due to intracranial aneurysms. Brain 1949;72:150–185.
13. Crompton MR. Intracerebral haematoma complicating ruptured cerebral berry aneurysm. J Neurol Neurosurg Psychiat 1962;25:378–386.
14. Reynolds AF, Shaw C-M. Bleeding patterns from ruptured intracranial aneurysms: an autopsy series of 205 patients. Surg Neurol 1981;15:232–235.
15. Mohr JP, Caplan LR, Melski JW, et al. The Harvard Cooperative Stroke Registry: a prospective registry. Neurology 1978;28:754–762.
16. Adams HP, Kassell NF, Boarini DJ, et al. The clinical spectrum of aneurysmal subarachnoid hemorrhage. J Stroke Cerebrovasc Dis 1991;1:3–8.
17. Stein BM, Wolpert SM. Arteriovenous malformations of the brain. I: current concepts and treatment. Arch Neurol 1980;37:1–5.

18. Peterson EW, Schulz DM. Amyloid in vessels of a vascular malformation in brain. Arch Pathol 1961;72:480–483.

19. Zellem RT, Buchheit WA. Multiple intracranial arteriovenous malformations: case report. Neurosurgery 1985;17:88–93.

20. King CR, Lovrien EW, Reiss J. Central nervous system arteriovenous malformations in multiple generations of a family with hereditary hemorrhagic telangiectasia. Clin Gen 1977; 12:372–381.

21. Eto RT, Harley JD, Chikos PM, et al. Subarachnoid hemorrhage in hereditary hemorrhagic telangiectasia: a report of two cases. Neuroradiology 1974;8:127–130.

22. Perret G, Nishioka H. Report on the cooperative study of intracranial aneurysms and subarachnoid hemorrhage. Section VI: arteriovenous malformations. J Neurosurg 1966; 25:467–490.

23. Crawford PM, West CR, Chadwick DW, et al. Arteriovenous malformations of the brain: natural history in unoperated patients. J Neurol Neurosurg Psychiat 1986;49:1–10.

24. Graf CJ, Perret GE, Torner JC. Bleeding from cerebral arteriovenous malformations as part of their natural history. J Neurosurg 1983; 58:331–337.

25. Abe M, Kjellberg RN, Adams RD. Clinical presentations of vascular malformations of the brain stem: comparison of angiographically positive and negative types. J Neurol Neurosurg Psychiat 1989;52:167–175.

26. Homan R, Devous MD, Stokely EM, et al. Quantification of intracerebral steal in patients with arteriovenous malformation. Arch Neurol 1986;43:779–785.

27. Awad IA, Little JR, Akrawi WP, et al. Intracranial dural arteriovenous malformations: factors predisposing to an aggressive neurological course. J Neurosurg 1990;72:839–850.

28. King WA, Martin NA. Intracerebral hemorrhage due to dural arteriovenous malformations and fistulae. Neurosurg Clin NA 1992;3:577–590.

29. Fults D, Kelly DL. Natural history of arteriovenous malformations of the brain: a clinical study. Neurosurgery 1984;15:658–662.

30. Batjer H, Samson D. Arteriovenous malformations of the posterior fossa: clinical presentation, diagnostic evaluation, and surgical treatment. J Neurosurg 1986;64:849–856.

31. Aminoff MJ, Kendall BE. Asymptomatic dural vascular anomalies. Br J Radiol 1973;46: 662–667.

32. Obrador S, Soto M, Silvela J. Clinical syndromes of arteriovenous malformations of the transverse-sigmoid sinus. J Neurol Neurosurg Psychiat 1975;38:436–451.

33. Houser OW, Campbell JK, Campbell RJ, et al. Arteriovenous malformation affecting the transverse dural venous sinus: an acquired lesion. Mayo Clin Proc 1979;54:651–661.

34. Malik GM, Pearce JE, Ausman JI, et al. Dural arteriovenous malformations and intracranial hemorrhage. Neurosurgery 1984;15:332–339.

35. Lasjaunias P, Chiu M, Ter Brugge K, et al. Neurological manifestations of intracranial dural arteriovenous malformations. J Neurosurg 1986;64:724–730.

36. Waga S, Fujimoto K, Morikawa A, et al. Dural arteriovenous malformation in the anterior fossa. Surg Neurol 1977;8:356–358.

37. Houser OW, Baker HL, Rhoton AL, et al. Intracranial dural arteriovenous malformations. Radiology 1972;105:55–64.

38. Solis OJ, Davis KR, Ellis GT. Dural arteriovenous malformation associated with subdural and intracerebral hematoma: a CT scan and angiographic correlation. Comput Tomogr 1977;1:145–150.

39. Grady MS, Pobereskin L. Arteriovenous malformations of the dura mater. Surg Neurol 1987;28:135–140.

40. Crawford JV, Russell DS. Cryptic arteriovenous and venous hamartomas of the brain. J Neurol Neurosurg Psychiat 1956;19:1–11.

41. Wakai S, Ueda Y, Inoh S, et al. Angiographically occult angiomas: a report of thirteen cases with analysis of the cases documented in the literature. Neurosurgery 1985;17: 549–556.

42. McCormick WF, Nofzinger JD. "Cryptic" vascular malformations of the central nervous system. J Neurosurg 1966;24:865–875.

43. Sand JJ, Biller J, Corbett JJ, et al. Partial dorsal mesencephalic hemorrhages: report of three cases. Neurology 1986;36:529–533.

44. Sano K. Spontaneous brain stem haematoma. Neurosurg Rev 1983;6:71–77.

45. Kempe LG. Surgical removal of an intramedullary haematoma simulating Wallenberg's syndrome. J Neurol Neurosurg Psychiat 1964;27:78–80.

46. Ropper AH, Davis KR. Lobar cerebral hemorrhages: acute clinical syndromes in 26 cases. Ann Neurol 1980;8:141–147.

47. Margolis G, Odom GL, Woodhall B, et al. The role of small angiomatous malformations in the production of intracerebral hematomas. J Neurosurg 1951;8:564–575.

48. Krayenbühl H, Siebenmann R. Small vascular malformations as a cause of primary intracerebral hemorrhage. J Neurosurg 1965;22:7–20.

49. Becker DH, Townsend JJ, Kramer RA, et al. Occult cerebrovascular malformations: a series of 18 histologically verified cases with negative angiography. Brain 1979;102:249–287.

50. Steiger HJ, Tew JM. Hemorrhage and epilepsy in cryptic cerebrovascular malformations. Arch Neurol 1984;41:722–724.

51. Kramer RA, Wing SD. Computed tomography of angiographically occult cerebral vascular malformations. Radiology 1977;123:649–652.

52. Bell BA, Kendall BE, Symon L. Angiographically occult arteriovenous malformations of the brain. J Neurol Neurosurg Psychiat 1978;41:1057–1064.

53. Kucharczyk W, Lemme-Pleghos L, Uske A, et al. Intracranial vascular malformations: MR and CT imaging. Radiology 1985;156:383–389.

54. New PFJ, Ojemann RG, David KR, et al. MR and CT of occult vascular malformations of the brain. Amer J Radiol 1986;147:985–993.

55. Gomori JM, Grossman RI, Goldberg HI, et al. Occult cerebral vascular malformations: high-field MR imaging. Radiology 1986;158:707–713.

56. Sze G, Krol G, Olsen WL, et al. Hemorrhagic neoplasms: MR mimics of occult vascular malformations. Am J Neuroradiol 1987;8:795–802.

57. Stahl SM, Johnson KP, Malamud N. The clinical and pathological spectrum of brain-stem vascular malformations: long-term course simulates multiple sclerosis. Arch Neurol 1980;37:25–29.

58. Yeates A, Enzmann D. Cryptic vascular malformations involving the brainstem. Radiology 1983;146:71–75.

59. Kashiwagi S, van Loveren HR, Tew JM, et al. Diagnosis and treatment of vascular brainstem malformations. J Neurosurg 1990;72:27–34.

60. Kilpatrick TJ, Davis SM, Tress BM, et al. Lateral tegmental pontine haemorrhage due to vascular malformations. Cerebrovasc Dis 1991;1:108–112.

61. Simard JM, Garcia-Bengochea F, Ballinger WE, et al. Cavernous angioma: a review of 126 collected and 12 new clinical cases. Neurosurgery 1986;18:162–172.

62. Yamasaki T, Handa H, Yamashita J, et al. Intracranial and orbital cavernous angiomas: a review of 30 cases. J Neurosurg 1986;64:197–208.

63. Tagle P, Huete I, Méndez J, et al. Intracranial cavernous angioma: presentation and management. J Neurosurg 1986;64:720–723.

64. Weber M, Vespignani H, Bracard S, et al. Les angiomes caverneux intracérébraux. Rev Neurol 1989;145:429–436.

65. Requena I, Arias M, López-Ibor L, et al. Cavernomas of the central nervous system: clinical and neuroimaging manifestations in 47 patients. J Neurol Neurosurg Psychiat 1991;54:590–594.

66. Otten P, Pizzolato GP, Rilliet B, et al. A propos de 131 cas d'angiomes caverneux (cavernomes) du S.N.C., repérés par l'analyse rétrospective de 24 535 autopsies. Neurochirurgie 1989;35:82–83.

67. Zimmerman RS, Spetzler RF, Lee KS, et al. Cavernous malformations of the brain stem. J Neurosurg 1991;75:32–39.

68. Giombini S, Morello G. Cavernous angiomas of the brain: account of fourteen personal cases and review of the literature. Acta Neurochir 1978;40:61–82.

69. Vaquero J, Salazar J, Martínez R, et al. Cavernomas of the central nervous system: clinical syndromes, CT scan diagnosis, and prognosis after treatment in 25 cases. Acta Neurochir 1987;85:29–33.

70. McCormick WF, Hardman JM, Boulter TR. Vascular malformations ("angiomas") of the brain with special reference to those occurring in the posterior fossa. J Neurosurg 1968;28:241–251.

71. Voigt K, Yaşargil MG. Cerebral cavernous haemangiomas or cavernomas: incidence, pathology, localization, diagnosis, clinical features and treatment. Neurochirurgia 1976;19:59–68.

72. Rigamonti D, Drayer BP, Johnson PC, et al. The MRI appearance of cavernous malformations (angiomas). J Neurosurg 1987;67:518–524.

73. Clark JV. Familial occurrence of cavernous angiomata of the brain. J Neurol Neurosurg Psychiat 1970;33:871–876.

74. Rigamonti D, Hadley MN, Drayer BP, et al. Cerebral cavernous malformations: incidence and familial occurrence. N Engl J Med 1988;319:343–347.

75. Hayman LA, Evans RA, Ferrell RE, et al. Familial cavernous angiomas: natural history

and genetic study over a 5-year period. Am J Med Genet 1982;11:147–160.

76. Jonutis AJ, Sondheimer FK, Klein HZ, et al. Intracerebral cavernous angioma with angiographically demonstrated pathologic vasculature. Neuroradiology 1971;3:57–63.

77. Kjellberg RN, Hanamura T, Davis KR, et al. Bragg-peak proton-beam therapy for arteriovenous malformations of the brain. N Engl J Med 1983;309:269–274.

78. Saito Y, Kobayashi N. Cerebral venous angiomas: clinical evaluation and possible etiology. Radiology 1981;139:87–94.

79. Rigamonti D, Spetzler RF, Medina M, et al. Cerebral venous malformations. J Neurosurg 1990;73:560–564.

80. Michels LG, Bentson JR, Winter J. Computed tomography of cerebral venous angiomas. J Comp Assist Tomogr 1977;1:149–154.

81. Tannier C, Pons M, Treil J. Les angiomes veineux encéphaliques 12 cas personnels et revue de la littérature. Rev Neurol 1991;147:356–363.

82. Malik GM, Morgan JK, Boulos RS, et al. Venous angiomas: an underestimated cause of intracranial hemorrhage. Surg Neurol 1988; 30:350–358.

83. Fierstien SB, Pribram HW, Hieshima G. Angiography and computed tomography in the evaluation of cerebral venous malformations. Neuroradiology 1979;17:137–148.

84. Moritake K, Handa H, Mori K, et al. Venous angiomas of the brain. Surg Neurol 1980; 14:95–105.

85. Valavanis A, Wellauer J, Yaşargil MG. The radiological diagnosis of cerebral venous angioma: cerebral angiography and computed tomography. Neuroradiology 1983;24:193–199.

86. Agnoli AL, Hildebrandt G. Cerebral venous angiomas. Acta Neurochir 1985;78:4–12.

87. Scotti LN, Goldman RL, Rao GR, et al. Cerebral venous angioma. Neuroradiology 1975;9: 125–128.

88. Wendling LR, Moore JS, Kieffer SA, et al. Intracerebral venous angioma. Radiology 1976; 119:141–147.

89. Malik GM. Surg Neurol 1989;31:482 (letter).

90. Spetzler RF. Surg Neurol 1989;31:412–413 (letter).

91. Wolf PA, Rosman NP, New PFJ. Multiple small cryptic venous angiomas of the brain mimicking cerebral metastases. Neurology 1967;17:491–501.

92. Rigamonti D, Spetzler RF. The association of venous and cavernous malformations: report of four cases and discussion of the pathophysiological, diagnostic, and therapeutic implications. Acta Neurochir 1988;92:100–105.

93. Senegor M, Dohrmann GJ, Wollmann RL. Venous angiomas of the posterior fossa should be considered as anomalous venous drainage. Surg Neurol 1983;19:26–32.

94. Biller J, Toffol GJ, Shea JF, et al. Cerebellar venous angiomas: a continuing controversy. Arch Neurol 1985;42:367–370.

95. Inagawa T, Taguchi H, Yamada T. Surgical intervention in ruptured venous angioma: case report. Neurol Med Chir 1985;25:559–563.

96. Courville CB. Morphology of small vascular malformations of the brain: with particular reference to the mechanism of their drainage. J Neuropath Exp Neurol 1963: 22:274–284.

97. Yamamoto M, Inagawa T, Kamiya K, et al. Intracerebral hemorrhage due to venous thrombosis in venous angioma: case report. Neurol Med Chir 1989;29:1044–1046.

98. Teilmann K. Hemangiomas of the pons. Arch Neurol Psychiat 1953;69:208–223.

99. Girard P, Tommasi M, Chatelain R. Cavernomes de télangiectasies de l'encéphale. Arch Anat Path 1969;17:167–178.

100. McConnell TH, Leonard JS. Microangiomatous malformations with intraventricular hemorrhage: report of two unusual cases. Neurology 1967;17:618–620.

101. Girard PF, Garde A, Devic M. Télangiectasies confluentes du IIIe ventricule. Rev Neurol 1952;86:232–236.

102. Farrell DF, Forno LS. Symptomatic capillary telangiectasis of the brainstem without hemorrhage: report of an unusual case. Neurology 1970;20:341–346.

# Chapter 9
# Cerebral Amyloid Angiopathy

## Carlos S. Kase

Cerebral amyloid angiopathy (CAA), also known as "congophilic" angiopathy, is a condition that selectively affects the cerebral vasculature, in the absence of amyloidosis elsewhere in the body.[1] Deposits of amyloid occur in the walls of small and medium-sized arteries and veins, preferentially affecting vessels of the cerebral cortex and leptomeninges; involvement of vessels in the deep portions of the cerebral hemispheres, as well as the brainstem and cerebellum, is distinctly rare in this condition.[2] The amyloid is deposited in the media and adventitia of the vessels, where it has an amorphous, deeply eosinophilic character on hematoxylin and eosin staining. The presence of amyloid in vessel walls can be confirmed with various histological techniques, the most commonly employed being the Congo red stain, which produces a salmon pink color under ordinary light, and a typical yellow-green ("apple green") birefringence under polarized light (Figure 9.1A, B).[3] The deposits of amyloid have a tendency to concentrate more heavily in areas of vascular bifurcations, a feature that can be demonstrated after staining of vessels stripped from the leptomeningeal covering of the cerebral hemispheres (Figure 9.1C). Affected vessels in cross section frequently have intramural clefts in areas of heavy amyloid deposition, leading to a "double-barreled" appearance (Figure 9.1D). Amyloid can also be identified with thiofla-

vin T and S, which produce fluorescence under ultraviolet light. Under the electron microscope, vascular amyloid appears as randomly distributed, nonramified fibrils of 8.5 to 9.5 nm in width, an aspect common to all forms of amyloid deposits, cerebral and systemic.[4]

The distribution of amyloid-laden blood vessels in CAA favors the superficial portions of the cerebral hemispheres, with characteristic sparing of basal ganglia, thalamus, cerebellum, and brainstem, the latter explaining the clinical observation of virtual absence of cases of primary brainstem intracerebral hemorrhage (ICH) due to CAA.[1] In the cerebral hemispheres, all lobes are probably involved to a similar degree, although some authors have reported a heavier concentration of affected vessels in the posterior, parieto-occipital, areas,[5,6] while others[7] have detected a frontoparietal predominance of the angiopathy. When this is translated into the clinical effects of rupture of amyloid-laden blood vessels, with production of ICH, a predominance of frontoparietal hematoma locations has been noticed.[1,2] This suggests that the mere presence of CAA may not be the single factor causing ICH, and other features must operate in the occurrence of vascular rupture.[1]

A characteristic feature of CAA is its increase in frequency with advancing age. In an autopsy study, Vinters and Gilbert[2]

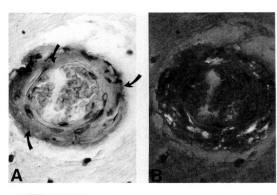

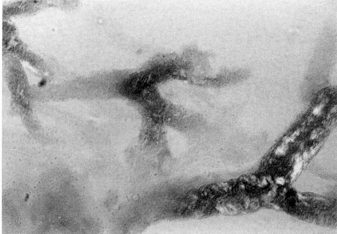

C

**Figure 9.1.** (A) Cortical vessel with amyloid deposits in the wall (arrows). (Congo red, ×200.) (B) Same vessel as in A, showing birefringence of amyloid deposits under polarized light. (Congo red, ×200.) (From Kase CS, Vonsattel J-P, Richardson EP. Case records of the Massachusetts General Hospital (Case 10-1988). N Engl J Med 1988;318:623–631, reproduced with permission.) (C) Amyloid deposits at sites of vascular bifurcation in leptomeningeal vessels. (Congo red, ×200.) (Courtesy of Dr. J-P Vonsattel, Neuropathology Laboratory, Massachusetts General Hospital, Boston, MA.) (D) Leptomeningeal arteriole with eosinophilic amyloid deposits in the vessel wall, and intramural clefts ("double-barrel" appearance). (H&E, ×200.) (From Kase CS, Vonsattel J-P, Richardson EP. Case records of the Massachusetts General Hospital (Case 10-1988). N Engl J Med 1988;318:623–631, reproduced with permission.)

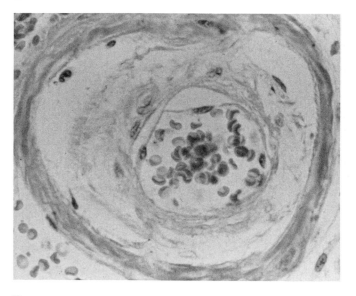

D

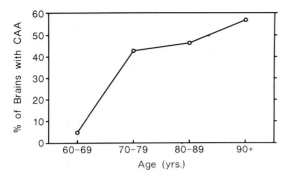

**Figure 9.2.** Frequency of CAA in relation to age, in autopsy study (Drawn from data from Vinters HV, Gilbert JJ. Cerebral amyloid angiopathy: incidence and complications in the aging brain. II. The distribution of amyloid vascular changes. Stroke 1983;14:924–928.)

systematically searched for histological features of CAA in eighty-four brains of individuals 60 to 97 years of age. CAA was documented in only 5% of those in the seventh decade, but the frequency rose steadily in subsequent decades, reaching values over 50% in persons over age 90 (Figure 9.2). Almost identical figures on frequency of CAA in different decades were reported in the autopsy studies of Tomonaga[7] and Masuda et al.[8] (Table 9.1). The latter authors[8] found CAA in 18.3% of men and 28.0% of women in a group of 400 consecutive autopsies in individuals between ages 40 and 90+. CAA was not documented in any of the specimens from patients in the 40- to 49-year-old age group in either sex. The low frequency of CAA in middle-aged adults results in the rarity of ICH due to this condition in individuals under age 55.[9]

CAA as a histological entity has been associated with a number of clinical and histological correlates, some of which are probably coincidental,[1] whereas others are causally or pathogenetically related to the angiopathy. Among the latter, ICH is by far the most consistent clinical effect of CAA, whereas Alzheimer's disease, cerebral infarcts, and leukoencephalopathy occur as less well-defined associations.

## Intracerebral Hemorrhage

This manifestation of CAA has been well known to pathologists for several decades, but its importance as a clinical entity only became widely recognized in the 1970s, when a number of authors [10-14] documented the association of CAA and ICH in various clinical settings. Jellinger[10] studied an autopsy series of 1010 brains of demented individuals over age 55, and 400 consecutive cases of nontraumatic ICH, and found fifteen instances of CAA, ten of which had multiple small ("miliary") hemorrhages, while eight brains showed massive recent ICH. The latter were predominantly located in the frontal and temporal lobes (three cases each), and only one hemorrhage occurred in the basal ganglia. The eight examples of massive ICH were related to widespread cortical and leptomeningeal CAA, and represented a frequency of 2% among the 400 consecutive cases of nontraumatic ICH. Regarding the histological features of the fifteen cases with CAA, Jellinger commented on the association of CAA with hypertensive "hyaline" angiopathy in eight of them, at times both changes appearing in closely related, contiguous segments of the same vessel. Based on these observations, he regarded CAA as an important cause of ICH in the elderly. Ulrich et al.[12] reported the autopsy findings of five patients with CAA between ages 52 and 74, three of whom (ages 58, 58, and 74) had presented clinically with ICH, which was the immediate cause of death in one of the three;

**Table 9.1.** Frequency of CAA in Relation to Age, Autopsy Series

| Age Group (yr) | Series | | | |
|---|---|---|---|---|
| | Vinters and Gilbert[2] | Tomonaga[7] | Masuda et al.[8] | |
| | | | Men | Women |
| 60–69 | 4.7% | 8.0% | 9.3% | 13.6% |
| 70–79 | 42.8% | 23.0% | 18.3% | 23.3% |
| 80–89 | 46.4% | 37.0% | 38.0% | 36.1% |
| 90+ | 57.0% | 58.0% | 42.8% | 45.8% |

this patient had at autopsy a fresh left frontoparietal ICH and an old right frontal hemorrhage. The other two patients with ICH had their hematoma surgically evacuated eleven months and nine days before their deaths due to a mesenteric infarct and to renal failure, respectively. Torack[13] reported three autopsy observations of recent ICH associated with CAA in patients who had been subjected to surgical procedures: two of them (Cases 1 and 3) had brain biopsy at the time of ventricular shunt insertion for normal-pressure hydrocephalus, whereas Case 2 died after reaccumulation of a spontaneous right temporal ICH drained surgically one day before. His Case 1 was particularly striking in that a large right parietal ICH was demonstrated along the shunt tract, extending from the cortical surface into the ventricular space. In Case 3, the hemorrhagic event occurred one month after ventriculoatrial shunt placement, and took the form of a subdural hematoma that proved fatal despite surgical evacuation. The postmortem brain examination disclosed residual subdural and epidural hematomas, as well as "extensive hemorrhagic infarction" in the posterior aspect of the right hemisphere. These observations have been frequently cited as suggestive of the potential role of surgical trauma in the pathogenesis of some cases of CAA-related ICH. The observations of Gudmundsson et al.[14] on the familial variety of CAA with ICH are discussed later in this chapter.

Since these early observations, the spectrum and varieties of CAA-related ICH have been further delineated, including the distinction of a common, sporadic, age-related form, from a rare, familial, geographically distinct variety of the condition. These two clinical forms are discussed separately.

### Sporadic Form of Cerebral Amyloid Angiopathy–related ICH

The *frequency* of the association between CAA and ICH is difficult to establish in clinical series, since the prevalence of the angiopathy in the population is impossible to establish for a condition that can only be diagnosed histologically. In an autopsy series of seventy-five consecutive ICH cases in individuals ages 35 to 86, Lee and Stemmermann[15] found CAA as the underlying cause in seven (9.3%) of the cases. However, all seven cases with CAA were in individuals in the 60- to 90-year-old group, which in turn accounted for forty-seven of the seventy-five ICH, thus resulting in a 15% (seven of forty-seven) rate of cerebral hemorrhage for the age groups in which CAA is known to occur. This figure is higher than the 2% frequency reported by Jellinger,[10] but this author did not provide an age distribution for his group of 400 cases of nontraumatic ICH, thus making direct comparisons between these two autopsy series impossible.

A large number of publications over the last decade have analyzed the clinical and radiological features of ICH in the setting of CAA. The summary of these studies is provided in Table 9.2.[1,16–33] The most consistent anatomical feature of CAA-related ICH is its *lobar location*, resulting from the superficial (cortical, leptomeningeal) distribution of the angiopathy. As a result, the majority of these hemorrhages occur in the subcortical white matter of the cerebral lobes (Figure 9.3), at a distance from the deep hemispheric structures that are the common site of hypertensive ICH. The consistent lack of CAA-related ICH in the deep hemispheric locations has been documented in a number of autopsy[6,26,29,34] and clinical[24,25,32] series. Although occasionally observed,[5,8,15,28] cerebellar hemorrhage is equally exceptional in the setting of CAA.[6,10,13,24,26,27] The superficial location of the angiopathy has rarely been associated with examples of pure subarachnoid or subdural bleeding.[13,29,35] A more common observation is the presence of local subarachnoid hemorrhage (SAH) in the immediate vicinities of a superficial, lobar ICH.[36] This feature, in combination with other smaller "satellite" areas of intraparenchymal hemorrhage surrounding the

**Table 9.2.** Clinical and Anatomical Features of Sporadic CAA-related ICH[1,17]

| Author | No. of Pts. | Mean Age (Range) | ICH Features | Comment |
|--------|-------------|------------------|--------------|---------|
| Ulrich et al.[12] | 3 | 63 (58–74) | Massive | Head trauma in 2 pts. |
| Torack[13] | 3 | 70 (62–76) | 2 ICH 1 SDH | 1 ICH and 1 SDH after ventricular shunt |
| Jellinger[10] | 15 | 74 (64–86) | Massive, 8/15 | F,T > P,O |
| Bruni et al.[16] | 3 | 77 (75–82) | 1 with SDH | 1 ICH in BG |
| Mandybur and Bates[18] | 1 | 58 | Massive | Occipital |
| Tucker et al.[19] | 2 | 67,74 | Lobar | Multiple |
| Regli et al.[20] | 1 | 75 | Massive | Multiple |
| Ackerman et al.[21] | 1 | 62 | Lobar | Multiple, recurrent |
| Tyler et al.[22] | 1 | 63 | Massive | Multiple |
| Gilbert and Vinters[6] | 11 | 75 (61–87) | Lobar | F-P > F > O |
| Finelli et al.[23] | 1 | 66 | Lobar | Multiple, recurrent |
| Wagle et al.[24] | 7 | 71 (62–84) | Lobar | 1 ICH in corpus callosum |
| Patel et al.[25] | 2 | 72 | Lobar | Multiple, recurrent |
| Gilles et al.[26] | 11 | 69 (60–81) | Lobar | Multiple, recurrent |
| Ishii et al.[27] | 7 | 77 (66–94) | Lobar | F,T > P,O |
| Kalyan-Raman and Kalyan-Raman[28] | 10 | 69 (54–88) | Lobar, BG, cerebellar | 1 on AC, 2 after head trauma |
| Cosgrove et al.[29] | 16 | 74 (58–88) | Lobar | F-P = P-O |
| Roosen et al.[30] | 1 | 59 | Lobar | Occipital, recurrent |
| Sobel et al.[31] | 2 | 72,67 | Lobar | Multiple, recurrent |
| Brown et al.[32] | 12 | 73 (62–89) | Lobar | 1 on AC, 4/12 recurrent |
| Kase et al.[3] | 1 | 73 | Lobar | Multiple, recurrent |
| Greene et al.[33] | 9 | 73 (62–82) | Lobar | Head trauma in 5, all 9 operated |

Abbreviations: SDH = subdural hematoma, F = frontal, T = temporal, P = parietal, O = occipital, BG = basal ganglia, AC = anticoagulants.

main focus of ICH, confers at times an irregular, variegated character to this type of hemorrhage (Figure 9.4). This aspect contrasts with the usually deep, single, and homogeneous focus of parenchymal hemorrhage (that does not communicate with the convexity subarachnoid space) seen in the setting of hypertension.

Any of the cerebral lobes can be affected by CAA-related ICH. Although the distribution of the angiopathy tends to favor the posterior aspects of the cerebral hemispheres,[2] with a frequently exclusive occipital (calcarine) location in cases with minimal involvement,[21,34] the hemorrhages are distributed more evenly among the cerebral lobes, with a suggested predominance for the frontoparietal areas.[2] From a combined tabulation of 171 hemorrhages related to CAA from the literature, Vinters[1] calculated the relative frequency for

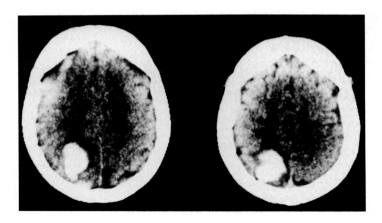

**Figure 9.3.** Left occipital lobar hemorrhage.

the various cerebral sites as follows: frontal 35.1%, parietal 26.3%, occipital 18.7%, temporal 14.0%, deep gray nuclei 4.1%, and cerebellum 1.8%. He pointed to the unexplained discrepancy between the posterior anatomical predominance of the angiopathy and the higher frequency of more anteriorly placed

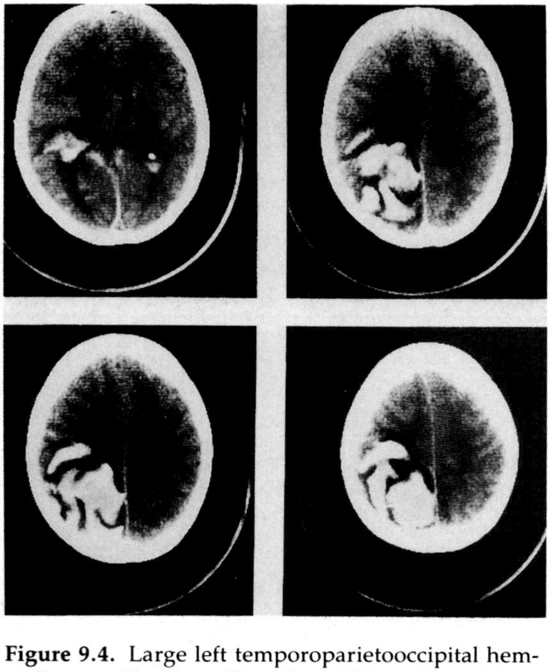

**Figure 9.4.** Large left temporoparietooccipital hemorrhage, with mass effect (A and B) and extension into the adjacent cortical subarachnoid space (B, C, and D).

hemorrhages, adding that factors other than the mere presence of CAA are likely to be implicated in the vascular rupture that leads to ICH in some of these cases.

The other distinctive characteristic of CAA-related ICH is its tendency to *recurrence*, a feature that also distinguishes it from hypertensive ICH, a variety of hemorrhage that rarely recurs.[17,37] The recurrent episodes of ICH in the setting of biopsy-documented CAA can be at times separated by periods of two or more years,[32] and multiple episodes of lobar hemorrhages can occur over prolonged periods, as in the remarkable patient reported by Finelli et al.[23] in whom eight separate episodes of ICH occurred over eight years, and that of Michel et al.[38] who had five lobar hematomas over a 27-month period. These recurrent ICH can thus appear on gross pathological examination as multiple lobar intracerebral hematomas of different ages, as well as simultaneous ICH in both cerebral hemispheres (Figure 9.5). The latter is also a very uncommon feature of hypertensive ICH: in a consecutive series of 600 cases of ICH diagnosed on CT scan, Weisberg[39] found only twelve examples (2%) of multiple simultaneous nontraumatic hematomas, in ten of which there was no clinical evidence of hypertension. These data, and the documented observation of multiple, at times simultaneous, intracerebral hematomas in patients with CAA stress the need for strongly considering this diagnosis in individuals with

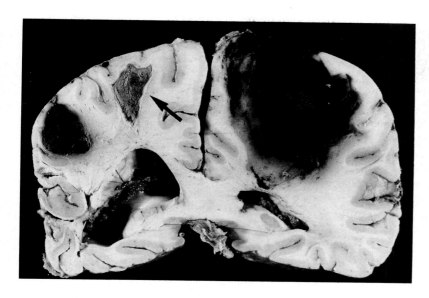

**Figure 9.5.** Multiple lobar ICH due to CAA in a 67-year-old man, two of them recent (one on each hemisphere), one old and partially organized (arrow) (Courtesy of Drs. David E. Burdette and Flaviu C.A. Romanul, Boston VA Medical Center, Boston, MA.)

multiple, recurrent, lobar ICH, especially in those over age 60.

The *mechanism of bleeding* in CAA-related ICH has not been clearly established. As mentioned above, occasional examples of ICH have followed head trauma[12,28,33] or neurosurgical procedures[13] in patients subsequently shown to have CAA. However, it is clear that in the majority of patients with CAA-related ICH the event is truly "spontaneous," without a documented precipitating event of traumatic character. As a result of this, attention has been directed at the angiopathy itself, in an effort at defining the features that may determine vascular rupture and hemorrhage. The concept that the amyloid-laden arteries have intrinsically weak walls, thus constituting mechanically "brittle" vessels, has been held as a possible explanation for vascular rupture,[18,24] although there is no anatomic evidence for such mechanical difference between affected and normal cerebral vessels. A more plausible mechanism for bleeding of amyloid-laden vessels is the association of CAA with other forms of vascular disease, either related to hypertension or coincidental with CAA. Among these associated vascular lesions, formation of microaneurysms[5,8] and "hya-line" degeneration of the vessel wall[10] are thought to be related to arterial rupture. Okazaki et al.[5] pointed to the common finding of microaneurysms in amyloid-laden blood vessels, but their presence at the rupture site has not been confirmed by serial section studies of specimens containing intracerebral hematomas.[3] A more consistent observation has been the presence of fibrinoid necrosis of the vessel wall at rupture sites,[40] a vascular change recognized since the initial observations that linked CAA to the occurrence of ICH.[10] Vonsattel et al.[40] examined at autopsy the brains of sixty-six elderly (age range: 75 to 107) patients from a general hospital and seventy patients (age range: 27 to 96) with various neuropsychiatric disorders but without ICH, as well as those of seventeen patients with CAA and ICH. CAA was found in 50% of those without ICH, and comparison of the features of the angiopathy in those with and without ICH showed severity of the angiopathy and concomitant fibrinoid necrosis to be the factors most closely correlated with the occurrence of ICH. These authors estimated the severity of CAA by the degree of involvement of the vessel wall rather than by the number of vessels involved, a feature that in turn correlated with the frequency of associated changes, in particular the formation of microaneurysms. They found fibrinoid necrosis as a prominent change in twelve of the seventeen (71%) brains with ICH; insufficient sampling in two patients without fibrinoid necrosis may have underestimated its frequency. In two of their ICH cases, serial histological sections revealed rupture of the vascular wall at the site of foci of fibrinoid necrosis, as well as formation of microaneurysms at sites involved by fibrinoid necrosis. These observations suggest that both the severity of the angiopathy and its association with fibrinoid necrosis may be of primary importance in promoting rupture of vessels affected by CAA.[40] Similarly, Mandybur[34] found a number of secondary changes in vessels affected by CAA, among which hyaline arteriolar degeneration and fibrinoid necrosis were both associated with histological evidence of past or recent bleeding. Other vascular changes, such as perivascular or transmural inflammatory infiltrates, on occasion resembling "rheumatoid vasculitis,"[41] bear a less clear relationship with vascular rupture and bleeding. The association of fibrinoid necrosis and CAA in cases with ICH led Vinters[1] to suggest a possible role of hypertension in increasing the risk of bleeding in the setting of CAA, supported by a reported incidence of hypertension in over 30% of patients with CAA-related ICH,[1] although such frequency of hypertension is within the range observed in the general elderly population.[42] In subsequent publications,[36,43] however, Vinters has held the view that hypertension does not appear to be an additional risk factor in causing ICH or infarcts in patients with age-related CAA. Finally, the potential role of iatrogenic factors in promoting ICH in elderly patients with CAA has been suggested by the report of this complication in the setting of thrombolytic treatment of acute myocardial infarction with streptokinase[44] and with tissue plasminogen activator.[45,45a] In view of the widespread use of these thrombolytic agents, generally combined with aspirin and intravenous heparin,

it is proper to raise concern about their potential for causing ICH when used in elderly or demented, or both, patients at risk of harboring CAA.[44-46]

These aspects of the pathogenesis of CAA-related ICH have been in part translated into the issue of conservative versus surgical *treatment* of this condition. Several authors[1,21,22,27,30,47,48] have questioned the safety of surgical drainage of large ICH related to CAA, based on the notion that "brittle" or fragile amyloid-laden vessels are likely to continue to bleed throughout and after the surgery, leading to reaccumulation of the hematoma. Based on this observation, some authors[21,27,30] have recommended a nonsurgical approach to the treatment of CAA-related ICH. However, Greene et al.[33] have recently offered a different view after analyzing a group of eleven patients with CAA who underwent either evacuation of an ICH (nine patients) or a surgical procedure for the evaluation or treatment of a dementing illness (two patients). They recorded no instances of postoperative hematoma formation, and the two postoperative deaths (surgical mortality, 22%) were due to cardiopulmonary arrest, unrelated to intracranial postsurgical complications. Follow-up information on eight patients, ranging between one week and seventy-four months, documented progressive neurological improvement in four patients, three of whom returned to independence in activities of daily living. These data on surgical safety suggest a less dismal prognosis for this condition, in comparison with previous reports of 75% surgical mortality[29] and 90% to 94% overall mortality[28,29] for CAA-related ICH. Similar data on surgical hemorrhagic risk in patients with CAA were reported by Matkovic et al.[49] These authors encountered one example of rebleeding two days after drainage of an occipital hemorrhage among eight patients operated during the acute phase of their ICH, whereas recurrent ICH at a different site and between one week and ten months from the surgery occurred in three other patients. The latter occurrence, in addition to two instances of recurrent bleeding among eight patients with CAA-related ICH who did not undergo surgery, led the authors to conclude that surgical evacuation of these hemorrhages does not increase the natural tendency of this angiopathy to promote recurrent ICH. This, in turn, suggested that hematoma evacuation is not contraindicated in the presence of CAA.[49] Our own experience with over a dozen operated patients with CAA-related ICH is similar to that reported by these authors,[33,49] since we have not observed a single instance of uncontrollable intraoperative bleeding or postoperative reaccumulation of the hematomas. As a result, our policy is to proceed with surgical evacuation of hematomas in patients with medium-sized or large lobar ICH that are causing significant mass effect, regardless of the potential for CAA as the underlying mechanism.

### Familial Form of Cerebral Amyloid Angiopathy–related ICH

The first detailed description of a high concentration of cases of CAA-related ICH within a family group was that of Gudmundsson et al.[14] in Iceland. These authors studied a family of 117 individuals in three generations, twenty-three of whom had ICH. The diagnosis of ICH was confirmed by either autopsy or detailed neurological examination in eight patients, whereas in ten it was determined by death certificate examination. In the remaining five patients the cause of death was listed as a different condition (eclampsia, heart failure), but the clinical details of the case suggested ICH as a most likely cause of death. The autopsy examinations in five cases documented recent ICH, as well as widespread amyloid deposition in intracerebral arteries, without systemic amyloidosis (with the exception of one case, in whom generalized amyloidosis coexisted, in the setting of "chronic tuberculous infection"). A more extensive distribution of the vascular amyloid deposition in comparison with the sporadic variety of CAA was noted in their

cases, with involvement not only of cortical and leptomeningeal vessels, but also those of the basal ganglia, brainstem, and cerebellum. An additional remarkable feature of these Icelandic familial cases was the early occurrence of ICH, affecting individuals in their 20s, 30s, or 40s, with a mean age at death of 44 years for the first and second generations, 29.6 years for the third, and 22.5 years for the fourth generation. Their youngest patient died from ICH at age 15. The pattern of inheritance of the condition was thought to be autosomal dominant. The authors commented on at least one more family from the same area of northwestern Iceland with a strikingly high incidence of ICH at a young age. They could not find a relationship with the family they had previously reported, after tracing the family's ancestry back to the beginning of the eighteenth century.

Following the clinical description of the Icelandic hereditary CAA-related ICH, a number of laboratories became interested in the biochemical analysis of the amyloid fibrils from such cases. Cohen et al.[50] determined that the amino acid sequencing of this amyloid protein was similar to the microprotein "gamma-trace," which is a hormone-like molecule with high concentrations in the pancreas, pituitary, and brain, with cerebrospinal fluid (CSF) concentrations that are fivefold those in serum. Subsequently, Grubb et al.[51] documented abnormally low CSF concentrations of "gamma-trace," later referred to as "cystatin C" (which is an inhibitor of lysosomal cysteine proteases), in patients with Icelandic hereditary ICH with CAA. In addition, they documented the same CSF abnormality in asymptomatic family members who went on to develop ICH later in life. Using immunohistochemical techniques, these same authors[52] demonstrated the widespread presence of cystatin C in the walls of arteries of the cerebrum, cerebellum, and leptomeninges. Recently, Ghiso et al.[53] showed that the amyloid protein of the Icelandic form of hereditary CAA-related ICH was a variant of cystatin C, that was ten residues shorter than cystatin C, with one amino acid substitution (glutamine instead of leucine) at residue 58. These authors[54] recently reported a mutation in the gene encoding cystatin C as the likely cause of amyloid fibril formation and deposition in the walls of blood vessels in patients with this form of hereditary ICH and CAA.

Since the detailed description of the Icelandic cases, a second form of hereditary CAA-related ICH was reported from the Netherlands,[55] from two fishing villages (Scheveningen and Katwijk) in the North Sea coast of Holland. These cases present clinically in a slightly different manner from the Icelandic cases, since the age of onset of ICH tends to be delayed in comparison, occurring mainly in the fifth to seventh decades (between ages 45 and 65) in the Dutch cases.[56] About two-thirds of the cases have died as a result of the first episode of ICH, and the survivors have shown recurrent hemorrhages between three weeks and fourteen years later (average, 4.5 years).[57] Luyendijk et al.[57] recently described 136 patients with this variety of hereditary ICH from the Dutch village of Katwijk. The family pedigrees were found to have no ancestral connections with those from Scheveningen (where all characteristics of the ICH are identical with those from Katwijk) and Iceland, and the mode of inheritance was autosomal dominant. The intracerebral hematomas were of lobar location, and predominated in the parietal subcortical white matter. In a more recent series,[58] one-half of the acute hematomas were multiple, and the mortality for the group of twenty-four patients was 33%. A substantial number of these patients have reported recurrent episodes of severe headache of short duration over the years that precede the first ICH.[59] Their mechanism is unknown, but it is conceivable that some may represent episodes of small ICH without accompanying neurologic dysfunction. Microscopically, the amyloid-laden vessels are encountered in the cerebral cortex and leptomeninges, being absent from the basal ganglia, brainstem, and spinal cord, rarely being found in the cerebellar cortex, thus following the general pattern of distribution of the sporadic, rather than that of the Icelandic familial form of CAA. In a recent communication, Haan et al.[60] reported nine Dutch patients with prior history of ICH studied with single-photon-emission computed tomography (SPECT), in order to correlate changes in cerebral blood flow (CBF) with CT evidence of prior ICH. They found SPECT to be less sensitive than CT scan in detecting the chronic sequelae from old ICH, implying that changes in CBF may not necessarily accompany such residual lesions. On the other hand, in one asymptomatic individual at risk for familial CAA they documented a focal left occipital CBF defect by SPECT, while the CT was normal. Three months later, he developed a small ICH in that same location, suggesting that there may be a role for SPECT in the detection of CBF abnormalities related to CAA, prior to the development of ICH. This finding, if confirmed in cases of sporadic CAA, could add significantly to the diagnostic suspicion of CAA in elderly patients with cognitive impairment and/or ICH.

The characterization of the amyloid protein in the Dutch cases has shown a further difference with the Icelandic cases, since it is not related to cystatin C, but rather to the amyloid beta-protein (Alzheimer A4 or β-peptide) of Alzheimer's disease and Down's syndrome.[61] The main features of the Icelandic and Dutch forms of hereditary CAA-related ICH are shown in Table 9.3. Recent studies have indicated that the likely genetic defect in the Dutch form of CAA is in the amyloid beta-protein precursor (APP) gene located in chromosome 21.[63] The single point mutation for this genetic defect has been identified as resulting in the substitution of glutamine for glutamic acid at position 22 of the amyloid protein.[64]

## Other Cerebral Amyloid Angiopathy–related Conditions

A number of conditions have been reported in association with CAA, some in high

**Table 9.3.** Familial Forms of CAA-related ICH

|  | **Icelandic** | **Dutch** |
|---|---|---|
| Mode of inheritance | Autosomal dominant | Autosomal dominant |
| Age of onset of ICH | Early (mean: 30 yrs.) | Later (mean: 55 yrs.) |
| Distribution of amyloid angiopathy | Extensive (cerebral, cerebellar, brainstem arteries) | More limited (cerebral cortex, leptomeninges) |
| Type of amyloid protein, molecular weight | Cystatin C (gamma-trace), 11,000–12,000 Da* | Beta-peptide, 4,200 Da |
| Peripheral lymphocyte function[†] | Abnormal | Normal |

*Da = Dalton.
[†]Measured by assessment of concanavalin A capping.[62]

enough frequency to suggest a pathogenic link to the angiopathy, others as rare, probably coincidental occurrences. Among the former are histological and clinical features of Alzheimer's disease, cerebral infarcts, and leukoencephalopathy, whereas the latter group include entities that are discussed later in this chapter in the "miscellaneous" group of CAA-related conditions.

### Alzheimer's Disease

It is well established that in cases with sporadic CAA, histological brain examination discloses neuritic plaques and neurofibrillary tangles with a frequency that is well above that of the age-matched general population.[1,2,6,65] It is estimated that at least 40% of patients with sporadic CAA-related ICH show Alzheimer's histological changes in autopsy examination,[1] and similar figures (30% to 40%) of clinically-documented dementia preceding the ICH have been reported.[1,26,34] However, there is not a good correlation between the severity of both processes, and it is known that neuritic plaques can occur in the absence of CAA, and CAA can be present without coexistent neuritic plaques.[1,66,67] Furthermore, the same lack of close correlation applies to the presence of Alzheimer's histological changes and the presence and severity of clinically-documented dementia.[1,66]

The familial forms of CAA with ICH are also different in this regard from the sporadic form, in that no histological features of Alz-

heimer's disease have been described in the young Icelandic patients dying with ICH,[14] and those with the Dutch variety have shown "primitive" neuritic plaques lacking the typical amyloid core seen in Alzheimer's disease, and neurofibrillary tangles have not been observed.[58,61] Furthermore, although the comparatively older patients with the Dutch form of the hereditary disease are known to develop a progressive dementia, its mechanism is not thought to relate to Alzheimer's changes, but rather to the occurrence of recurrent strokes or leukoencephalopathy, or both.[68]

The coexistence of CAA with histological features of Alzheimer's disease, with neuritic plaques with amyloid cores seen both in the sporadic form of CAA and in Alzheimer's disease and Down's syndrome,[69,70] has generated a great deal of speculation about a common metabolic origin for both conditions. This view has been further suggested by the documentation of the biochemical similarity of the abnormal protein (Alzheimer A4 or β-peptide) that characterizes the amyloid of the sporadic form of CAA and the Dutch variety of familial CAA with that of Alzheimer's disease and Down's syndrome.[61,71] These findings have prompted Coria et al.[72] to propose a common metabolic origin for Alzheimer's disease and the sporadic and Dutch forms of CAA, and they have grouped these conditions under the rubric of "beta-protein deposition diseases."[72]

Although the sharing of a common link between Alzheimer's disease, Down's syndrome, and CAA (sporadic and Dutch types) through the accumulation of an identical amyloid beta-protein is well established, the origin and mechanism of the abnormal amyloid deposits are still unknown.[73] It has been postulated that the deposited amyloid beta-proteins may derive from a common circulating precursor that penetrates the central nervous system via injured capillaries with abnormal blood-brain barrier permeability, with deposition of amyloid in vessel walls and in the core of neuritic plaques.[74,75] This hypothesis, however, does not fully explain the fact that CAA and neuritic plaques do not always coexist, and either one can occur in isolation.[1] Levy et al.[64] have recently pointed to the observation that in both forms of hereditary CAA, the Icelandic and Dutch types, the biochemically different amyloid precursor proteins (cystatin C and beta-protein, respectively) are circulating protease inhibitors with a gene substitution that involves the same amino acid, glutamine. The relationship between this particular amino acid substitution and the deposition of amyloid in CAA remains unknown. Of added interest is the recent report by Vinters et al.[76] and Yong et al.[77] of immunohistochemical staining of amyloid-laden cortical vessels in brains with sporadic CAA by *both* beta-protein and cystatin C antibodies. This co-localization may suggest that the reported distinct biochemical separation of the sporadic and familial (Icelandic) forms of CAA may not be as clear as previously held. These observations of Vinters et al.[76] have been recently confirmed by Maruyama et al.[78] However, these findings have to be interpreted with caution, as they were obtained with immunohistochemical techniques, and a definite confirmation of this observation should await further biochemical analysis of the amyloid proteins involved in both forms of the disease.

## Cerebral Infarcts

Since the early pathological descriptions of CAA, it has been pointed out that the angi-

opathy is not only associated with ICH, but also with small cortical infarcts.[5,7,34] These tend to occur in areas of particularly severe vascular amyloid deposits, at times correlating with marked thickening of the vessel walls with luminal occlusions.[34] However, some authors have questioned the association between CAA and cerebral infarcts. Vonsattel et al.[40] found infarcts with equal frequency in their patients with (25 of 68, or 36.8%) and without (30 of 68, or 44.1%) CAA, and commented on the generally patent lumens of affected arteries, regardless of the severity of involvement of the wall by CAA. Aside from this issue of frequency, the occurrence of small and superficial CAA-related cerebral infarcts does not result in presentations with stroke syndromes in the distribution of single large cerebral arteries.[9] This observation raises doubts regarding the cause and effect relationship between CAA and reported presentations with transient ischemic attacks.[77,79] Although the available information in this regard is scanty, it is more likely that any potential contribution of multiple small cortical cerebral infarcts to neurological morbidity in CAA may be mediated by their addition to other more obvious causes of neurological dysfunction, such as Alzheimer's changes, the effects of repeated episodes of ICH, and a leukoencephalopathy, possibly leading to progressive dementia.[68]

## Leukoencephalopathy

A leukoencephalopathy characterized by bilateral hemispheric white matter lesions is being increasingly recognized as another radiological and histological concomitant of CAA. Gray et al.[80] reported the pathological analysis of twelve brains with CAA, eight of which showed diffuse changes in the hemispheric white matter. These abnormalities included macroscopic diffuse or patchy pallor of the white matter on whole-brain sections stained for myelin, with maximal involvement of the centrum semiovale, sparing the subcortical U fibers, corpus callosum, internal capsules, optic radiations, and temporal lobe white matter. Histologically, the white matter loss was characterized by vacuolation leading to a spongy aspect, accompanied by swelling of oligodendrocytes, dilatation of perivascular spaces, astrocytic proliferation, and occasional Rosenthal fibers. In all twelve instances, CAA was documented in cortical and leptomeningeal vessels, but no consistent large areas of infarction or specific angiopathy in vessels of the affected white matter were present. This lack of involvement of white matter vessels is a commonplace observation in CAA in general[8] (with or without leukoencephalopathy), and Fisher[81] has commented on a remarkable abrupt termination of the amyloid deposits in involved cortical vessels as they leave the gray matter to enter the white matter. CT scans performed in three of the patients reported by Gray et al.[80] showed bilateral hypodensity of the hemispheric white matter. These authors explained the leukoencephalopathy as developing in a manner similar to Binswanger's subcortical encephalopathy, suggesting that the white matter changes represent chronic ischemia secondary to hypoperfusion via amyloid-laden cortical penetrating arteries. They favored this explanation over that of white matter changes secondary to multiple cortical lesions (either infarcts or small petechial hemorrhages, both found routinely in autopsies of patients with CAA) because of the lack of histological features suggestive of wallerian degeneration. Rather, the presence of spongiosis, swollen oligodendrocytes, and enlarged perivascular spaces were felt to be consistent with subacute edema, which eventually leads to loss of myelin and astrocytosis. The mechanism of this subacute edema was interpreted as ischemic, due to stenosis of amyloid-laden cortical perforators in the leukoencephalopathy of CAA,[80] and to hypertension-induced stenosis of perforator arteries in Binswanger's encephalopathy.[82]

In recent reports,[58,83–85] the leukoencephalopathy has been demonstrated by CT and MRI scans in a number of patients with CAA. Loes et al.[83] documented white matter hyperintensities on T2-weighted MRI sequences in three of four patients with histologically documented, sporadic CAA. The distribution of the white matter changes paralleled the pathological descriptions of Gray et al.[80] The abnormalities predominated in the centrum semiovale, and spared the corpus collosum, subcortical U fibers, and internal capsules (Figure 9.6). These authors[83] also favored chronic hypoperfusion of the white matter as a result of the amyloid angiopathy as the explanation for the leukoencephalopathy. Hendricks et al.[84] and DeWitt and Louis[85] documented leukoencephalopathy and multiple cortical petechial hemorrhages by MRI in patients with biopsy-proved CAA, in the absence of preceding clinical episodes of ICH. Both Loes et al.[83] and Hendricks et al.[84] suggested that CAA should enter in the differential diagnosis of MRI-documented T2 hyperintensities of the hemispheric white matter.

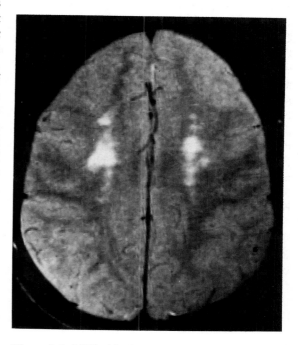

**Figure 9.6.** MRI of leukoencephalopathy associated with CAA, with confluent areas of white matter hyperintensity in the periventricular white matter, T2-weighted sequence (TR: 2500 msec, TE: 45 msec).

In addition to these sporadic varieties of CAA with leukoencephalopathy, patients with the Dutch form of hereditary ICH with amyloidosis have been found to show white matter abnormalities on CT and MRI scans in a high proportion of cases. Haan et al.[58] found such CT abnormalities in twenty of twenty-four patients, in eighteen of them bilaterally. No clinical correlation between white matter hypodensity and dementia was found, as the CT changes occurred in both demented and nondemented individuals. In an MRI study of seven patients, Haan et al.[86] documented periventricular white matter hyperintensities on T2-weighted sequences in all patients, who in addition showed variable combinations of recent and old hemorrhagic lesions. Neuropsychological deficits were present in all seven patients, with documentation of progression in the two patients who had repeated testing after three-and-a-half- and two-year intervals, respectively. Neuropathological examination revealed CAA, neuritic plaques without amyloid cores, absence of neurofibrillary tangles, and extensive areas of demyelination of the deep hemispheric white matter. The latter abnormality was thought to represent "incomplete infarction" secondary to chronic hypoperfusion of the white matter by perforating cortical vessels affected by CAA.[86] On the basis of these latter observations, as well as the documentation of progressive dementia by neuropsychological testing in some of their Dutch patients, Haan et al.[68] have suggested that such gradual and progressive cognitive changes are unlikely to be only due to the effects of repeated strokes, and commented on the possibility of other contributing factors, such as the Alzheimer's disease changes and the leukoencephalopathy, in the pathogenesis of dementia in these cases.

At present, it is apparent that leukoencephalopathy is probably a frequent feature of the sporadic and Dutch familial forms of CAA. Its pathogenesis, as well as its potential role in the production of clinically detected neurological and cognitive deficits, remains to be established, pending the systematic clinical, neuropsychological, and radiological or pathological evaluation of well-defined groups of patients with CAA.

### Miscellaneous Conditions

A large number of disease entities have been described in association with CAA (Table 9.4). Some of these are rarely seen in patients with CAA and are probably coincidental, whereas others (such as Down's syndrome) may represent associations that imply a potential common pathogenesis. In two patients with *Down's syndrome* who died in their sixth decade, Alzheimer's disease changes coexisted with CAA,[89] in one of them associated with ICH,[89] the other displaying vascular cerebral changes consistent with giant-cell arteritis.[88] The latter, however, had the atypical histological feature of giant cells located in the media rather than in the internal elastic lamina. This feature raised the possibility that giant cells formed as a reaction to the presence of amyloid, rather than as part of a primary vasculitis, a phenomenon that has

**Table 9.4.** Conditions Reported in Association with CAA

| Condition | References |
|---|---|
| Down's syndrome | 87–90 |
| Vasculitis | |
|    Giant-cell arteritis | 88 and 91 |
|    Rheumatoid vasculitis | 41 |
|    Granulomatous angiitis of the CNS | 92–95 |
| Familial ataxia with dementia | 96–98 |
| Postcerebral irradiation | 16 and 99 |
| Vascular malformations | 16 and 100–102 |
| Spongiform encephalopathy | 103 and 104 |
| Dementia pugilistica | 105 |
| "Mass lesion" | 106 |
| Demyelinating disorder | 107 |
| Oculoleptomeningeal amyloidosis | 108–110 |

CNS = central nervous system.
(Modified from Vinters HV. Cerebral amyloid angiopathy: a critical review. Stroke 1987;18:311–324. With permission of the publisher.)

been commented on by Vinters.[1] The presence of CAA in patients with Down's syndrome is thought to be more common than generally reported,[90] and is probably more likely to occur in the older groups of the population with Down's syndrome. The link between CAA, Alzheimer's disease changes, and Down's syndrome is likely to be the common biochemical origin of the abnormal amyloid protein (beta-protein) in the three conditions.[61,71] This connection is further suggested by the high frequency of association between Down's syndrome and Alzheimer's disease.[87]

As mentioned above, some reports[88] on the association of *giant-cell arteritis* with CAA may not represent the combination of the two different types of angiopathy, but rather a giant-cell reaction to the abnormal vascular amyloid deposits.[1] However, one report[91] documented the apparently true association of both forms of vascular disease, with chronic inflammatory changes in cortical and subarachnoid vessels, with multinucleated giant cells in areas of disrupted elastic membranes. A further unusual feature of this case was the description of amyloid-laden vessels not only in the subarachnoid and cortical vessels, but also in those of the subcortical white matter. The patient presented clinically with a four-week history of headache, nausea, vomiting, and unsteady gait, and examination showed a left homonymous hemianopia and a gait disturbance. CT scan demonstrated a mass lesion in the right temporo-parietal area with prominent surrounding edema. At craniotomy, the resected tissue corresponded histologically to infarction of various ages, without evidence of ICH. The single report by Mandybur[41] of CAA in vessels affected by an inflammatory reaction akin to that of *rheumatoid vasculitis* raises the possibility that in some instances the pathogenesis of CAA may relate to chronic local vascular inflammation,[1] a situation possibly also applicable to the rare reports of CAA associated with giant-cell arteritis.[88,91] The same applies to the reported instances of CAA coexisting with examples of *granulomatous angiitis of the*

*central nervous system* (CNS).[92–95] In the two cases reported by Probst and Ulrich,[92] a close topographical association between the two types of angiopathy suggested a pathogenic relationship between them rather than a mere coincidental occurrence. The authors were of the opinion that the two may have been causally related, and suggested that amyloid formation could have occurred as a reaction to the chronic vasculitis. The patients' courses were chronic and progressive, without episodes of clinically-apparent large ICH, but postmortem examinations showed multiple small intracortical hemorrhages of different ages in both cases. The single case reported by Shintaku et al.[93] presented with a fresh left occipital ICH in the setting of a history of headache and physical findings that included "anisocoria, severe nuchal rigidity, and bilateral choked discs." The vascular changes of granulomatous angiitis of the CNS coexisted with those of CAA, and both were abundant near the occipital ICH. The authors commented on the possibility that the two forms of angiopathy could be either coincidental or pathogenically related through "a common background of immunological abnormality." The association between CAA and granulomatous angiitis of the CNS, and their response to treatment, have been further analyzed in recent case reports.[94,95] Ginsberg et al.[94] reported the case of a 73-year-old woman who presented with progressive cognitive deterioration, aphasia, gait apraxia, elevated sedimentation rate, and CT evidence of swelling and hypodensity in the white matter of the hemispheres, predominantly posteriorly. No areas of ICH were present. Brain biopsy documented prominent changes of chronic granulomatous angiitis involving leptomeningeal and superficial cortical small arteries and arterioles, along with widespread CAA in vessels with and without granulomatous inflammation. Treatment with dexamethasone followed by prednisolone resulted in marked clinical improvement, the patient being described as symptom-free on maintenance steroids after over one year from onset.

Mandybur and Balko[95] reported a 62-year-old woman who developed progressive cognitive deterioration, apraxia, left hemiparesis, and homonymous hemianopia with neglect, along with partial motor seizures on the left side of the body. CT scan showed nonenhancing "white matter edema" of the right posterior parietal lobe, and MRI revealed both cortical and white matter involvement in the area. Biopsy of the lesion showed the combination of CAA and granulomatous angiitis, without Alzheimer's disease changes. Following treatment with prednisone and cyclophosphamide, a "marked improvement in neurologic function" was detected, but the patient died eight months after onset of symptoms as a result of opportunistic cytomegalovirus bronchopneumonia and hemorrhagic enteritis. Autopsy study demonstrated a virtual resolution of the features of granulomatous angiitis, as well as a reduction in the severity of CAA, as compared with the biopsy material. This led the authors to speculate that the treatment may have resulted in both suppression of vascular inflammation and amyloid formation, recommending consideration of immunosuppressive treatment in instances of documented association of granulomatous angiitis and CAA.

A familial condition characterized by the association of CAA with a progressive neurologic disorder featuring *dementia, spasticity, and ataxia* with onset in the fifth decade was first described by Worster-Drought et al.[96,97] Recently, Plant et al.[98] have further extended the original clinical and pathological data on the pedigree of two families related by a common ancestor. Despite the presence of profuse generalized CAA (in leptomeninges, cerebral and cerebellar cortex and white matter, basal ganglia, diencephalon, brainstem, and spinal cord) and the occurrence of "stroke-like" episodes in several members of the families, no cases of ICH have been recorded in association with this condition, which is inherited with an autosomal dominant pattern. The one instance of recorded fatal ICH was due to the rupture of an incidental intracranial aneurysm in a 48-year-old

man who had no neurological symptoms before the SAH.

Mandybur and Gore[99] described two patients who developed *postirradiation necrosis* of the brain several years after receiving high-dose local radiation therapy for basal-cell carcinoma of the scalp. In both instances, the onset of focal seizures and neurological deficits, four and three years after the last course of radiation treatment, respectively, was accompanied by local signs of mass effect that led to surgery with resection of focally abnormal brain tissue. The biopsy materials, as well as subsequent postmortem brain examination in Case 1, documented postirradiation demyelination, angionecrosis, thrombosis, and ischemic necrosis, along with bizarre hypertrophic astrocytes, but without evidence of local tumor spread. Histological examination in addition showed abundant amyloid deposits, both as irregular masses within the necrotic brain parenchyma, as well as in the walls of blood vessels, at times with focal perivascular extensions of amyloid into the adjacent brain substance. A review of their cases and others from the literature led the authors to conclude that parenchymal necrosis is a prerequisite for vascular amyloid deposition after brain irradiation; however, an exception to that notion was subsequently reported in a patient who developed postirradiation vascular amyloid deposits in the absence of brain necrosis.[16] Mandybur and Gore[99] speculated about the presence of a circulating alpha-globulin that gained access to the necrotic brain via abnormally permeable vessels, allowing for its combination with the necrotic tissue, resulting in the formation of amyloid.

*Vascular malformations* of the brain have rarely been found to develop amyloid deposition. Neumann[100] described a 45-year-old patient who died from a left hemispheric lobar ICH. In addition to the fatal hemorrhage, scars from smaller ICH were present in both hemispheres, and widespread abnormalities in blood vessels were seen histologically in relationship to these hemorrhages, as well as in areas not affected by cerebrovascular lesions. The vascular abnormalities consisted of "malformed" blood vessels, but without demonstration of an arteriovenous or cavernous pattern, along with extensive amyloid deposits. An additional histological feature was the presence of abundant neuritic plaques, without neurofibrillary tangles. The episodes of ICH were interpreted as secondary to rupture of "a small vascular malformation," and the author also alluded to the possibility of "weakening" of blood vessels by the amyloid deposits as a factor in causing ICH. Other authors[16,101,102] have reported the rare observation of dense amyloid deposits within vessels of an arteriovenous malformation, even in the absence of overt episodes of bleeding.[16,101] Hart et al.[102] observed widespread and dense amyloid deposits in only two of eighty-five surgical specimens of arteriovenous malformations, and both occurred in elderly individuals (ages 85 and 74), leading the authors to conclude that amyloid deposition in the setting of an arteriovenous malformation reflects the pre-existing vascular anomaly and it occurs over prolonged periods of time.

The association of CAA with the *spongiform encephalopathies* has been reported as a rare occurrence, although parenchymal amyloid deposition in plaque form is a frequent observation in Creutzfeldt-Jakob disease and kuru.[103] Vascular amyloid deposits are occasionally seen in the Gerstmann-Sträussler variety of slowly-progressive, predominantly cerebellar spongiform encephalopathy,[104] but they are always less prominent than in the parenchyma,[1] and no case of ICH has been reported in this setting.

An isolated autopsy report documented widespread CAA and a fatal right hemispheric hemorrhage at age 51, in a boxer with history of "parkinsonian symptoms" and progressive dementia since age 38, labeled *"dementia pugilistica."*[105] In addition to CAA, microscopic brain examination disclosed abundant neuritic plaques and neurofibrillary degeneration. A single case report of CAA presenting as a *"mass lesion"*[106] described a 55-year-old woman with focal seizures in relation to a CT-documented expanding hypodense lesion in the right frontal lobe. On craniotomy for biopsy, no local abnormalities were detected, and histological examination showed prominent CAA in leptomeningeal and cortical vessels, a few of which also contained mononuclear perivascular infiltrates and rare giant cells. The authors interpreted the histological findings as CAA combined with an inflammatory vasculopathy. The significance of these rare presentations of CAA,[106] or its occasional association with other neurological disorders,[103] is difficult to establish. In the latter situation in particular, it is likely that the two conditions represent a mere coincidental occurrence, rather than one with a causal link. The same probably applies to instances of CAA in association with a *demyelinating disorder*. Although five such cases were collected by Heffner et al.,[107] the association has not been further reported. The demyelinating white matter lesions were consistent with multiple sclerosis plaques, but a profuse vascular and perivascular amyloid deposition in the vicinities of the plaques separated these cases from routine examples of multiple sclerosis. In all but one of the cases the amyloid deposits were restricted to the cerebral vasculature. No instances of ICH, grossly or microscopically, were detected in the five pathologically studied cases, all of whom were in their 40s and 50s, making unlikely that they had a combination of multiple sclerosis and sporadic CAA.

A rare familial condition has been reported in Japan[108,109] and in a U.S. family of German origin,[110] in which profuse *oculoleptomeningeal amyloidosis* is associated with systemic amyloidosis, leading to loss of vision, autonomic abnormalities, and episodes of cerebral infarction, the latter as a result of occlusion of branches of the middle cerebral artery by a process of intimal proliferation coincident with heavy adventitial amyloid deposits.[108,109] No instances of ICH were recorded in any of these families, in which the disorder has a dominant pattern of inheritance. Uitti et al.[111] have recently reported a new family of Italian origin with this condition. Their three cases were unusual in that they became symptomatic at an early age, generally in the third decade, with recurrent hemiplegic migraine, seizures, visual impairment, progressive myelopathy, and peripheral neuropathy. Two of the three patients developed ICH, in one of them massive at age 28. Autopsy studies in two patients showed extensive amyloidosis in the leptomeninges of the brain and spinal cord, as well as in the cerebral and systemic vasculature, with severe amyloid deposits in the viscera and connective tissue. Analysis of the amyloid in these cases revealed the prealbumin transthyretin as its main component.

## References

1. Vinters HV. Cerebral amyloid angiopathy: a critical review. Stroke 1987;18:311–324.
2. Vinters HV, Gilbert JJ. Cerebral amyloid angiopathy: incidence and complications in the aging brain. II. The distribution of amyloid vascular changes. Stroke 1983;14:924–928.
3. Kase CS, Vonsattel J-P, Richardson EP. Case records of the Massachussets General Hospital (Case 10-1988). N Engl J Med 1988;318:623–631.
4. Okoye MI, Watanabe I. Ultrastructural features of cerebral amyloid angiopathy. Hum Pathol 1982;13:1127–1132.
5. Okazaki H, Reagan TJ, Campbell RJ. Clinicopathologic studies of primary cerebral amyloid angiopathy. Mayo Clin Proc 1979;54:22–31.
6. Gilbert JJ, Vinters HV. Cerebral amyloid angiopathy: incidence and complications in the aging brain. I. Cerebral hemorrhage. Stroke 1983;14:915–923.
7. Tomonaga M. Cerebral amyloid angiopathy in the elderly. J Amer Geriatr Soc 1981;29:151–157.
8. Masuda J, Tanaka K, Ueda K, et al. Autopsy study of incidence and distribution of cerebral amyloid angiopathy in Hisayama, Japan. Stroke 1988;19:205–210.
9. Kase CS. Intracerebral hemorrhage: nonhypertensive causes. Stroke 1986;17:590–595.
10. Jellinger K. Cerebrovascular amyloidosis with cerebral hemorrhage. J Neurol 1977;214:195–206.
11. Jellinger K. Cerebral hemorrhage in amyloid angiopathy. Ann Neurol 1977;1:604 (letter).
12. Ulrich G, Taghavy A, Schmidt H. Zur Nosologie und Ätiologie der kongophilen Angiopathie (Gefässform der cerebralen Amyloidose). J Neurol 1973;206:39–59.
13. Torack RM. Congophilic angiopathy complicated by surgery and massive hemorrhage: a light and electron microscopic study. Am J Pathol 1975;81:349–366.
14. Gudmundsson G, Hallgrimsson J, Jonasson TA, et al. Hereditary cerebral haemorrhage with amyloidosis. Brain 1972;95:387–404.
15. Lee S-S, Stemmermann GN. Congophilic angiopathy and cerebral hemorrhage. Arch Pathol Lab Med 1978;102:317–321.
16. Bruni J, Bilbao JM, Pritzker KPH. Vascular amyloid in the aging central nervous system: clinico-pathological study and literature review. Can J Neurol Sci 1977;4:239–244.
17. Kase CS, Mohr JP. General features of intracerebral hemorrhage. In: Barnett HJM, et al. eds. Stroke: Pathophysiology, Diagnosis, and Management. Vol. 1. New York: Churchill-Livingstone, 1986;497–523.
18. Mandybur TI, Bates SRD. Fatal massive intracerebral hemorrhage complicating cerebral amyloid angiopathy. Arch Neurol 1978;35:246–248.
19. Tucker WS, Bilbao JM, Klodawsky H. Cerebral amyloid angiopathy and multiple intracerebral hematomas. Neurosurgery 1980;7:611–614.
20. Regli F, Vonsattel J-P, Perentes E, et al. L'angiopathie amyloïde cérébrale. Une maladie cérébro-vasculaire peu connue: étude d'une observation anatomo-clinique. Rev Neurol 1981;137:181–194.
21. Ackerman RH, Richardson EP, Heros RC. Case Records of the Massachusetts General Hospital (Case 49-1982). N Engl J Med 1982;307:1507–1514.
22. Tyler KL, Poletti CE, Heros RC. Cerebral amyloid angiopathy with multiple intracerebral hemorrhages. J Neurosurg 1982;57:286–289.
23. Finelli PF, Kessimian N, Bernstein PW. Cerebral amyloid angiopathy manifesting as recurrent intracerebral hemorrhage. Arch Neurol 1984;41:330–333.
24. Wagle WA, Smith TW, Weiner M. Intracerebral hemorrhage caused by cerebral amyloid

angiopathy: radiographic-pathologic correlation. Am J Neuroradiol 1984;5:171–176.

25. Patel DV, Hier DB, Thomas CM, et al. Intracerebral hemorrhage secondary to cerebral amyloid angiopathy. Radiology 1984;151:397–400.

26. Gilles C, Brucher JM, Khoubesserian P, et al. Cerebral amyloid angiopathy as a cause of multiple intracerebral hemorrhages. Neurology 1984;34:730–735.

27. Ishii N, Nishihara Y, Horie A. Amyloid angiopathy and lobar cerebral haemorrhage. J Neurol Neurosurg Psychiat 1984;47:1203–1210.

28. Kalyan-Raman UP, Kalyan-Raman K. Cerebral amyloid angiopathy causing intracranial hemorrhage. Ann Neurol 1984;16:321–329.

29. Cosgrove GR, Leblanc R, Meagher-Villemure K, et al. Cerebral amyloid angiopathy. Neurology 1985;35:625–631.

30. Roosen N, Martin J-J, De La Porte C, et al. Intracerebral hemorrhage due to cerebral amyloid angiopathy: case report. J Neurosurg 1985;63:963–969.

31. Sobel DF, Baker E, Anderson B, et al. Cerebral amyloid angiopathy associated with massive intracerebral hemorrhage. Neuroradiology 1985; 27:318–321.

32. Brown RT, Coates RK, Gilbert JJ. Radiographic-pathologic correlation in cerebral amyloid angiopathy. J Can Assoc Radiol 1985;36:308–311.

33. Greene GM, Godersky JC, Biller J, et al. Surgical experience with cerebral amyloid angiopathy. Stroke 1990;21:1545–1549.

34. Mandybur TI. Cerebral amyloid angiopathy: the vascular pathology and complications. J Neuropath Exp Neurol 1986;45:79–90.

35. Ohshima T, Endo T, Nukui H, et al. Cerebral amyloid angiopathy as a cause of subarachnoid hemorrhage. Stroke 1990;21:480–483.

36. Vinters HV, Duckwiler GR. Intracranial hemorrhage in the normotensive elderly patient. Neuroimag Clin NA 1992;2:153–169.

37. Douglas MA, Haerer AF. Long-term prognosis of hypertensive intracerebral hemorrhage. Stroke 1982;13:488–491.

38. Michel B, Gastaut JL, Gambarelli D, et al. Hématomes intracérébraux lobaires récidivants au cours de l'angiopathie amyloïde cérébrale. Rev Neurol 1988;144:503–507.

39. Weisberg L. Multiple spontaneous intracerebral hematomas: clinical and computed tomographic correlations. Neurology 1981;31:897–900.

40. Vonsattel JP, Myers RH, Hedley-Whyte ET, et al. Cerebral amyloid angiopathy without and with cerebral hemorrhages: a comparative histological study. Ann Neurol 1991;30:637–649.

41. Mandybur TI. Cerebral amyloid angiopathy: possible relationship to rheumatoid vasculitis. Neurology 1979;29:1336–1340.

42. Roberts J. Blood pressure levels of persons 6–74 years, United States, 1971–1974. Vital and health statistics, Series 11, National Health Survey no. 203. Hyattsville, Maryland, 1977;72.

43. Ferreiro JA, Ansbacher LE, Vinters HV. Stroke related to cerebral amyloid angiopathy: the significance of systemic vascular disease. J Neurol 1989;236:267–272.

44. Ramsay DA, Penswick JL, Robertson DM. Fatal streptokinase-induced intracerebral haemorrhage in cerebral amyloid angiopathy. Can J Neurol Sci 1990;17:336–341.

45. Pendlebury WW, Iole ED, Tracy RP, et al. Intracerebral hemorrhage related to cerebral amyloid angiopathy and t-PA treatment. Ann Neurol 1991;29:210–213.

45a. Wijdicks EFM, Jack CR. Intracerebral hemorrhage after fibrinolytic therapy for acute myocardial infarction. Stroke 1993;24:554–557.

46. Kase CS, Pessin MS, Zivin JA, et al. Intracranial hemorrhage after coronary thrombolysis with tissue plasminogen activator. Am J Med 1992;92:384–390.

47. Leblanc R, Preul M, Robitaille Y. Cerebral amyloid angiopathy: surgical considerations. Stroke 1991;22:28 (abstract).

48. Feldmann E, Tornabene J. Diagnosis and treatment of cerebral amyloid angiopathy. Clin Geriat Med 1991;7:617–630.

49. Matkovic Z, Davis S, Gonzales M, et al. Surgical risk of hemorrhage in cerebral amyloid angiopathy. Stroke 1991;22:456–461.

50. Cohen DH, Feinder H, Jensson O, et al. Amyloid fibril in hereditary cerebral hemorrhage with amyloidosis (HCHWA) is related to the gastroentero-pancreatic neuroendocrine protein, gamma trace. J Exp Med 1983;158: 623–628.

51. Grubb A, Jensson O, Gudmundsson G, et al. Abnormal metabolism of γ-trace alkaline mi-

croprotein: the basic defect in hereditary cerebral hemorrhage with amyloidosis. N Engl J Med 1984;311:1547–1549.

52. Löfberg H, Grubb AO, Nilsson EK, et al. Immunohistochemical characterization of the amyloid deposits and quantitation of pertinent cerebrospinal fluid proteins in hereditary cerebral hemorrhage with amyloidosis. Stroke 1987;18:431–440.

53. Ghiso J, Pons-Estel B, Frangione B. Hereditary cerebral amyloid angiopathy: the amyloid fibrils contain a protein which is a variant of cystatin C, an inhibitor of lysosomal cysteine proteases. Biochem Biophys Res Comm 1986; 136:548–554.

54. Levy E, Lopez-Otin C, Ghiso J, et al. Stroke in Icelandic patients with hereditary amyloid angiopathy is related to a mutation in the cystatin C gene, an inhibitor of cysteine proteases. J Exp Med 1989;169:1771–1778.

55. Luyendijk W. Intracerebral haematoma. In: Vinken PJ, Bruyn GW, eds. Handbook of Clinical Neurology. Vol 11. Amsterdam: North Holland, 1972;660–719.

56. Wattendorf AR, Bots GTAM, Went LN, et al. Familial cerebral amyloid angiopathy presenting as recurrent cerebral haemorrhage. J Neurol Sci 1982;55:121–135.

57. Luyendijk W, Bots GTAM, Vegter-van der Vlis M, et al. Hereditary cerebral haemorrhage caused by cortical amyloid angiopathy. J Neurol Sci 1988;85:267–280.

58. Haan J, Algra PR, Roos RAC. Hereditary cerebral hemorrhage with amyloidosis—Dutch type: clinical and computed tomographic analysis of 24 cases. Arch Neurol 1990;47:649–653.

59. Haan J, Roos RAC, Briët PE, et al. Hereditary cerebral hemorrhage with amyloidosis—Dutch type. Clin Neurol Neurosurg 1989;91:285–290.

60. Haan J, van Kroonenburgh MJPG, Algra PR, et al. Hereditary cerebral hemorrhage with amyloidosis—Dutch type: Tc-99 HM-PAO single photon emission computed tomography. Neuroradiology 1990;32:142–145.

61. Van Duinen SG, Castaño EM, Prelli F, et al. Hereditary cerebral hemorrhage with amyloidosis in patients of Dutch origin is related to Alzheimer disease. Proc Natl Acad Sci USA 1987;84:5991–5994.

62. Haan J, Demmers RT, Buruma OJS, et al. Lymphocyte concanavalin A capping in hereditary cerebral haemorrhage with amyloidosis—Dutch type. J Neurol 1990;237:117–119.

63. Van Broeckhoven C, Haan J, Bakker E, et al. Amyloid β-protein precursor gene and hereditary cerebral hemorrhage with amyloidosis (Dutch). Science 1990;248:1120–1121.

64. Levy E, Carman MD, Fernandez-Madrid IJ, et al. Mutation of the Alzheimer's disease amyloid gene in hereditary cerebral hemorrhage, Dutch type. Science 1990;248:1124–1126.

65. Mandybur TI. The incidence of cerebral amyloid angiopathy in Alzheimer's disease. Neurology 1975;25:120–126.

66. Mountjoy CQ, Tomlinson BE, Gibson PH. Amyloid and senile plaques and cerebral blood vessels: a semi-quantitative investigation of a possible relationship. J Neurol Sci 1982;57:89–103.

67. Richardson EP. Amyloid in the human brain. West J Med 1985;143:518–519 (editorial).

68. Haan J, Lanser JBK, Zijderveld Z, et al. Dementia in hereditary cerebral hemorrhage with amyloidosis—Dutch type. Arch Neurol 1990;47:965–967.

69. Miyakawa T, Shimoji A, Kuramoto R, et al. The relationship between senile plaques and cerebral blood vessels in Alzheimer's disease and senile dementia. Virchows Arch [Cell Pathol] 1982;40:121–129.

70. Miyakawa T, Uehara Y. Observations of amyloid angiopathy and senile plaques by the scanning electron microscope. Acta Neuropathol 1979;48:153–156.

71. Coria F, Castaño EM, Frangione B. Brain amyloid in normal aging and cerebral amyloid angiopathy is antigenically related to Alzheimer's disease beta-protein. Am J Pathol 1987;129:422–428.

72. Coria F, Prelli F, Castaño EM, et al. Beta-protein deposition: a pathogenetic link between Alzheimer's disease and cerebral amyloid angiopathies. Brain Res 1988;463:187–191.

73. Selkoe DJ. Biochemistry of altered brain proteins in Alzheimer's disease. Ann Rev Neurosci 1989;12:463–490.

74. Wong CW, Quaranta V, Glenner GG. Neuritic plaques and cerebrovascular amyloid in Alzheimer disease are antigenically related. Proc Natl Acad Sci USA 1985;82:8729–8732.

75. Glenner GG. On causative theories in Alzheimer's disease. Hum Pathol 1985;16:433–435.

76. Vinters HV, Secor DL, Pardridge WM, et al. Immunohistochemical study of cerebral amyloid angiopathy. III. Widespread Alzheimer A4 peptide in cerebral microvessel walls colocalizes with gamma trace in patients with

leukoencephalopathy. Ann Neurol 1990;28: 34–42.

77. Yong WH, Robert ME, Secor DL, et al. Cerebral hemorrhage with biopsy-proved amyloid angiopathy. Arch Neurol 1992;49:51–58.

78. Maruyama K, Ikeda S, Ishihara T, et al. Immuno-histochemical characterization of cerebrovascular amyloid in 46 autopsied cases using antibodies to beta protein and cystatin C. Stroke 1990;21:397–403.

79. Smith DB, Hitchcock M, Philpott PJ. Cerebral amyloid angiopathy presenting as transient ischemic attacks: case report. J Neurosurg 1985;63:963–964.

80. Gray F, Dubas F, Roullet E, et al. Leukoencephalopathy in diffuse hemorrhagic cerebral amyloid angiopathy. Ann Neurol 1985;18: 54–59.

81. Fisher CM. Binswanger's encephalopathy: a review. J Neurol 1989;236:65–79.

82. Mikol J. Maladie de Binswanger et formes apparentées. Rev Neurol 1968;118:111–132.

83. Loes DJ, Biller J, Yuh WTC, et al. Leukoencephalopathy in cerebral amyloid angiopathy: MR imaging in four cases. Am J Neuroradiol 1990;11:485–488.

84. Hendricks HT, Franke CL, Theunissen PHMH. Cerebral amyloid angiopathy: diagnosis by MRI and brain biopsy. Neurology 1990;40:1308–1310.

85. DeWitt LD, Louis DN. Case records of the Massachusetts General Hospital (Case 27-1991). N Engl J Med 1991;325:42–54.

86. Haan J, Roos RAC, Algra PR, et al. Hereditary cerebral haemorrhage with amyloidosis—Dutch type: magnetic resonance imaging findings in 7 cases. Brain 1990;113:1251–1267.

87. Glenner GG, Wong CW. Alzheimer's disease and Down's syndrome: sharing of a unique cerebrovascular amyloid fibril protein. Biochem Biophys Res Commun 1984;122: 1131–1135.

88. Reid AH, Maloney AFJ. Giant cell arteritis and arteriolitis associated with amyloid angiopathy in an elderly Mongol. Acta Neuropathol 1974;27:131–137.

89. Belza MG, Urich H. Cerebral amyloid angiopathy in Down's syndrome. Clin Neuropathol 1986;5:257–260.

90. Schwartz P. Amyloidosis of the nervous system in the aged. In: Minckler J, ed. Pathology of the Nervous System. Vol. 3. New York: McGraw-Hill, 1971;2832–2833.

91. Murphy MN, Sima AAF. Cerebral amyloid angiopathy associated with giant cell arteritis: a case report. Stroke 1985;16:514–517.

92. Probst A, Ulrich J. Amyloid angiopathy combined with granulomatous angiitis of the central nervous system: report on two patients. Clin Neuropathol 1985;4:250–259.

93. Shintaku M, Osawa K, Toki J, et al. A case of granulomatous angiitis of the central nervous system associated with amyloid angiopathy. Acta Neuropathol 1986;70:340–342.

94. Ginsberg L, Geddes J, Valentine A. Amyloid angiopathy and granulomatous angiitis of the central nervous system: a case responding to corticosteroid treatment. J Neurol 1988;235:438–440.

95. Mandybur TI, Balko G. Cerebral amyloid angiopathy with granulomatous angiitis ameliorated by steroid-Cytoxan treatment. Clin Neuropharmacol 1992;15:241–247.

96. Worster-Drought C, Greenfield JG, McMenemey WH. A form of familial presenile dementia with spastic paralysis (including the pathological examination of a case). Brain 1940;63:237–254.

97. Worster-Drought C, Greenfield, JG, McMenemy WH. A form of familial presenile dementia with spastic paralysis. Brain 1944; 67:38–43.

98. Plant GT, Révész T, Barnard RO, et al. Familial cerebral amyloid angiopathy with non-neuritic amyloid plaque formation. Brain 1990;113:721–747.

99. Mandybur TI, Gore I. Amyloid in late post-irradiation necrosis of brain. Neurology 1969; 19:983–992.

100. Neumann MA. Combined amyloid vascular changes and argyrophilic plaques in the central nervous system. J Neuropath Exp Neurol 1960;19:370–382.

101. Peterson EW, Schulz DM. Amyloid in vessels of a vascular malformation in brain. Arch Pathol 1961;72:480–483.

102. Hart MN, Goeken J, Schelper RL, et al. Amyloid in cerebrovascular malformations. J Neuropath Exp Neurol 1986;45:348 (abstract).

103. Masters CL, Gajdusek DC, Gibbs CJ. Creutzfeldt-Jakob disease virus isolations from the Gerstmann-Sträussler syndrome: with an analysis of the various forms of amyloid plaque deposition in the virus-induced spongiform encephalopathies. Brain 1981; 104:559–588.

104. Adam J, Crow TJ, Duchen LW, et al. Familial cerebral amyloidosis and spongiform encephalopathy. J Neurol Neurosurg Psychiat 1982;45:37–45.

105. Brandenburg W, Hallervorden J. Dementia pugilistica mit anatomischem Befund. Virchows Arch [Path Anat Phys] 1954;325:680–709.

106. Briceno CE, Resch L, Bernstein M. Cerebral amyloid angiopathy presenting as a mass lesion. Stroke 1987;18:234–239.

107. Heffner RR, Porro RS, Olson ME, et al. A demyelinating disorder associated with cerebrovascular amyloid angiopathy. Arch Neurol 1976;33:501–506.

108. Okayama M, Goto I, Ogata J, et al. Primary amyloidosis with familial vitreous opacities: an unusual case and family. Arch Int Med 1978;138:105–111.

109. Ogata J, Okayama M, Goto I, et al. Primary familial amyloidosis with vitreous opacities: report of an autopsy case. Acta Neuropath 1978;42:67–70.

110. Goren H, Steinberg MC, Farboody GH. Familial oculoleptomeningeal amyloidosis. Brain 1980;103:473–495.

111. Uitti RJ, Donat JR, Rozdilsky B, et al. Familial oculoleptomeningeal amyloidosis: report of a new family with unusual features. Arch Neurol 1988;45:1118–1122.

# Chapter 10
# Drugs

## Louis R. Caplan

Drug abuse is a very serious and common problem. The illicit use of drugs has dramatically increased during the second half of the twentieth century, as has our knowledge of the effects and complications of drug use and abuse. Strokes had occasionally been recognized in the past in drug users, but recent studies show that stroke is a common, life-threatening, and often disabling complication of the use of many different street drugs.[1,2,3] Because of man's never-ending search for ways to induce pleasurable feelings, stimulants and hallucinogens make up a high proportion of drugs used. Stimulants often have catecholaminergic effects, raise blood pressure, and precipitate intracranial bleeding. Hemorrhages into the brain and subarachnoid space account for a high percentage of all drug-related strokes and drug-related hemorrhages now account for a significant and growing proportion of all intracranial hemorrhages (ICH), especially in individuals under age 35.[1] Not only is drug-related ICH an important public health problem, but it may offer an opportunity for insights into the pathogenesis of ICH in general. Drug-related ICH is one variety of hemorrhage in which cause, time of drug administration, course, and pathology are potentially able to be defined.

Although drug-related brain hemorrhage and stroke are fruitful grounds for research, the details of drug use are not always easy to clarify. Drug takers often use more than one substance. They do not always honestly report their usage or the source of their drugs, and often are not available for follow-up examinations and testing. Street drugs are not always as they are characterized by their sellers. Drugs are mixed with a host of different diluents. Drugs are often also shared, and users, when high, are poor at estimating the amount used. When drugs are injected, sterile precautions are seldom followed. These features make it difficult to assess the role of an individual drug or adulterant and to determine the effect of dose, foreign body or infectious contamination, and the frequency of long-term effects. Drug users are characteristically unconcerned about their health, so they often refuse investigation such as arteriography or follow-up imaging tests.

Drugs implicated in causing stroke can be divided into three general groups. *Group 1 drugs* are *stimulants* ("uppers") and *hallucinogenic* drugs. The *amphetamines* are the prototypic drug in this group. Stimulants generally have sympathomimetic effects and raise the blood pressure, quicken the pulse, and cause arterial contraction and constriction. *Methamphetamine* ("speed") is taken in pill form or injected. Recently, a new solid form of d-methamphetamine base that can be smoked ("ice") has appeared on the streets. A number of other pills are often sold on the streets designed to resemble amphetamines ("look-alike pills"), or are available over the counter as anorectants or sleep-preventative agents. *Phenylpropanolamine, ephedrine,* and *methylphenidate* (Ritalin), are some examples of widely available agents with amphetamine-like effects. Some of the hallucinogenic agents, *phencyclidine* ("angel dust"), *lysergic acid diethylamide* (LSD) and *mescaline* have similar stimulant properties as amphetamines. By far the most important stimulant that has been implicated in drug-related stroke is *cocaine.* Cocaine was traditionally used as cocaine hydrochloride powder, which could be taken orally, snorted or inhaled nasally, or injected intravenously. More recently, the alkaloidal form of cocaine ("crack") has become more popular. Crack is a more potent form of cocaine that is readily accessible in large cities around the world and is usually smoked.

*Group II drugs* are stimulants and other agents that are manufactured as pills but are mashed and injected intravenously by abusers. Included in this group are *methylphenidate* (Ritalin), *pentazocine* (Talwin), and *tripelennamine* (Pyribenzamine), the last two are often combined in a preparation called "T's and blues."[4] These pills contain binders like cornstarch, talc and microcrystalline cellulose which hold the drug in pill form. These drugs are injected into peripheral or neck veins and sometimes accidentally are injected directly into arteries in the neck and limbs.

*Group III drugs* are the opiates among which *heroin* is the most popular. When sold on the street, heroin is diluted ("cut") with different white powder adulterants, including amphetamines, talc, starch, curry powder, vim, ajax, caffeine, quinine, and even heparin.[2,3,5] Although heroin has often been implicated in causing stroke, nearly all heroin-related strokes have been ischemic.

Drug-related hemorrhages have been explained by different pathogenetic mechanisms. *(1) Pharmacologically mediated changes in blood pressure and flow.* Amphetamines, cocaine, methylphenidate, phencyclidine, mescaline, and LSD all have potential pres-

sor effects. Cocaine sensitizes vessels to the effects of epinephrine and norepinephrine by preventing the uptake of sympathomimetic neurotransmitters by nerve terminals.[6] Phencyclidine stimulates directly alpha adrenergic receptors.[7] Phencyclidine, LSD, and mescaline all produce potent contractile responses when applied to isolated brain arteries.[8] Methylphenidate and the amphetamines induce potent catecholamine-like responses. Sudden changes in blood pressure and blood flow cause rupture of arterioles and capillaries. The topic of sudden changes in blood pressure has been discussed in detail in Chapter 6. *(2) Endocarditis.* Narcotic addicts and those who inject drugs intravenously are especially likely to develop endocarditis.[9,10] Embolization of bacterial vegetations can involve the arterial wall leading to development of mycotic aneurysms that rupture, or the infective material can lead to vascular necrosis and hemorrhage.[11] In drug users, the organisms causing endocarditis are often coagulase positive staphylococci or fungi. The tricuspid valve is often involved and usually there is no underlying congenital or rheumatic valvular lesion; the bacteria cause an acute valvulitis with vegetations and microabcesses. Mortality is high. *(3) Vascular damage with subsequent bleeding.* Arterial injury can result from embolization of foreign materials such as talc and microcrystalline cellulose, from bacterial invasion as in endocarditis, and from immunologically mediated vascular damage ("arteritis"). Drug users often have evidence of immunological abnormalities. Hypergammaglobulinemia, circulating immune complexes, positive Coombs' test, antibodies to smooth muscles and lymphocyte membranes, and false-positive serology and lupus anticoagulant have been described.[2,3,12–14] Morphine binding by gammaglobulin has also been noted in addicts.[15] It is also possible that beading of arteries, found in users of amphetamines, could represent a direct response of the arterial wall to vasoconstriction. *(4) Coagulopathy.* Although seldom documented, ICH can be due to blood changes related to the drugs or secondary organ damage. Alcohol especially is known to affect platelets and can cause hypoprothrombinemia related to its hepatic toxicity. Liver and kidney damage are known to complicate various types of drug abuse and could lead to coagulopathies. In one patient, heparin was apparently a contaminant in heroin.[5]

## Amphetamines

Amphetamines were introduced into clinical medicine in the 1930s and were used to treat narcolepsy, hypotension, obesity, depression, and behavioral disorders in children. The first report of intracranial hemorrhage was by Gericke in 1945.[16] A 36-year-old man who was a drug abuser developed headache, confusion, and right limb weakness after an intentional overdose of oral amphetamine. He died within twenty-four hours and autopsy showed subarachnoid and subdural bleeding.[16] Since then, there have been numerous reports of intracranial bleeding after amphetamine use.[17–41]

We reviewed thirty reported, well documented instances of intracranial hemorrhage after use of amphetamines.[16–41] Among these, twenty-four were known drug abusers and some had taken other drugs and often also used alcohol. The remainder used amphetamines for diet control or to spark energy levels, or overdosed on the drugs. The three most frequently used preparations were amphetamine, methamphetamine, and dextroamphetamine. Recognized use before the hemorrhage was characterized as: oral amphetamine (nine patents), intravenous methamphetamine (eight patients), intravenous amphetamine (four patients), and nasal amphetamine (one patient). In all, seventeen patients took oral amphetamines, twelve used drugs intravenously, and one inhaled the amphetamine nasally. Infarction has also been described following nasal inhalation of methamphetamine crystals[42,43] but is unusual after oral or intravenous administration. Amphetamine (fourteen patients) and

methamphetamine (twelve patients) were implicated more often than dextroamphetamine (four patients) in causing intracranial bleeding. Dosage varied and was often unknown, but intracranial hemorrhage followed doses as small as 20 mg of oral amphetamine.[35] Among the thirty patients, twenty-two were men and eight were women. Ages ranged from 16 to 51 with an average age of 25.4. Most patients were drug abusers in their late teens or early 20s. In seven cases the bleeding was only subarachnoid; none of these patients had a berry aneurysm, but one patient had irregular arterial beading and luminal irregularity and a 2-mm fusiform aneurysmal dilatation of an anterior temporal branch of the middle cerebral artery.[33] One patient had a primary intraventricular hemorrhage after intravenous injection of a large dose of amphetamine.[41] In the other twenty-two patients, bleeding was intracerebral and often both intracerebral and subarachnoid. When localization of the hematoma was defined, four ICH were deep (one thalamic, three ganglionic) and nine were lobar. Frontal, central, parietal, and temporal lobes were about equally represented in this small sample, but none were limited to the occipital lobe. Among patients with ICH, thirteen incidents followed oral amphetamine use, eight followed intravenous use, and one followed nasal use. In only one patient with ICH was a vascular malformation found. This patient was a 28-year-old chronic heroin and amphetamine abuser who developed a right superficial temporal hematoma within twenty minutes of an intravenous injection of methamphetamine. Computed tomography (CT) showed a large draining vein and angiography showed a right Sylvian arteriovenous malformation (AVM) which was removed.[32] Among the twenty-nine patients with amphetamine-related intracranial hemorrhage, seven died and nine had surgical treatment of their hematomas.

Symptoms usually began with headache minutes after amphetamine use. Nausea, dizziness, and vomiting were also frequent accompaniments of the headache. Most patients had some reduction in level of consciousness ranging from minor drowsiness to frank coma. Examination usually showed an increased blood pressure when the patients were seen shortly after onset. Stiff neck, drowsiness, restlessness, and often stupor were the most frequent findings. Although focal neurological signs were often noted, the clinical picture was dominated by generalized alteration in behavior and alertness. Frank hemiplegia was less common than minor motor, reflex, sensory, or visual asymmetry. Amphetamines probably produce a multifocal encephalopathy with areas of edema, petechial hemorrhages, and microinfarcts in addition to intracerebral and subarachnoid bleeding. CT showing a large lobar ICH often came as a surprise considering the minor degree of focal findings on neurological examination. CT also often showed subarachnoid blood and brain swelling.

Angiography, when performed, has often shown striking abnormalities in chronic amphetamine users and patients with amphetamine related ICH.[23,25-27,30,31,33,35,36,38,39] The most common abnormalities are segmental areas of constriction, irregularity, and occasionally fusiform dilatation. These focal regions of abnormality usually involve mostly superficial branches and are often referred to as "beading." The changes have been reported to disappear on subsequent studies.[30] Angiography of systemic arteries in one methamphetamine user who also had hepatitis B showed multiple small aneurysms in the branches of the celiac and hepatic arteries.[44] Citron et al.[45] studied fourteen polydrug abusers, all of whom admitted to methamphetamine use. None had cerebral hemorrhages or infarcts recognized clinically, but some had neuropathy. Arterial lesions were found in the brain and in a host of other organs including skeletal muscle, spleen, pancreas, intestinal tract, kidney, and coronary arteries. Medium-sized and small arteries and arterioles were involved but elastic arteries, capillaries, and veins were spared. In acute lesions, fibrinoid necrosis involving the intima and media was prominent; the inflammatory infiltrate included neutrophils, eosinophils, lymphocytes, and histiocytes. Occlusive thrombi were also often found. Subacute arterial lesions were characterized by intimal proliferation and luminal narrowing. Older lesions showed marked destruction of muscular and elastic elements and replacement by collagen with resulting marked luminal narrowing. In some areas, a defective area of the vascular wall showed a nodular ("nodose") bulge of aneurysmal dilatation.[45]

During the era of maximal amphetamine abuse, Rumbaugh et al. studied the angiographic and pathological findings in human drug abusers[46] and experimental animals given methamphetamine.[47] In the patients, most of whom were young polydrug abusers who used methamphetamine, angiography showed segmental changes in vessel caliber, beading, and regions of slow flow.[46] The monkeys given intravenous methamphetamine during a two-week period had similar segmental changes and beading.[47] Necropsy in the animals showed microaneurysms, vascular degeneration, small hemorrhages, and zones of infarction. Because of the experimental and observational findings of Rumbaugh et al. and the frequent presence of segmental changes on angiography, many now diagnose "arteritis" when segmental changes are found. However, in recent years, series of patients with segmental vasoconstriction and beading have been described in whom the pathogenesis is likely to be reversible vasoconstriction ("spasm") rather than arteritis.[48] Similarly, in drug abusers, amphetamines are known to be potent vasoconstrictors. The segmental changes in some, perhaps even most, of the patients, may reflect reversible vasoconstriction rather than arteritis. Oral and intravenous amphetamine use declined in the 1980s, but the prospect of an "ice" epidemic (smoked crystalline d-methamphetamine) that could parallel the "crack" cocaine rage, may loom in the 1990s and beyond. If so, "ice" is even more likely than other forms of amphetamine to produce rapid changes in blood pressure and intracranial bleeding.

## Amphetamine-like Substances and Hallucinogens

Intracranial bleeding has been described after the use of a number of amphetamine-like preparations. The most commonly implicated agent is *phenylpropanolamine* (PPA), a popular decongestant, appetite depressant, and stimulant. It has been estimated that as many as five billion doses of pills containing PPA are taken annually.[49] PPA is available in many over-the-counter pills, and is also a frequent constituent of pills sold on the street to look like amphetamines. Most often, PPA is included among other drugs in popular combination pills used for colds, dieting, and as "pick-me-ups," or to suppress drowsiness. In decongestants, PPA is often combined with an antihistamine and anticholinergic agent; in anorexant pills, PPA is usually combined with caffeine.[50] PPA is also sometimes called norephedrine; it is primarily a partial alpha-adrenergic agonist and has little if any beta-adrenergic agonist activity.[51] PPA has a negligible effect on the release of norepinephrine from adrenergic nerve terminals but does inhibit reuptake of norepinephrine by nerve terminals.[51] PPA is well absorbed orally and is rapidly excreted in the urine. Lasagna has reviewed in detail the chemistry, pharmacokinetics, and pharmacology of PPA.[51]

Table 10.1 lists cases reported as intracranial bleeding putatively attributed to the use of PPA-containing compounds.[52–64] Women predominate; only seven of twenty-one patients were men. The average age was 33 and eleven of the twenty-one patients were under age 30 at the time of the event. In some, PPA compounds were taken in large doses in suicide attempts. A broad range of compounds was used, and most contained other drugs, most commonly caffeine or ephedrine. The most common reason for using PPA was as a diet aid appetite suppressant. Two patients

had subarachnoid bleeding only. Nineteen patients had ICH and two patients had multiple hematomas (one had two[54] and the other had four hematomas[55]) (Figure 10.1). Twelve hematomas were lobar, nine were putaminocapsular, and two were thalamic. Of note, blood pressures recorded on initial examination were usually within normal range. Only three of twenty-one patients had clearly hypertensive blood pressure recordings, 210/130,[53] 160/104,[55] 210/110.[62] The temporal relationship of the blood pressure measurements, the intake of PPA-containing pills, and the onset of symptoms were usually not recorded or not known. Fifteen patients had angiography. In three, the angiograms were normal; in twelve there were segmental abnormalities that included focal constriction, beading, irregularity, and minor dilatations and occlusions of small arteries (Figure 10.2). In one patient[61] the segmental changes had cleared after one month of abstinence of PPA-containing pills. Histological analysis of tissue removed at surgical drainage of the hematoma or at autopsy was available in four patients. In three, there were no signs of vascular disease on light microscopy; only one had histological evidence of necrotizing vasculitis.[56]

The small number of reported examples of intracranial bleeding pales in proportion to the widespread use of PPA. In some patients, PPA use was probably incidental. An example is Case 4 of McDowell and LeBlanc[61] of a 59-year-old woman with known vascular disease who had been taking one diet pill a day for years. In others, coincidental use of other drugs or substances may have potentiated the effects of PPA. Monoamine oxidase (MAO) inhibitors are known to enhance sympathomimetic effects. At least one reported patient took Nardil[61] and others have been noted to be depressed or suicidal and could have been taking MAO inhibitors. Use of nonsteroidal analgesics can also potentiate blood pressure changes or bleeding. Alcohol use, heavy use of coffee and colas have been mentioned and could add to the risk of intracranial bleeding. In two patients,[56,59]

**Table 10.1.** Reported Instances of Intracranial Hemorrhage Related to PPA Use

| Author | Age and Sex | Hypertension | | PPA Ingestion | | Δ Ingest. and Symptoms | Type Hem. | A-gram |
|---|---|---|---|---|---|---|---|---|
| | | Hist. | Adm. | First | Amt.* | | | |
| King[60] | 37/F | No | No | ? | 170 | Hours | ICH | ND |
| Bernstein and Diskant[58] | | | | | | | | |
| Pt.2 | 26/M | No | No | ? | 100 | 3–4 h. | SAH | ND |
| Pt.3 | 17/M | No | No | ? | 100 | 6 h. | ICH | ND |
| Fallis and Fisher[53] | 20/F | No | 210/130 | No | ?50 | ? | ICH | Beading |
| Kikta et al.[54] | | | | | | | | |
| Pt.1 | 56/F | No | 140/100 | Yes | 150 | 1 h. | ICH | ND |
| Pt.2 | 45/F | No | No | No | 50 | 1 h. | SAH | No ANR,AVM |
| McDowell and LeBlanc[61] | | | | | | | | |
| Pt.1 | 18/F | No | No | ? | 400 | Hours | ICH | ND |
| Pt.2 | 45/F | No | 150/? | Yes | 100 | Hours | ICH | ND |
| Pt.3 | 23/F | No | ? | ?Yes | 50 | Hours | ICH | Beading |
| Pt.4 | 59/F | No | No | No | 75 | Hours | ICH | Beading |
| Stoessl et al.[52] | | | | | | | | |
| Pt.1 | 20/F | No | No | Yes | ? | 2 h. | ICH | Beading |
| Pt.2 | 23/M | No | No | Yes | ? | 1 h. | ICH | Beading |
| Kase et al.[55] | | | | | | | | |
| Pt.1 | 39/F | Yes | 160/104 | Yes | 75 | Hours | ICH | Beading |
| Pt.2 | 32/M | No | No | Yes | 150 | 8 h. | ICH | Normal |
| Glick et al.[56] | 35/F | No | ? | No | ? | 90 m. | ICH | Beading† |
| Maher[59] | 30/F | No | No | No | ? | 30 m. | ICH | Beading |
| Maertens et al.[62] | 27/M | No | 210/110 | ? | 585 | 1 h. | ICH | Beading |
| Le Coz et al.[63] | | | | | | | | |
| Pt.2 | 61/F | No | 150/80 | Yes | ? | Hours | ICH | Beading |
| Forman et al.[57] | 17/F | No | No | No | 375 | 5 h. | ICH | Beading |
| Barinagarrementeria et al.[64] | | | | | | | | |
| Pt.1 | 36/M | No | No | ? | 300 | 3 h. | ICH | Normal |
| Pt.2 | 29/M | No | No | ? | 240 | 6 h. | ICH | Beading |

Abbreviations: Hist. = history, Adm. = admission, PPA = phenylpropanolamine, First = first time, Δ = time between, Ingest. = ingestion, Hem. = hemorrhage, A-gram = angiogram, Pt. = patient, M = male, F = female, h. = hour, m. = minutes, ICH = intracerebral hemorrhage, SAH = subarachnoid hemorrhage, ND = not done, ANR = aneurysm, AVM = arteriovenous malformation.

*Amount ingested in mg.

† Corresponding to vasculitis on histological examination of biopsy material.

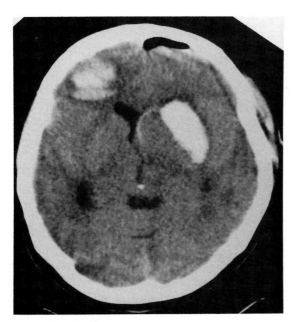

**Figure 10.1.** Bilateral ICH, lobar and basal ganglionic, in a young patient after ingestion of PPA. (From Kase CS, Foster TE, Reed JE, et al. Intracerebral hemorrhage and phenylpropanolamine use. Neurology 1987;37:393–404, with permission.)

intracranial hemorrhages occurred three weeks post partum, a time of vulnerability for blood pressure and blood volume changes. Not all patients have been fully investigated for other causes of intracranial bleeding, such as bleeding diathesis, trauma, or vascular malformation.

Studies of groups of patients have not revealed important adverse cardiovascular effects of PPA. In one study, 881 healthy individuals were given PPA or placebo.[65] A statistically significant but clinically unimportant pressor effect was noted for the short-term administration of PPA. Blood pressure increased 2 to 4 mm on average and pulse rate increased 1 to 3 beats a minute compared to the placebo treated group. Diastolic blood pressure, weight, and other drug use affected frequency of blood pressure increases after PPA.[65] Population-based studies of the risk of cerebral hemorrhage[66] or hospitalization[67] attributable to taking PPA

containing compounds indicates that the risk, if present at all, is very small. It seems reasonable to conclude that reactions to PPA containing compounds are considerably idiosyncratic. Higher than recommended dosage, prior hypertension, overuse of alcohol or caffeine, concomitant use of MAO inhibitors and possibly nonsteroidal analgesics, and use in the postpartum period probably compound the risk of intracerebral hemorrhage after PPA use.

Intracerebral hemorrhage has also been reported after ephedrine use.[68] The patient, a 20-year-old man, was an amphetamine addict who bought "speed" on the street. While hospitalized for a subarachnoid hemorrhage, blood analysis showed the presence of ephedrine and not other amphetamines. Skin biopsies showed deposits of immune substances about the lumina of small dermal blood vessels. Another patient, a 60-year-old man, had been taking *diethylpropion hydrochloride*, a prescription anorexant drug with sympathomimetic activity.[35] After four or five tablets of diethylpropion, he developed a right parietal lobe hematoma. Angiography showed segmental irregularities of intracranial arteries.

Another drug with sympathomimetic capabilities that can be quite hazardous is *phencyclidine*. Phencyclidine hydrochloride was originally developed as an anesthetic and analgesic agent. Now it is sold on the street and is referred to by users variously as PCP, angel dust, angel mist, and hog. PCP has a profound effect on mental state, often causing disorientation, violence, and seizures.[7,8,69] PCP is used primarily for its hallucinogenic activity, though "bad trips" are well known to users. Street sellers often sell it to teenagers as "acid" substituting it for LSD, mescaline, psilocybin, or THC.[7] Marijuana is often "dusted" with PCP and smoked. PCP can be taken orally, intravenously, as an inhalant, or smoked with marijuana.

PCP causes a slight increase in systolic and diastolic blood pressure. The drug enhances the pressor effects of epinephrine, norepinephrine, levarterenol, and serotonin,

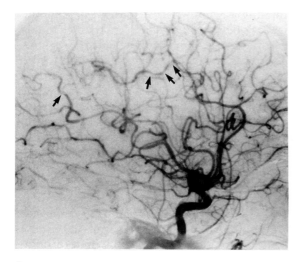

A

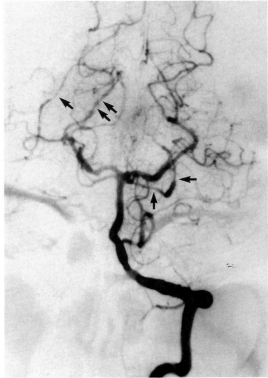

B

**Figure 10.2.** Multiple areas of arterial constriction and dilatation ("beading") (arrows) in the carotid (A) and vertebrobasilar territories (B), following ingestion of PPA. (From Kase CS, Foster TE, Reed JE, et al. Intracerebral hemorrhage and phenylpropanolamine use. Neurology 1987;37:399–404, with permission.)

and the pressor effect is not blocked by hexamethonium.[7,69] PCP probably has a sympathomimetic effect due to stimulation of alpha-adrenergic receptors but it also may affect peripheral catecholamine storage.[7] There have been two reported cases of ICH after phencyclidine use. A 13-year-old boy developed marked hypertension (220/130) and ICH and died after PCP use.[69] A 20-year-old man collapsed and became comatose after smoking what he thought was marijuana.[70] Blood pressure was 180/100. He had markedly increased intracranial pressure and subarachnoid and intraventricular bleeding that proved fatal. Toxic analysis revealed PCP.[70] Another patient, an 18-year-old polydrug abuser had hypertensive encephalopathy without intracranial bleeding after taking pills that contained phencyclidine.[69] *Lysergic acid diethylamide* (LSD) and *mescaline*, two other hallucinogens sold on the street, can elevate blood pressure and each, in addition to PCP, can cause vasoconstriction when applied to isolated arteries.[8] To our knowledge, intracranial bleeding has not been reported after use of mescaline or LSD.

Now commonly appearing on the streets are a host of new "designer drugs." Many are derivatives of phenylethylamines and are mescaline analogs.[71] These drugs have psychoactive and sympathomimetic effects. The two most commonly used of the designer phenylethylamine derivatives are 3-4-methylenedioxyamphetamine (MDA) and 3-4-methylenedioxymethamphetamine (MDMA).[71] Clinical effects are similar to those of amphetamine abuse and include tachycardia, hypertension, fever, sweating, mydriasis, and agitation.[71] Although we are unaware of reports of ICH after the use of MDA and MDMA, it is quite likely that such have and will occur.

## Cocaine

Abuse of cocaine has increased recently into epidemic proportions. Undoubtedly, cocaine is now widely recognized as one of the most dangerous illicit drugs in common use.[72,73] In 1986, it was estimated that 30 million Americans had used cocaine at some time, five million use it regularly, and that each day another five thousand used it for the first time.[72] Patterns of cocaine use in the 1970s usually involved social-recreational doses of crystalline cocaine hydrochloride snorted nasally.[72] From 1978 to 1982 doses for recreational use increased. In the 1980s, episodes of frequent binges became more common as did the introduction of "crack" cocaine. Crack cocaine is made by mixing aqueous cocaine hydrochloride with ammonia and sometimes baking soda.[74] The chemical reaction converts the hydrochloride to a volatile form of the drug, almost pure cocaine. The basic cocaine alkaloid is inhaled or smoked after the cocaine is mixed in the alkaline solution and precipitated as alkaloidal cocaine.[74] Smoked freebase cocaine ("crack") provides a rapid intense euphoria because of high blood concentrations. Crack cocaine is absorbed quickly and gets to the brain in less than ten seconds.[74]

In recent years, cocaine-related deaths have risen steadily. Cocaine dealers prefer to sell crack instead of cocaine hydrochloride powder because of its high addiction potential, low unit cost, and ease of handling.[73] Crack use has been associated with a greater incidence of medical and neurological complications, including death. Cocaine hydrochloride is taken orally, vaginally, sublingually, rectally, nasally, and by subcutaneous, intramuscular, or intravenous injection. Crack is usually smoked or inhaled. Cardiovascular effects begin immediately after cocaine use and include an increase in pulse, blood pressure, temperature, and metabolism.[74] Acute effects subside about thirty minutes after intravenous use and about one hour after nasal use. Cocaine and amphetamines are neuropharmacologically similar.[73] The pressor effect of cocaine is probably mediated through a peripheral catecholamine mechanism.[74] Vasospasm may occur and myocardial,[75] renal, intestinal, and brain ischemia have been reported.[2,3,74] Myocardial infarction, cardiac arrhythmia, and myocarditis are important and serious complications of cocaine use.[72,73,75]

The first reported cocaine-related stroke was in 1977 in a man who became aphasic and hemiparetic from a left cerebral infarction an hour after injecting cocaine hydrochloride intravenously.[2] Recently, reports of both occlusive and hemorrhagic stroke have increased because of the widespread availability and toxicity of crack cocaine.[76] Amphetamine-related strokes are almost exclusively hemorrhagic. Cocaine-related strokes have been predominantly hemorrhagic but infarction is also very common. We will review herein only cocaine-related intracranial hemorrhage.

Subarachnoid hemorrhage is an important and frequent complication of cocaine use. We reviewed thirty-one reported cases.[77,79–84,86–93] SAH occurred irrespective of route of intake. Nine instances occurred after smoking crack, nine after nasal snorting of cocaine hydrochloride, four after intravenous injection of cocaine, and in nine, the route of intake was not known. Symptoms might begin immediately during the use of cocaine or could be delayed for hours.[97] Severe headache, vomiting, and loss of consciousness were the most frequent symptoms, but sudden death was also common. The thirty-one cases included sixteen men and fifteen women; ages ranged from 22 to 63, with an average age of 31.6. In some, cocaine was injected with heroin[77,79] or taken with alcohol.[82,86,92] One patient was pregnant when she developed SAH after crack use.[91] The two most important and distinctive features were the *very high mortality* and the *high frequency of aneurysm detection*. Fifteen of the thirty-one cases of cocaine-related SAH died (48.4%). In twenty-five of the thirty-one patients with SAH, aneurysms were discovered during angiography or at necropsy; three patients had normal angiography, one had no aneurysm at autopsy, and two had no angiography or autopsy. Thus, among twenty-nine patients studied by angiography or autopsy, twenty-five (86%) had aneurysms (Figure 10.3). Recall that in sharp contrast, no patient with PPA-related intracranial hemorrhage and only one with amphetamine-related ICH had an AVM shown. The reason for this discrepancy is not known, but the high incidence of aneurysms in patients with cocaine-related SAH makes angiography mandatory in this group of patients.

Intracerebral hemorrhage has also been common after cocaine use. Table 10.2 outlines forty-five reported cases.[3,76–85,89,92,93,95–97] There were twenty-eight men (62%) and only seventeen women (38%). Male predominance was also a feature of amphetamine-related intracranial hemorrhage but PPA-related bleeding was primarily in women. Age at time of ICH ranged from 22 to 57, average age 33.6 years, figures comparable to those in cocaine-related SAH. Most reports did not note the time of onset of symptoms in relationship to cocaine use, but in the series of Levine et al., ICH often occurred immediately or shortly after drug use.[97] Headache, focal signs, and sudden loss of consciousness were the most common symptoms. Sudden death was also reported and some of the patients were coroner's cases.[92,93] In some patients, coexistent medical conditions (hypertension,[84] pregnancy,[97] postpartum period,[78] renal dialysis[77]) were present that could pre-

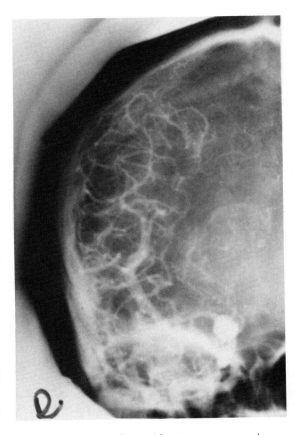

**Figure 10.3.** Internal carotid artery aneurysm in patient who presented with SAH after use of crack cocaine. (Courtesy of Steven R. Levine, M.D., Henry Ford Hospital, Detroit, MI.)

dispose to ICH. Concurrent use of alcohol was also common. Mortality was also high; fourteen of the forty-five (31%) patients died of cocaine-related ICH. Intracerebral hemorrhage followed use by any route: fifteen patients used crack, fourteen snorted cocaine nasally, and eleven injected the drug intravenously, and in 5, the method of cocaine use was unknown.

The most common location of cocaine-related ICH was lobar. Twenty-six (57%) were lobar with no obvious predilection for one cerebral lobe versus the other. In eight, bleeding was into the lateral ganglionic area (putaminal or capsular) (Figure 10.4), three were primarily intraventricular, three tha-

**Table 10.2.** Cocaine-related ICH

| Author | Age | Sex | Route | Location | Vascular Lesion | Other-Outcome |
|---|---|---|---|---|---|---|
| Nolte and Gelman[76] | 29 | F | IV | lobar, massive | aut-no vasc lesion | sudden death |
| Mangiardi[77] | 33 | M | IV+heroin | lobar | no angio | death |
| | 41 | F | IV+heroin | lobar | angio-no vasc lesion | death |
| | 22 | M | IV+heroin | capsular | angio-aneurysm | death-SBE |
| | 32 | M | IV+heroin | lobar | angio-no vasc lesion | alcohol-renal dial |
| | 35 | F | IV | intravent | angio-ependymal AVM | death |
| | 34 | F | crack | intravent | angio-thalamic AVM | rebled |
| | 24 | F | nasal | lobar | angio-AVM | |
| | 30 | M | nasal | lobar | angio-no vasc lesion | |
| | 22 | M | nasal | lobar | angio-no vasc lesion | |
| Mercado et al.[78] | 25 | F | crack | lobar | angio-no vasc lesion | postpartum day four |
| Jacobs et al.[79] | 29 | F | IV+heroin | putaminal | angio-no vasc lesion | |
| | 44 | M | crack | putaminal | no angio | |
| | 45 | M | crack | thalamic | no angio | |
| | 34 | M | IV | lobar | angio-AVM | |
| Klonoff et al.[80] | 29 | F | crack | putaminal | angio-segmental changes | 120/80 |
| | 32 | M | nasal | lobar | angio-aneurysm | 220/110 |
| | 34 | M | IV | hemispheral | aut-no vasc lesion | 170/110, death |
| | 56 | M | crack | thalamic | angio-no vasc lesion | 240/140, death |
| Lichtenfeld et al.[81] | 24 | F | nasal | lobar | angio-AVM | |

**Table 10.2.** *Continued*

| Author | Age | Sex | Route | Location | Vascular Lesion | Other-Outcome |
|---|---|---|---|---|---|---|
| Wojak and Flamm[84] | 34 | M | IV | caud-vent | angio-no vasc lesion | hx hypertension, 210/120 |
| | 22 | M | nasal | lobar | | |
| | 42 | M | ? | lobar-recurrent | | |
| | 51 | M | nasal | lobar | | |
| Green et al.[85] | 36 | M | crack and alcohol | multiple lobar | no angio | 148/88 |
| Caplan et al.[3] | 22 | M | nasal | lobar | angio-no vasc lesion | |
| Lehman[94] | 30 | F | nasal | lobar | angio-AVM, 2 aneurysms | |
| Lowenstein et al.[89] | 32 | M | IV | lobar | angio-AVM | |
| | 57 | M | nasal | ganglionic | no angio | |
| Mody et al.[96] | 34 | M | crack | lobar | angio-no vasc lesion | 140/90 |
| | 30 | M | crack | lobar | angio-segmental changes | 142/90 |
| | 32 | M | crack | lobar | angio-AVM | 130/82 |
| Tardiff et al.[92] | 33 | M | ? | massive | autopsy-no vasc lesion | death |
| | 28 | F | ? | massive | autopsy-no vasc lesion | death |
| Schwartz and Cohen[82] | 30 | M | nasal | lobar | angio-no vasc lesion | |
| Rowley et al.[97] | 23 | F | nasal | thal and midbrain | no angio | |
| Mittleman[93] | 50 | M | nasal | lobar | aut-no vasc lesion | death |
| | 35 | M | nasal | ganglionic | aut-no vasc lesion | death |
| | 26 | F | ? | lobar | aut-AVM | death |
| | 28 | F | ? | lobar | aut-AVM | death |
| Levine et al.[97] | 49 | M | crack | intravent | no angio | 310/140,death |
| | 36 | F | crack | massive | no angio | 140/70 |
| | 28 | M | crack | ganglionic | no angio | |
| | 23 | F | crack | lobar | angio-AVM | pregnant |
| | 46 | F | crack | ganglionic | no angio | |

Abbreviations: M = male; F = female; IV = intravenous; intravent = intraventricular; aut = autopsy; vasc = vascular; angio = angiogram; AVM = arteriovenous malformation; SBE = subacute bacterial endocarditis; dial = dialysis; caud-vent = cuadate-ventricular; thal = thalamus; hx = history of.

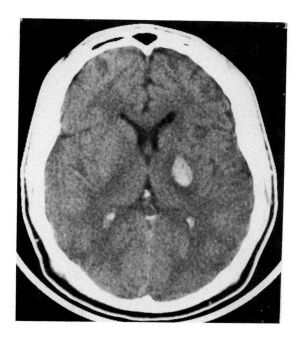

**Figure 10.4.** Small basal ganglionic-capsular hemorrhage after use of crack cocaine (Courtesy of Steven R. Levine, M.D., Henry Ford Hospital, Detroit, MI.)

lamic, one of which extended into the midbrain and one began in the caudate nucleus and spread to the ventricle. In four patients, the hemorrhage was very large (Figure 10.5) and involved one hemisphere, but a site of origin was not designated. An underlying potential bleeding lesion was also common in cocaine-related ICH, just as it had been in the cocaine-related SAH patients. Twelve patients with ICH had underlying AVM, three had aneurysms (Figure 10.6), and one had a glioma with recurrent hemorrhage into the tumor. Ten of the forty-five patents did not have angiography or autopsy examination, so that sixteen of the thirty-five patients studied (46%) had pre-existing lesions, a very high frequency. Among the twelve patients with AVM, ten had lobar hemorrhages and two had intraventricular bleeding. Underlying vascular lesions were rare when the ICH was ganglionic, thalamic or caudate, since only one of these patients had an abnormality, a

single instance of aneurysm.[77] One patient with a lobar hemorrhage after snorting cocaine nasally had an AVM and two had aneurysms on angiography. *Clearly, cocaine-related ICH is also an indication for angiography especially if the bleeding is lobar.* In only two patients with cocaine-related hemorrhage[80,95] were angiographic segmental beading and narrowing noted. Recall that segmental changes on angiography were very frequently found in users of amphetamine and in patients with PPA-related ICH. The reason for this discrepancy is also uncertain.

The type of cocaine used and route of administration affect the likelihood of brain hemorrhage versus infarction, and the likelihood of having an underlying vascular lesion as the cause of cocaine-related hemorrhage. A recent study compared strokes after cocaine hydrochloride use (nasal and intravenous) versus strokes after use of alkaloidal "crack" cocaine.[98] The great majority of strokes after cocaine hydrochloride were hemorrhages (69% after nasal and 97% after parenteral use) but only 55% of strokes after alkaloidal cocaine use were hemorrhages.[98] The chances of harboring an aneurysm were less in alkaloidal cocaine-related ICH (22%) compared with 39% of ICH after nasal cocaine hydrochloride and 57% after intravenous cocaine hydrochloride.[98]

Most authors have attributed cocaine-related hemorrhage to the sympathomimetic effects of the drug. Blood pressures were frequently not reported, and when reported, the time since drug use was not noted. In some patients, blood pressure was strikingly high (240/140,[80] 220/110,[80] 210/120,[84] 300/140[97]) but the elevation might have been affected by the presence of ICH and increased intracranial pressure. Vasculitis has been mentioned but has only recently been documented after cocaine-related intracranial hemorrhage.[98a] Two patients with multifocal neurological signs and brain ischemia who smoked crack have had biopsy-proven vasculitis.[99] Bleeding diatheses have not been found with cocaine-related SAH or ICH. Seizures and acidosis are known to complicate cocaine over-

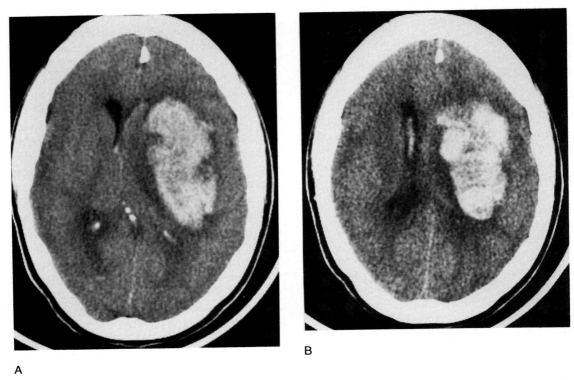

A
B

**Figure 10.5.** Large basal ganglionic ICH (A) with upward extension into the frontoparietal white matter (B) after use of crack cocaine (Courtesy of Steven R. Levine, Henry Ford Hospital, Detroit, MI.)

doses[100] and can potentiate bleeding. Acidosis has not been noted in patients with cocaine-related intracranial bleeding. Much research still needs to be done to explain the striking differences in amphetamine-, PPA-, and cocaine-related bleeding.

### Alcohol

Alcohol is undoubtedly the most frequently used and abused of all drugs. Statistics on alcohol and disease are truly staggering. Perhaps between 20% and 50% of hospital admissions, probably 50% of emergency room visits, and nearly half of all accidental deaths, suicides, and homicides are in some way related to alcohol.[101] Alcohol has its major desired effect, intoxication and relaxation, by its effect on the nervous system, and many of its toxicities also relate to damage to

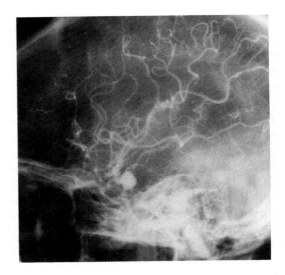

**Figure 10.6.** Anterior communicating artery aneurysm in patient who presented with ICH after use of crack cocaine (Courtesy of Steven R. Levine, M.D., Henry Ford Hospital, Detroit, MI.)

the central and peripheral nervous systems. Cardiovascular effects are also well known. Understandably, there has been great interest in the relation between alcohol use, both chronic and acute, and stroke.

The literature and data on stroke and alcohol consumption are very different than those cited already on other drugs. Data on cocaine, amphetamine, and amphetamine-like drugs and stroke came mostly from anecdotal reports on series of patients who had stroke in some relationship to drug use. In contrast, alcohol and stroke studies and reviews consist mostly of epidemiological reports. Alcohol use is so ubiquitous that in any single incidence of stroke, abuse of alcohol within twenty-four hours or chronically might very well be coincidental and have little causal relationship to the stroke. The only way to be certain of a relationship would be studies of large groups of patients that would give statistically valid results. Such studies are difficult since patients notoriously underestimate or understate alcohol use and often accurate data are not available. Wolf,[102] Camargo,[103] and Gorelick[101,104] reviewed the literature on alcohol and stroke and discussed some of the pitfalls and problems in the existing data.

There are a number of mechanisms by which alcohol could contribute to intracranial bleeding. Hypertension is probably more prevalent among chronic drinkers, and acute rise in blood pressure sometimes accompanies acute alcohol use or withdrawal.[101,105] Liver injury by alcohol leads to decreased levels of coagulation factors such as prothrombin, abnormal fibrinogens, and increased fibrinolysis.[100,105,106] With moderate alcohol consumption, the bleeding time is prolonged and platelet function can be impaired. There are also effects of alcohol that could lead to an increased risk for ischemic stroke.[101,105]

Many studies do not divide stroke into various subtypes. Gill et al. reported a case-control retrospective study of 230 stroke patients.[107] In men, the relative stroke risk was reduced in light drinkers compared with nondrinkers, but was four times higher in heavy drinkers. The data on women in this study were insufficient. The relation between alcohol and stroke was studied in women in the Nurses' Health Study, a prospective investigation of female nurses.[108] There was reduced incidence of stroke in light drinkers and increased incidence in heavy drinkers. SAH was positively associated with alcohol intake with a relative risk of 3.7 associated with intake of 5 to 14 grams of alcohol per day.[108]

Several epidemiological studies specifically consider the relationship between alcohol use and hemorrhagic stroke. Hillbom and Kaste in Finland studied consecutive patients presenting with SAH.[109,110] Among 172 patients (eighty-eight men, eighty-four women; ages 15 to 55), in thirty-seven (22%) alcohol intoxication was present in the twenty-four hours before the onset of SAH.[110] Heavy drinkers accounted for 19% of the patients. Alcohol intoxication preceding SAH was two to three times more common in men and two to thirteen times as common in women than in the general Finnish population matched for age and sex.[110] Tanaka et al. studied the relationship of alcohol to cerebral hemorrhage in a rural Japanese community.[111] A cohort of 772 men and 901 women, all stroke-free, were followed prospectively for ten years. High alcohol intake increased the risk of stroke, the relative risk being 3.02.[111] The Honolulu Heart Program followed 8006 men.[112] During twelve years of follow-up, 197 drinkers and 93 nondrinkers had strokes. Although there was no significant relationship between alcohol and thromboembolic stroke, the risk of hemorrhagic stroke more than doubled for light drinkers and nearly tripled for heavy drinkers.[112] In this study, both SAH and ICH had an increased incidence in heavy drinkers. Klatsky et al. recently prospectively studied 107,137 patients receiving health examinations in a prepaid health plan during a six-year period.[113] Daily intake of three or more drinks but not lighter drinking was associated with higher hospitalization rates for intracranial bleeding, especially ICH. In this study, the authors concluded that higher blood pressure was an important, but only partial, mediator of the relation between alcohol use and subsequent intracranial hemorrhage.[113]

The epidemiological evidence relating alcohol use to ICH is for us impressive, although clearly more work and data are necessary. There is no information about the location, size, and outcome of ICH in those who use alcohol compared with nonusers. In our experience, ICH related to alcohol and liver disease tend to be lobar and large. There may be a special predilection for hematomas in the superior parietal lobule and posterior parietal regions. Many of these patients have abnormalities of platelet and clotting functions.

## Other Miscellaneous Drugs

Although opiates, especially heroin, are frequently abused, hemorrhagic stroke has rarely been attributable directly to their use. The vast majority of heroin-related strokes are ischemic.[2,3] When ICH occurs in an heroin user, it is most often an indirect effect caused by a medical complication of heroin addiction. Brust and Richter included two patients with brain hemorrhage in their original report of stroke in heroin addicts.[114] One patient with ICH had heroin nephropathy and malignant hypertension. The other patient had a fatal massive putaminal hemorrhage three days after starting methadone detoxification. He developed seizures, had normal blood pressure, and had an autopsy by the medical examiners, but the intracranial arteries were not studied. The cause of the ICH was not determined.[114] Possible causes of ICH in heroin users include endocarditis with mycotic aneurysms and septic embolization,[9,11] lacing of heroin with heparin or heparin-like substances,[5] nephropathy related to hypertension,[114] and immune-related vasculopathy with bleeding from an arteritic vessel.[2,3,13]

Some people intravenously inject mashed pills manufactured for oral consumption. Methylphenidate (Ritalin) and pentazocine and tripelennamine (Talwin and Pyribenzamine—"T's and blues") are the best known. At times, when arm veins are obliterated, addicts use the jugular vein and can mistakenly inject these drugs into a carotid artery.[115] Methylphenidate does have a sympathomimetic effect and so could cause ICH by abruptly increasing blood pressure, but such has not been reported. One patient had a large frontal ICH develop after taking "T's and blues."[4] In that patient, angiography showed obliteration of branch arteries, beading and segmental changes, and extravasation of dye. The posited mechanism of bleeding was immune-mediated vasculopathy. ICH has been described in patients with vasculitis of diverse causes.[4]

Although inhalants are frequently abused and the incidence of "glue sniffing" is increasing, these drugs have not been associated with ICH or stroke. Liver and renal toxicity could, however, predispose to ICH.

The coming years will undoubtedly broaden our knowledge of drug-related ICH, its wide spectrum and mechanisms. This information may yield clues to spontaneously occurring ICH in nonusers of drugs.

## References

1. Kaku DA, Lowenstein DH. Emergence of recreational drug abuse as a major risk factor for stroke in young adults. Ann Intern Med 1990; 113:821–827.
2. Brust JCM. Stroke and drugs. In: Toole, J. F., ed. Handbook of Clinical Neurology. Vol II(55). Vascular Disease Part III. Amsterdam: Elsevier Science, 1989;517–531.
3. Caplan LR, Hier DB, Banks G. Stroke and drug abuse. Stroke 1982;13:869–872.
4. Caplan LR, Thomas C, Banks G. Central nervous system complications of addiction to "T's and Blues." Neurology 1982;32:623–628.
5. Maqbool Z, Billett HH. Unwitting heparin abuse in a drug addict. Ann Intern Med 1982;96:790–791 (letter).

6. Brust JCM, Richter RW. Stroke associated with cocaine abuse? NY State J Med 1977;77:1473–1475.

7. Stratton MA, Witherspoon JM, Kirtley T. Hypertensive crises and phencyclidine abuse. Virginia Med 1978;105:569–572.

8. Altura BT, Altura BM. Phencyclidine, lysergic acid diethylamide, and mescaline: cerebral artery spasms and hallucinogenic activity. Science 1981;212:1051–1052.

9. Louria DB, Hensle T, Rose J. The major medical complications of heroin addiction. Ann Intern Med 1967;67:1–22.

10. Banks T, Fletcher R, Ali N. Infective endocarditis in heroin addicts. Amer J Med 1973;55:444–451.

11. Davenport J, Hart RG. Prosthetic valve endocarditis: 1976–1987. Stroke 1990;21:993–999.

12. Becker CE. Medical complications of drug abuse. Adv Intern Med 1979;24:183–202.

13. Ortona L, Laghi V, Cauda R. Immune function in heroin addicts. N Engl J Med 1979. 300:45 (letter).

14. Toler KA, Anderson B. Stroke in an intravenous drug user secondary to the lupus anticoagulant. Stroke 1988;19:274 (letter).

15. Ryan JJ, Parker CW, Williams RC. Gammaglobulin binding of morphine in heroin addicts. J Lab Clin Med 1972;80:155–164.

16. Gericke OL. Suicide by ingestion of amphetamine sulfate. JAMA 1945;128:1098–1099.

17. Poteliakhoff A, Roughton BC. Two cases of amphetamine poisoning. Br Med J 1956;1:26–27.

18. Lloyd JTA, Walker DRH. Death after combined dexamphetamine and phenelzine. Br Med J 1965;2:168–169 (letter).

19. Coroner's Report, Amphetamine overdose kills boy. Pharmaceut J 1967;198:172.

20. Kane FJ, Keeler MH, Reifler CB. Neurological crisis following methamphetamine. JAMA 1969;210:556–557 (letter).

21. Goodman SJ, Becker DP. Intracranial hemorrhage associated with amphetamine abuse. JAMA 1970;212:480 (letter).

22. Weiss SR, Raskind R, Morganstern NL, et al. Intracerebral and subarachnoid hemorrhage following use of methamphetamine ("speed"). Int Surg 1970;53:123–127.

23. Margolis MT, Newton TH. Methamphetamine ("speed") arteritis. Neuroradiology 1971;2:179–182.

24. Hall CD, Blanton DE, Scatliff JH, et al. Speed kills: fatality from the self-administration of methamphetamine intravenously. South Med J 1973;66:650–652.

25. Chynn KY. Acute subarachnoid hemorrhage. JAMA 1975;233:55–56.

26. Olsen ER. Intracranial hemorrhage and amphetamine usage: review of the effects of amphetamines on the central nervous system. Angiology 1977;28:464–471.

27. Kessler JT, Jortner BS, Adapon BD. Cerebral vasculitis in a drug abuser. J Clin Psychiat 1978;39:559–564.

28. LoVerme S. Complications of amphetamine abuse. In: Culebras A, ed. Clini-Pearls. Syracuse: Creative Medical Publishers, 1979;2(8):5.

29. Delaney P, Estes M. Intracranial hemorrhage with amphetamine abuse. Neurology 1980;30:1125–1128.

30. Cahill DW, Knipp HJ, Mosser J. Intracranial hemorrhage with amphetamine abuse. Neurology 1981;31:1058–1059 (letter).

31. Edwards KR. Hemorrhagic complications of cerebral arteritis. Arch Neurol 1977;34:549–552.

32. Lukes SA. Intracerebral hemorrhage from an arteriovenous malformation after amphetamine injection. Arch Neurol 1983;40:60–61.

33. Matick H, Anderson D, Brumlik J. Cerebral vasculitis associated with oral amphetamine overdose. Arch Neurol 1983;40:253–254.

34. D'Souza T, Shraberg D. Intracranial hemorrhage associated with amphetamine use. Neurology 1981;31:922–923 (letter).

35. Harrington H, Heller HA, Dawson D, et al. Intracerebral hemorrhage and oral amphetamine. Arch Neurol 1983;40:503–507.

36. Yarnell PR. "Speed": headache and hematoma. Headache 1977;17:69–70.

37. Shukla D. Intracranial hemorrhage associated with amphetamine use. Neurology 1982;32:917–918 (letter).

38. Yu YJ, Cooper DR, Wellenstein DE, et al. Cerebral angiitis and intracerebral hemorrhage associated with methamphetamine abuse: case report. J Neurosurg 1983;58:109–111.

39. Salanova V, Taubner R. Intracerebral haemorrhage and vasculitis secondary to amphetamine use. Postgrad Med J 1984;60:429–430.

40. Yatsu FM, Wesson DR, Smith DE. Amphetamine abuse In: Richter RW, ed. Medical Aspects of Drug Abuse. Hagerstown: Harper and Row, 1975;50–56.

41. Imanse J, Vanneste J. Intraventricular hemorrhage following amphetamine abuse. Neurology 1990;40:1318–1319.

42. Sachdeva K, Woodward KG. Caudal thalamic infarction following intranasal methamphetamine use. Neurology 1989;39:305–306.

43. Rothrock JF, Rubenstein R, Lyden PD. Ischemic stroke associated with methamphetamine inhalation. Neurology 1988;38:589–592.

44. Koff RS, Widrich WC, Robbins AH. Necrotizing angiitis in a methamphetamine user with hepatitis B–angiographic diagnosis, five month follow-up results and localization of bleeding site. N Engl J Med 1973;288:946–947.

45. Citron BP, Halpern M, McCarron M, et al. Necrotizing angiitis associated with drug abuse. N Engl J Med 1970;283:1003–1011.

46. Rumbaugh CL, Bergeron RT, Fang, HCH, et al. Cerebral angiographic changes in the drug abuse patient. Radiology 1971;101:335–344.

47. Rumbaugh CL, Bergeron RT, Scanlan RL, et al. Cerebral vascular changes secondary to amphetamine abuse in the experimental animal. Radiology 1971;101:345–351.

48. Call GK, Fleming MC, Sealfon S, et al. Reversible cerebral segmental vasoconstriction. Stroke 1988;19:1159–1170.

49. Morgan JP. Phenylpropanolamine: a critical analysis of reported adverse reactions and overdosage. Fort Lee, NJ: Jack K. Burgess, 1986.

50. Pentel P. Toxicity of over-the-counter stimulants. JAMA 1984;252:1898–1903.

51. Lasagna L. Phenylpropanolamine: A review. New York: John Wiley, 1988.

52. Stoessl AJ, Young GB, Feasby TE. Intracerebral haemorrhage and angiographic beading following ingestion of catecholaminergics. Stroke 1985;16:734–736.

53. Fallis RJ, Fisher M. Cerebral vasculitis and hemorrhage associated with phenylpropanolamine. Neurology 1985;35:405–407.

54. Kikta DG, Devereaux MW, Chandar K. Intracranial hemorrhages due to phenylpropanolamine. Stroke 1985;16:510–512.

55. Kase CS, Foster TE, Reed JE, et al. Intracerebral hemorrhage and phenylpropanolamine use. Neurology 1987;37:399–404.

56. Glick R, Hoying J, Cerullo L, et al. Phenylpropanolamine: an over-the-counter drug causing central nervous system vasculitis and intracerebral hemorrhage. Neurosurgery 1987;20:969–974.

57. Forman HP, Levin S, Stewart B, et al. Cerebral vasculitis and hemorrhage in an adolescent taking diet pills containing phenylpropanolamine: case report and review of literature. Pediatrics 1989;83:737–741.

58. Bernstein E, Diskant BM. Phenylpropanolamine: a potentially hazardous drug. Ann Emerg Med 1982;11:311–315.

59. Maher LM. Postpartum intracranial hemorrhage and phenylpropanolamine use. Neurology 1987;37:1686 (letter).

60. King J. Hypertension and cerebral haemorrhage after Trimolets ingestion. Med J Aust 1979;2:258 (letter).

61. McDowell JR, LeBlanc HJ. Phenylpropanolamine and cerebral hemorrhage. West J Med 1985;142:688–691.

62. Maertens P, Lum G, Williams JP, et al. Intracranial hemorrhage and cerebral angiopathic changes in a suicidal phenylpropanolamine poisoning. South Med J 1987;80:1584–1586.

63. Le Coz P, Woimant F, Rougemont D, et al. Angiopathies cérébrales bénignes et phénylpropanolamine. Rev Neurol 1988;144:295–300.

64. Barinagarrementería F, Méndez A, Vega F. Hemorragia cerebral asociada al uso de fenilpropanolamina. Neurología 1990;5:292–295.

65. Blackburn GL, Morgan JP, Lavin PT, et al. Determinants of the pressor effect of phenylpropanolamine in healthy subjects. JAMA 1989;261:3267–3272.

66. Jick H, Aselton P, Hunter JR. Phenylpropanolamine and cerebral haemorrhage. Lancet 1984;1:1017 (letter).

67. Aselton P, Jick H, Hunter JR. Phenylpropanolamine exposure and subsequent hospitalization. JAMA 1985;253:977 (letter).

68. Wooten MR, Khangure MS, Murphy MJ. Intracerebral hemorrhage and vasculitis related to ephedrine abuse. Ann Neurol 1983;13:337–340.

69. Eastman JW, Cohen SN. Hypertensive crisis and death associated with phencyclidine poisoning. JAMA 1975;231:1270–1271.

70. Bessen HA. Intracranial hemorrhage associated with phencyclidine abuse. JAMA 1982;248:585–586.

71. Buchanan JF, Brown CR. "Designer drugs": a problem in clinical toxicology. Med Toxicol 1988;3:1–17.

72. Cregler LL, Mark H. Medical complications of cocaine abuse. N Engl J Med 1986;315:1495–1500.

73. Gawin FH, Ellinwood EH. Cocaine and other stimulants. N Engl J Med 1988;318:1173–1182.

74. Levine SR, Welch KMA. Cocaine and stroke. Stroke 1988;19:779–783.

75. Isner J, Estes NAM, Thompson PO, et al. Acute cardiac events temporally related to cocaine abuse. N Engl J Med 1986;315:1438–1443.

76. Nolte KB, Gelman BB. Intracerebral hemorrhage associated with cocaine abuse. Arch Pathol Lab Med 1989;113:812–813.

77. Mangiardi JR, Daras M, Geller ME, et al. Cocaine-related intracranial hemorrhage: report of nine cases and review. Acta Neurol Scand 1988;77:177–180.

78. Mercado A, Johnson G, Calver D, et al. Cocaine, pregnancy and postpartum intracerebral hemorrhage. Obstet Gynecol 1989;73:467–468.

79. Jacobs IG, Roszler MH, Kelly JK, et al. Cocaine abuse: neurovascular complications. Radiology 1989;170:223–227.

80. Klonoff DC, Andrews BT, Obana WG. Stroke associated with cocaine use. Arch Neurol 1989;46:989–993.

81. Lichtenfeld PJ, Rubin DB, Feldman RS. Subarachnoid hemorrhage precipitated by cocaine snorting. Arch Neurol 1984;41:223–224.

82. Schwartz KA, Cohen JA. Subarachnoid hemorrhage precipitated by cocaine snorting. Arch Neurol 1984;41:705 (letter).

83. Levine SR, Washington JM, Jefferson MF, et al. "Crack" cocaine–associated stroke. Neurology 1987;37:1849–1853.

84. Wojak JC, Flamm ES. Intracranial hemorrhage and cocaine use. Stroke 1987;18:712–715.

85. Green RM, Kelly KM, Gabrielsen T, et al. Multiple intracerebral hemorrhages after smoking "crack" cocaine. Stroke 1990;21:957–962.

86. Lundberg GD, Garriott JC, Reynolds PC, et al. Cocaine-related death. J Forensic Sci 1977;22:402–408.

87. Rogers JN, Henry TE, Jones AM, et al. Cocaine-related deaths in Pima County, Arizona, 1982–1984. J Forensic Sci 1986;31:1404–1408.

88. Cregler LL, Mark H. Relation of stroke to cocaine abuse. NY State J Med 1987;87:128–129 (letter).

89. Lowenstein DH, Massa SM, Rowbotham MC, et al. Acute neurologic and psychiatric complications associated with cocaine abuse. Am J Med 1987;83:841–846.

90. Altés-Capellá J, Cabezudo-Artero JM, Forteza-Rei J. Complications of cocaine abuse. Ann Int Med 1987;107:940 (letter).

91. Henderson CE, Torbey M. Rupture of intracranial aneurysm associated with cocaine use during pregnancy. Am J Perinatol 1988;5:142–143.

92. Tardiff K, Gross E, Wu J, Stajic M, Millman R. Analysis of cocaine-positive fatalities. J Forensic Sci 1989;34:53–63.

93. Mittleman RE, Wetli CV. Cocaine and sudden "natural" death. J Forensic Sci 1987;32:11–19.

94. Lehman LB. Intracerebral hemorrhage after intranasal cocaine use. Hosp Physician 1987;7:69–80.

95. Mody CK, Miller BL, McIntyre HB, et al. Neurologic complications of cocaine abuse. Neurology 1988;38:1189–1193.

96. Rowley HA, Lowenstein DH, Rowbotham MC, Simon RP. Thalamomesencephalic strokes after cocaine abuse. Neurology 1989;39:428–430.

97. Levine SR, Brust JCM, Futrell N, et al. Cerebrovascular complications of the use of the "crack" form of alkaloidal cocaine. N Engl J Med 1990;323:699–704.

98. Levine SR, Brust JCM, Futrell N, et al. A comparative study of cerebrovascular complications of cocaine: alkaloidal versus hydrochloride—a review. Neurology 1991;41:1173–1177.

98a. Tapia JF, Golden JA. Case records of the Massachusetts General Hospital (Case 27-1993). N Engl J Med 1993;329:117–124.

99. Krendel DA, Ditter SM, Frankel MR, et al. Biopsy-proven cerebral vasculitis associated with cocaine abuse. Neurology 1990;40:1092–1094.

100. Jonsson S, O'Meara M, Young JB. Acute cocaine poisoning: importance of treating seizures and acidosis. Am J Med 1983;75:1061–1064.

101. Gorelick PB. The status of alcohol as a risk factor for stroke. Stroke 1989;20:1607–1610 (editorial).

102. Wolf PA. Cigarettes, alcohol and stroke. N Engl J Med 1986;315:1087–1089 (editorial).

103. Camargo CA. Moderate alcohol consumption and stroke: the epidemiologic evidence. Stroke 1989;20:1611–1626.

104. Gorelick PB. Alcohol and stroke. Stroke 1987;18:268–271.

105. Wolf PA, Kannel WB, Verter J. Current status of risk factors for stroke. Neurol Clin 1983;1:317–343.

106. Cowan DH. Effect of alcoholism on hemostasis. Semin Hematol 1980;17:137–147.

107. Gill JS, Zezulka AV, Shipley MJ, et al. Stroke and alcohol consumption. N Engl J Med 1986;315:1041–1046.

108. Stampfer MJ, Colditz GA, Willett WC, et al. A prospective study of moderate alcohol consumption and the risk of coronary disease and stroke in women. N Engl J Med 1988;319:267–273.

109. Hillbom M, Kaste M. Does alcohol intoxication precipitate aneurysmal subarachnoid haemorrhage? J Neurol Neurosurg Psychiat 1981;44:523–526.

110. Hillbom M, Kaste M. Alcohol intoxication: a risk factor for primary subarachnoid hemorrhage. Neurology 1982;32:706–711.

111. Tanaka H, Ueda Y, Hayashi M, et al. Risk factors for cerebral hemorrhage and cerebral infarction in a Japanese rural community. Stroke 1982;13:62–73.

112. Donahue RP, Abbott RD, Reed DM, et al. Alcohol and hemorrhagic stroke. JAMA 1986; 255:2311–2314.

113. Klatsky AL, Armstrong MA, Friedman GD. Alcohol use and subsequent cerebrovascular disease hospitalizations. Stroke 1989; 20:741–746.

114. Brust JCM, Richter RW. Stroke associated with addiction to heroin. J Neurol Neurosurg Psychiat 1976;39:194–199.

115. Chillar RK, Jackson AL. Reversible hemiplegia after presumed intracarotid injection of Ritalin. N Engl J Med 1981;304:1305 (letter).

# Chapter 11

# Head Trauma and Related Intracerebral Hemorrhage

## Louis R. Caplan

## Historical Review

Head injuries have fascinated medical personnel since the earliest recorded history. Injuries to the skull related to warfare were described in the Edwin Smith Papyrus written approximately 17 centuries B.C., and note was made that injuries often involved the "marrow of the head" as well as the skull.[1] Hippocrates, writing about 400 years B.C., included a chapter on head injuries.[2] Skull fractures and depressed bone elements were known to Hippocrates, who described the effects of different weapons and advised about trephination. The Hippocratic writings were especially concerned with prognostication. Observation of the wounded and the wounds was emphasized. Hippocrates made observations on the clinical effects of injuries and knew that paralysis or apoplexy could follow head injury "and, for the most part, convulsions seize the other side of the body; for if the wound be situated on the left side, the convulsions will seize the right side of the body; or if the wound be on the right side of the head, the convulsion attacks the left side of the body. And some become apoplectic."[2] Most early descriptions emphasized the skull injuries. Hemorrhage in the brain and dural compartments was given scant attention until the work of Carpi, who in 1518 described what he considered were signs of injury to the dura mater, pia, and brain.[1] Carpi's text also noted that brain damage could occur without skull fracture and that brain hemorrhage could be inferred by the clinical signs.[1] Fabry, a Swiss surgeon practicing in the sixteenth century, wrote a compilation of his own surgical cases that included patients with head and spine injuries.[1,3] Fabry described patients with intracranial hemorrhage and emphasized that unexpected death and collapse could follow a relatively minor head injury.[1,3]

The first major work dedicated solely to head injury was a monograph by the British surgeon, Sir Percival Pott, published first in 1768.[4] Pott wrote of contusions and "extravazations" outside and inside the dura mater and inside the brain. Pott wrote "violent and even fatal commotions of the brain happen when no injury has been done to the skull. . . ."[4] Pott also noted traumatic hematomas. In his Case 38: "a woman came to my house complaining that her husband had kicked her downstairs and had broke her skull. . . . I took her into the hospital where she was taken all possible care of; but she became first paralytic and then comatose, and so died. The ventricles of the brain were full of extravasated serum, and near the origin of the medulla oblongata was a large lump of firmly coagulated blood."[4] In another case, "there was no injury done to the skull; no extravasation of either blood or serum, either upon or between the membranes, nor any unnatural appearances in the cavities of the brain. But upon the plexus choroides was a lump of coagulated blood, nearly as big as half a small chestnut."[4]

O'Halloran, in another monograph on head trauma published shortly after Pott's book, pointed out the phenomenon of "compression" or mass effect related to traumatic hematomas.[5] He noted that symptoms of hemorrhagic compression were often delayed for days after the head injury. Benjamin Bell, writing in his multivolume *System of Surgery* in 1804, outlined the symptoms of compression: "giddiness; dimness of sight; stupefaction; loss of voluntary motion; vomiting; and apoplectic stertor in the breathing; convulsive tremors in different muscles; a dilated state of the pupils, even when the eyes are exposed to clear light; paralysis of different parts, especially of the side of the body opposite to the injured part of the head; involuntary evacuation of the urine and feces; an oppressed and in many cases an irregular pulse."[1] This description is clearly a prelude to Cushing's work on increased intracranial pressure. The phenomenology and presence of compression in cases of head injury became a controversial topic in the nineteenth century; important clinicians such as Abernathy and Gama did not accept the idea of compression and intracranial pressure as being important in producing the signs described by Bell.[1]

Undoubtedly, one of the most extensive and influential writings on head injury was the very long and detailed monograph by Henri Duret.[6] This work was begun in the early 1870s when Duret was working in the laboratory of Charcot in Paris, but the monograph was not published until over forty years later. The great bulk of the book was devoted to various fractures and skull injuries and their mechanism, but Duret also discussed intracerebral hemorrhage (ICH), "les foyers de contusion intra-cérébraux (héma-

tomes céntraux)," and "la compréssion cérébrale," and "l'hypertension intra-craniènne" in detail. Duret introduced the concept of chemical effects caused by the intracranial blood which he dubbed "l'intoxication hematique" which was "empoisonment et un altération des élements des centres nerveux." Duret's major contributions were the description of hemorrhages in the brainstem due to rapid increase in intracranial pressure, and descriptions of the anatomy of penetrating arteries in the brainstem and cerebral hemispheres (Figure 11.1). He also recognized that hematomas could occur on the opposite side of that injured, and described the clinical findings in patients with hematomas in the various cerebral lobes.

Bollinger is generally given credit for describing sudden-onset delayed deterioration, so called "spät apoplexy," in patients after head injury.[7] He defined the conditions necessary for the diagnosis of spät apoplexy as the absence of pre-existing vascular disease, a definite history of trauma, an asymptomatic interval, and a subsequent apoplectiform onset. Bollinger noted that at necropsy, the apoplexy could be foci of softening in the cerebrum or brainstem, or ICH. Bollinger's cases all had Duret hemorrhages in the brainstem.[7,8] The concept of spät apoplexy remains controversial today, especially its frequency and mechanisms.

The modern era of knowledge about head trauma care and traumatic intracranial hemorrhages began with the studies of Harvey Cushing. Cushing emphasized the frequency of traumatic brain hemorrhages, "almost all severe cases of concussion are probably associated with minute lesions of this sort (cortical hemorrhages) which may be so small as to escape notice, or on section of the brain, may be visible to the naked eye as punctate foci of extravasation."[9] "Cranial injuries which have led to serious contusions or lacerations of the brain may lead to a regular and widespread extravasation arising from the vascular cortical layer" (Figure 11.2). In Keen's textbook of surgery, Cushing wrote of his ideas on brain compression. He had

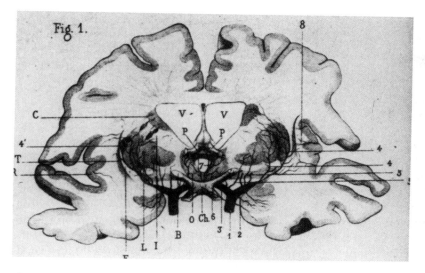

**A**

**Figure 11.1.** (A) Henry Duret's drawings of the distribution of supply of the lenticulostriate arteries. (B) Duret's drawing of the penetrating branches of the vertebral and basilar arteries. (Reprinted with permission from McHenry L, ed. Garrison's History of Neurology. Springfield, IL: Charles C Thomas, 1969, p. 385, Figure 152.)

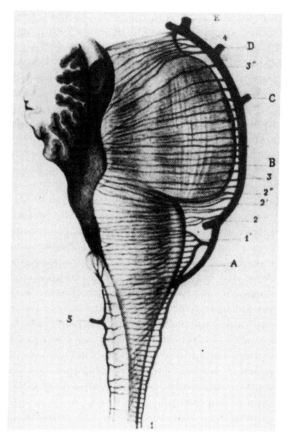

**B**

previously made experimental and clinical observations on animals and patients with head injury and other space taking lesions.[10] Cushing noted that compressive effects were of two types—local compression and a more widespread disturbance, "general increase in intracranial tension."[9] Compression injured tissue by its effect on blood vessels and brain perfusion. "Insofar as the brain is a vascular organ, it may be made smaller by having some of its blood supply squeezed out through pressure."[9] Of focal compression he wrote, "the compressive effects of such a local disturbance diminish with the distance from the primary seat of pressure, and only in case they are of high degree are they felt throughout the entire chamber." Ultimately, general increase in intracranial pressure led to venous stasis and also decreased arterial and capillary perfusion of the medulla. Medullary dysfunction led to increased arterial pressure, slowing of the pulse, and abnormalities of respiration. Cushing also wrote of the possibility of surgical drainage of traumatic and spontaneous hematomas. Cushing wrote "Is it possible that by surgical measures a capsular clot may be evacuated? Would there be a fatal continuance of bleeding after such an evacuation? Can fatal com-

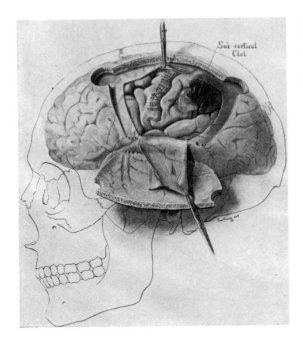

**Figure 11.2.** Harvey Cushing's sketch of an operation on a patient with a traumatic subcortical hematoma. The patient had ataxia and a right hemianesthesia. (Reprinted with permission from Cushing H. Surgery of the Head. The Classics of Neurology and Neurosurgery Library, Birmingham: Gryphon Editions Ltd., 1983, p. 211, Figure 112.)

pression be thus warded off? Is the life of a patient with a serious capsular hemorrhage worth prolonging in view of his future mental and physical incapacities?"[9]

Perhaps even more than in other causes of hematomas, the advent of computed tomography (CT) led to a dramatic change in the care of patients with traumatic brain hemorrhages. Previously, only skull x-rays and A-mode echoencephalography were available routinely for study of head injury patients. Angiography or pneumoencephalography were the only means of defining intracranial changes more definitively. However, because many traumatic contusions and lacerations were located near the basal surfaces of the frontal and temporal lobes, imaging by CT was suboptimal. Magnetic resonance imaging (MRI), introduced in the 1980s, allowed better definition and imaging of traumatic

lesions of all types. Better diagnostic capability has led to advances in our knowledge of the frequency, location, and nature of intracranial hemorrhages after various types of head injury.

## Pathology

The pathology of traumatic ICH differs considerably from other causes of brain hemorrhage. Invariably, when a head injury is severe enough to cause a traumatic hematoma, there are other brain injuries. Probably the most common lesions are *contusions*, which represent bruising of brain tissue at points of impact. Contusions are most frequently found along the orbital frontal surfaces, along the base of the brain, and on the inferior and medial surfaces of the basal part of the temporal lobes. The pia mater and very superficial cortical layers are often denuded and at times, successive crowns of adjacent gyri are involved, but the valleys of the same gyri are spared. Contusions probably represent direct injury due to contact impact and then a bouncing back or reflection of the intracranial contents forces the basal brain surfaces against the rough, irregular, craggy surfaces of the anterior fossa and the knife-like edge of the lesser wing of the sphenoid bone. The rough, bony surfaces bruise or lacerate the brain in motion.[11] Contusions often contain petechial hemorrhage or foci of frank larger hematomas. *Lacerations* of vessels and brain tissue, and small and large regions of *edema* are also often found in traumatized brains at necropsy. Some specimens also contain *infarcts* presumably caused by associated injury to feeding arteries. Since injury to the head is often accompanied by other body injuries, including chest wounds and neck injuries, hypoxic-ischemic changes in the brain result from cardiovascular complications of the trauma.

Bleeding sites are often not limited to brain parenchyma. Often accompanying the brain hematomas are bleeding sites related to other brain compartments. Scalp hematomas may overlie the point of impact. Skull fractures and injury to the meningeal arteries cause *epidural collections* of blood. *Subdural blood collections* can develop acutely if large veins are injured or may develop more insidiously. Some degree of *subarachnoid bleeding* occurs in nearly every patient with serious head injury. Many patients have both extracerebral and intracerebral bleeding. In several large series of patients with head injuries compiled by Teasdale, Jennett, and Galbraith,[12,13] subdural and intracerebral hematomas often occurred in the same patients (Table 11.1). The only other mechanisms of ICH that frequently cause subdural, subarachnoid, and intracerebral bleeding are coagulopathies and bleeding diatheses which can lead to hemorrhages at multiple sites. Skull fractures and epidural hemorrhages are diagnostic of traumatic injury.

Intracerebral hematomas can be single, but more often are multiple and scattered. Figure 11.3 shows a brain specimen from a patient dying after a motor vehicle accident with multiple hematomas. Multiple sites of hemorrhage within the brain suggest the presence of trauma or a bleeding tendency. By far, the temporal lobe is the most common site for traumatic hematomas. Among a group of 208 cases of traumatic hematomas reviewed by De Vet, 169 (81%) involved the temporal lobes. In thirty-one (15%) the frontal lobes were involved, and only eight (4%) involved the parietal or occipital lobes.[14] In De Vet's own series of eighty-seven patients with traumatic ICH, sixty (70%) were entirely confined to the temporal lobe, another eleven involved the temporal lobe but extended also into the frontal or inferior parietal regions, eleven were confined to the frontal lobes, and five involved the parietal lobes.[14] The hematomas are often located near the basal surfaces within the orbital frontal lobes, or the inferomedial temporal lobes. Another favorite location is in the paramedian frontal lobe above the cingulum, or within the corpus callosum. Basal ganglionic, intraventricular, brainstem and cerebellar hematomas also occur and will be considered in more detail in the clinical section.

The impact of the injury can also traumatize the extracranial carotid and vertebral

**Table 11.1.** Incidence of Different Types of Traumatic Hematoma

| Source of Data | Total Cases | Extradural Only (%) | Extradural and Intradural (%) | Subdural Only (%) | Subdural and Intracerebral (%) | Intracerebral (Discrete) (%) |
|---|---|---|---|---|---|---|
| London McKissock et al. | 298 | 42 | | | 58 | |
| Cincinnati McLaurin et al. | 137 | 11 | 9 | 3 | 10 | |
| Brisbane Jamieson and Yelland | 763 | 13 | 11 | 34 | 36 | 6 |
| Richmond Becker et al. | 62 | 19 | | 42 | 39 | |
| International Collaborative Study Glasgow, Rotterdam, Groningen, Los Angeles | 487 | 16 | 7 | 22 | 34 | 20 |
| Glasgow Teasdale and Galbraith | 180 | 24 | 9 | 31 | 23 | 13 |
| Giessen Pia et al. | 980 | 20 | | 70 | | 10 |

(From: Jenett B. Teasdale, G. Management of Head Injuries. F. A. Davis, Philadelphia, 1981. p. 158, with permission.)

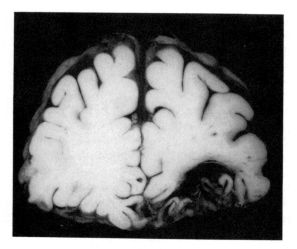

A

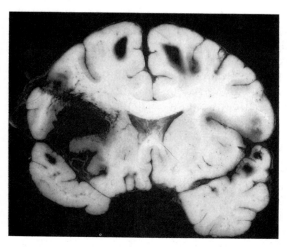

B

**Figure 11.3.** (A) Acute hematomas in patient in a fatal automobile accident. Lesion involves orbital surface of frontal lobe. The pia and surface cortex are injured. (B) More posterior coronal section from same patient showing multiple intracerebral hematomas. Symmetric small hematomas involve the temporal lobes and the medial frontal lobes.

arteries leading to occlusions, pseudoaneurysms, and traumatic dissections, all of which can lead to brain infarction. Injury to pial and intraparenchymatous small blood vessels are almost invariably found in necropsy studies of patients dying after head injury.

Evans and Scheinker have studied the vessels extensively in specimens from head injured patients.[15,16] Smaller veins and capillaries often show extreme distention and engorgement and luminal contents show evidence of hemolysis and homogenization of red blood cells indicating stasis of blood flow.[16] The vessel walls have increased permeability as evidenced by distention of the perivascular spaces with extravasated serum and erythrocytes. The small blood vessels, especially veins, also show degenerative changes if the patient has survived for some time after the injury. Tissue elements of the walls of these veins are more difficult to define and the vessel wall becomes looser in texture.[16] Necrosis of vessel walls with invasion of leukocytes is occasionally found. Study of patients that have survived serious head trauma for years reveals chronic vascular changes. Vessel walls often show homogenization, loss of stainability, and thinning. Elastic tissue may be fragmented, muscular elements are replaced by connective tissue, and the adventitia is thickened. The perivascular spaces are widened and may contain fibroblasts and macrophages. Edema and ischemic changes may surround the thrombosed vessels acutely and in the chronic state, loss of tissue and gliosis predominate. Scheinker and Evans have attributed the acute vascular changes to "vasoparalysis," mechanical irritation causing episodic vasoconstriction followed by paralytic dilatation of distal vessel segments while proximal segments remain contracted.[15,16] Certainly, acute vascular tearing and injury causes hematoma formation and petechial hemorrhages.

## Clinical Findings

In most patients with traumatic brain hematomas, ICH is only one part of a complex of medical problems related to the injury. Hypoventilation results from increased intracranial pressure and stupor and/or from cardiopulmonary injury, or reduced chest motion due to paralysis caused by head or neck injuries or to injuries to the chest wall. Loss of blood and body fluids from abdominal, limb, and chest injuries can lead to shock, hypotension, and reduced cerebral perfusion. Traumatic occlusion or dissection of extracranial vessels can lead to brain infarction. Injury to the skull, epidural and subdural hemorrhages, and brain edema, contusions, and lacerations add to the patient's clinical deficits. The multiplicity of brain and extracerebral hemorrhages also complicates the clinical picture. Headache, vomiting, stiff neck, reduction of consciousness and seizures, are common general findings in patients with head injuries whether or not they also harbor brain hematomas.

At times, it is not clear on presentation that the brain lesions are traumatic. The impact of the injury produced concussion or more serious injury, impairing the laying down of memories. Retrograde amnesia, clouding of consciousness, and cognitive deficits often limit the patient's ability to tell the medical staff what happened. Superficial injuries may not be present or evident. There may be no observers. We have even encountered observers or friends who have deliberately given wrong information so as not to incriminate themselves. A young woman was admitted to the Boston City Hospital in the pre-CT era with aphasia and a right hemiplegia. The man with whom she lived said that she had suddenly developed the signs while they were eating breakfast together. Spinal fluid was bloody and angiography showed a well circumscribed avascular mass (hematoma) but no aneurysm or malformation. The staff noted that each time the man visited, she became very agitated. Skull x-rays showed a small crack in the region adjacent to the hematoma. After recovery, the woman was able to tell us that the man had hit her in the head with a gavel. In another circumstance, a nurse at a nursing home reported that she had found one of her elderly charges unresponsive and hemiplegic on her morning rounds. When necropsy showed skull fractures, an epidural hematoma, and multiple brain hematomas, she confessed

that the patient had been left unattended and fell downstairs. She found him unconscious and fearing that her supervisor would blame the injury on her neglect, she and her paramour put the patient back into bed and "found him there" the next morning. In other patients who are brought into emergency facilities with an injury and focal neurological deficits, it is difficult to tell if a stroke had preceded and, in fact, caused the accident, or if the neurological deficit resulted from injury during the accident. This chicken-egg issue is usually not able to be settled by history unless observers are present. Now, modern imaging technology often clarifies these instances of inapparent or hidden trauma. Small skull fractures, small epidural or subdural collections, and the subpial location and shape of the hemorrhages often lead to recognition that they have been caused by trauma.

On CT or MRI, several imaging characteristics help identify a traumatic etiology. We have already noted the importance of looking for skull fractures on scans taken with "bone windows." Small collections of blood in the dural spaces and subarachnoid hemorrhage are also helpful. Traumatic hematomas are often multiple, predominantly temporal and frontal, emphasize the orbital and basal surfaces, are often adjacent to the cortical surface, often have mixed densities due to edema and ischemic necrosis within contusion, are located in a path that might suggest coup and contre-coup injuries, and are often irregular in shape as compared with the round shape of acute hypertensive ICH. MRI is clearly superior to CT in detecting hematomas along the basal surfaces since these lesions are often obscured on CT by the bony margins.

Hematomas may take time to attain full size and may even develop after the injury (spät apoplexy). Brain edema is often seen contiguous to the hematoma or surrounding it and is probably more prevalent than in other causes of brain hemorrhage since some of the edema results from the injury and is a reaction to the hematomas. Schneider studied the development and evolution of traumatic ICH using serial CT scans.[17] Hematoma size and edema were both monitored. Hematoma formation usually attained its maximal size by the fourth post-trauma day. Edema formation was bimodal with some patients having little early edema and others had a large border of edema when first studied.[17] From the eighth day after trauma on, the two edema groups merged so that the hematoma/edema ratio was equal at 0.3. Patients with large hematomas (greater than 37 cm) often had stupor, anisocoria, and a bad outcome.[17] Single-photon-emission computed tomography (SPECT) scans often show perfusion defects larger than the traumatic hematomas; at times, there is poor retention of isotope in the entire hemisphere ipsilateral to the hematoma.[18] These findings indicate more widespread damage and a poor prognosis for recovery.[18]

In the past, traumatic intracranial hematomas have been characterized as acute, subacute, or chronic.[13] This classification referred to epidural and subdural as well as intracerebral hematomas. In the pre-CT period, it was often hard to distinguish among these loci, and more than one compartment was often involved. Mostly, these time frames relate to subdural collections. Parenchymatous hematomas fit better into two categories— acute, that is, present on admission, and delayed, or spät hematomas, which seem to develop later. We will first discuss general aspects of acute hematomas and then discuss the late lesions separately.

Head injury can lead to defibrinization, intravascular coagulation, and a coagulopathy. Defibrinization is common after brain tissue injury and occurs early.[19–22] Goodnight and colleagues studied twenty-six patients admitted to a neurosurgical intensive care unit within twelve hours of injury.[19] Defibrinization was not found in thirteen patients who had lost consciousness but had no evidence of brain tissue destruction. In the other thirteen who had brain damage, defibrinization was shown by hypofibrinogenemia, elevated fibrinogen and fibrin-related

antigens, reduced levels of factors V and VIII, and reduced platelet counts. Positive protamine tests, thrombocytopenia, reduced coagulation factors and, at times, prolonged prothrombin times were evidence that intravascular coagulation did occur.[19] Active defibrinization did not persist but could have contributed to the extent of early bleeding. There are several likely mechanisms of the coagulopathy found after head injury. The brain is very rich in thromboplastin and release of this substance into the circulation activates the extrinsic coagulation pathway.[20] Endothelial and vessel wall injury could also activate the intrinsic pathway of coagulation. Fibrinolytic activity is increased because of the clotting. Consumption of platelets and proteins active in coagulation lead to disseminated intravascular coagulation (DIC).[20] It is not known how often, and to what degree, these coagulation changes contribute to new hematoma formation or increase in size of existent hematomas. Perivascular clotting probably causes the stasis seen histologically by Evans and Scheinker and attributed to vasoparalysis by these authors.[15,16]

Some have analyzed whether studies of coagulation or catecholamine levels are good predictors of outcome after severe head injury.[22,23] Crone and colleagues measured fibrin degradation products in thirty-three patients with severe closed head injuries.[22] Patients with higher concentrations of fibrin degradation products had poorer functional outcomes. Among the twenty-two patients with levels of fibrin degradation products less than 64 mcg/ml, only one developed early respiratory failure while nine of eleven with concentrations above this level had the "adult respiratory distress syndrome." High levels predicted poor functional outcome and respiratory failure, and systemic injury did not affect the results.[22] In another study, Hamill et al. measured catecholamines after traumatic brain injury.[23] The levels of norepinephrine and dopamine at forty-eight hours and one week correlated very well with the severity of injury and outcome. Norepinephrine and epinephrine levels increased four to five times above normal in those with the most severe brain injuries.[23] Both signs of fibrin degradation and catecholamine outpouring correlated well with the degree of brain damage.

Acute seizures and post-traumatic epilepsy are common sequelae of head injury. In one series of 219 civilian patients with head injury, investigators correlated the findings on CT scans taken within three days of admission.[24] Among the thirteen patients who developed post-traumatic epilepsy, twelve had intracerebral hematomas, in seven also accompanied by extracerebral hematomas. Edema often surrounded the intracerebral lesions. The presence of an intracerebral hematoma was the only factor that correlated significantly with the later development of seizures.[24]

## Hemispheral Hematomas

The most common location for traumatic hematomas is the cerebral lobes. As has been noted, the most common loci are the temporal lobes, followed by the frontal lobes. Parietal and occipital lesions are far less frequent. Since traumatic hematomas are often accompanied by contusions, edema, extracerebral blood collections, and other hematomas, it is often difficult to know what clinical phenomena relate to which lesions.

### Frontal

Signs depend on the size of the hematomas and the location within the frontal lobe. Hematomas tend to involve the orbital, basal surface and also to occur just above the corpus callosum near the cingulate gyri. Some affect the frontal pole region. In our experience, orbital frontal hematomas often cause a disinhibited, aggressive state in which patients are argumentative, uncooperative, and sometimes physically and sexually aggres-

sive. Difficulty in concentration and poor confrontation memory are also common features. During the acute stage, patients may be disoriented, claiming that they are home, back in the war, shopping, or any other place or activity that they are dreaming about at the time. Unlike the patients with Wernicke-Korsakoff syndrome or other amnestic states, patients with frontal lobe damage do not look around to figure out where they might be; they simply report what is in their minds. Answers vary from day to day and from minute to minute. Patients with large frontal hematomas are often abulic. They show diminished spontaneity, decreased amount of speech and motor activity, prolonged latency in responding to directions or queries, and a lack of ability to persevere with tasks. Traumatic hematomas are usually anterior or inferior to the motor cortex and pyramidal projections so more often than not there is no weakness or motor signs.

### Temporal

The temporal lobe is by far the most common site for traumatic hematomas. Large hematomas cause shifting of intracranial contents and herniation of medial temporal lobe structures against the midbrain. Third nerve palsies and coma with decerebration can result and prove fatal. The so-called "pulped temporal lobe syndrome," in which the anterior temporal lobe is badly contused, swollen, and hemorrhagic, is one situation in which the temporal lobe swells dramatically, pushing out of the confines of the middle cranial fossa. Anterior temporal lobectomy is often performed as a life-saving measure in this situation. Smaller lesions often affect limbic structures and memory. Involvement of limbic structures within the temporal lobes often causes a change in behavior and personality. Aggressiveness or unaccustomed hostility may result. Some patients become quite irascible and argumentative and curse and become abusive physically and verbally. Changes in food and sexual appetites are common. Often, memory is also affected, even in unilateral lesions, so that patients are unable to make new memories and often have a retrograde amnesia for events prior to the injury. In unilateral temporal lobe injuries, the amnesia is usually reversed after a period of six months or longer. Abnormalities of taste and smell are also very common after injuries to either the temporal lobe structures subserving these functions, or after orbital frontal lesions that affect the olfactory pathways leading to the temporal lobes. Lesions of the dominant, usually left temporal lobe, often produce an anomic aphasia. A Wernicke aphasia–like syndrome is less common but occurs in large hematomas or those that involve the posterior, superior and lateral aspects of the temporal lobe. Seizures are probably more common after temporal lobe and frontal lobe traumatic hematomas than injuries at other sites. Figure 11.4 shows a cavity resulting from an old temporal lobe traumatic hematoma.

## Parietal

Parietal lobe hematomas occur in regions just under blunt skull injuries or represent contre-coup injuries. The findings are predominantly sensory-motor, cognitive, and behavioral, and do not differ from those of parietal hematomas of other causes.

## Occipital

Occipital lobe hematomas are rare. They cause predominantly visual field abnormalities, occasionally accompanied by somatosensory abnormalities when the hematoma spreads into the parietal lobe.

## Basal Ganglionic, Deep Hemispheral Hematomas

Deep hematomas result from shearing and tearing of lenticulostriate and anterior chor-oidal arterial penetrating branches. These lesions are most often found after motor vehicle injuries. In a large series of 2000 patients admitted to the Glasgow Neurosurgical Center with head injuries, sixty-one (3%) had basal ganglionic hematomas, 83% due to traffic accidents.[25] In a series from a Boston area rehabilitation hospital, again 3% of severe head injury patients had basal ganglionic traumatic hematomas.[26] Basal ganglionic location of hematomas may be more common in the pediatric age group and adolescents.[27] In the Glasgow series, forty-one (68%) were isolated while in twenty patients other hematomas (eleven lobar, five subdural, four extradural) were also present.[25] In twenty-eight of the sixty-one patients (46%) a skull fracture was detected radiographically.

The size of the hematoma is of course, variable, but more often than not the hematomas are large and are often associated with considerable mass effect.[25] The clinical abnormalities are generally motor, cognitive, and behavioral and do not differ greatly from other causes of putaminal hemorrhage. Nearly all patients have a hemiparesis when initially seen. When the lesions involve the posterior limb of the internal capsule, a persistent hemiparesis results.[26] Patients with more anterior lesions or hematomas that spare the capsule have better recovery of weakness. Speech abnormalities are very common after dominant hemisphere basal ganglionic hematomas. Muteness was present initially in two of the three patients with left hematomas in the Boston area series.[26] Reduced verbal fluency and naming difficulties were common sequelae. Typical nondominant hemisphere syndromes with left neglect, visuospatial abnormalities, flat affect, dysprosody, and lack of awareness of the deficit were common after right-sided deep hematomas.[26]

In the large Glasgow series, the prognosis in patients with traumatic basal ganglionic hematomas was very poor: 68% of the isolated and 60% of the multiple lesion group were either dead, vegetative, or severely disabled six months after the injury.[25]

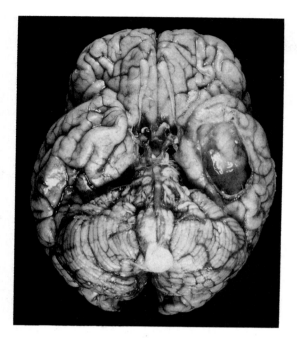

**Figure 11.4.** (A) View from basal surface showing large left temporal lobe cavity at site of a healed traumatic hematoma. Note that pia and superficial cortex are gone. (B) Coronal section of same patient showing location of the cavity which is limited to the basal surface but communicates with the temporal horn of the lateral ventricle.

A

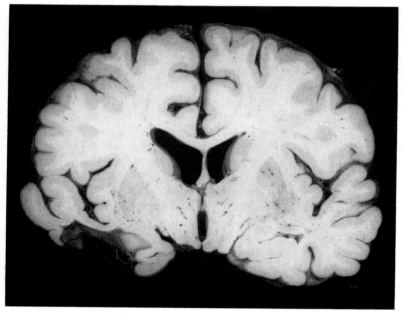

B

The worst outcome occurred in the group with large hematomas and raised intracranial pressure. Among the six patients in the Boston series, the prognosis was better, but the series included only patients that referring physicians believed would profit from rehabilitation.[26]

## Intraventricular Hemorrhage

Intraventricular hemorrhage is a common finding among patients with severe head injuries who have CT scans.[28–33] The finding may, like basal ganglionic hemorrhage, be more common in children and adolescents.[30] Among one very large series of 7075 severely head-injured patients studied in Japan, twenty-six had significant intraventricular bleeding found on CT.[33] In fifteen patients among these twenty-six (58%) there were hemispheral hemorrhagic lesions that presumably dissected into the ventricular system. Contusions in the frontal or temporal lobes (six patients), caudate region hemorrhages (five patients), and thalamic hematomas (four patients) were the primary location of injury. Drainage into the ventricular system was sometimes delayed. In six patients, the trauma had caused concomitant brainstem injuries and the outcome was very poor in this group. Only a small number, five patients, had primary intraventricular bleeding. The amount of ventricular blood was often small, and other injuries, such as subdural effusions, were also present.[33] Intraventricular bleeding probably most often results from spread of contiguous hemorrhagic contusions or hematomas especially in relation to the basal brain surfaces and the caudate nucleus and thalamus. In some patients, vessels of the choroid plexus are torn.

## Brainstem Hematomas

Brainstem injury had been considered an uncommon event in head trauma except in very severe fatal injuries. LeCount and Apfelbach, in 1920, described brainstem hematomas found at necropsy and emphasized their frequency in patients with skull fractures involving the posterior fossa and skull base.[34] Courville, however, deserves great credit for emphasizing the frequency of contusions and hematomas in the upper pons and midbrain in patients with head injuries, and in explaining the mechanism of their development.[35] The advent of CT and later MRI has now made detection of brainstem hemorrhage easier and has proven that brainstem lesions are relatively common in head injury.

Courville, in 1945, described four basic mechanisms of brainstem injury and hemorrhage.[35] (1) General effects of the injury. By this term was meant petechial hemorrhages secondary to diffuse cerebral edema and hypoxia or related to air or fat embolism to small arteries. (2) Direct focal injury to the brainstem. These often were found in association with basal skull fractures. Contusions, hematomas, or frank lacerations of the brainstem could result. (3) Contre-coup injury. Almost invariably, this type of injury occurred in trauma in which the occiput hit an immobile object, such as the ground. Usually subfrontal and temporal contusions were also present (see Figure 11.4). The configuration of the hematomas was usually linear, extending from the aqueduct towards the base involving the midbrain tegmentum (Figure 11.5). In the pons, the bleeding was more widespread and involved the tegmentum and the basis pontis (Figure 11.6). (4) Duret-type hemorrhages secondary to brainstem distortion. Distortion could arise because of a rapid downward pressure cone related to supratentorial bleeding, from lateral compression due to temporal lobe herniation, or from local distortion of the brainstem due to an adjacent collection of subdural or subarachnoid blood.

Courville's patients were mostly comatose and the clinical descriptions were sparse.[35] Kremer et al. a few years later amplified on the clinical neurological signs in nine patients who probably had direct brainstem injury.[36] Dysarthria, ataxia, dizziness, ptosis, oculomotor dysfunction, and abnormal

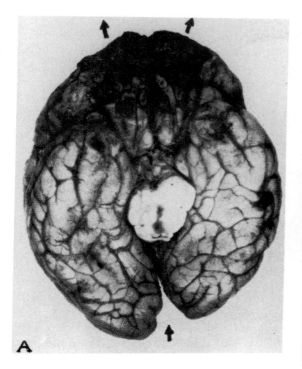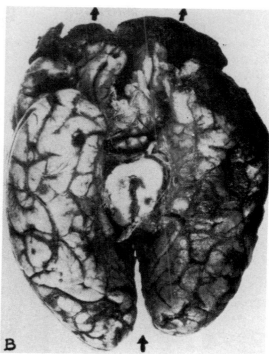

**Figure 11.5.** (A and B) Contre-coup injuries of the midbrain. A and B each show patients injured after falling on back of head (arrows indicate lines of force). Each had extreme frontal contusions and linear midbrain hemorrhages. (From Courville, Effects of Closed Cranial injuries on the Midbrain and Upper Pons, in Trauma of the Central Nervous System, Res. Publ. Assoc. Res. Nerv Ment Dis., Vol XXIV, Baltimore: Williams & Wilkins, 1945, p. 137, figures 86A and B. With permission.)

pupils were common findings. Clearly, survival could occur despite relatively severe rostral brainstem damage, mostly limited to the tegmental region.

Anthony Jefferson, in 1961, pointed out that brainstem lesions and hematomas could occur even in seemingly minor head injuries.[37] He described four patients, all of whom had head injury without loss of consciousness. Three had sports injury, two during soccer and one during rugby, and the fourth case was a miner who was hit on the helmet by a large piece of stone. Each noted dizziness and diplopia, sometimes delayed until hours after the injury. The findings included dilated or small poorly reactive pupils, ptosis, vertical gaze palsies, ocular

skewing, and nystagmus. Motor abnormalities were usually absent or minor, but some patients had extensor plantar responses. The clinical findings suggested tegmental injuries to the rostral midbrain.[37] Jefferson believed this area was injured directly by displacement of the brainstem against the tentorium or by injury to the blood vessels in this area with secondary brainstem ischemia. No imaging or pathology was available. In some patients, the oculomotor signs disappeared and in others they remained.

Ropper and Miller in the CT era, described five patients with presumed direct single acute traumatic midbrain hemorrhages.[38] Four of the patients had hematomas on CT usually in the tegmentum at or near the

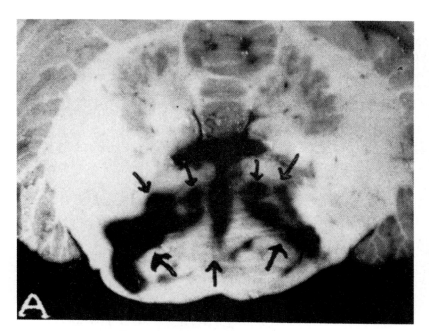

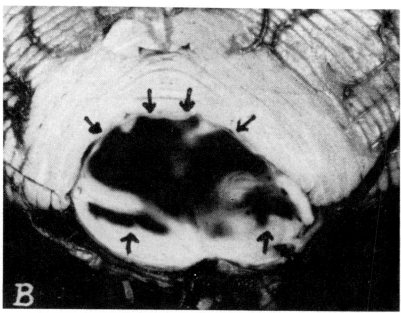

**Figure 11.6.** A and B. Examples of traumatic coup, contre-coup injuries to the pons. Hemorrhages are relatively symmetric and mostly tegmental. Arrows point to symmetric lesions. (From Courville, Effects of Closed Cranial injuries on the Midbrain and Upper Pons, in Trauma of the Central Nervous System, Res. Publ. Assoc. Res. Nerv Ment Dis., Vol XXIV, Baltimore: Williams & Wilkins, 1945, p. 137, Figures 87A & B. With permission.)

midbrain-diencephalic junction, and in two the findings were confirmed at necropsy. The clinical findings were rather stereotyped and included deep coma, large round pupils not reactive to light, reduced tone in all limbs especially the arms, absent horizontal eye movements on oculocephalic stimulation and lack of ocular adduction on caloric stimulation, decerebrate posturing after stimulation but little spontaneous movement, asymmetrical diminished corneal responses, extensor plantar reflexes, and shallow respirations.[38] The outlook was poor; four died and the other patient had persistent dysphonia, third nerve palsies, and poor memory.

The vast majority of the brainstem hematomas and contusions discussed so far were bilateral and mostly tegmental. Lesions however, can be unilateral and either basal or tegmental. Herskowitz et al. described a patient who developed a unilateral injury to the cerebral peduncle area after a minor injury without loss of consciousness.[39] The patient was a 25-year-old man who was struck from behind while playing rugby. Almost immediately, he noted ataxia of the left arm and leg, and examination showed a left ataxic hemiparesis with a left Babinski sign. MRI showed a hematoma near the red nucleus in the cerebral peduncle on the right (Figure 11.7). One of us (LRC) recently cared for a patient with a unilateral midbrain tegmental hematoma after head injury. The patient fell on the back of his head and then noted headache, diplopia, dizziness, and ataxia. Findings included ocular skewing, nystagmus, bilateral

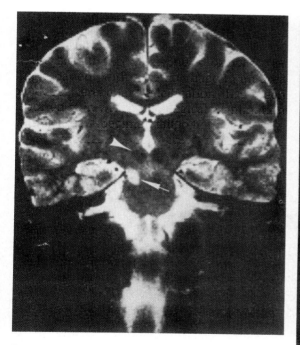

A

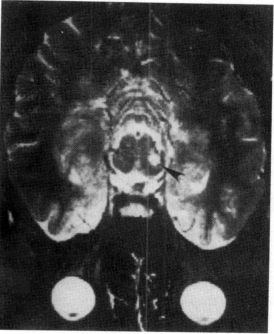

B

**Figure 11.7.** Patient with midbrain hemorrhage from minor head trauma during rugby. (A) T2 weighted axial section. Hemorrhage (arrow) inferior to red nucleus (arrowhead). (B) T2 weighted coronal section showing lesion (arrow) near the peduncle. (From Hershkowitz N, Bergey CK, Joslyn J, Evans D. Isolated midbrain lesion resulting from closed head injury: a unique presentation of ataxic hemiparesis. Neurology 1989;39:452–453. With permission.)

limb ataxia, and a hemisensory loss. MRI showed a unilateral midbrain tegmental hemorrhage (Figure 11.8A and B). Frontal and temporal contusions were also present (Figure 11.8C). The midbrain hemorrhage was probably due to contre-coup injury to the midbrain and shows that the lesions can be quite asymmetrical.

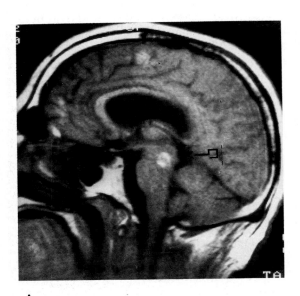

A

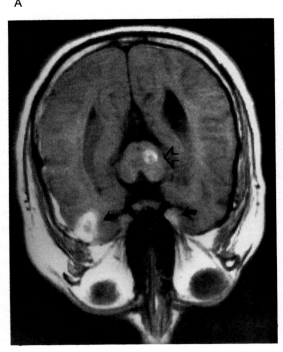

B

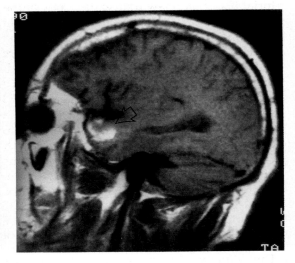

C

Figure 11.8. MRI from patient who fell on back of head. (A) Sagittal section. T2-weighted large midbrain hematoma (arrow). Small parasagittal medial frontal lesion also seen above the corpus callosum. (B) Transverse axial—T2 weighted. Midbrain tegmental lesion seen (open arrow), closed black arrows point to bitemporal contusions. (C) Sagittal section showing large temporal contusion and hematoma (arrow).

Duret hemorrhages in the upper brainstem probably result from distortion of the upper brainstem with traction on the paramedian vessels. They are especially apt to develop if the supratentorial or extracerebral clot or pressure-producing lesions are large and when the lesions have developed quickly, overwhelming the adaptive capacity of the system. In 1977, Caplan and Zervas reported two patients with signs of midbrain dysfunction that they attributed to Duret hemorrhages.[40] Each patient had a large subdural hematoma that was rapidly drained surgically. Postoperative findings included bilateral third nerve dysfunction (asymmetrical in one patient) and decerebrate rigidity on one side. Pneumoencephalography showed no supratentorial lesion. The midbrain lesion was secondary to a rapidly developing pressure cone related to the subdural hemorrhage. Removal of the subdural collections allowed survival with severe midbrain dysfunction but preserved intellect and hemispheral functions.[40]

Duret hemorrhages can develop later in the course of traumatic or spontaneous supratentorial hematomas or injuries. Herbstein and Schaumburg effectively proved the development of delayed brainstem hematomas by injecting erythrocytes tagged with chromium-51 in patients one to five hours after presentation of hypertensive supratentorial ICH.[41] No new uptake occurred supratentorially, but uptake did appear within Duret hemorrhages that developed after the injection of tagged red blood cells. Figure 11.9 shows a Duret hemorrhage in the midbrain and pons in the patient whose lesions are illustrated in Figure 11.3. Figure 11.10 shows a Duret hemorrhage secondary to a subdural hematoma and illustrates the relation of the brainstem to the hemispheres. Chapter 14 also includes several illustrations of Duret hemorrhages in patients with large, rapidly evolving putaminal hemorrhages.

## Cerebellar Hematomas

The literature on traumatic intracerebral hemorrhages is very sparse since these le-

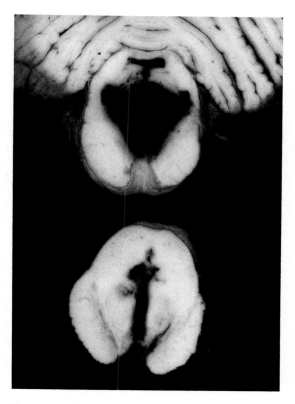

**Figure 11.9.** Duret hemorrhages in patient with fatal supratentorial hematoma. Midbrain lesions on bottom are linear and below aqueduct. Pontine lesion is broader in the tegmentum.

sions are uncommon and rarely recognized ante mortem. Ataxia is probably most commonly due to brainstem injury rather than a cerebellar lesion.[42] Acute cerebellar injuries most often occur after gunshot wounds.[43,44] In other patients with closed head injury, headache, stiff neck, drowsiness, and ataxia are noted before the rapid onset of coma. Coma and usually death are due to brainstem compression by the enlarging cerebellar hematoma.[44] This chain of events is less likely to occur now since intracerebellar hematomas should be readily detected by CT or MRI. Cystic cerebellar lesions can develop gradually after head injury and can present as an expanding posterior fossa mass.[44] The clinical signs are identical to those described in Chapter 20 on cerebellar hemorrhage.

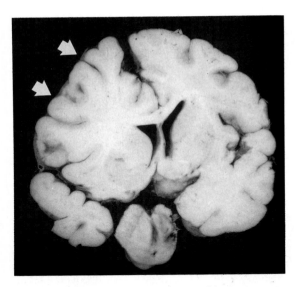

**Figure 11.10.** Patient died of subdural hematoma which was located over the left cerebral hemisphere (arrow). Midbrain is distorted with a Kernohan's notch in the right cerebral peduncle and a midline midbrain Duret hemorrhage.

## Delayed Development of Hematomas ("Spät" Apoplexy)

Bollinger had in the late nineteenth century called attention to "traumatische spät apoplexie," in which even a slight head injury could be followed by softenings in the cerebrum or medulla, blood vessel injury, and intracranial bleeding.[7] Necropsy examination of the four patients described by Bollinger revealed brainstem lesions in the form of Duret-type hemorrhages in all.[7,8] The deterioration in his cases was likely due to mass effect with herniation. In the pre-CT era, it was often difficult to determine the mechanism of delayed worsening in traumatized patients. Enlargement of extracerebral and intracerebral hematomas and brain edema were probably common. Infarction might occur secondary to direct injury to extracranial or intracranial arteries with dissection of the arterial wall or thrombosis. Ischemia is often delayed after vascular dissection. Mass effects with displacement of arteries can also cause infarction.[45,46] Displacement of the an-

teromedial frontal lobe under the falx impinges on the anterior cerebral artery and leads to a contralateral parasagittal infarct. Pressure on the posterior cerebral artery at the tentorial notch causes occipital and temporal lobe infarction. Occasionally, even compression of the middle cerebral artery in the Sylvian fissure can lead to a lateral convexity infarct.[47] Delayed hemorrhage can also occur, and will be the focus of interest here.

DeJong, in 1942, reviewed prior concepts and reports of delayed hematoma formation and described two patients studied clinically and at post mortem.[8] The first patient was a 27-year-old who was struck with a board behind the right ear. Headache occurred for one hour, then abated. But twenty-four hours later, headache recurred, he became weak, and after six days, right hemiplegia, aphasia, and papilledema were found. Necropsy showed subdural and subarachnoid hemorrhages and massive softening and edema of the left frontal lobe with herniation. In the second patient, there was a four-day delay in onset of a left hemiplegia after a fall downstairs. A massive right temporoparietal hematoma was found with surrounding ischemic changes and softening. DeJong interpreted the findings as due to "vascular spasm" caused by the trauma, causing first infarction and in case two, hemorrhage, into the area of softening. It is possible, however, that the softening around the hemorrhage was due to the pressure effects of the hematoma itself. Prior authors had attributed delayed hematomas to prior vascular disease or vascular injury. Before the CT era, it was impossible to know if the hematomas appeared de novo, represented enlargement of hematomas already present initially after the injury, or were the result of bleeding into areas of contusion or edema.

Recent studies utilizing modern neuroimaging technology convincingly show that spät hematomas are common and that they represent bleeding into areas of contused or edematous injured brain tissue. Fukamachi et al. reported a large series including eighty-four traumatic intracerebral hematomas all of whom had CT scans within six hours of injury, thirty-nine within one hour.[48] On sequential scanning, twenty hematomas had developed in an area in which no lesion was visible on the initial scan. In twenty-two other patients, new hematomas appeared in a region in which the initial CT scan had shown a flecked pattern of high-density small foci. Thus forty-two of the eighty traumatic hematomas (50%) developed after a delay and would qualify as delayed traumatic ICH.[48] Nearly three-fourths of the delayed hematomas were visible by forty-eight hours postinjury. Extracerebral and especially epidural hematomas were common in patients with delayed hematomas, and in eleven patients new ICH lesions appeared only after surgical drainage of the epidural hematomas.

In another study, CT scans were obtained within two hours of head injury followed immediately by T2-weighted MR images.[49] Two findings in relation to the clinical features and results of the initial CT predicted the development of new delayed hematomas on later CT scans. When the initial CT showed an intracranial but extracerebral hemorrhage and when the focal clinical signs were more severe than explained by the initial CT, delayed development of hematoma was predicted. Among the six patients with either of these two findings, four had MR images that showed areas of increased signal intensity interpreted as focal regions of edema. The lesions were all ipsilateral and near or contre-coup to the area of impact. All four of these patients developed hematomas in the area of abnormal MR signal on CT scans, eighty, twenty, fourteen, and twenty-five hours after injury. In the two patients with no parenchymal lesion on MRI, no hematoma developed.[49]

From these and other studies, a chain of events leading to delayed hematoma formation can be outlined. The initial head injury causes a focal contusive injury. This injury consists of brain softening and edema and injury to small arteries. The vessel injury and release of substances that activate clotting lead to thrombosis and retraction of the blood

vessels in the area of injury. Local edema or general increase in pressure (as might result from an extracerebral hematoma), or both, help to compress and tamponade the injured vessels, acting to prevent bleeding. With time, fibrinolytic activity increases[19,21] and vasospasm diminishes. Improvement in local edema, removal of a compressive hematoma, or the use of systemic diuretics reduces the local compressive pressure. Under these circumstances, the injured arteries, no longer thrombosed, bleed freely into the area of contusion. This idea takes into consideration the known facts revealed by neuroimaging studies of patients with "spät apoplexy." No doubt this phenomenon is very common but not sufficiently appreciated. Most often, the spät hematomas remain small, but can be very large. In other cases of delayed worsening, hematomas initially present enlarge on subsequent scans, a finding in nine of the patients described by Fukamachi et al.[49]

## References

1. Mettler FA, Mettler CC. Historic development of knowledge relating to cranial trauma. In: Trauma of the Central Nervous System. Res. Publ. Assoc. Res. Nerv. Ment. Dis. Vol. 24. Baltimore: Williams & Wilkins, 1945;1–47.
2. Adams F. The Genuine Works of Hippocrates. Baltimore: Williams & Wilkins, 1939;142–156.
3. Fabry W. Observationum et curationum chirurgicarum. Basel, 1606.
4. Pott P. Observations on the nature and consequences of those injuries to which the head is liable from external violence. London: Hawes, Clarke, Collins, 1768. Reprinted by Classics of Neurology and Neurosurgery Library. Birmingham: Gryphon Editions, 1989.
5. O'Halloran S. A new treatise on the different disorders arising from external injuries of the head. Illustrated by eight-five (selected from above fifteen hundred) practical cases. London, 1793.
6. Duret H. Traumatismes Cranio-Cérébraux. Paris: Librarie Felix Alcan, 1919.
7. Bollinger O. Ueber Traumatische Spät-Apoplexie: Ein Beitrag zur Lehre von der Hirnschütterung. In: Internationale Beiträge

zur wissenschütterung Medicin, Festschrift, Rudolf Virchow Gewidmet zur Vollendung seines 70. Vol. 2. Lebensjahres. Berlin: A. Hirschwald, 1891;457–470.

8. DeJong RN. Delayed traumatic intracerebral hemorrhage. Arch Neurol Psychiat 1942;48: 257–266.

9. Cushing H. Surgery of the head. In: Keen WW. Surgery: Its Principles and Practice. Vol. III. 1908;1–276. Reprinted by the Classics of Neurology and Neurosurgery Library, Birmingham: Gryphon Editions, 1983.

10. Cushing H. Concerning a definite regulatory mechanism of the vaso-motor centre which controls blood pressure during cerebral compression. Bull Johns Hopkins Hosp 1901; 12:290–292.

11. Gurdjian ES, Webster JE. Experimental and clinical studies on the mechanisms of head injury. In: Trauma of the Central Nervous System. Res Publ Assoc Res Nerv Ment Dis. Vol. 24. Baltimore: Williams & Wilkins, 1945; 48–97.

12. Teasdale G, Galbraith S. Acute traumatic intracranial haematomas. In: Progress in Neurological Surgery. Vol. 10. Basel; Karger, 1980.

13. Jennett B, Teasdale G. Management of Head Injuries. Philadelphia: F. A. Davis, 1981;158.

14. de Vet AC. Traumatic intracerebral haematoma. In: Vinken PJ, Bruyn GW, eds. Handbook of Clinical Neurology. Vol. 24. Injuries of the Brain and Skull, Part II. Amsterdam: North-Holland Publ Co., 1976; 351–368.

15. Evans JP, Scheinker IM. Histologic studies of the brain following head trauma. II: Posttraumatic petechial and massive intracerebral hemorrhage. J Neurosurg 1946;3:101–113.

16. Scheinker IM, Evans JP. Histologic studies of the brain following head trauma. V: Alterations in the vessels of the central nervous system following trauma. In: Trauma of the Central Nervous System. Res Publ Assoc Res Nerv Ment Dis. Vol. 24. Baltimore: Williams & Wilkins, 1945;98–130.

17. Schneider T. Verlaufsbeobachtung computertomographischer Befunde bei traumatischen intrazerebralen Hämatomen. Neurochirurgia. 1989;32:105–109.

18. Choksey MS, Costa DC, Iannotti F, et al. $^{99}$TC$^m$-HMPAO SPECT studies in traumatic intracerebral haematoma. J Neurol Neurosurg Psychiat 1991;54:6–11.

19. Goodnight SH, Kenoyer G, Rapaport SI, et al. Defibrination after brain-tissue destruction: a serious complication of head injury. N Engl J Med. 1974;290:1043–1047.

20. Kaufman HH, Mattson JC. Coagulopathy in head injury. In: Becker DP, Povlishock JT, eds. Central Nervous System Trauma Status Report 1985. Bethesda: National Institutes of Neurological and Communicative Disorders and Stroke, 1985;187–206.

21. Kaufman HH, Moake JL, Olson JD, et al. Delayed and recurrent intracranial hematomas related to disseminated intravascular clotting and fibrinolysis in head injury. Neurosurgery 1980;7:445–449.

22. Crone KR, Lee KS, Kelly DL. Correlation of admission fibrin degradation products with outcome and respiratory failure in patients with severe head injury. Neurosurgery 1987; 21:532–536.

23. Hamill RW, Woolf PD, McDonald JV, et al. Catecholamines predict outcome in traumatic brain injury. Ann Neurol 1987;21:438–443.

24. D'Alessandro R, Ferrara R, Benassi G, et al. Computed tomographic scans in posttraumatic epilepsy. Arch Neurol 1988;45:42–43.

25. MacPherson P, Teasdale E, Dhaker S, et al. The significance of traumatic haematoma in the region of the basal ganglia. J Neurol Neurosurg Psychiat 1986;49:29–34.

26. Katz DI, Alexander MP, Seliger GM, et al. Traumatic basal ganglia hemorrhage: clinicopathologic features and outcome. Neurology 1989;39:897–904.

27. Levin HS, Benton AL, Grossman RG. Neurobehavioral consequences of closed head injury. New York: Oxford University Press, 1982.

28. Cordobés F, de la Fuente M, Lobato RD, et al. Intraventricular hemorrhage in severe head injury. J Neurosurg 1983;58:217–222.

29. Kim CH, Tanaka R, Kawakami K, et al. Traumatic primary intraventricular hemorrhage. Surg Neurol 1981;16:415–417.

30. Kobayashi S, Nakazawa S, Otsuka T. Acute traumatic intraventricular hemorrhage in children. Child's Nerv Syst 1985;1:18–23.

31. Oliff M, Fried AM, Young AB. Intraventricular hemorrhage in blunt head trauma. J Comput Assist Tomogr 1978;2:625–629.

32. Zuccarello M, Iavicoli R, Pardatscher K, et al. Posttraumatic intraventricular haemorrhages. Acta Neurochir 1981;55:283–293.

33. Fujitsu K, Kuwabara T, Muramoto M, et al. Traumatic intraventricular hemorrhage: report of twenty-six cases and consideration of the pathogenic mechanism. Neurosurgery 1988; 23:423–430.

34. LeCount ER, Apfelbach CW. Pathologic anatomy of traumatic fractures of cranial bones and concomitant brain injuries. JAMA 1920; 74:501–511.

35. Courville CB. Effects of closed cranial injuries on the midbrain and upper pons. In: Trauma of the Central Nervous System. Res Publ Assoc Res Nerv Ment Dis. Vol. 24. Baltimore: Williams & Wilkins, 1945;131–150.

36. Kremer M, Ritchie Russell W, et al. A midbrain syndrome following head injury. J Neurol Neurosurg Psychiat 1947; 10:49–60.

37. Jefferson A. Ocular complications of head injuries. Trans Opthalml Soc UK 1961; 81: 595–612.

38. Ropper AH, Miller DC. Acute traumatic midbrain hemorrhage. Ann Neurol 1985;18:80–86.

39. Hershkowitz N, Bergey GK, Josyln J, et al. Isolated midbrain lesion resulting from closed head injury: a unique presentation of ataxic hemiparesis. Neurology 1989;39:452–453.

40. Caplan LR, Zervas NT. Survival with permanent midbrain dysfunction after surgical treatment of traumatic subdural hematoma: the clinical picture of a Duret hemorrhage? Ann Neurol 1977;1:587–589.

41. Herbstein DJ, Schaumburg HH. Hypertensive intracerebral hematoma: an investigation of the initial hemorrhage and rebleeding using chromium Cr51-labelled erythrocytes. Arch Neurol 1974;30:412–414.

42. Symonds C. Concussion and contusion of the brain and their sequellae. In: Brock S, ed. Injuries of the Brain and Spinal Cord and their coverings. Fourth Edition. New York: Springer, 1960;69–117.

43. Holmes G. Clinical symptoms of cerebellar disease and their interpretation. Lancet 1922; 1:1177–1182, 2:59–65.

44. Gurdjian ES, Webster JE. Traumatic intracranial hemorrhage. In: Brock S, ed. Injuries of the Brain and Spinal Cord and their coverings. Fourth Edition. New York: Springer, 1960;127–186.

45. Evans JP, Scheinker IM. Histologic studies of the brain following head trauma: VI. Posttraumatic central nervous system changes interpreted in terms of circulatory disturbances. In: Trauma of the Central Nervous System. Res Publ Assoc Res Nerv Ment Dis. Baltimore: Williams & Wilkins, 1945;254–273.

46. Lindenberg R. Compression of brain arteries as pathogenetic factor for tissue necroses and their areas of predilection. J Neuropathol Exp Neurol 1955;14:223–243.

47. Caplan LR, Hier D, Goodwin J, et al. Subdural hematoma mimicking other stroke syndromes. Trans Am Neurol Assoc 1980; 105: 167–169.

48. Fukamachi A, Nagaseki Y, Kohno K, et al. The incidence and developmental process of delayed traumatic intracerebral haematomas. Acta Neurochir 1985;74:35–39.

49. Tanaka T, Sakai T, Uemura K, et al. MR imaging as predictor of delayed posttraumatic cerebral hemorrhage. J Neurosurg 1988;69: 203–209.

# Chapter 12
# Intracranial Tumors

## Carlos S. Kase

Hemorrhage into brain tumors is relatively uncommon: in large surgical[1,2] and pathological[3-6] series of central nervous system (CNS) tumors, hemorrhage as a form of presentation is reported with a frequency of 0.6% to 1.3%[1,2] and 5.1% to 6%,[3-6] respectively. These figures are even lower (0.5%,[1] 0.7%,[3] 0.7%,[4] 1.4%,[5] and 2.5%[6]) if one considers those patients who present with a "spontaneous" intracerebral hemorrhage (ICH) in the setting of a previously unknown brain tumor. On the other hand, series of patients presenting with ICH report the finding of an underlying brain tumor in 6% to 10% of the cases.[1,7,8] The latter figures indicate that, on occasion, a search for a brain tumor is appropriate in patients with ICH, the former lesion being suggested by atypical clinical or radiological features of the hemorrhage.

The occurrence of ICH within a brain tumor is largely confined to the malignant varieties,[1-9] although rare instances of hemorrhage into benign tumors are documented.[4,10-12] Wakai et al.[3] reported a series of 1861 cases of brain tumor, 94 (5.1%) of whom presented with hemorrhage. Forty-nine of the hemorrhages occurred in their 311 cases of pituitary adenomas, corresponding to a frequency of bleeding of 15.8%. The distribution of cases by histological diagnosis and frequency of hemorrhage is shown in Table 12.1. The authors found hemorrhage into a brain tumor to occur more frequently

**Table 12.1.** Incidence of Tumoral Hemorrhage in Relation to Tumor Type[3]

| Tumor Type* | Total Cases | Hemorrhage | |
| --- | --- | --- | --- |
| | | No. Cases | % |
| Glioblastoma multiforme | 129 | 10 | 0.8 |
| Astrocytoma | 178 | 8 | 0.4 |
| Oligodendroglioma | 43 | 3 | 7.0 |
| Mixed glioma | 5 | 1 | 20.0 |
| Medulloblastoma | 62 | 1 | 1.6 |
| Ependymoma | 57 | 5 | 8.8 |
| Choroid plexus papilloma | 12 | 2 | 1.7 |
| Meningioma | 310 | 4 | 1.3 |
| Craniopharyngioma | 91 | 3 | 3.3 |
| Pituitary adenoma | 311 | 49 | 15.8 |
| Metastases | 104 | 3 | 2.9 |

*No instances of tumoral hemorrhage were documented in the following tumor types (number of cases in brackets): ganglioglioma [2], neuroblastoma [2], neurinoma [193], sarcoma [12], lymphoma [12], hemangioblastoma [34], germinoma [62], teratoma [27], chordoma [6], and chondroma [3].

(5.3%) in patients younger than age 14 as compared with those older (2.3%). All of their eight examples of hemorrhage into posterior fossa tumors occurred in patients younger than age 14. Among possible precipitating factors for hemorrhage into a brain tumor, Wakai et al.[3] identified ventricular drainage, ventriculoperitoneal shunt, carotid

**Table 12.2.** Incidence of Intratumoral Hemorrhage in Relation to Tumor Histology[4]

| Tumor Histology* | Total Cases | Macroscopic Hemorrhage | |
|---|---|---|---|
| | | No. Cases | % |
| Glioblastoma multiforme | 264 | 17 | 6.4 |
| Astrocytoma | 64 | 7 | 10.9 |
| Oligodendoglioma | 14 | 2 | 14.3 |
| Mixed oligo/ astrocytoma | 24 | 7 | 29.2 |
| Meningioma | 219 | 1 | 0.5 |
| Sarcoma | 3 | 2 | 66.7 |
| Lymphoma | 19 | 1 | 5.3 |
| Metastatic melanoma | 14 | 5 | 35.7 |
| Metastatic adenocarcinoma | 70 | 2 | 2.9 |
| Metastatic anaplastic carcinoma | 43 | 2 | 4.7 |
| Epidermoid cyst | 5 | 1 | 20.0 |

*No instances of intratumoral hemorrhage were observed in the following tumor types (number of cases in brackets): ependymoma [12], medulloblastoma [8], gliosarcoma [6], primitive neuroectodermal tumor [1], malignant meningioma [3], schwannoma [45], choroid plexus papilloma [2], germinomas [2], chordoma [5], hemangioblastoma [10], craniopharyngioma [9], metastatic squamous-cell carcinoma [16], and metastatic small-cell carcinoma [4].

angiography, and head injury in seven patients, all of them younger than age 14. Kondziolka et al.[4] reported a series of 905 consecutive brain tumors (with exclusion of pituitary adenomas and recurrent tumors), forty-nine (5.4%) of which developed macroscopic hemorrhage. The histological types and frequency of macroscopic hemorrhage within each group are listed in Table 12.2. These two large series[3,4] showed some differences in the frequency of tumors and their hemorrhage rates, probably reflecting in part a different age distribution of the populations studied. They both found a generally high rate of bleeding into gliomas (especially oligodendroglioma and mixed glioma). The high frequency of hemorrhage within metastatic melanoma reported by Kondziolka

et al.[4] is in agreement with most reported series.[1,13,14]

In addition to the histological type of tumor involved, other factors related to the presence of a malignancy may play a role in the pathogenesis of ICH: in an autopsy series of 500 patients with systemic (non-CNS) cancer, Graus et al.[15] reported 244 instances of intracranial hemorrhage, 56.5% of which had been symptomatic (Table 12.3). Among the cases of ICH (157 patients), intratumoral hemorrhage (38%) was second to coagulopathy (56%) as the mechanism of bleeding, the remaining 6% being due to a non-cancer-related cause, hypertension. Between two-thirds and three-fourths of these patients had been symptomatic as a result of the ICH, 42.6% of them presenting with an acute stroke-like onset. All sixty instances of intratumoral hemorrhage occurred into metastases of solid tumors, whereas the ICH secondary to coagulopathy (eighty-eight patients) were most often (78%) seen in the setting of leukemia associated with thrombocytopenia or diffuse intravascular coagulation. The extracerebral forms of hemorrhage, subdural and subarachnoid, were due in about equal proportion of cases to leukemia or metastases of solid tumors. All cases with supratentorial subdural hematoma due to carcinoma had tumoral infiltration of the dura at the site of the hematoma; in ten cases, the subdural hematomas were spinal

**Table 12.3.** Causes of Intracranial Hemorrhage in Patients with Systemic, Non-CNS Cancer, Autopsy Data[15]

| Type of Hemorrhage | No. Patients | % Symptomatic |
|---|---|---|
| Intracerebral hematomas | | |
| Intratumoral | 60 | 78% |
| Due to coagulopathy | 88 | 65% |
| Hypertensive | 9 | 89% |
| Subdural hematoma | 63 | 25% |
| Subarachnoid hemorrhage | 24 | 42% |
| Total | 244 | 56.5% |

in location, all following a lumbar puncture in thrombocytopenic patients. The symptomatic subarachnoid hemorrhages were most often due to either incidental congenital aneurysms or coagulopathy, rarely to bleeding from a periventricular metastasis.

## Tumor Types Associated with Intracerebral Hemorrhage

The various tumor types have different incidences, and different rates of presentation with ICH, thus frequency distributions differ in series that report brain tumors in general,[3,4] as opposed to those that report on the specific clinical and pathological aspects of bleeding into brain tumors.[1,7] Although a large variety of brain tumors can at times present with intratumoral hemorrhage (see Tables 12.1 and 12.2), for many of them it is an exceptional occurrence, while others do so with a clinically relevant frequency. The latter group includes gliomas, metastases, pituitary adenomas, and meningiomas, and they will be discussed separately.

### Gliomas

In this group of primary brain tumors there are at least four varieties that frequently show areas of bleeding on pathological examination, leading occasionally to large ICH with a stroke-like presentation. These include, in an increasing order of frequency of hemorrhage, the astrocytomas, glioblastoma multiforme, oligodendroglioma, and the mixed astrocytoma/oligodendroglioma variety.[3,4] These tumors as a group were found to have "gross hemorrhage . . . with or without attendant clinical symptoms," in thirty-one of 832 (3.7%) cases belonging to Cushing's series, reported by Oldberg[16] in 1933. Clinical symptoms in the form of acute stroke-like presentations only occurred in seven of the thirty-one patients, amounting to 0.84% of the total group of 832 patients.[16]

*Astrocytomas* of low grade (I, II) of malignancy are rarely associated with intratumoral hemorrhage. The true frequency is, however, difficult to establish from the literature due to either lack of uniformity in the classification of the tumors or poor description of their histological character. Only a handful of cases of bleeding into low-grade astrocytomas has been reported.[1,2,16,17] Scott[1] operated on a 46-year-old patient with a previously treated (radiation therapy, ten years before), recurrent grade II astrocytoma that presented with intracerebral hemorrhage, followed by a twelve-year survival. De Waele et al.[17] discussed a 61-year-old man who had a fatal hemorrhage into a basal ganglionic astrocytoma that corresponded histologically to a low-grade, "protoplasmic" form. The tumor was made of isomorphic, small glial cells with scarce fibers, with multiple small cystic cavities, without prominent vasculature or endothelial proliferation, necrosis, or abundant mitoses. The authors speculated that in instances in which the histological aspects of the tumor lack features indicative of bleeding potential, such as prominent vascularity with endothelial proliferation or foci of necrosis, additional factors, such as head trauma, may provoke intratumoral hemorrhage. Head trauma, however, was found to be a potential factor in intratumoral bleeding in only one of nine cases studied at autopsy by Globus and Sapirstein,[18] and the tumor corresponded to a clearly malignant variety (cerebral metastases of Wilms' tumor). Gross and Bender[19] reported preceding "trivial" head trauma, without loss of consciousness, in one of their four patients with massive hemorrhage into brain tumors. The histological diagnosis was "hemangioendothelioma." Other potential risk factors for intratumoral bleeding, such as use of anticoagulants, although occasionally reported in bleeding into metastatic tumors,[6] have not been found to promote hemorrhage into gliomas.[20,21] Oldberg[16] reported bleeding in three of 255 (1.2%) patients with either fibrillary or protoplasmic astrocytomas; however, this frequency may even be lower for this variety of astrocytoma, since his detailed description of one of the three cases (Case 1), suggests a diagnosis of malignant, high-grade astrocytoma, as it is described as "a soft, necrotic, markedly-degenerated tumor . . . removed nearly in entirety by suction. Histologically, the tumor was difficult to classify, but it was finally placed among the fibrillary astrocytomas."

In conclusion, well-documented instances of large, clinically significant bleeding into low-grade astrocytomas are exceptionally rare in the literature, and the potential role of precipitating events, such as head trauma, remains unclear.

*Glioblastoma multiforme* or *"malignant" astrocytomas* are more often found as the underlying mechanism in instances of ICH. Although the brain tumor is generally symptomatic prior to the ICH, in rare occasions the latter has been the first manifestation of the malignancy,[7,9,22,23] at times causing sudden death.[24] The hemorrhages into malignant astrocytomas generally occur within a single tumor focus, but rare examples of multiple, recurrent hemorrhages at different sites in a diffusely infiltrating glioblastoma multiforme[25] (Figure 12.1), and a cerebellar hemorrhage into a presumed "multicentric" (cerebellar vermian and temporal-basal ganglionic) malignant astrocytoma[26] have been described. The mechanism of bleeding in this setting is thought to be related to necrosis and rupture of either the "glomeruloid" tumoral blood vessels of glioblastoma multiforme or the parenchymal vessels infiltrated by tumor.[8,27] These abnormal tumoral vessels have been considered responsible for tumor necrosis, vascular thrombosis, and hemorrhage.[28] Their ultrastructural features include fenestration of capillaries, widened intercellular junctions, and increased pinocytosis,[29] presumably resulting in breakdown of the blood-brain barrier as well as fragility with potential for rupture and bleeding.[25] Recently, Liwnicz et al.[30] analyzed the vascular histological features in 160 cases of brain tumor, five of which (three glioblastoma multiforme, two oligodendro-

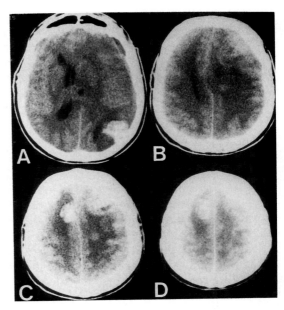

**Figure 12.1.** Multiple intracerebral hemorrhages in a patient with a diffusely infiltrating glioblastoma multiforme. (A) Small right parieto-occipital ICH, with a disproportionate degree of midline shift due to the presence of the diffusely infiltrating hemispheric tumor. (B) Anterior-superior right frontal hemorrhage with mass effect (shift of the midline, herniation of the gyrus cingulum under the falx). (C) Left frontal parasagittal hemorrhage. (D) Extension of the latter hemorrhage upwards. In all these locations, hemorrhage occurred at sites of infiltration of the brain substance by glioblastoma multiforme. (From Kase CS, Louis DN. Case records of Massachusetts General Hospital (case 26-1990). N Engl J Med 1990;322:1866–1878, with permission.)

glioma) had clinically significant hemorrhages. They classified the tumor vessels into "axial," "retiform," and "glomeruloid" types, finding that all five cases with large hemorrhage contained the retiform variety of capillary, and such capillary type was also correlated with microhemorrhages, found in over half of their ninety glioblastomas and thirty oligodendrogliomas; in the latter group the correlation was positive only when calcification of the retiform capillaries was also present.

*Oligodendrogliomas* are thought to have a higher tendency to bleed than astrocytomas and glioblastoma multiforme,[3,4,7] but their lower frequency among the gliomas results in the reporting of relatively few cases in the literature. Harada et al.[31] reported a case of massive frontal ICH in a 32-year-old man with an oligodendroglioma, and reviewed seven other cases reported in the literature, two of which corresponded to subarachnoid hemorrhage caused by tumors that were either intraventricular or immediately adjacent to the ventricular system. The pathogenesis of these hemorrhages is similar to that of glioblastoma multiforme, in that the abnormal tumor vasculature (made up of delicate branching vessels, primarily corresponding to calcified retiform capillaries, according to Liwnicz et al.[30]) is prone to rupture and hemorrhage. In a rare instance, subarachnoid hemorrhage occurred in the setting of an intraventricular oligodendroglioma and a cortical arteriovenous malformation, the bleeding having been caused by the former, as determined by CT scan on presentation and the observation of an intact, unruptured arteriovenous malformation at the time of surgery.[32]

*Mixed gliomas*, made up of a combination of astrocytoma and adjacent oligodendroglioma, are an uncommon variety of gliomas, which appear to have a particularly high tendency (20% to 30%) to develop intratumoral hemorrhage.[3,4] In a unique and well studied case of a massive, fatal cerebellar hemorrhage in a mixed glioma in a child, Specht et al.[33] documented the origin of the bleeding from the oligodendroglioma component of the tumor; its other component, a juvenile pilocytic astrocytoma, showed no evidence of bleeding at post-mortem examination. The oligodendroglioma portion of the tumor contained the typical delicate, thin-walled, branching vessels of this tumor, but in areas it also had foci of extensive vascular endothelial proliferation (of the type seen in glioblastoma multiforme), thought to be the likely source of the spontaneous intratumoral hemorrhage.

## Metastases

Systemic malignant tumors metastasize to the brain with different degrees of predilection depending on their primary site (Table 12.4).[34] In Posner's series of 225 patients with cerebral metastases (out of a pool of 2088 cancer patients) a high frequency of secondary cerebral tumors was found for melanoma (40%), followed by lung and kidney (21% each), breast and osteogenic sarcoma (10% each), and ovary and colon (5% each). Due to the different frequency of these primary tumors, the distribution of the primary site in a series of 572 patients with cerebral metastases from the same institution[34] showed lung to be the most common primary site (26%), followed by melanoma (21%), breast (14%), testicle (9%), and kidney (5%). Other features that characterize the various primary tumors relate to the single or multiple character of their metastases: in Posner's series,[34] only 14% to 35% of metastases were single, a more likely occurrence with breast and renal-cell primary tumors, whereas lung and melanoma were more often associated with multiple lesions.

Hemorrhage into metastatic brain tumors has been estimated to occur in about 14% of the cases, a frequency substantially higher than that of bleeding into gliomas (3.7%),

**Table 12.4.** Rate of Cerebral Metastases of Different Primary Malignancies

| Primary Tumor | No. Pts. | Brain Metastases | |
| --- | --- | --- | --- |
| | | No. Pts. | % |
| Breast | 324 | 33 | 10 |
| Lung | 297 | 62 | 21 |
| Melanoma | 125 | 50 | 40 |
| Kidney | 52 | 11 | 21 |
| Ovary | 60 | 3 | 5 |
| Colon | 130 | 6 | 5 |
| Osteogenic sarcoma | 39 | 4 | 10 |

(From Posner JB. Brain metastases: a clinician's view. In: Weiss L, Gilbert HA, Posner JB (eds). Brain Metastasis. Boston: GK Hall, 1980, pp 2–29, with permission.)

and is also dependent on the type of primary malignancy involved, the ones most commonly associated with hemorrhagic metastases being melanoma, choriocarcinoma, lung, and renal-cell carcinoma.[35] Rare instances of hemorrhagic metastases have been described in tumors of lower frequency, such as adrenal carcinoma,[7] laryngeal carcinoma,[35] carcinoid tumor,[35] hepatocellular[36] and hepatobiliary[37] carcinoma, osteogenic sarcoma,[38] carcinoma of the colon, bladder, thyroid, testicle, and endometrium,[39] carcinoma of the breast,[15] and rhabdomyosarcoma.[39]

Hemorrhage into brain metastases from *melanoma* occurs in about 30% of the cases.[15] Since these metastases are often multiple, a presentation with several simultaneous hemorrhagic lesions is occasionally seen[35] (Figure 12.2). The tumors can be of variable size, and their location favors the corticosubcortical areas of the cerebral hemispheres, where small blood-borne particles generally tend to become arrested in the cerebral circulation (Figure 12.3). In CT studies of metastatic mel-

anoma the majority of lesions (78% to 100%) are hyperdense in comparison with normal brain, and about one-third of the cases show evidence of frank hemorrhage in noncontrast studies.[14,40] A substantial proportion of the hyperdense lesions that are not overtly hemorrhagic on CT are shown on neuropathological examination to contain hemorrhage within the tumor, whereas isodense lesions lack hemorrhagic components.[14] In MRI studies, the various forms of metastatic melanoma are identified with greater precision than with CT scan. This technique permits the distinction of melanotic from amelanotic metastatic melanoma, and is also accurate in documenting the presence and stage of evolution of intratumoral hemorrhage,[41] through changes in signal intensity with "short" (T1-weighted) and "long" (T2-weighted) spin-echo sequences (Table 12.5). Angiography in metastatic melanoma generally shows an avascular mass, but occasionally a vascular "blush" is demonstrated, the latter aspect corresponding with lesions without hemorrhagic character on noncontrast CT scan.[14]

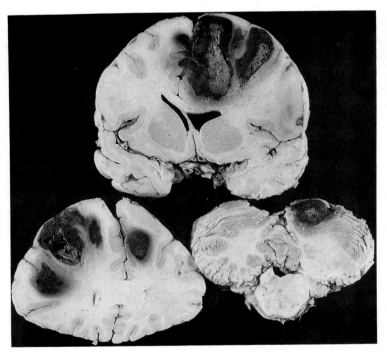

**Figure 12.2.** Multiple hemorrhagic metastases of melanoma, in both cerebral hemispheres and cerebellum (Courtesy of Dr. Flaviu CA Romanul, Boston VA Medical Center, Boston, MA.)

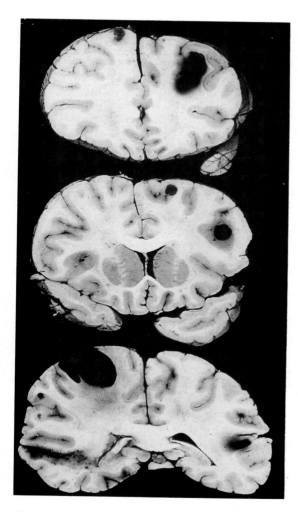

**Figure 12.3.** Multiple, densely hemorrhagic metastases of melanoma, predominantly located in the corticosubcortical area of the cerebral hemispheres.

Cerebral metastases of *choriocarcinoma* are common, with an estimated frequency of about 20%,[42] the highest among all cancers arising in the female genital system. Its frequency is particularly high in Asian populations of Southeast Asia and Taiwan; in a series of cerebral metastases from Thailand, Shuangshoti et al.[43] reported choriocarcinoma only second to lung cancer as the most common primary tumors, and it accounted for 12% of all secondary intracranial malignancies. From their series of twenty patients with cerebral metastases from choriocarcinoma, three (15%) presented with an acute, stroke-like onset, without prior symptoms from the primary or metastatic tumors. Two of these patients had large hemorrhages into metastatic lesions, while the third patient had tumor emboli to the brain. The hemorrhages were large, of lobar location, and the clots contained islands of choriocarcinoma, with malignant cells also present in the lumen and walls of local blood vessels. The authors suggested that the possibility of metastatic choriocarcinoma should be raised in the setting of a stroke-like event in an Asian woman of child-bearing age and with a history of pregnancy during the preceding year.[43] A similar recommendation by Watanabe and Smoker[44] was based on a report of a young woman presumably non-Asian (race not stated), who developed a total of five ICH in the postpartum period, the first hemorrhage occurring fourteen weeks after delivery. Cerebral angiography demonstrated the avascular mass effect of the hemorrhages as well as multiple areas of segmental arterial dilatation and narrowing, vascular occlusion, and contrast medium extravasation, all

**Table 12.5.** Signal Intensity Changes in MRI of Cerebral Metastatic Melanoma

| Type of Lesion | Short TR/TE (T1-weighted) | Long TR/TE (T2-weighted) |
|---|---|---|
| Amelanotic melanoma | Mildly hypointense or isointense | Mildly hyperintense or isointense |
| Melanotic melanoma | Markedly hyperintense | Mildly hyperintense or isointense |
| Subacute hemorrhage (early) | Markedly hyperintense | Markedly hypointense |
| Subacute hemorrhage (late) | Markedly hyperintense | Markedly hyperintense |

(From Atlas SW, Grossman RI, Gomori JM, et al. MR imaging of intracranial metastatic melanoma. J Comput Assist Tomogr 1987;11:577–582, with permission.)

suggesting widespread arterial lesions presumed secondary to metastatic choriocarcinoma. The diagnosis was based on the presence of choriocarcinoma in the spleen, which was removed in order to control severe thrombocytopenia that developed *after* the onset of ICH, and no cerebral tissue was available for histologic study, as the patient recovered without surgical treatment of her cerebral hemorrhages. Van den Doel et al.[45] reported the case of a young woman who developed two ICH in the setting of unsuspected metastatic choriocarcinoma, the diagnosis being suggested by cytological examination of the bloody aspirate from craniotomy for drainage of one of the hematomas. The diagnosis was subsequently confirmed at autopsy. The authors stressed the value of cytological examination of surgical aspirates of ICH for making the diagnosis of an underlying tumor.

Other cerebral metastatic tumors known to be complicated by local bleeding are bronchogenic carcinoma and renal-cell carcinoma. *Bronchogenic carcinoma* metastases are thought to have a lower frequency of bleeding, on the order of 5%,[15] in comparison with melanoma[15] and choriocarcinoma.[43] Bleeding has been reported more often in instances of metastatic anaplastic carcinoma or adenocarcinoma,[4,5] but small-cell tumors have been implicated as well.[46] In *renal-cell carcinoma*, a very high frequency (70%) of hemorrhagic metastases was reported in one study,[46] but the low frequency of this systemic malignancy results in relatively few cases of hemorrhagic metastatic cerebral tumors reported in the literature. On occasion, cerebral metastases of renal-cell carcinoma have presented a cystic appearance, and bleeding into them has produced blood-fluid levels within the lesions.[47] The cystic character of the lesions was interpreted as due to tumor necrosis, with secondary bleeding into the partially liquefied necrotic tumor producing the blood-fluid levels.

The *mechanisms of bleeding* into cerebral metastases, some of which are shared by malignant gliomas, are probably multiple (Table

**Table 12.6.** Mechanisms of Bleeding into Malignant Brain Tumors

1. Rupture of tumoral blood vessels with abnormal permeability and increased fragility (metastases, gliomas).
2. Tumoral infiltration of parenchymal vessels, leading to increased fragility, formation of pseudoaneurysms (metastases, especially choriocarcinoma).
3. Tumor emboli, leading to vascular occlusion and necrosis of vessel wall with rupture (metastatic choriocarcinoma).
4. Tumor necrosis, with necrosis of blood vessels (metastases, gliomas).
5. Coincidental factors: head trauma, anticoagulant treatment, disseminated intravascular coagulation.

12.6). The main factor in promoting bleeding in malignant brain tumors is thought to be the abnormal character of the tumoral/peritumoral blood vessels.[28,29,35] These are particularly abundant at the advancing edge of an infiltrating tumor, leading at times to a bleeding pattern in the form of a ring of hemorrhage that separates the tumor from the adjacent parenchyma (Figure 12.4). In specific tumor types, such as choriocarcinoma, vascular invasion by tumor either from local metastases or by blood-borne tumor emboli, is particularly prominent, presumably due to the biologic propensity of trophoblastic tissue to invade vascular structures.[42,43] This aspect of the tumor invasion leads to vascular occlusion and necrosis, as well as the possible formation of pseudoaneurysms, both lesions having the potential for vascular rupture and bleeding.[42–44,48] In other instances, hemorrhages into tumors of high growth rates are related to central tumor necrosis, as a result of insufficient blood supply to the rapidly growing neoplasm. The role of coincidental factors in promoting intratumoral bleeding remains speculative. Head trauma has been infrequently related to tumoral ICH,[8,19,35] and it probably is not a significant risk factor for this complication of brain tumors. Anticoagulant treatment for

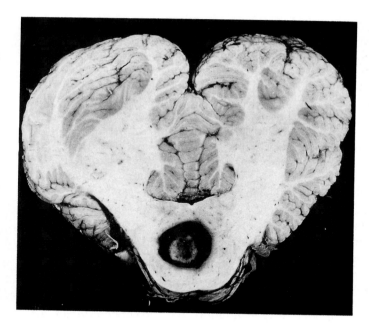

**Figure 12.4.** Metastasis from adenocarcinoma of the lung in the basis pontis, surrounded by a ring of fresh hemorrhage.

concomitant deep-vein thrombosis has likewise been thought not to increase the risk of tumoral hemorrhage in patients with cerebral gliomas.[20,21] However, in a group of sixtynine patients with cerebral metastases, two (3%) developed intratumoral hemorrhage while receiving heparin by continuous intravenous infusion.[49] Both patients had metastatic lung carcinomas, received intravenous heparin for prevention of pulmonary embolism, and developed intratumoral hemorrhages during anticoagulant treatment, with aPTT in the therapeutic range (69.2 seconds) in one and excessively prolonged (more then 120 seconds) in the other. Decreased coagulability may predispose to intratumoral hemorrhage, as excessively prolonged aPTT or PT was documented in six of eight patients reported by So et al.[50] These authors reported a case of bleeding into a metastatic melanoma, and reviewed seven prior reported cases of bleeding into various CNS lesions, including pituitary adenoma, pineal cyst, cerebral abscess, meningioma, and spinal cord ependymoma. These patients were receiving either heparin or warfarin for prevention of pulmonary or systemic emboli, or progression of

cerebral ischemia. A unique case of bleeding into a cerebellopontine angle schwannoma in the setting of cocaine use has been reported,[51] raising the issue of sympathomimetic drug use as a potential risk factor for intratumoral hemorrhage in this era of increasing illicit drug use. The role of disseminated intravascular coagulation in producing hemorrhage into brain metastases of solid carcinomas is probably insignificant, but this coagulation disorder was found to be a substantial contributor to intracranial bleeding in patients with leukemia.[15]

### Pituitary Adenomas

Pituitary adenomas are known to frequently undergo secondary changes, mainly necrosis and hemorrhage, thought to be the result of the tumor outgrowing its vascular supply.[52] These changes occur in approximately 9% to 16% of pituitary adenomas,[53–55] although occasional figures as high as 25.7%[56] have been reported. However, it is apparent that a substantial number of these lesions are asymptomatic, mainly representing surgical findings, whereas the remainder (approximately 5% to 7% of pituitary adenomas[53,55,56]) present with the acute syndrome "pituitary apoplexy." This condition refers to an acute increase in size of a pituitary adenoma or, rarely, a normal pituitary gland, as a result of hemorrhage or ischemic necrosis within their substance.[52,57] The majority of the reported cases correspond to acute intratumoral hemorrhage in an adenoma (Figure 12.5). A proportion of these cases (approximately 1% to 2% of pituitary adenomas[53]) present with the acute syndrome of "apoplexy" as the initial clinical manifestation of a previously unsuspected sellar tumor.

The *clinical picture* of pituitary apoplexy includes the sudden onset of headache, frequently with nausea and vomiting, accompanied by decreased level of consciousness, ophthalmoplegia, and various patterns of decreased visual acuity.[52,53,55,56,58] The symptoms are due to compression of the oculomotor nerves at the cavernous sinus level, and of the optic chiasm by the upward (suprasellar) extension of the lesion. At times, the presentation is that of sudden coma (from presumed hypothalamic compression by the rapidly enlarging hemorrhagic tumor), or even sudden death.[52] The headache of pituitary "apoplexy" has generally been described as an early symptom. The most common location is bilateral and frontotemporal,[53,58] at times with subsequent diffuse radiation, the latter generally in the setting of associated bleeding into the subarachnoid space.[58] On initial examination, most patients show an abnormal level of consciousness, although occasionally patients are reported as "alert and coherent" in the face of an acute intratumoral hemorrhage that has led to visual loss or ophthalmoplegia.[58] The latter findings have the highest diagnostic value, since ophthalmoplegia (unilateral or bilateral third nerve palsies more often than sixth nerve palsies) and unilateral or bilateral visual deficits are present in 90% to 100% of the patients.[53,58] The visual deficits can occur as either unilateral amblyopia secondary to optic nerve com-

pression, or visual field changes due to compression of the optic chiasm, the most common pattern being bitemporal hemianopic defects.[53]

It is unclear whether there are defined *risk factors* for massive bleeding into pituitary adenomas. The initial suggestion that histological type was important, in that "secretory" adenomas (associated with acromegaly or with Cushing's syndrome) were more likely to bleed massively than "nonsecretory" adenomas[52] was not substantiated in subsequent large series of pituitary tumors.[54,55,58] A large size of the tumor was thought to relate to an increased frequency of bleeding by some,[56] but size was not a factor in the large series of Wakai et al.[55] A concomitant coagulation defect, either drug-induced thrombocytopenia[54] or therapeutic anticoagulation,[54,58,59] has been documented in isolated instances, suggesting caution in the use of anticoagulants in patients with known pituitary tumors.[54] The preceding use of tumor radiotherapy was suggested as a risk factor for intratumoral bleeding by Weisberg,[53] as ten of his fourteen cases developed hemorrhage in close association with this form of treatment. He postulated that patients at particularly high risk of bleeding are those with pre-existing hemorrhagic, necrotic, and cystic changes in the tumor, as opposed to those with solid, homogeneous tumors. Since the former is thought to be less radiosensitive, Weisberg[53] suggested that patients with cystic and hemorrhagic tumors, as defined by CT scan or trans-sphenoidal tumor biopsy, should be treated surgically, avoiding radiotherapy altogether, or reserving it for postoperative treatment of remnants of solid tumor.

The *diagnosis* of pituitary "apoplexy" used to rely in the past on the documentation of an enlarged sella on plain skull x-rays or hemorrhagic, xanthochromic CSF, followed by imaging studies (angiography, pneumoencephalography) confirmatory of a sellar-suprasellar mass. Since the advent of CT scan and MRI, the diagnosis has been greatly simplified. Noncontrast CT scans done

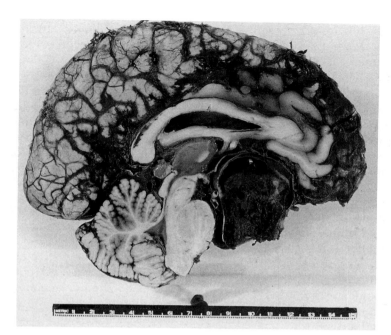

**Figure 12.5.** Massive hemorrhage into large pituitary adenoma with marked suprasellar extension, with clinical presentation as "pituitary apoplexy." (A) Midsagittal cut. (B) Coronal view.

A

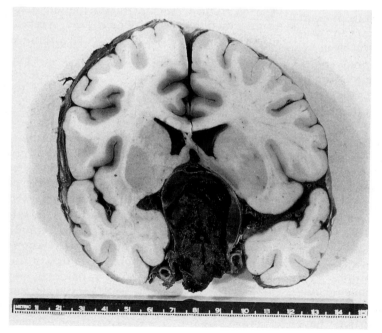

B

acutely, within seventy-two hours of onset, invariably document high-density areas within the sellar/suprasellar tumor mass.[53,57,60] The results of contrast-enhanced CT scans are more variable, depicting either no enhancement at all, or partial uptake of contrast, at times in a ring-like pattern.[60] Occasionally, pituitary "apoplexy" appears on acute CT scan as an area of blood density with a "fluid-blood level,"[61] presumably representing acute hemorrhage into a partially cystic adenoma. The more difficult radiological diagnosis of subacute or remote hemorrhage into a pituitary adenoma cannot be resolved by CT scan, as imaging shows only variable degrees of hypodensity (at times with ring-like postcontrast enhancement) within the tumor mass.[57] This diagnosis can now be made with MRI, which shows hyperintense signal changes in T1-weighted spin-echo sequences[57] (Figure 12.6).

The differential diagnosis of pituitary "apoplexy" includes hemorrhage from a giant carotid artery aneurysm (which can produce unilateral, but very rarely *bilateral*, ophthalmoplegia[58]) and mesencephalic hemorrhage (in which ophthalmoplegia is generally accompanied by hemiplegia, the latter not being a feature of pituitary "apoplexy"). The diagnosis of these conditions is greatly facilitated by the use of cerebral angiography and, in particular, CT and MRI scans, the brain imaging studies generally establishing the diagnosis upon acute presentation.

## Meningiomas

These generally benign tumors are rarely associated with acute hemorrhage. However, rare examples of both intratumoral and subdural or subarachnoid hemorrhage have been described as a cause of a stroke-like syndrome in patients with (generally previously asymptomatic) meningiomas (Table 12.7). The majority of patients had meningiomas of benign character, but abundant vascularity[10,11] and an angioblastic pattern with prominent capillaries and mitoses[12] were felt to have contributed to the tumoral bleeding in some cases. In only one instance[65] did a potential extrinsic factor promote bleeding, in the form of an excessive level of anticoagulation used to prevent pulmonary embolism.

The clinical presentation of these cases was invariably with sudden onset of headache and decreased level of consciousness, less commonly with new onset of seizures. The radiological diagnosis in most pre-CT cases was based on cerebral angiography, which generally showed an avascular mass, rarely with a prominent external carotid (meningeal) artery in the area, suggestive of an underlying meningioma.[65] The current availability of CT and MRI should facilitate the diagnosis of bleeding into, or adjacent to, such tumor prior to its confirmation at surgery. However, a meningioma with acute bleeding may be at times indistinguishable by MRI from a vascular malformation (cavernous angioma),[66] in which case cerebral angiography may be valuable in the differential diagnosis.

## Miscellaneous Tumors

A number of other tumors, primary or systemic, occur in the brain and, in rare instances, can be complicated by intratumoral hemorrhage. In *non-Hodgkin's lymphoma*, cerebral involvement usually takes the form of leptomeningeal infiltration, leading to progressive cranial and spinal nerve compromise, rather than to intraparenchymal tumor masses.[67,68] However, in "primary CNS lymphoma," a B-cell lymphoma that favors the immunocompromised host,[69] parenchymal cerebral involvement is well known. It can occur as a multicentric primary brain tumor, and bleeding into it is rarely present.[8,15,70–72] The diagnosis of primary CNS lymphoma can be suggested by imaging studies that reveal a primarily deep (in basal ganglia, corpus callosum) and generally isodense (in noncontrast CT) hemispheric neoplasm, with homogeneous postcontrast enhance-

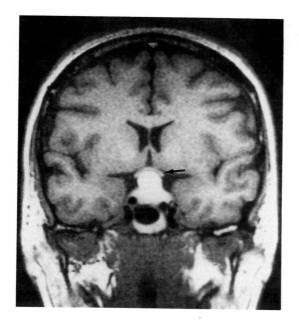

A

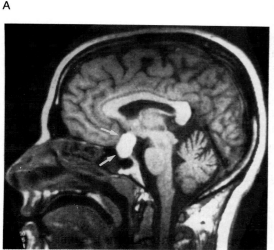

B

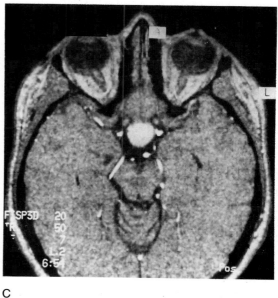

C

**Figure 12.6.** MRI (T1-weighted) of pituitary "apoplexy" in a 26-year-old woman, with confirmation of tumoral bleeding at surgery. (A) Coronal view; note upward displacement and compression of the optic chiasm (arrow). (TR = 350 msec; TE = 15 msec.) (B) Midsagittal view; intrasellar and suprasellar hemorrhagic tumor (arrows). (TR = 400 msec; TE = 15 msec.) (C) Axial view of suprasellar hemorrhagic tumor. (TR = 50 msec; TE = 7 msec.)

ment.[73–76] Primary (nonmetastatic) *posterior fossa tumors* can rarely present with spontaneous bleeding, an event virtually limited to the pediatric population. The tumor types most commonly implicated have been astrocytoma,[77] ependymoma,[78,79] and medulloblastoma.[16,80] In several of these cases,[77,78] the placement of a ventriculoperitoneal shunt or ventriculostomy preceded the intra-

tumoral hemorrhage, an occurrence documented in seven of forty cases (17.5%) of bleeding into posterior fossa tumors recorded from the literature by Reinchenthal et al.[79] The same authors reviewed six reported cases of bleeding into posterior fossa ependymomas, and added a seventh case of their own. All these patients were younger than age 11 (mean age 5.8). In three of the

**Table 12.7.** Cases of Acute Hemorrhage Related to Meningiomas

| Authors | Type of Hemorrhage | Type of Meningioma |
|---|---|---|
| El-Banhawy and Walter[62] | SAH | Endotheliomatous |
| Goran et al.[10] (5 cases) | SDH+ICH | Endotheliomatous |
| | IT | Endotheliomatous |
| | IT | Endotheliomatous |
| | ICH | Meningothelial with sarcomatous changes |
| | IT | Endotheliomatous |
| Skultety[63] | SDH+ICH+IT | Fibroblastic |
| Gruszkiewicz et al.[64] | ICH+IT | Fibroblastic |
| Modesti et al.[11] (4 cases) | SDH+ICH | Meningoendotheliomatous |
| | SDH+ICH | Meningoendotheliomatous |
| | SDH+IT | Angioblastic |
| | SDH | Meningoendotheliomatous |
| Nakao et al.[12] | ICH | Angioblastic* |
| Everett et al.[65] | SDH+ICH+IT | Syncytial, with transitional areas† |

*Patient with recurrent angioblastic meningioma, after total removal and high-dose radiotherapy. Histologically with high cellularity, abundant capillaries and mitoses.
†Patient on anticoagulants for deep-vein thrombosis, with PT 4× control and aPTT 2.5× control.
Abbreviations: SAH = subarachnoid hemorrhage, SDH = subdural hematoma, IT = intratumoral.

seven cases the hemorrhagic event was the first manifestation of the tumor in a previously well child. A recent report by Gordon et al.[81] documented the unusual occurrence of recurrent episodes of SAH during a one-year period, in the setting of an undiagnosed thalamic ependymoma. The last event was a massive, fatal right thalamic intratumoral hemorrhage. A unique case of bleeding into two intraparenchymal *plasmacytomas* (in the cerebellum and frontal lobe) was reported by Husain et al.[82] The patient had been symptomatic twelve years previously owing to systemic plasmacytomas, but had no evidence of intracranial involvement until the acute presentation with two ICH. At autopsy, the two hemorrhages occurred at sites of parenchymal infiltration by plasmacytomas, and no evidence of leptomeningeal, dural, or bony tumor was present. The authors pointed to the rarity of ICH into plasmacytomas in the absence of thrombocytopenia or other coagulation defects. They mentioned only two other reported cases of this occurrence,[83,84] one of which involved hemorrhage into an intracranial but extracerebral (i.e., dural) tumor.[84]

## Features Suggestive of Intracerebral Hemorrhage in a Tumor

Based on the various issues discussed above, it is possible to list a number of circumstances in which the clinical and radiological features of a patient with ICH should justify a search for an underlying primary or metastatic tumor. These include:[13,85] (1) history of preceding chronic headache and/or focal neurological deficit and/or personality change for days or weeks before the onset of ICH; (2) finding of papilledema on initial presentation with ICH; (3) multiple separate foci of ICH occurring simultaneously; (4) an area of "ring-like" hemorrhage with a low-density center in noncontrast CT (see Figure 12.4); (5) an ICH that on CT scan appears as an irregular, mottled, high-density, and involves structures rarely affected in primary "hypertensive" ICH, such as the corpus callosum (which is more often affected in malignant gliomas and lymphoma); (6) a disproportionate amount of edema and mass effect around an acute hematoma (Figure 12.7); (7) presence of postcontrast nodular enhancement near an acute ICH. In addition, Iwama

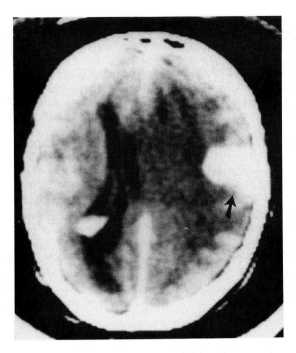

**Figure 12.7.** CT scan of acute left lobar frontoparietal ICH of moderate size (arrow), with extensive low-density edema of most of the hemisphere, and marked midline shift, due to bleeding into metastases of bronchogenic carcinoma.

et al.[86] have observed a low-density indentation at the periphery of an ICH as a distinctive CT sign of a tumoral nodule as the cause of the hemorrhage.

The MRI distinctions between tumoral and nontumoral ICH have been reviewed in detail.[87–89] Using spin-echo imaging, Atlas et al.[87] found the following features to be suggestive of hemorrhage into a tumor: (1) A heterogeneous and complex pattern of signal changes within the brain: heterogeneity is explained by different areas showing either different stages of hemoglobin change or adjacent foci of hemorrhagic and nonhemorrhagic (i.e., tumor) tissue, by the presence of signal intensity "levels" from layering of blood breakdown products within cystic, necrotic, or fluid-filled cavities, and by mixed signal intensities surrounded by high-signal edema on T2-weighted sequences. (2) A

delayed temporal evolution of hemoglobin changes in comparison with nontumoral ICH: this occurred as unusually long persistence (up to sixteen days) of signal change corresponding to intracellular deoxyhemoglobin and delayed (up to two months) methemoglobin presence at the periphery of the lesion. The differences between tumoral and nontumoral ICH were most marked in regards to hemosiderin formation, a consistent and predictable change in nontumoral ICH,[88] which was absent, decreased, or fragmented in cases of intratumoral ICH. This MRI feature of intratumoral hemorrhage is, however, rather inconsistent, since Destian et al.[39] reported the frequent observation of the peripheral hypointense hemosiderin rim in hemorrhagic intracranial neoplasms. (3) The presence of marked and persistent peritumoral edema; this bright-signal abnormality on T2-weighted sequences persisted into the subacute and chronic stages of the lesion, unlike its transient character in nontumoral ICH.[88]

The CT and MRI differential diagnosis between hemorrhagic tumors and vascular malformations may at times be difficult.[66,89] In MRI, both lesions can present with similar signal intensity changes: the "typical" aspect of vascular malformation, with a high-intensity center and peripheral rim of hypointensity on T2-weighted sequences,[90] can at times be seen in hemorrhagic cerebral tumors.[66] Useful, but not definite, differential points in favor of intratumoral hemorrhage (into metastatic lesions), as opposed to vascular malformations, include the multiplicity of lesions and the presence of prominent surrounding edema.[66,89] However, these features are not always diagnostic, since vascular malformations can be multiple in up to 50% of the cases,[66] and a similar percentage of malformations can be associated with adjacent edema.[91] On occasion, CT scan is helpful in this differential diagnosis by documenting calcification, a feature strongly against metastatic tumor, which on the other hand is found in 20% to 33% of vascular malformations.[92–94]

## Prognosis of Intratumoral Hemorrhage

Bleeding into an intracranial tumor is, in general, a grave event, associated with high mortality; in addition, the malignant or benign character of the underlying neoplasm further influences the vital prognosis in an individual case. Early (thirty-day) mortality after intratumoral bleeding was 77% (ten of thirteen patients) in the series of Little et al.,[7] with only one patient (with metastatic renal-cell carcinoma) surviving for one year; the remaining two patients died after five weeks and two months, respectively, from the hemorrhagic event. Although the selection of therapy was not randomized, two of three patients treated surgically left the hospital, while none of those treated medically survived longer than four weeks. A similar short-term beneficial effect of surgical treatment was reported by Albert,[9] but he did not include figures on mortality and duration of survival. In Mandybur's series[35] seven of fifteen (47%) patients with hemorrhage into metastatic tumors died within thirty days of the event; the average survival time for the whole group was sixty-five days. Only one patient, with metastatic choriocarcinoma, was still alive at the time of the report, and the longest reported survival in the group was nine months, in a patient with metastatic melanoma. In the group of twenty patients with hemorrhagic metastatic tumors reported by Weisberg,[46] three of six with solitary lesions underwent surgical treatment, and their survival was six to fourteen months, death being due to the effects of the systemic metastatic malignancies, without evidence of CNS recurrence. For the rest of the group, with single or multiple lesions treated with corticosteroids but without radiotherapy, survival was no longer than two months.

## References

1. Scott M. Spontaneous intracerebral hematoma caused by cerebral neoplasms: report of eight verified cases. J Neurosurg 1975;42:338–342.

2. Bitoh S, Hasegawa H, Ohtsuki H, et al. Cerebral neoplasms initially presenting with massive intracerebral hemorrhage. Surg Neurol 1984;22:57–62.

3. Wakai S, Yamakawa K, Manaka S, et al. Spontaneous intracranial hemorrhage caused by brain tumor: its incidence and clinical significance. Neurosurgery 1982;10:437–444.

4. Kondziolka D, Bernstein M. Resch L, et al. Significance of hemorrhage into brain tumors: clinicopathological study. J Neurosurg 1987; 67:852–857.

5. Niizuma H, Nakasato N, Yonemitsu T, et al. Intracerebral hemorrhage from a metastatic brain tumor: importance of differential diagnosis preceding stereotaxic hematoma aspiration. Surg Neurol 1988;29:232–236.

6. Padt JP, De Reuck J, vander Eecken H. Intracerebral hemorrhage as initial symptom of a brain tumor. Acta Neurol Belg 1973;73: 241–251.

7. Little JR, Dial B, Belanger G, et al. Brain hemorrhage from intracranial tumor. Stroke 1979;10:283–288.

8. Kothbauer P, Jellinger K, Flament H. Primary brain tumour presenting as spontaneous intracerebral haemorrhage. Acta Neurochir 1979;49:35–45.

9. Albert F. Spontaneous haemorrhage in intracranial tumours—a clinical report of 50 cases. Acta Neurochir 1982;62:143–144 (abstract).

10. Goran A, Ciminello VJ, Fisher RG. Hemorrhage into meningiomas. Arch Neurol 1965; 13:65–69.

11. Modesti LM, Binet EF, Collins GH. Meningiomas causing spontaneous intracranial hematomas. J Neurosurg 1976;45:437–441.

12. Nakao S, Sato S, Ban S. Massive intracerebral hemorrhage caused by angioblastic meningioma. Surg Neurol 1977;7:245–248.

13. Gildersleeve N, Koo AH, McDonald CJ. Metastatic tumor presenting as intracerebral hemorrhage: report of 6 cases examined by computed tomography. Radiology 1977;124: 109–112.

14. Enzmann DR, Kramer R, Norman D, Pollock J. Malignant melanoma metastatic to the central nervous system. Radiology 1978; 127:177–180.

15. Graus F, Rogers LR, Posner JB. Cerebrovascular complications in patients with cancer. Medicine 1985;64:16–35.

16. Oldberg E. Hemorrhage into gliomas. Arch Neurol Psychiat 1933;30:1061–1073.

17. De Waele JW, De Reuck J, Vanderkerckhove T. An unusual case of a spontaneous intracerebral haematoma. Acta Neurol Belg 1986;86: 145–151.

18. Globus JH, Sapirstein M. Massive hemorrhage into brain tumor: its significance and probable relationship to rapidly fatal termination and antecedent trauma. JAMA 1942;120: 348–352.

19. Gross SW, Bender MB. Massive hemorrhage in brain tumors. Arch Neurol Psychiat 1948; 60:612–617.

20. Choucair AK, Silver P, Levin VA. Risk of intracranial hemorrhage in glioma patients receiving anticoagulant therapy for venous thromboembolism. J Neurosurg 1987;66: 357–358.

21. Olin JW, Young JR, Graor RA, et al. Treatment of deep vein thrombosis and pulmonary emboli in patients with primary and metastatic brain tumors: anticoagulants or inferior vena cava filter? Arch Intern Med 1987;147:2172–2179.

22. Richardson RR, Siqueira EB, Cerullo LJ. Malignant glioma: its initial presentation as intracranial haemorrhage. Acta Neurochir 1979;46:77–84.

23. Weisberg LA. Hemorrhagic primary intracranial neoplasms: clinical-computed tomographic correlations. Comput Radiol 1986; 10:131–136.

24. Schultz OT. Sudden death due to hemorrhage into silent cerebral gliomas. Am J Surg 1935;30:148–153.

25. Kase CS, Louis DN. Case Records of the Massachusetts General Hospital (Case 26-1990). N Engl J Med 1990;322:1866–1878.

26. Misra BK, Steers AJW, Miller JD, et al. Multicentric glioma presenting with hemorrhage. Surg Neurol 1988;29:73–76.

27. Zülch KJ. Neuropathology of intracranial haemorrhage. Prog Brain Res 1968;30:151–165.

28. Hardman J. The angioarchitecture of the gliomata. Brain 1940;63:91–118.

29. Hirano A, Matsui T. Vascular structures in brain tumors. Hum Pathol 1975;6:611–621.

30. Liwnicz BH, Wu SZ, Tew JM. The relationship between the capillary structure and hemorrhage in gliomas. J Neurosurg 1987; 66:536–541.

31. Harada K, Kiya K, Matsumura S, et al. Spontaneous intracranial hemorrhage caused by oligodendroglioma—a case report and review of the literature. Neurol Med Chir 1982; 22:81–84.

32. Martinez-Lage JF, Poza M, Esteban JA, et al. Subarachnoid hemorrhage in the presence of cerebral arteriovenous malformation and an intraventricular oligodendroglioma: case report. Neurosurgery 1986;19:125–128.

33. Specht CS, Pinto-Lord C, Smith TW, et al. Spontaneous hemorrhage in a mixed glioma of the cerebellum: case report. Neurosurgery 1986;19:278–281.

34. Posner JB. Brain metastases: a clinician's view. In: Weiss L, et al., eds. Brain Metastasis. Boston: G K Hall, 1980;2–29.

35. Mandybur TI. Intracranial hemorrhage caused by metastatic tumors. Neurology 1977; 27:650–655.

36. Otsuka S, Fukumitsu T, Yamamoto T, Komori H, Shirane H. Brain metastasis of hepatocellular carcinoma presenting with hemorrhage. Neurol Med Chir 1987;27:654–657.

37. Davis JM, Zimmerman RA, Bilaniuk LT. Metastases to the central nervous system. Radiol Clin N Amer 1982;20:417–435.

38. Zimmerman RA, Bilaniuk LT. Computed tomography of acute intratumoral hemorrhage. Radiology 1980;135:355–359.

39. Destian S, Sze G, Krol G, et al. MR imaging of hemorrhagic intracranial neoplasms. Amer J Radiol 1989;152:137–144.

40. Solis OJ, Davis KR, Adair LV, et al. Intracerebral metastatic melanoma: CT evaluation. Comput Tomogr 1977;1:135–143.

41. Atlas SW, Grossman RI, Gomori JM, et al. MR imaging of intracranial metastatic melanoma. J Comput Assist Tomogr 1987;11: 577–582.

42. Vaughan HG, Howard RG. Intracranial hemorrhage due to metastatic chorionepithelioma. Neurology 1962;12:771–777.

43. Shuangshoti S, Panyathanya R, Wichienkur P. Intracranial metastases from unsuspected choriocarcinoma. Neurology 1974;24:649–654.

44. Watanabe AS, Smoker WRK. Computed tomography and angiographic findings in metastatic choriocarcinoma. J Comput Assist Tomogr 1989;13:319–322.

45. van den Doel EMH, van Merriënboer FJJM, Tulleken CAF. Cerebral hemorrhage from unsuspected choriocarcinoma. Clin Neurol Neurosurg 1985;87:287–290.

46. Weisberg LA. Hemorrhagic metastatic intracranial neoplasms: clinical-computed tomo-

graphic correlations. Comput Radiol 1985;9: 105–114.

47. Kaiser MC, Rodesch G, Capesius P. Blood-fluid levels in multiloculated cystic brain metastasis of a hypernephroma. Neuroradiology 1983;25:339–341.

48. Montaut J, Hepner H, Tridon P, et al. Aspects pseudo-vasculaires des métastases intracraniennes des chorio-épithéliomes. Neurochirurgie 1971;17:119–128.

49. Wolfe MW. Intracranial hemorrhage during systemic anticoagulation in patients with cerebral metastasis. Arch Intern Med 1988; 148:1878–1879 (letter).

50. So W, Hugenholtz A, Richard MT. Complications of anticoagulant therapy in patients with known central nervous system lesions. Can J Surg 1983;26:181–183.

51. Yapor WY, Gutierrez FA. Cocaine-induced intratumoral hemorrhage: case report and review of the literature. Neurosurgery 1992;30: 288–291.

52. Brougham M, Heusner AP, Adams RD. Acute degenerative changes in adenomas of the pituitary body—with special reference to pituitary apoplexy. J Neurosurg 1950;7: 421–439.

53. Weisberg LA. Pituitary apoplexy: association of degenerative change in pituitary adenoma with radiotherapy and detection by cerebral computed tomography. Am J Med 1977; 63:109–115.

54. Mohr G, Hardy J. Hemorrhage, necrosis, and apoplexy in pituitary adenomas. Surg Neurol 1982;18:181–189.

55. Wakai S, Fukushima T, Teramoto A, et al. Pituitary apoplexy: its incidence and clinical significance. J Neurosurg 1981;55:187–193.

56. Mohanty S, Tandon PN, Banerji AK, et al. Haemorrhage into pituitary adenomas. J Neurol Neurosurg Psychiat 1977;40:987–991.

57. Ostrov SG, Quencer RM, Hoffman JC, et al. Hemorrhage within pituitary adenomas: how often associated with pituitary apoplexy syndrome? Am J Neuroradiol 1989;10:503–510.

58. Rovit RL, Fein JM. Pituitary apoplexy: a review and reappraisal. J Neurosurg 1972;37: 280–288.

59. Nourizadeh AR, Pitts FW. Hemorrhage into pituitary adenoma during anticoagulant therapy. JAMA 1965;193:623–625.

60. Post MJD, David NJ, Glaser JS, Safran A. Pituitary apoplexy: diagnosis by computed tomography. Radiology 1980;134:665–670.

61. Fujimoto M, Yoshino E, Ueguchi T, et al. Fluid blood density level demonstrated by computerized tomography in pituitary apoplexy: report of two cases. J Neurosurg 1981;55: 143–144.

62. El-Banhawy A, Walter W. Meningiomas with acute onset. Acta Neurochir 1962;10:194–206.

63. Skultety F M. Meningioma simulating ruptured aneurysm. J Neurosurg 1968;28: 380–382.

64. Gruszkiewicz J, Doron Y, Gellei B, et al. Massive intracranial bleeding due to supratentorial meningioma. Neurochirugia 1969;12: 107–111.

65. Everett BA, Kusske JA, Pribram HW. Anticoagulants and intracerebral hemorrhage from an unsuspected meningioma. Surg Neurol 1979;11:233–235.

66. Sze G, Krol G, Olsen WL, et al. Hemorrhagic neoplasms: MR mimics of occult vascular malformations. Am J Neuroradiol 1987;8:795–802.

67. Young RC, Howser DM, Anderson T, et al. Central nervous system complications of non-Hodgkin's lymphoma: the potential role for prophylactic therapy. Am J Med 1979; 66:435–443.

68. MacKintosh FR, Colby TV, Podolsky WJ, et al. Central nervous system involvement in non-Hodgkin's lymphoma: an analysis of 105 cases. Cancer 1982;49:586–595.

69. Snider WD, Simpson DM, Aronyk KE, et al. Primary lymphoma of the nervous system associated with acquired immune-deficiency syndrome. N Engl J Med 1983;308:45 (letter).

70. Helle TL, Britt RH, Colby TV. Primary lymphoma of the nervous system: clinicopathological study of experience at Stanford. J Neurosurg 1984;60:94–103.

71. Bogdahn U, Bogdahn S, Mertens HG, et al. Primary non-Hodgkin's lymphomas of the CNS. Acta Neurol Scand 1986;73:602–614.

72. Hochberg FH, Miller DC. Primary central nervous system lymphoma. J Neurosurg 1988; 68:835–853.

73. Enzmann DR, Krikorian J, Norman D, et al. Computed tomography in primary reticulum cell sarcoma of the brain. Radiology 1979; 130:165–170.

74. Tadmor R, Davis KR, Roberson GH, et al. Computed tomography in primary malignant lymphomas of the brain. J Comput Assist Tomogr 1978;2:135–140.

75. Kazner E, Wilske J, Steinhoff H, et al. Computed tomography in primary malignant

lymphomas of the brain. J Comput Assist Tomogr 1978;2:125–134.

76. Hardwidge C, Diengdoh JV, Husband D, et al. Primary cerebral lymphoma—a clinicopathological study. Clin Neuropathol 1990;9: 217–223.

77. Epstein F, Rasagopalah M. Pediatric posterior fossa tumors: hazards of "preoperative" shunt. Neurosurgery 1978;3:348–350.

78. Zuccarello M, Dollo C, Carollo C. Spontaneous intratumoral hemorrhage after ventriculoperitoneal shunting. Neurosurgery 1985;16: 245–246.

79. Reichenthal E, Rubinstein AB, Cohen ML. Infratentorial intratumoral hemorrhage. Mt Sinai J Med 1989;56:309–314.

80. McCormick WF, Ugajin K. Fatal hemorrhage into medulloblastoma. J Neurosurg 1967;26: 78–81.

81. Gordon DL, Biller J, Moore SA, et al. Thalamic ependymoma presenting as recurrent subarachnoid hemorrhage. J Stroke Cerebrovasc Dis 1992;2:106–109.

82. Husain MM, Metzer S, Binet EF. Multiple intraparenchymal brain plasmacytomas with spontaneous intratumoral hemorrhage. Neurosurgery 1987;20:619–623.

83. McCarthy J, Proctor SJ. Cerebral involvement in multiple myeloma: case report. J Clin Pathol 1978;31:259–264.

84. Harper L, LeBlanc HJ, McDowell JR. Intracranial extension and spontaneous hemorrhage of a sphenoid plasmacytoma. Neurosurgery 1982;11:797–799.

85. Kase CS. Intracerebral hemorrhage: nonhypertensive causes. Stroke 1986;17:590–595.

86. Iwama T, Ohkuma A, Miwa Y, et al. Brain tumors manifesting as intracranial hemorrhage. Neurol Med Chir 1992;32:130–135.

87. Atlas SW, Grossman RI, Gomori JM, et al. Hemorrhagic intracranial malignant neoplasms: spin-echo MR imaging. Radiology 1987;164:71–77.

88. Gomori JM, Grossman RI, Goldberg HI, et al. Intracranial hematomas: imaging by high-field MR. Radiology 1985;157:87–93.

89. Leeds NE, Sawaya R, Van Tassel P, et al. Intracranial hemorrhage in the oncologic patient. Neuroimaging Clin N Amer 1991;2: 119–136.

90. Gomori J, Grossman R, Goldberg H, et al. Occult cerebral vascular malformations: high-field MR imaging. Radiology 1986;158: 707–713.

91. Kramer R, Wing S. Computed tomography of angiographically occult cerebral vascular malformations. Radiology 1977;123:649–652.

92. Kucharczyk W, Lemme-Pleghos L, Uske A, et al. Intracranial vascular malformations: MR and CT imaging. Radiology 1985;156:383–389.

93. Lemme-Pleghos L, Kucharczyk W, Brant-Zawadzki M, et al. MR imaging of angiographically occult vascular malformations. Am J Neuroradiol 1986;7:217–222.

94. New P, Ojemann R, Davis K, et al. MR and CT of occult vascular malformations of the brain. Am J Neuroradiol 1986;7:771–779.

# Chapter 13
# Vasculitis and Other Angiopathies

## Carlos S. Kase

A large number of heterogeneous conditions that affect the cerebral blood vessels can result in their rupture and hemorrhage. Some of these are inflammatory (vasculitis), while others are of less clear pathogenesis (moyamoya disease, arterial dissection, vascular changes related to migraine). The discussion that follows emphasizes the various forms of vascular disease, inflammatory and noninflammatory, that are known to cause intracranial hemorrhage, especially intracerebral hemorrhage (ICH).

## Vasculitis

Vasculitis is characterized by inflammation of blood vessels, which usually results in vascular occlusion and cerebral infarction, and less often leads to vessel rupture and hemorrhage. Vascular inflammation can produce necrosis of vessel walls, at times with pseudoaneurysm formation, both lesions having the potential for rupture with resulting hemorrhage, either subarachnoid or intracerebral.

The causes of vasculitis are multiple. Some correspond to the cerebral manifestation of a systemic disorder, others occur as primary cerebral vasculitis, while others are the result of secondary foci originating from bacterial or fungal infections elsewhere in the body. The causes of vasculitis, as outlined by

Cohen and Biller,[1] are listed in Table 13.1. Among the multiple vasculitic disorders, some have been associated with intracranial hemorrhage in isolated instances, while others often have hemorrhagic complications as a feature of their clinical course. This discussion addresses the latter group of diseases.

### Necrotizing Vasculitis

#### Polyarteritis Nodosa

Polyarteritis nodosa (PAN) is a systemic disorder characterized by necrotizing vasculitis of medium and small arteries. Its clinical manifestations are protean due to the widespread character of the vasculitis, which affects virtually all organs, with the exception of the lung and spleen.[2] Common clinical findings include fever, malaise, weight loss, headache, abdominal pain and gastrointestinal hemorrhage, arthralgias, skin rash, hypertension, congestive heart failure, and renal failure. Laboratory evaluation often shows anemia, leukocytosis, eosinophilia, elevated sedimentation rate, hematuria, and proteinuria. Arkin[3] listed the frequency of involvement of the various organs as follows: kidneys 80%, heart 70%, liver 65%, gastrointestinal tract 50%, pancreas 25%, mesenteric artery 30%, muscles 30%, periph-

**Table 13.1.** Vasculitic Syndromes

Primary Necrotizing Vasculitides
  Polyarteritis nodosa*
  Allergic granulomatosis and angiitis
  Necrotizing systemic vasculitis overlap syn-
    drome
  Wegener's granulomatosis*
  Lymphomatoid granulomatosis

Vasculitis Associated with Systemic Disease
  Systemic lupus erythematosus*
  Rheumatoid arthritis*
  Sjögren's syndrome
  Scleroderma
  Dermatomyositis-polymyositis
  Sarcoidosis*
  Behçet's syndrome*
  Ulcerative colitis
  Relapsing polychondritis
  Kohlmeier-Degos disease
  X-linked lymphoproliferative syndrome

Giant Cell Arteritides
  Takayasu's arteritis
  Temporal (cranial) arteritis

Hypersensitivity Vasculitides
  Henoch-Schönlein purpura
  Drug-induced vasculitides†
  Chemical vasculitides
  Essential mixed cryoglobulinemia
  Vasculitis associated with malignancy

Vasculitis Associated with Infection
  Bacterial*
  Treponemal
  Fungal*
  Rickettsial
  Viral*

Other Noninfectious Vasculitides
  Cogan's syndrome
  Eale's syndrome
  Thromboangiitis obliterans

Primary Central Nervous System Vasculitis*

(From Cohen BA, Biller J. Hemorrhagic stroke due to cerebral vasculitis and the role of immunosuppressive
  therapy. Neurosurg Clin NA 1992;3:611–624, with
  permission.)
*Conditions in which intracranial hemorrhage is either a
  likely complication or has been well documented in
  the literature.
†This group of drug-related hemorrhages are described
  separately in Chapter 10.

eral nerves 20%, central nervous system
(CNS) 8%. The higher frequency of peripheral nerve involvement, in comparison with
CNS involvement, has been since amply
documented. In fact, peripheral neuropathy
is the most common neurological feature of
PAN.[2]

CNS involvement, alone or in combination with peripheral neuropathy, occurs in
29%[4] to 46%[5] of the patients. Common symptoms of brain dysfunction include headache,
mental changes (delirium, hallucinations,
delusions, mania, paranoia; cognitive impairment; decreased level of consciousness,
often fluctuating), hemiparesis, brainstem
signs, and convulsions, with prominent
changes of acute retinopathy with hemorrhages and exudates on funduscopic examination.[5] The frequency of intracranial hemorrhagic complications is difficult to assess
from the literature. Instances of purely subarachnoid hemorrhage (SAH) have been
documented.[4–6] Summers[6] reported a 35-
year-old man with a fatal SAH due to a ruptured aneurysm of the left posterior cerebral
artery. The diagnosis of PAN with multisystem involvement was only made at autopsy,
which also showed occlusion of the right
middle cerebral artery (MCA). Although it
was implied that the cerebral vasculitis was
responsible for the occurrence of the aneurysm with SAH, there was no microscopic
description of the vasculitis and its relationship to the aneurysm. Griffith and Vural[4]
found one patient with "subarachnoid and
intracerebral" hemorrhage among nine patients with PAN who had postmortem examinations. Although the gross brain pathological findings were not described, the history
was suggestive of acute intracranial hemorrhage (SAH and ICH), assumed secondary to
cerebral vasculitis, without mention of aneurysm or other focal vascular lesion at the site
of the hemorrhage. A more detailed description of intracranial hemorrhagic events in patients with PAN was provided by Ford and
Siekert.[5] They found cerebrovascular lesions,
either infarcts or hemorrhages, in fifteen

(13%) of 114 patients. These included one example of SAH, three recent ICH (frontal lobar, basal ganglionic, and cerebellar, one each), and one old parietal lobar ICH, all documented at postmortem examination. Another patient had a clinical picture compatible with fulminant intracranial hemorrhage, but there was no autopsy performed. A single example of a massive, fatal parietal lobar ICH in a 46-year-old woman with PAN was described in detail by Hiller.[7] The patient had a large (4 cm by 4 cm by 10 cm) superficial clot in the right parietal lobe, and widespread necrotizing vasculitis with profuse inflammatory exudates that extended from the vessel wall into the adjacent brain parenchyma. Although the patient had developed hypertension at the time of the onset of CNS symptoms five days before death, postmortem examination failed to show vascular changes suggestive of hypertensive arteriopathy. The author concluded that the patient's fatal ICH was most likely secondary to rupture of small cortical arteries damaged by the necrotizing arteritis.

In conclusion, cerebrovascular manifestations in PAN are common, as either infarction or hemorrhage, the latter occurring in the brain parenchyma more often than in the subarachnoid space. The likely sources of bleeding are ruptured arteries whose walls have been rendered necrotic by PAN. The additional contribution of other factors, such as hypertension and formation of pseudoaneurysms, in causing hemorrhages is currently unclear.

*Wegener's Granulomatosis*

This form of necrotizing vasculitis is similar to PAN, although its clinical manifestations are more restricted. It involves the upper (nasal cavity, paranasal sinuses) and lower (lungs, bronchi, trachea) respiratory tract and the kidneys by a process of necrotizing vasculitis that affects both arteries and veins.[2] Neurological involvement in Wegener's granulomatosis favors the peripheral and cranial nerves, although cerebrovascular lesions secondary to the vasculitis are well recognized. These can take the form of arterial or venous occlusions resulting in infarction[8,9] or, more often, intracranial hemorrhages. Clinically symptomatic hemorrhages have been described in the subarachnoid space and in the parenchyma. Tuhy et al.[8] reported a 39-year-old man who died as a result of SAH four months after onset of upper respiratory and systemic symptoms of Wegener's granulomatosis. The terminal neurological event began suddenly and was characterized by headache, vomiting, neck stiffness, and progressive decline in level of consciousness into coma, with hemorrhagic CSF. Postmortem findings included extensive SAH, and a large volume of blood (150 ml) "in the posterior fossa," without further description, except for "some hemorrhage within the cerebellar substance as well." No vascular malformations were present. It is possible that hemorrhage occurred at various sites intracranially (in the meninges and cerebellar parenchyma) as well as systemically, since multiple hemorrhagic foci were also described in other areas of the body. A second patient reported by Tuhy et al.,[8] a 46-year-old man, died one year after onset of symptoms, without having clinical episodes suggestive of stroke. At postmortem examination however, multiple "foci of acute hemorrhage" in the right frontal pole and left parietal area were present in the brain surface. These lesions coexisted with multiple small foci of brain infarction of different ages, some of them apparently with hemorrhagic features. MacFadyen[10] described a 42-year-old man with large, fatal bilateral thalamic hemorrhages. The patient died after several months of illness, after suddenly developing signs of apparently bihemispheric lesions (aphasia, left hemiplegia) that rapidly resulted in coma and death. Bilateral, "massive" thalamic hemorrhages at necropsy were associated with the finding of fibrinoid necrosis and perivascular inflammation in adjacent small blood vessels. The author attributed the hemorrhages to the combined effects of Wegener's vasculitis and hypertension, the latter resulting from the renal involvement ("glomerulitis") that was also present.

In an extensive review of the neurological complications of Wegener's granulomatosis, Drachman[11] emphasized the high frequency (54%, or 56 of 104 reported patients) of involvement of the peripheral and central nervous system. He added one personal observation of a 30-year-old man who died after ten months of symptoms. The patient had an episode of disorientation and confusion, and hypertension (220/120), with CSF under high pressure (300 mm of water) and with 100 red blood cells, three months before death. Although he recovered from that episode without residual neurological deficits, he continued to have occasional episodes of confusion. At postmortem examination, a focal area of SAH was found in the right frontal parasagittal area, next to a branch of the anterior cerebral artery that contained a recent thrombus and severe infiltration of its wall by inflammatory cells. Multiple other smaller foci of infarction, some of them hemorrhagic, were described throughout the cerebral hemispheres and brainstem. The focal right frontal SAH was thought to be due to rupture of an adjacent superficial artery affected by severe vasculitis, whereas the multiple foci of infarction were likely the result of vasculitis and fibrinoid necrosis of adjacent small arteries.[11] Drachman estimated that vasculitis is the most frequent cause of neurological complications in Wegener's granulomatosis. In a recent review of 324 patients with Wegener's granulomatosis, Nishino et al.[12] reported neurologic complications in 109 (33.6%), only thirteen of whom had cerebrovascular events. These corresponded to cerebral infarction in twelve patients, and a subdural hematoma (SDH) without obvious trauma in one patient.

In conclusion, SAH and ICH are rare complications of Wegener's granulomatosis, are often a late occurrence in the course of the disease, and can occasionally be the cause of death.

## Vasculitis Associated with Systemic Disease

### Systemic Lupus Erythematosus

Systemic lupus erythematosus (SLE) can affect virtually any organ of the body, and CNS involvement is frequent. The mechanism of the CNS lesions is still difficult to document in a given patient, but the frequent finding of vascular lesions in autopsy series[13,14] suggests that a vascular pathogenesis is the likely cause of some neurological presentations. The actual frequency of "true" vasculitis (defined as inflammatory cells invading vessel walls) as opposed to mere perivascular collections of inflammatory cells (which can be secondary to adjacent processes of necrosis, infection, or inflammation), is probably low in SLE. In autopsy studies, CNS vasculitis occurred in three of the twenty-four (12.5%) patients reported by Johnson and Richardson,[13] and in four of fifty-seven (7%) in the series of Ellis and Verity.[14] Other vascular lesions, including perivascular inflammation, vascular hyalinization, endothelial proliferation, and fibrin thrombi formation, occur more frequently. Some of these changes, which generally affect small blood vessels, may account for the frequent finding of multiple microinfarcts in brains of patients with SLE.[13,14]

Intracranial hemorrhage in SLE has been a relatively frequent finding in autopsy series, and isolated examples have also been reported clinically. Ellis and Verity[14] found CNS hemorrhage in twenty-four of fifty-seven (42%) patients, the most common type being SAH (seventeen patients, or 30%), whereas ICH occurred in six (10%) patients. These authors found a strong correlation between the presence of vasculitis and the occurrence of both types of hemorrhage: five instances of SAH occurred among seven patients (71%) with vasculitis, whereas the remaining twelve examples of SAH occurred among the fifty patients (24%) who did not have vasculitis. A similar relationship existed for ICH, as three hemorrhages were found among the seven patients (43%) with vasculitis, while the other three hemorrhages occurred in the fifty patients (6%) without vasculitis. Johnson and Richardson,[13] in a detailed postmortem study of twenty-four patients with SLE, found three examples of large hemispheric ICH (12.5%), one with multiple pontine hemorrhages, two with multiple small hemorrhages, and one with an incidental small subpial hemorrhage. Among the four patients with large hemorrhages, all of whom presented clinically with a stroke-like syndrome prior to death, two had evidence of vasculitis and the other two showed vascular necrosis, these lesions being the likely explanation for the hemorrhages. Although vasculitis was found in only three of twenty-four (12.5%) patients in this series, two of the three large, clinically relevant hemispheric ICHs occurred in patients with vasculitis, further suggesting that this vascular lesion is strongly correlated with this complication of SLE.

The examples of intracranial hemorrhage in SLE have been generally attributed to vascular lesions affecting small intraparenchymal or meningeal vessels, including arterioles and capillaries.[13] On occasion, however, focal inflammatory involvement of medium or large extraparenchymal vessels has been documented, leading to massive extracerebral hemorrhage. Harvey et al.,[15] in discussing causes of death in patients with SLE, briefly described a patient who died "with a massive cerebral hemorrhage when a small aneurysm associated with lupus arteritis ruptured." Kelley et al.[16] reported a 29-year-old woman with SLE nephropathy and hypertension, who developed SAH secondary to rupture of a fusiform aneurysm of the left posterior communicating artery, a vessel that also showed angiographic irregularity suggestive of vasculitis. She developed right hemiparesis and aphasia on day 4, presumed secondary to post-SAH vasospasm with infarction in the left MCA territory. Despite partial resolution of the subarachnoid blood on computed tomography (CT), she died three weeks after onset of the SAH. Postmortem examination demonstrated a ruptured

fusiform aneurysm at the junction of the left internal carotid and posterior communicating arteries. Extensive transmural, and to a lesser degree perivascular, inflammation was present focally at the site of aneurysmal rupture, with associated fragmentation of the internal elastic lamina and focal subintimal proliferation. No organisms were demonstrated histologically or on culture. Similarly, Sasaki et al.[17] reported two patients with SLE, one with SAH, the other with a SDH, which were caused by pathologically documented ruptured aneurysms at sites of transmural angiitis. The patient with SAH, a 22-year-old woman, died as a result of the hemorrhage, and postmortem examination showed five fusiform aneurysms (two in the left internal carotid artery, three in the left MCA), all of which showed extensive transmural inflammation of the arterial wall. The other patient presented with a right frontal SDH, and cerebral angiography revealed a small aneurysm of the right anterior cerebral artery. This lesion was removed at the time of surgical drainage of the SDH, and it showed transmural angiitis on histological examination. In neither patient was an infectious mechanism for the aneurysms found.

In summary, intracranial hemorrhage in patients with SLE can have different forms, either intracerebral from rupture of small intraparenchymal vessels affected by vasculitis, or subarachnoid as a result of rupture of aneurysms of larger extracerebral arteries at sites of focal transmural angiitis.

*Rheumatoid Arthritis*

The neurological complications of rheumatoid arthritis are usually the result of the bony abnormalities that characterize the disease, the most serious one being cervical cord compression from atlantoaxial subluxation. Intracranial complications are rare. Occasional patients develop cranial nerve or cerebral lesions secondary to adjacent rheumatoid nodules, usually in the meninges.[18] Steiner and Gelbloom[18] found these lesions associated with local subarachnoid and sub-dural blood collections at postmortem examination. However, the clinical significance of the areas of local bleeding and their relationship with findings of "active vasculitis" in subarachnoid space vessels is difficult to assess from that report, since the patient died with severe purulent meningitis, which could have been responsible for some of the vascular changes.

A clear example of ICH from rheumatoid vasculitis was reported by Watson et al.[19] A 54-year-old woman with a twenty-year history of rheumatoid arthritis suddenly developed signs of left cerebral hemisphere and left pontine involvement. After an initial partial improvement while on corticosteroids, she eventually died six months later, as a result of pneumonia. At postmortem examination, fresh right frontal lobar and basal pontine ICH were present, along with older, partially reabsorbed left frontal and basal pontine hematomas. Microscopically, necrotizing vasculitis of small and medium arteries was found in the areas of the hematomas. Similar vascular changes were present in other areas of cerebrum, brainstem, and cerebellum, which were not affected by hemorrhage. More recently, an example of a small ICH in a 48-year-old woman with rheumatoid arthritis was reported by Gobernado et al.[20] The patient developed a small right temporal lobe hemorrhage, with extensive post-contrast enhancement of the subarachnoid space over the cerebral convexities. Cerebral angiography showed multiple areas of segmental narrowing of medium size arteries in middle cerebral, posterior cerebral, and posterior-inferior cerebellar artery territories, interpreted as representing vasculitis. Her clinical deficits gradually resolved following a course of corticosteroid treatment.

In summary, rare instances of intracranial hemorrhage have been reported in patients with rheumatoid arthritis and cerebral vasculitis. This complication appears to be less common in this disease, in comparison with PAN and SLE.

## Sarcoidosis

Sarcoidosis is a granulomatosis that affects the lymphatic system as well as the lungs and other organs. Ocular involvement occurs in approximately 50% of the patients, whereas the CNS is affected in about 5% of the patients.[21] The CNS involvement generally occurs in the early phases of the disease, whereas sarcoidosis of the peripheral nervous system and skeletal muscle is seen in the chronic stage.[21] The main form of presentation of CNS sarcoidosis is with meningeal granulomas which preferentially affect the basal meninges, resulting in clinical presentations with cranial nerve and hypophyseal-hypothalamic involvement.

The occurrence of vasculitis in sarcoidosis is well known, but its true frequency, nosology, and clinical significance are debated. In pathological reports, the presence of non-caseating sarcoid granulomas in the adventitia of blood vessels (arteries and veins) is commonplace. At times, these granulomas involve the vessel wall as well, extending into the media and elastic layers, occasionally leading to vessel wall necrosis with occlusion and resulting infarction.[22] In instances in which the vessel wall is prominently affected by a granulomatous inflammation, a clear distinction between sarcoid vasculitis and "granulomatous angiitis of the CNS" becomes problematic.[23] Sarcoid vasculitis seems to preferentially involve veins, causing periphlebitis. In the retina, sheething of veins and exudates are manifestations of this periphlebitis. The labeling of a case as the "angiitic form of neurosarcoidosis" has to be based not only on the occurrence of adventitial granulomas, but also on the presence of inflammation and necrosis of the vessel wall, generally associated with occlusion.[24]

The occurrence of ICH as a complication of neurosarcoidosis is rare. No examples of stroke, ischemic or hemorrhagic, were encountered by Delaney[21] in his series of twenty-three patients with neurosarcoidosis. Rottino and Hoffman[25] reported an unusual

37-year-old man with Hodgkin's disease who developed a fatal left frontoparietal ICH, and was found at postmortem examination to have granulomatous lesions with a predilection for blood vessels and perivascular spaces. The vascular lesions varied in severity, but examples of panvasculitis with noncaseating granuloma formation were present, without features suggestive of Hodgkin's disease or infection by mycobacterial or fungal organisms. The blood vessels adjacent to the ICH were not described in detail, and no actual vascular bleeding site was identified. This report illustrates the difficulties in distinguishing "sarcoid angiitis" from "granulomatous angiitis of the CNS," the latter being an entity that can be associated with a systemic malignancy. In analyzing Rottino and Hoffman's patient,[25] a diagnosis of "neoplastic-associated granulomatous angiitis of the nervous system" was favored in the review of Cohen and Biller.[1]

A clear example of ICH related to sarcoid angiitis was reported by Caplan et al.[26] The patient, a 21-year-old man with sarcoidosis confirmed by lymph node biopsy, developed a left cerebellar hemorrhage (Figure 13.1) that rapidly led to coma and death. At postmortem examination, in addition to the finding of multiple meningeal epithelioid granulomas, similar lesions affected the adventitia of arteries and the entire walls of veins. These vascular lesions were the presumed mechanism of hemorrhage in the left cerebellar hemisphere and brachium pontis.

In conclusion, sarcoidosis of the CNS occasionally produces a true angiitis, most often a periphlebitis that is distinguishable from other forms of granulomatous CNS vasculitis, and this condition is rarely associated with ICH.

### Behçet's Disease

Behçet's disease is a multisystem disorder characterized by relapsing oral and genital "aphthous" ulcers and ocular inflammation. Frequently associated systemic features include arthritis, thrombophlebitis, colitis, and neurological disorders.[27] Neurological involvement occurs in approximately 25% to 30% of patients with Behçet's disease,[28,29] generally years after disease onset. This takes the form of recurrent episodes of meningoencephalitis, with prominent involvement of deep hemispheric and brainstem areas, where pathological examination shows tissue necrosis and adjacent foci of vasculitis affecting small arteries and venules (Figure 13.2). Occasional aneurysms are present in peripheral arteries,[30] but they have not been described in cerebral arteries.

The clinical presentation in neuro-Behçet's disease is with recurrent episodes of a febrile illness accompanied by cranial nerve involvement, pyramidal and cerebellar tract dysfunction, and CSF findings of increased protein, normal sugar, and predominantly mononuclear pleocytosis.[27–29] Stroke syndromes as a form of neurological presentation in Behçet's disease are rare, and no examples were reported in the series of Chajek and Fainaru[28] and O'Duffy and Goldstein,[29] which included the analysis of twelve and seven patients with neuro-Behçet's disease, respectively. Similarly, a 36-year-old man (Case 2) reported by Kozin et al.[27] had the acute onset of right hemiparesis and aphasia, possibly suggestive of a vascular mechanism, but work-up and stereotactic aspiration biopsy only suggested a necrotic left basal ganglionic lesion, with angiographic signs of avascular mass effect, without vascular occlusions or features suggestive of cerebral vasculitis being mentioned. The patient developed a syndrome of "toxic megacolon," and surgical biopsy documented multiple ulcerations of the mucosa, with "florid vasculitis" at the base of the ulcers.

Instances of ICH in Behçet's disease have been rarely reported. Nagata[31] described a 50-year-old Japanese man who carried the diagnosis of Behçet's disease since age 42, at which point he was also diagnosed as having hypertension. He presented to the hospital with the acute onset of left hemiataxia, with

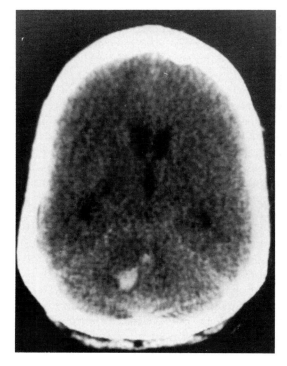

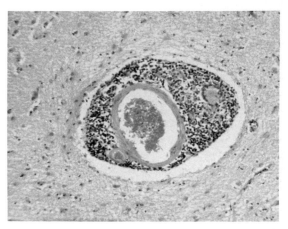

C

A

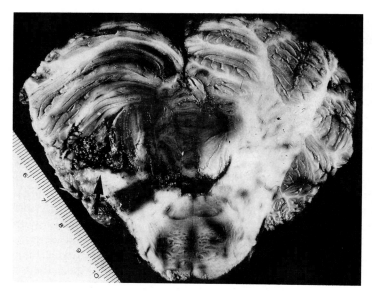

B

**Figure 13.1.** ICH in a 21-year-old man with neurosarcoidosis. (A) CT showing small left cerebellar hemorrhage with extension into the fourth ventricle. (B) Postmortem specimen showing hemorrhage in the left cerebellar hemisphere (arrow). (C) Cellular infiltration by lymphocytes and giant cells in the perivascular space of a small artery. (H&E, ×230.) (From Caplan L, Corbett J, Goodwin J, et al. Neuro-ophthalmologic signs in the angiitic form of neurosarcoidosis. Neurology 1983;33:1130–1135, with permission.)

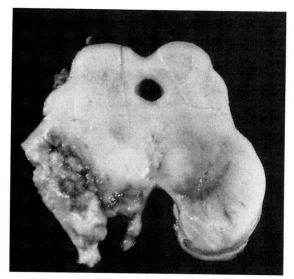

A

**Figure 13.2.** (A) Necrosis of the right cerebral peduncle, substantia nigra and red nucleus in a 35-year-old woman with Behçet's disease. (B) Mononuclear inflammatory infiltrate in the wall of a vein, with foamy macrophages in the perivascular space, near a focus of necrosis. (H&E, ×400.)

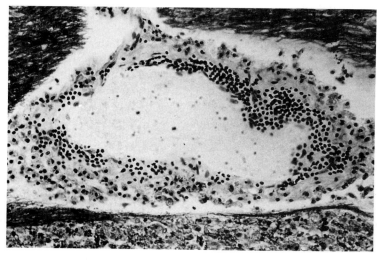

B

blood pressure of 240/120, and CT showed a large left cerebellar hemorrhage. He remained severely hypertensive despite treatment, and subsequently developed a left and then a right basal ganglia hemorrhage, seven and fifty-three days after onset of the cerebellar hemorrhage, respectively. He died sixty-five days after onset of the initial ICH. Postmortem examination revealed "slight lymphocytic infiltration around the small blood vessels in the cerebral white matter," along with "marked hypertensive arterial changes" in the form of thickening of the vessel walls, hyalinosis, and fibrinoid degeneration, most prominently in the small arteries in the basal ganglia. The author concluded that these findings indicated that the likely cause of the patient's unusual multiple hemorrhages was the presence of hypertensive cerebrovascular disease, rather than the vasculitis of Behçet's disease. Altinörs et al.[32] reported a 26-year-old normotensive man with Behçet's disease for about two years, who developed a right temporoparietal ICH, from which he had good recovery following nonsurgical treatment. Cerebral angiography was reported as normal, and fluorescein retinal angiography showed "findings of vasculitis." The ICH was interpreted as secondary to vasculitis, although no further proof of such mechanism was available.

With the use of MRI, Al Kawi et al.[33] showed that microhemorrhages may be observed in the evolution of patients with Behçet's disease. They documented the presence of a hypodense hemosiderin ring surrounding a central focus of hyperintensity in T2-weighted sequences in MRI performed after the acute phase of the illness. They interpreted this finding as indicative of small foci of hemorrhage or diapedesis of red blood cells in the acute stage, with the expected progression into hypodense areas in T2-weighted MRI images as a result of the formation of hemosiderin.

A more common cerebrovascular complication of Behçet's disease is venous occlusion. Among thirty-eight patients with angiographically documented cerebral venous thrombosis reported by Bousser et al.,[34] six (16%) had Behçet's disease. None of these patients presented with ICH or hemorrhagic venous infarcts however, but rather with syndromes of intracranial hypertension without hyper- or hypodense lesions on CT scan in the three patients who had this test performed. Among 250 patients with Behçet's disease from the same institution, twenty-five (10%) had cerebral venous thrombosis documented angiographically.[35] The dural sinuses were mainly involved, the most common clinical presentation was intracranial hypertension (twenty of twenty-five patients, or 80%), at times associated with either focal deficits (in eight patients, or 32%), or seizures (in five patients, or 20%), but no examples of ICH or hemorrhagic infarction were recorded in the twenty-two patients who had CT scans. Only one patient had MRI features suggestive of hemorrhagic infarction, without hyperdense areas on CT, while being treated with anticoagulants.

In summary, although Behçet's disease is frequently associated with CNS involvement and evidence of vasculitis, cerebrovascular events are rare, and the reported instances of ICH do not support a convincing causal relationship with the systemic disease. Venous occlusive phenomena, with involvement of intracranial dural sinuses and veins, are more common cerebrovascular findings in this disease, but patients with dural sinus occlusions often present with a syndrome of intracranial hypertension rather than with ICH or hemorrhagic infarction.

### Infectious Vasculitis

A number of organisms have a propensity to involve cerebral blood vessels, causing either thrombosis or rupture, the latter resulting in ICH or SAH. The infectious agents can be carried into the cerebral vasculature by septic embolization, generally secondary to bacterial endocarditis, or by spread from contiguous septic intracranial processes, such as meningitis, dural sinus thrombophlebitis, skull osteomyelitis, or after neurosurgical interventions. Bacteria, fungi, and viruses have all been known to cause intracranial hemorrhagic complications.

#### Bacterial Infections

Bacterial infections have been recognized as a source of secondary arterial involvement since Osler, in 1885, reported the findings of debris in an aortic arch aneurysm that were similar to those formed in the infected heart valves. He used the term "mycotic" only to refer to the infectious character of the endocarditis. Following this early description, an impressive body of information has been gathered on the vascular septic complications of bacterial infections, especially infectious endocarditis.

*Infectious endocarditis* is often associated with neurological complications. The frequency of neurological involvement has been estimated to be approximately 25% to 30%,[36–39] although some modern series have reported frequencies as high as 56%.[40] In bacterial endocarditis that occurs as a late (after sixty days) complication of prosthetic valve replacement, neurological complications have been documented in 40% of patients.[41] In 6% to 15% of patients with bacterial endocarditis, the neurological complication is the presenting feature of the disease.[42]

In the older literature, bacterial endocarditis was usually a complication of rheumatic heart disease, and the predominant responsible agent was the low virulence *Streptococcus viridans*, this combination resulting in most of the cases of subacute bacterial endocarditis.[36] Less often, acute bacterial endocarditis was caused by the more virulent *Staphylococcus aureus*. A number of changes have occurred in the presentation of bacterial endocarditis during the past two decades:[38,39] (1) rheumatic heart disease has become less common, while other cardiac disorders (congenital heart disease, malformed aortic valves, mitral valve prolapse, aortic sclerosis, mitral annulus calcification, prosthetic heart valves) are often the underlying pathology;[39] (2) intravenous drug use has dramatically increased as an important cause of heart valve infection;[39,43] (3) there is an increase in nosocomial sources of bacterial endocarditis, resulting from the widespread use of intravascular catheters and other devices, as well as manipulations of the gastrointestinal and genitourinary tracts;[38,39] (4) the organisms responsible for bacterial endocarditis have changed over the years with an increase in infections due to *Staphylococcus aureus*, fungi, and other agents, resulting in a proportionately lower frequency of *Streptococcus viridans* as the cause of the infection;[38–40] (5) despite an improvement in the bacteriological techniques of organism identification and antibiotic treatment, the mortality of bacterial endocarditis remains high, in particular for patients who develop neurological complications. The mortality for those with CNS signs

has been reported to be 50% to 83%, whereas for those without neurological complications it is 20% to 26%.[37,38,40] The overall mortality is 1.6 to 3.2 times greater in patients with neurological complications, especially intracranial hemorrhage and meningitis, and in those with infection caused by *Staphylococcus aureus*.[39,40]

The neurological complications of bacterial endocarditis occur more frequently with involvement of the mitral valve than the aortic valve.[38,40] Pruitt et al.[38] found neurological complications in 52% (forty-two patients) of eighty-one patients with mitral valve infection, as opposed to 28% (twenty-one of seventy-four patients) in those with aortic valve endocarditis. A similar predominance of mitral valve involvement has been observed in patients with late prosthetic valve endocarditis with neurological complications. Keyser et al.[41] found neurological complications in five of seven (71%) patients with mitral valve replacement, compared with three of twelve (25%) with aortic valve replacement. These authors also observed a higher frequency of neurological complications with mechanical valves (54.5% or six of eleven patients) as compared with those with bioprosthetic valves (22.2%, or two of nine patients). An additional feature that correlates with a high frequency of neurological complications in bacterial endocarditis, both native and prosthetic, is infection with *Staphylococcus* as opposed to *Streptococcus* species. In the series of Pruitt et al.,[38] neurological complications occurred in twenty-six of forty-nine (53%) patients with staphylococcal infection and in nine of ten (90%) patients with infection by enteric bacteria, as opposed to 37 of 122 (30%) patients with streptococcal infection. This predominance of staphylococcal infection in patients with neurological complications of bacterial endocarditis is in turn associated with an increased mortality in those infected with this agent. Among 110 patients with neurological complications of bacterial endocarditis, Jones et al.[37] observed a mortality of 77% (twenty of twenty-six patients) in those with staphylococcal infections compared with 36% (twenty-six of seventy-two patients) with streptococcal infections.

Cerebrovascular events (especially embolic infarctions) are a common and generally devastating complication of bacterial endocarditis, and they represent approximately 50% of the neurological complications of this disease.[37] Intracranial hemorrhage, both ICH and SAH, although less common than infarction (Table 13.2), carries a poor prognosis. Death was the outcome in ten of eleven (90%) patients with intracranial hemorrhage in the series of Jones et al.,[37] in thirteen of fifteen (87%) patients reported by Le Cam et al.,[40] and in all three (100%) patients with late prosthetic valve endocarditis reported by Keyser et al.[41]

ICH in patients with bacterial endocarditis is variable in its location and size (Figure 13.3), and this may in part reflect the mechanism of the hemorrhage, as well as the effect of anticoagulant treatment in its pathogenesis. Masuda et al.[44] studied sixteen patients with intracranial hemorrhage complicating bacterial endocarditis, twelve of whom presented with ICH. The hemorrhages were generally superficial (lobar) in location, involving cortical and subcortical regions, often in communication with the adjacent subarachnoid space. These features were thought to reflect the mechanism of ICH in bacterial endocarditis. Despite the almost universal assumption in the literature that ICH in bacterial endocarditis results from rupture of mycotic (or bacterial)

aneurysms,[37–39,45] Hart et al.[46] and Masuda et al.[44] found this lesion to be rare[46] or nonexistent[44] in their series. Hart et al.[46] studied seventeen patients with intracranial hemorrhage and bacterial endocarditis, and found mycotic aneurysms in only two patients (12%). The most common mechanisms of ICH were septic erosion of the arterial wall with rupture (but without aneurysm formation), and symptomatic bleeding into areas of embolic brain infarction. Septic vasculitis usually indicated infection with virulent agents, such as *Staphylococcus* species, and the predominantly lobar hemorrhages tended to occur early in the course of the illness, usually within forty-eight hours of admission. At postmortem examination, these examples of pyogenic arteritis were characterized by polymorphonuclear infiltration and necrosis of arterial walls, at times with an associated septic embolus (with abundant organisms enmeshed in fibrin) occluding the lumen. The other mechanism of ICH documented by Hart et al.,[46] in the absence of mycotic aneurysms on pathological or angiographic examination, was hemorrhagic transformation of embolic brain infarcts. Hemorrhagic transformation was more often symptomatic in patients receiving anticoagulants, whereas asymptomatic hemorrhagic infarction occurred in two patients not receiving anticoagulants. These authors thought that anticoagulant treatment contributed to intracranial hemorrhage in four of the seventeen patients (24%). They con-

**Table 13.2.** Type and Frequency of Cerebrovascular Complications of Bacterial Endocarditis

| | | Neurologic Complication | | | |
|---|---|---|---|---|---|
| | | **ICH** | **SAH** | **Mycotic ANR** | **Infarct** |
| **Author** | **N** | **No. Pts. (%)** | **No. Pts. (%)** | **No. Pts. (%)** | **No. Pts. (%)** |
| Jones et al.[37] | 385 | 8 (2.1) | 3 (0.8) | — | 44 (11.4) |
| Pruitt et al.[38] | 218 | 4 (1.8) | 5 (2.3) | 4 (1.8) | 34 (15.6) |
| Le Cam et al.[40] | 86 | 15 (17.5)* | | 4 (4.7) | 25 (29.0) |
| Pankey[36†] | 41 | 9 (22.0)* | | 5 (12.0) | — |

Abbreviations: N = number of patients with bacterial endocarditis, ANR = aneurysm, Pts. = patients.
*Patients labeled as having "intracranial hemorrhage," without distinguishing between ICH and SAH.
†Autopsy data

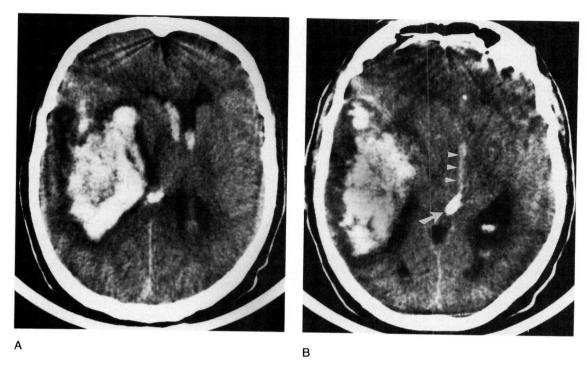

A

B

**Figure 13.3.** Massive fatal basal ganglionic hemorrhage in 65-year-old man with *streptococcus bovis* endocarditis of the aortic valve. (A) Marked midline shift, with ventricular extension of the hemorrhage. (B) Inferior extension of the hemorrhage, with shift of the calcified pineal gland (arrow), and blood in the third ventricle (arrowheads).

cluded that the common link to the three possible mechanisms of ICH in bacterial endocarditis—pyogenic arteritis, mycotic aneurysm, and hemorrhagic transformation of infarction—was septic embolism, which usually caused acute necrosis of the arterial wall in patients infected with virulent organisms (generally *Staphylococcus* species) or more indolent inflammation of the arterial wall that caused the formation of mycotic aneurysms in patients infected by less virulent organisms (*Streptococcus* species). Similar conclusions were reached by Masuda et al.,[44] who studied fifteen postmortem and one surgical patient with intracranial hemorrhage and bacterial endocarditis. Among twelve patients with ICH, no mycotic aneurysms were found, and the causes of ICH were either pyogenic arteritis (eight patients) or hemorrhagic transformation of embolic infarcts

(four patients). Pyogenic arteritis with rupture generally occurred in small cortical arteries localized to sulci and correlated with the predominant cortical or subcortical location of the ICH. These authors[44] found evidence of antecedent cerebral ischemic events in five of the twelve patients with ICH examined postmortem, and postulated that hemorrhagic transformation of ischemic infarction is the most common cause of ICH in patients with bacterial endocarditis, possibly through the mechanism of pyogenic arteritis. The importance of preceding cerebral embolic infarction and concomitant use of anticoagulants in the pathogenesis of ICH had previously been emphasized by Lieberman et al.[47] in an analysis of patients with prosthetic heart valve endocarditis. In two of their six patients, bacterial endocarditis under treatment with anticoagulants was associated with fatal ICH that occurred at the site of a preceding embolic infarct, two months and two days, respectively, before the ICH. In neither patient was the mechanism of ICH documented, since no cerebral angiography or postmortem examination were performed. In conclusion, pathological studies[44,46] have shown a low frequency of mycotic aneurysms as the cause of ICH in patients with bacterial endocarditis, suggesting that other mechanisms, such as hemorrhagic transformation of embolic infarcts and pyogenic arteritis with rupture are more common factors. The latter is probably the likely cause of ICH in patients who have cerebral angiograms that do not show arterial lesions, either mycotic aneurysm or embolic branch occlusions (Figure 13.4).

*Mycotic aneurysms* in bacterial endocarditis have been extensively reported in the literature, in part because of the ease of their demonstration by cerebral angiography. Their frequency varies among the bacterial endocarditis series (see Table 13.2), but they are considered to occur in approximately 2% to 12% of these patients.[36,38,42,45,48–50] On the other hand, mycotic aneurysms accounted for 2.6% (five patients) of a series of 191 patients with intracranial aneurysms reported by Roach and Drake,[50] and 4.4% (thirteen patients) of 296 patients in the series of Frazee et al.[49] However, the true frequency of this lesion is unknown, but is thought to be underestimated,[45,51,52,52a] since these aneurysms are probably often asymptomatic, and their documentation would necessitate the

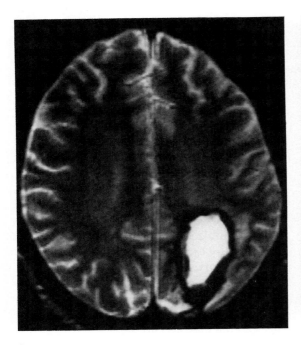

A

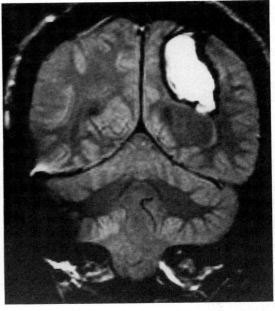

B

**Figure 13.4.** MRI of left superior parietal lobar hemorrhage in a 44-year-old HIV-positive drug abuser with *Actinomyces* bacterial endocarditis. Cerebral angiogram showed only avascular mass effect, without mycotic aneurysm or signs of vasculitis in the area of the hemorrhage. (A) Axial view of the high-signal hemorrhage surrounded by dark hemosiderin ring in T2-weighted image. (B) Coronal view of superior parietal hemorrhage, T2-weighted image (Courtesy of Judy Fine-Edelstein, M.D., Boston VA Medical Center, Boston, MA.)

performance of cerebral angiography in all patients with bacterial endocarditis, regardless of the presence or absence of neurological manifestations. Even routine angiography to detect cerebral mycotic aneurysms, which is neither practiced nor recommended, would be likely to miss detection of some aneurysms. Detection would depend on the timing of angiography, since these lesions are known to resolve during antibiotic treatment when they have been followed with repeated angiograms.[53,54]

Mycotic aneurysms generally occur in young patients, of mean ages in the 30s and 40s and with equal frequency in men and women.[48,49] They are commonly located at bifurcation sites of peripheral branches of the intracranial arteries, distal to the circle of Willis[38,39,46,48–52,55] (Figure 13.5), in comparison with congenital, berry aneurysms that are typically located proximally, in the circle of Willis. Their site of preference is the MCA, where 50% to 80% of these lesions have been described,[38,49,50,52a] the remainder occurring in the anterior and posterior cerebral arteries, the cerebellar arteries, and, rarely, the basilar artery. The majority of mycotic aneurysms are single, but multiple lesions are not rare, having been described in as many as 17.6%[52] and 25%[49] of patients.

The clinical presentation of ICH due to ruptured mycotic aneurysm is often sudden, without premonitory events, except for antecedent embolic cerebral infarction in up to 50% of the patients.[38,39] On occasion, however, prodromal events have been identified. Frazee et al.[49] recognized the importance of sudden severe headache and seizures as events preceding ICH, in two of their patients occurring a few hours before a massive hemorrhage. In other patients, these symptoms, as well as focal neurological deficits, occurred days before the ICH. Wilson et al.[56] also commented on the presence of severe localized headache prior to the onset of ICH in their eight patients with mycotic aneurysms. It is unclear whether these "prodromes" represent sentinel bleeding from a mycotic aneurysm or episodes of cerebral embolism. In the patients who have focal deficits and probably also in those who develop seizures several days prior to ICH, these events are likely to represent cerebral embolism, whereas in patients who present with sudden headache or seizures a short time (hours) before ICH, the event may represent sentinel bleeding from mycotic aneurysm. In both situations the cerebrospinal fluid is likely to be abnormal, with findings of either limited SAH (in the case of sentinel bleeding) or polymorphonuclear pleocytosis and elevated protein in patients with septic embolism, frequently accompanied by red blood cells that presumably are related to the hemorrhagic character of embolic infarction. The CT findings in ICH due to ruptured mycotic aneurysm are nonspecific, only showing high-density hematomas during the acute stage (Figure 13.6). Simmons et al.[57] reported a patient with acute ICH due to a ruptured mycotic aneurysm, in whom contrast CT examination suggested the presence of two mycotic aneurysms that were subsequently found on cerebral angiography, which also showed a third aneurysm not visualized by CT.

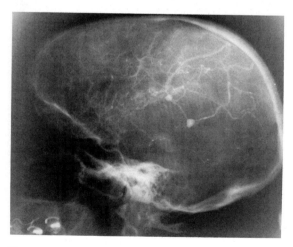

**Figure 13.5.** Lateral carotid angiogram showing two peripherally located mycotic aneurysms in branches of the MCA (Courtesy of Dr. Fernando Díaz, Trudeau Hospital, Santiago, Chile.)

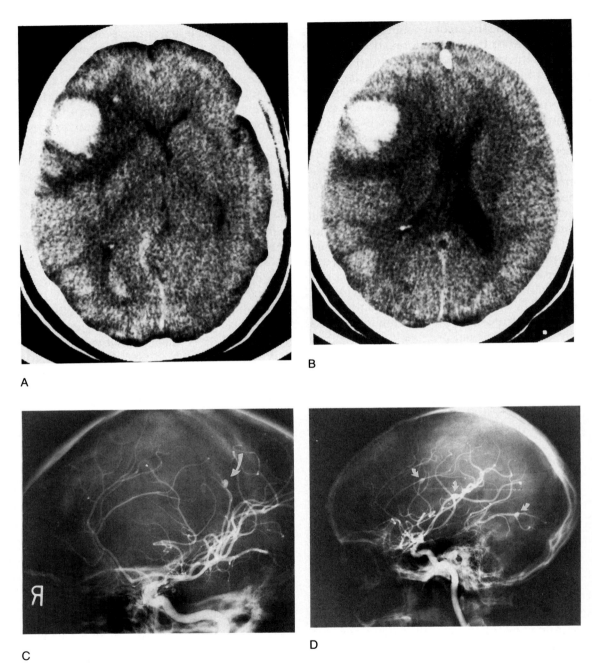

**Figure 13.6.** Intracerebral hemorrhage due to ruptured mycotic aneurysms. (A) Right frontal lobar hematoma with surrounding edema. (B) Superior extension of the hematoma with mass effect and midline shift. (C) Right carotid angiogram showing mycotic aneurysm in posterior temporoparietal branch of the MCA (arrow), in addition to avascular area in the frontal lobe. (D) Left carotid angiogram showing three additional unruptured mycotic aneurysms in MCA branches (arrows). (Courtesy of Shripad Tilak, M.D., Department of Radiology, Boston University Medical Center, Boston, MA.)

The pathogenesis of mycotic aneurysms is closely linked to septic cerebral embolism. In clinical series, the finding of mycotic aneurysms has been related to prior evidence of cerebral embolism in 50% of the patients.[38] The preceding ischemic event can occur several weeks before documentation of the aneurysm, and it can present as either a transient ischemic attack or a completed stroke.[38,58] On occasion, the coexistence of the septic embolus with the infectious aneurysm can be shown at necropsy by the presence of an intraluminal clot infiltrated by inflammatory cells and inflammation of the adventitia and media of the artery, along with thinning or interruption of the internal elastic lamina.[38,52a,59]

These pathological aspects of mycotic aneurysms were further studied by Molinari et al.[60] in an experimental model in dogs. After the intracarotid injection of silicone rubber emboli containing *Staphylococcus aureus* to sixteen dogs, eight animals not treated with penicillin were sacrificed in a moribund state two days later. The animals had developed subdural hematomas on the undersurface of the brain, adjacent to dilated and ruptured branches of the MCA, the silicone embolus being found within the subdural clot. Hemorrhage from ruptured bacterial aneurysms occurred as early as twenty-four hours after embolization. In two instances in which the embolic particle became fragmented, there were aneurysmal dilatations of the arterial wall at each site of lodging of emboli. Three animals treated with a single dose of 1.2 million units of procaine penicillin G and injected with penicillin-resistant organisms initially recovered from the anesthesia, remaining hemiplegic, and then deteriorated to a comatose or moribund state three to four days later. They all had hemorrhagic lesions similar to those found in the animals not treated with penicillin. Finally, five penicillin-treated animals given penicillin-sensitive organisms had the uneventful postoperative recovery of hemiplegic dogs, and were electively sacrificed seven or eight days later. All these animals had unruptured aneurysms.

These lesions appeared at sites of embolic occlusions, and were characterized by acute polymorphonuclear inflammation of the adventitia, with irregular infiltration of the outer layers of the muscularis, at times extending as far as the elastic membrane. The histological characteristics of the lesions were similar in the penicillin-treated and untreated animals, and in those given sensitive and resistant organisms, except for the finding of larger aneurysms with thicker and fibrotic walls in those who survived about one week after embolization. Molinari et al.[60] found two possible ways of explaining the formation of mycotic aneurysms as a result of septic inflammation proceeding from the adventitia inward: (1) extension of the infection from the intraluminal embolus to the adventitia via the vasa vasorum; however, this was rarely observed in the histological specimens, since vasa vasorum "were exceedingly rare" in the cerebral vessels of their animals, "as in higher species," and (2) spreading of the bacterial infection from the luminal embolus into the adventitia through the perivascular space of adjacent small penetrating arteries. These experimental findings corroborated the importance of preceding septic embolism in the pathogenesis of mycotic aneurysms, characterized this process as one that proceeds from the adventitia inward, and supported the role of penetrating vessels, rather than the vasa vasorum, in allowing the infectious agent to extend into the adventitia.

The importance of mycotic aneurysms derives from their tendency to rupture and cause ICH, a complication that is said to carry a mortality of 60% to 90%.[42,49] However, small modern series of patients with ICH due to ruptured mycotic aneurysms secondary to bacterial endocarditis (predominantly streptococcal) have shown improved survival rates.[55] In addition, diagnosis of mycotic aneurysm in a patient with bacterial endocarditis is followed by a number of management decisions, some of which are still controversial.[48,49,51,52,61] Controversy about treatment results in part from limited knowledge about the natural history of these lesions. On one hand, it is well recognized that rupture of mycotic aneurysms in patients with bacterial endocarditis is a major cause of mortality and morbidity, and such event can be the first manifestation of their presence. On the other hand, the intravenous use of the proper antibiotics can result in "cure" of mycotic aneurysms that progressively decrease in size on repeated angiograms until their disappearance. Cantu et al.[53] documented the peculiar course of these lesions in a 41-year-old man with streptococcal bacterial endocarditis who developed SAH. No aneurysm was detected angiographically at the time of the hemorrhage, but repeat angiography two months later, after completion of six weeks of intravenous antibiotics, showed a large left MCA mycotic aneurysm. This lesion was no longer present in a follow-up angiogram performed six months later. Similarly, Moskowitz et al.[54] documented the disappearance of single unruptured mycotic aneurysms on angiograms performed five months and three and one-half months after hospitalization in two young patients with streptococcal endocarditis. In both instances angiography showed the concomitance of an MCA mycotic aneurysm with embolic arterial occlusions, of MCA branches in one patient and of the supraclinoid internal carotid artery (ICA) in the other. At times the angiographic disappearance of mycotic aneurysms has been preceded by a period of aneurysm enlargement, and even by the appearance of new lesions, while under antibiotic treatment.[51] The whole process of change in the angiographic character of mycotic aneurysms evolved during a period of twenty-eight months in one of the patients reported by Morawetz and Karp.[51] This evolution of mycotic aneurysms has often occurred without rupture during the period of angiographic follow-up,[51,53,54] although there are well documented instances of rupture during appropriate antibiotic therapy,[62] as well as delayed rupture,[55] after as long as one year following a full course of treatment with intravenous antibiotics.[63]

Information on the course of mycotic aneurysms has led to a number of recommendations for their management. There is general agreement on the indications to perform cerebral angiography in patients with bacterial endocarditis who develop either ICH, sudden headache with red blood cells in the CSF, focal neurological deficits (transient or persistent) attributable to cerebral embolism, or seizures.[48,49,51,52,52a,55,61] Cerebral angiography has also been suggested in patients with nonfocal cerebral symptoms, if they are candidates for anticoagulant treatment.[48] In those with recent ICH and angiographic documentation of a mycotic aneurysm, surgery is recommended for drainage of the hematoma and clipping of the aneurysm.[49–52,55,56] On occasion, clipping of the aneurysm or its trapping preceded by extracranial-intracranial bypass has been made technically difficult because of the friable character of the acutely inflamed cerebral blood vessels.[51] In regard to the management of unruptured mycotic aneurysms, most authors agree on the value of repeated cerebral angiography during intravenous antibiotic treatment after the initial documentation of the lesion. Some[49,52] recommend serial angiograms every ten days to two weeks, others[48,51] perform the follow-up study at the completion of antibiotic treatment. In the event of persistence of an aneurysm after completion of antibiotic treatment, it is prudent to perform follow-up angiograms every three months thereafter,[51] in order to document its eventual disappearance, an event that is likely to be the result of thrombosis.[51] Most of the discrepancies in the management of these lesions relate to the indications for surgery in unruptured mycotic aneurysms. Some authors[49,50,52] recommend excision or clipping of any peripherally located mycotic aneurysms, based on their relatively easy surgical accessibility on one hand and their potential for rupture on the other. Others[51,55,61] argue that the demonstration of such lesions is not a clearcut indication for surgical repair, based on the possibility of their disappearing under antibiotic treatment. In patients treated only with antibiotics, persistence or progressive enlargement of the aneurysm is a factor generally considered to favor surgical treatment,[49,52,61] although in some instances even such a course has been followed by eventual disappearance of the aneurysm.[51] A more difficult surgical dilemma is posed by patients who develop either multiple aneurysms or aneurysms located in the proximal portions of the cerebral circulation (circle of Willis or trunk of major vessels, such as the MCA) where surgical accessibility is less favorable than more peripherally. In the latter case, it is recommended that surgical clipping be delayed beyond completion of antibiotic treatment and, in the event of persistence of the proximally located aneurysm on a follow-up angiogram, clipping of a less friable, fibrotic lesion should be attempted.[50,52,55] If clipping is not possible, treatment by carotid ligation or trapping preceded by extracranial-intracranial bypass have been suggested.[52] The management of multiple mycotic aneurysms that do not disappear after antibiotic treatment is even more difficult. Since they can evolve to disappearance over months after completion of antibiotic treatment, a nonsurgical approach with follow-up angiograms seems justified,[51] although in some neurosurgical centers[49,52] an aggressive approach with clipping, especially if all lesions are unilateral, is taken. In the event of bilateral lesions, the order in which they are surgically managed is generally dictated by aneurysm size, attempting repair of the larger lesions first, deferring treatment of the rest based on their presence or change in size on followup angiograms.[49]

An additional problem posed by patients with bacterial endocarditis and neurological complications (especially mycotic aneurysms) is the need for surgical repair of the infected heart valve. In the event of cardiac decompensation requiring emergency valve replacement, cardiac surgery is recommended before any consideration of surgical treatment of the mycotic aneurysm.[51] This approach has resulted in no instances of worsening of neurological deficits or periop-erative aneurysmal rupture in one large center, despite the heparinization necessary for cardiopulmonary bypass.[64] In the patient who requires valve replacement and is known to have a mycotic aneurysm, the use of bioprosthetic valves is preferred over mechanical valves in order to reduce the length of postoperative anticoagulation.[51]

Cerebral infectious aneurysms are known to develop as a result of *extravascular infections*, including meningitis[55,65,66] and cavernous sinus thrombophlebitis.[55,66] Bacterial meningitis (pneumococcal) without endocarditis was associated with the development of multiple fusiform aneurysms in peripheral branches of the anterior cerebral artery territory in a 46-year-old woman reported by Ojemann et al.[65] She had no clinical episodes indicative of ICH or SAH, and follow-up angiogram five weeks after the initial study showed disappearance of the lesions in association with evidence of occlusion or irregular narrowing of the vessel previously harboring the aneurysm, suggesting that the process of "healing" may be primarily the result of thrombosis. The formation of the aneurysms was thought to be due to direct spreading of infection from the meninges into the arterial wall. Similar observations were reported by Suwanwela et al.[66] in two patients, one with *Staphylococcus aureus* meningitis, the other with tuberculous meningitis. The former patient recovered with antibiotic treatment, resulting in angiographic disappearance of a single MCA aneurysm, whereas the patient with tuberculous meningitis died. Neither patient developed intracranial bleeding. Three patients with bacterial meningitis and aneurysms were reported by Barrow and Prats.[55] The locations of the aneurysms were relatively unusual, involving the basilar artery (in meningitis by *Pseudomona aeruginosa* in a 12-year-old immunocompromised patient with Burkitt's lymphoma), the intracavernous ICA (in a 48-year-old woman with streptococcal meningitis secondary to a tooth abscess), and the vertebral artery (in a 3-year-old child with pneumococcal meningitis). Intracranial hemorrhage occurred in one of these three patients, but the characteristics of the hemorrhage were not described in detail in the report.

The other extravascular mechanism of formation of infectious aneurysms involves thrombophlebitis of the cavernous sinus. This infection has generally been by *Staphylococcus aureus*,[66] rarely by *Streptococcus* species.[55] The patients have developed the classic ophthalmoparesis of cavernous sinus thrombophlebitis, with angiographic demonstration of an aneurysm of the adjacent intracavernous ICA.[55,56] In some instances,[66] the aneurysms have either decreased in size or disappeared on follow-up angiograms, but one that increased in size[55] required treatment by occlusion of the ICA by detachable balloon. None of these patients developed intracranial bleeding from aneurysmal rupture. These aneurysms are usually infraclinoid and extradural in location.

These instances of aneurysm formation as a result of local extravascular infection suggest that their pathogenesis may be the same as that of mycotic aneurysms secondary to bacterial endocarditis, that is, spreading of infection to the adventitia of affected arteries. In both situations, intravascular septic embolization in bacterial endocarditis and local intracranial extravascular infection, the initial process is likely to be spreading of infection to the adventitia, with subsequent involvement of the media of the artery, as documented by Molinari et al.[60] in their experimental model of bacterial mycotic aneurysms.

*Fungal Infections*

Fungal infections of the nervous system are becoming more frequent as a result of the expanding pool of immunocompromised hosts, in whom these infections are more likely to occur.[39] These include patients with cancer, frequently treated with chemotherapy, as well as those on chronic steroid therapy, hemodialysis, immunosuppression after organ transplant, and those with acquired immune deficiency syndrome (AIDS). Other less well defined conditions with impaired immune responses, such as alcoholism and liver failure, have also been associated with "opportunistic" fungal infections of the nervous system.[67] In the nonimmunocompromised host, fungal infections have at times followed neurosurgical operations and steroid treatment.[55,68,69] Most of the nervous system fungal infections produce subacute or chronic meningitis, but certain organisms have a propensity to involve the vascular system, resulting in acute cerebrovascular syndromes.

Cerebrovascular disorders caused by fungal infection of the nervous system are most commonly the result of infection by *Aspergillus fumigatus* species. The organism is characterized histologically by hyphae of uniform size that are septate, with acute angle (Y-shaped) branching, and staining with both routine (hematoxylin and eosin) and specific (methenamine silver) stains. *Aspergillus* has a marked tendency to invade the walls of blood vessels (Figure 13.7), resulting in both ischemic and hemorrhagic clinical presentations. Other less common fungal agents responsible for stroke syndromes, in particular intracranial hemorrhage, include *Petriellidium boydii* and *Pseudallescheria boydii*,[55] *Phycomycetes*,[70] *Candida albicans*,[68] and *Coccidioides immitis*.[71] Infections by *Aspergillus* have resulted in multiple examples of fatal intracranial hemorrhage, predominantly SAH secondary to rupture of mycotic aneurysms. On occasion, however, fatal SAH has resulted from rupture of necrotic and inflamed arteries that contain *Aspergillus* hyphae, but without formation of mycotic aneurysms.[72–74]

Examples of massive ICH secondary to *Aspergillus* mycotic aneurysms have been reported by Visudhiphan et al.[75] and by Horten et al.[76] The reported patients with *Aspergillus* mycotic aneurysms have shared a number of features: (1) frequent febrile course and coexistence with subacute or chronic basilar meningitis,[68,69,75,77] recent neurosurgical procedure,[55,68,69] signs of paranasal sinus infection,[78,79] or endocarditis,[76] (2) preceding use of steroids or cytotoxic drugs,[67,80] and (3) in-

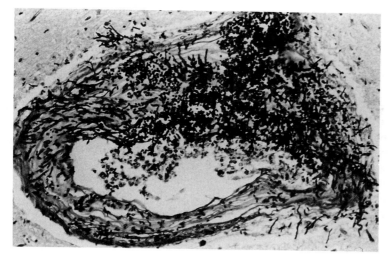

A

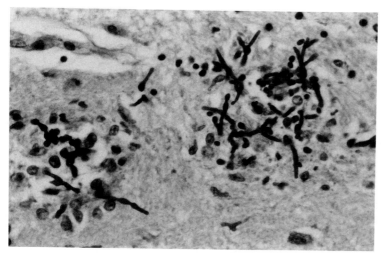

B

**Figure 13.7.** Cerebral blood vessel with invasion of its wall by *Aspergillus*. (A) Heavy infiltration of the vascular wall by septate fungal hyphae, with necrosis and mononuclear inflammatory infiltration. (H&E, ×250.) (B) Detail of fungal hyphae in the adjacent brain parenchyma, showing the typical Y-shaped branching pattern of *Aspergillus*. (H&E, ×400.)

variably fatal outcome.[55,67–69,75–82] The aneurysms are generally large and their locations favor the more proximal portions of the cerebral vasculature, in the circle of Willis, in contrast with the more peripheral locations of the smaller bacterial mycotic aneurysms secondary to bacterial endocarditis: among thirteen reported patients with a total of seventeen *Aspergillus* mycotic aneurysms, their locations were in the basilar artery (six); vertebral artery (three); MCA (three); ICA and anterior cerebral artery (ACA) (two each);

posterior cerebral artery (PCA) (one) (Table 13.3). Ten of the twelve hemorrhagic strokes were SAH, only two were ICH. Fungal mycotic aneurysms may have more propensity to bleed than bacterial aneurysms, and their prognosis is poorer, since there are no reports of suspected fungal aneurysms that have disappeared during antifungal treatment (amphotericin B). The histological appearance of the mycotic aneurysms includes profuse inflammatory infiltration and necrosis of all the arterial layers, at times with

**Table 13.3.** Examples of *Aspergillus* Mycotic Aneurysms Reported in the Literature

| Author | Age/Sex | Mycotic aneurysm | | | |
|---|---|---|---|---|---|
| | | Location | Size (mm.) | Presentation | Outcome |
| Davidson and Robertson[81] | 75/M | BA | 15 | SAH | Death |
| Visudhiphan et al.[75] | 13/M | BA | ? | SAH | Death |
| (2 pts.) | 5/F | ? MCA | ? | ICH | Death |
| Horten et al.[76] | 17/F | MCA | 6 | ICH | Death |
| (2 aneurysms) | | ACA | ? | | |
| Ahuja et al.[78] | 18/M | ICA | 8 | SAH | Death |
| Mielke et al.[68] | 58/F | BA | ? | SAH | Death |
| Fernando and Lauer[82] | 56/M | MCA | ? | SAH | Death |
| Walsh et al.[67] | 64/F | PCA | ? | SAH | Death |
| Vu et al.[77] | 62/M | ACA | 9 | SAH | Death |
| Kowall and Sobel[80] | 27/M | BA | 5 | | |
| (3 aneurysms) | | VA | ? | SAH | Death |
| | | VA | ? | | |
| Iihara et al.[79] | 78/F | BA | ? | SAH | Death |
| Barrow and Prats[55] | 4/M | VA | ~9 | SAH | Death |
| (2 aneurysms) | | BA | ~13 | | |
| Komatsu et al.[69] | 61/F | ICA | 15 | SAH | Death |

Abbreviations: M = male, F = female, BA = basilar artery, VA = vertebral artery, ICA = internal carotid artery, MCA = middle cerebral artery, ACA = anterior cerebral artery, PCA = posterior cerebral artery, SAH = subarachnoid hemorrhage, ICH = intracerebral hemorrhage, pts. = patients, ? = information not stated in report, ~ = approximate reading from published photograph.

multinucleated giant cells, with abundant dichotomously branching hyphae with septations.

The nervous system fungal infection most often originates from the paranasal sinuses, usually as a result of chronic sinusitis. At times, the sinus infection spreads to the orbit first, causing ophthalmoparesis and optic nerve involvement prior to extending intracranially, where meningitis and vascular compromise follow.[68,73,79,82] In two reported instances the intracranial infection followed the trans-sphenoidal resection of a pituitary area lesion,[68,69] and another patient developed fatal *Aspergillus* infection after removal of a posterior fossa astrocytoma.[55] These instances of focal spreading of infection from an adjacent site are virtually always accompanied by a basilar fungal meningitis. This infection may in turn serve as the source of fungal involvement of the vessels. A less common form of nervous system infection is hematogenous spread from a focus of fungal endocarditis,[76] a condition more likely to result from *Candida albicans* than from *Aspergillus* infection.[68]

Another feature that characterizes the vascular invasion by *Aspergillus* is the frequent development of arterial thrombosis with cerebral infarction, which is often hemorrhagic. Even in patients who succumb to massive SAH from proximal arterial rupture, postmortem examination often documents large vessel thrombotic occlusion, either locally or at a distance from the intracranial infectious focus, of arteries affected by *Aspergillus* infiltration of the wall.[68,77–79,82] In immunosuppressed patients with nervous system involvement in disseminated aspergillosis, Beal et al.[83] documented a high frequency (eleven of twelve patients) of cerebral abscess formation and vascular invasion, the latter associated with foci of hemorrhagic infarction. In two of these patients, a massive ICH involved a large portion of one cerebral hemisphere. The usual portal of entry for disseminated aspergillosis is the lung.[67,83] Early detection of pulmonary infection in the appropriate host is important in order to provide specific treatment to prevent the development of neurological complications, which generally have devastating consequences, despite antifungal therapy.

*Viral Infections*

Viral infections of the CNS generally involve the meninges or the brain parenchyma, causing meningitis or encephalitis, respectively. Some varieties of viral encephalitis, such as that caused by herpes simplex Type I virus, have a tendency to produce necrotic and hemorrhagic brain lesions, but examples of ICH or SAH are distinctly uncommon. This relates in part to a general lack of predilection of viruses for involving vascular structures directly, causing vasculitis. However, there are exceptions to this rule, since the varicella zoster (VZ) and, probably also the human immunodeficiency virus (HIV), have been shown to be associated with focal or generalized infection of the cerebral vasculature, respectively.[84,85]

The VZ virus has been implicated as the cause of a focal arteritis in patients with trigeminal distribution herpes zoster who developed ipsilateral cerebral infarction.[86,87] The brain infarction resulted from arteritic involvement of the intracranial ICA or its branches,[86] and herpes virus particles were demonstrated by electron microscopy of the affected vessels.[87] Viral particles in the muscularis layer were identified by electron microscopy in a basilar artery affected by granulomatous angiitis in a 20-year-old man with Hodgkin's disease who developed generalized VZ infection that started in the right ophthalmic branch of the trigeminal nerve.[88] The authors postulated direct viral invasion of the vessel wall by the virus, via trigeminal nerve branches, with location in the outer layers of the artery, without the presence of viral particles in the endothelium, a finding that would have been expected if the spread of the virus to the vessel wall had been by the hematogenous route. A unique example of intracranial hemorrhage caused by this

mechanism was reported by Fukumoto et al.,[84] who reported a patient with fatal SAH due to rupture of a basilar artery aneurysm caused by VZ virus infection of the artery. The patient was a 70-year-old man who developed herpes zoster infection of the C2 dermatome and died suddenly as a result of massive SAH seventy days after the onset of the viral infection. Postmortem examination identified a ruptured aneurysm in the midportion of the basilar artery. Microscopically, this lesion corresponded to a form of arteritis with infiltration of the vessel wall by lymphocytes, histiocytes, and multinucleated giant cells, with destruction of the internal elastic lamina. With immunohistochemical techniques, VZ virus antigen was identified in the nuclei and cytoplasm of histiocytes in areas of granulomatous inflammation of the basilar artery. This observation was further corroborated by the demonstration of intracytoplasmic viral particles in histiocytes by electron microscopy.

Infection of the CNS with the HIV virus has been associated with a large variety of processes, including progressive dementia and encephalitis; opportunistic infections by bacterial, viral, and parasitic agents; malignancies such as Kaposi's sarcoma and lymphoma; and subacute myelopathy.[89] Cerebrovascular complications in HIV-infected patients have been estimated to occur in 0.5% to 7% of patients in clinical series,[89–92] and in 11% to 34% of patients in autopsy series.[85,93–95] The predominant cerebrovascular lesions in HIV-infected patients are cerebral infarcts,[85,96] which are usually small and mediated by cerebral embolism, as a result of nonbacterial thrombotic (or marantic) endocarditis and disseminated intravascular coagulation.[89,90,94] In the autopsy series of Mizusawa et al.,[85] however, such mechanism was not documented in any of their twenty-three patients, the main source of infarction being apparent in situ thrombosis of cerebral vessels and embolism originated in bacterial endocarditis, prosthetic heart valve, or atherosclerotic cerebrovascular lesions. Instances of intracranial hemorrhage were documented in three of fifty (6.0%) patients with AIDS by Snider et al.,[90] in five of eighty-three (6.0%) patients in the autopsy series of Mizusawa et al.,[85] and in three of 154 (1.9%) patients in the series of Berger et al.[96] Of these eleven hemorrhages, four were clinically significant ICH, three were SAH, and four were small incidental hemorrhages found at postmortem examination. The mechanisms of the hemorrhages are probably multiple (Table 13.4). Instances of brain vasculitis have been documented in HIV-infected patients,[97–100] but no patients with ICH due to this mechanism have been reported. One unique example of a frontal (lobar) ICH in a 31-year-old patient with AIDS was due to histologically documented cerebral toxoplasmosis.[101]

### Primary Central Nervous System Vasculitis

Primary CNS vasculitis, also referred to as "isolated angiitis of the CNS,"[102] or "granulomatous angiitis of the CNS,"[103] is a form of vasculitis limited to the cerebral vessels, without systemic involvement.[2,102–105] It is characterized by inflammation of small and medium intracranial arteries, which develop segmental inflammation and necrosis of the intima and adventitia, with relative sparing of the media. The inflammatory infiltrates are made of lymphocytes, plasma cells, histiocytes, epithelioid cells, and multinucleated giant cells, with variable degree of granuloma formation. Eosinophils are not present in the granulomas, which do not develop necrosis. The vasculitis can also affect veins, but the brunt of the inflammation is sustained by arteries, which may either thrombose or rupture, the latter usually as a result of the formation of micro-aneurysms.[106]

Clinically, primary CNS vasculitis most often has a subacute course of progressive headache, mental status changes, and development of focal cerebral neurological deficits or signs of spinal cord involvement.[2,105] The occurrence of hemiparesis, aphasia, or visual field defects is usually the result of brain infarction, but occasionally the mechanism of such focal deficits is an episode of intracranial hemorrhage. The diagnosis is suggested by features of segmental narrowing, alternating with dilatations ("beading") in small and medium arteries in cerebral angiography.[2,102,105] However, an abnormal angiogram is only found in slightly over 50% of patients, since the affected vessels are usually 500 µm or less in diameter, thus being too small to be detected angiographically.[105] The definitive diagnosis rests in the pathological documentation of the angiopathy by biopsy of cortical and leptomeningeal vessels. This condition is treatable, with resolution of the angiopathy with the use of immunosuppressants, generally with a combination of prednisone and cyclophosphamide.[2]

The cause of primary CNS vasculitis is unknown, but it is thought to be either infectious or immunological. The infectious agents that have been implicated are the VZ virus,[84,107] HIV,[97] and *Mycoplasma*.[108] On the other hand, the lack of consistent specific infections prior to the onset of the neurological disease, as well as the absence of microscopic demonstration of an infectious agent at the site of granulomatous inflammation, has led to the suggestion that the disorder may have an immunological basis.[104]

Intracranial hemorrhages, both ICH and SAH, are relatively frequent in patients with primary CNS vasculitis. In some instances, multiple small hemorrhagic foci are found

**Table 13.4.** Causes of Intracranial Hemorrhage in HIV-infected Patients

1. Thrombocytopenia
   a. Autoimmune
   b. Drug-induced
   c. DIC
   d. Other
2. Intracranial Malignancy
3. Vasculitis
4. Ruptured Mycotic Aneurysm

Abbreviations: HIV = human immunodeficiency virus, DIC = disseminated intravascular coagulation.
(From Berger JR, Harris JO, Gregorios J, et al. Cerebrovascular disease in AIDS: a case-control study. AIDS 1990;4:239–244. With permission.)

only at postmortem examination,[109–111] while in others the hemorrhagic events are clinically significant (Table 13.5). The latter have often been in the form of large and fatal ICH in the basal ganglia or lobar white matter, at times even multiple and recurrent. The intracranial hemorrhage has occasionally been the first manifestation of the primary CNS vasculitis.[121] The youngest patient described with intracranial hemorrhage and primary CNS vasculitis was 15 years old[115] and the oldest was 70 years old.[121] In at least six of the twelve patients reported, a preceding subacute myelopathy was the main associated feature. On pathological examination, De Reuck et al.[117] demonstrated that the myelopathy was due to ischemia of the spinal cord resulting from a chronic primary CNS vasculitis, with prominent replacement of the vascular wall by fibrous tissue, contrasting with a more acute form of vasculitis intracranially, which was responsible for fatal ICH. A

**Table 13.5.** Cases of Intracranial Hemorrhage due to Primary CNS Vasculitis

| Author | Age/Sex | Type of Hemorrhage | Associated Features | Treatment | Outcome |
|--------|---------|--------------------|---------------------|-----------|---------|
| Harbitz[112] (Case III) | 26/F | ICH | ?Myelopathy | None | Death* |
| Peison and Padleckas[113] | 45/M | ICH, multiple | Subacute HA, personality changes | Supportive measures | Death* |
| Kolodny et al.[104] (Case 3) | 21/M | ICH, cerebellar | Myelopathy; HA, mental decline, papilledema | Corticosteroids | Death* |
| Magidson et al.[114] | 40/F | SAH, 2° to angiitis and aneurysm | R trigeminal VZ infection | Surgery (subarachnoid clot removal) | †Survived |
| Shuangshoti[115] | 15/F | SAH, ICH, 2° to angiitis and aneurysm | Papilledema | Corticosteroids | Death* |
| Rawlinson & Braun[116] | 19/M | ICH | Myelopathy | Corticosteroids | Death* |
| De Reuck et al.[117] | 69/M | ICH | Myelopathy, VZ infection | Corticosteroids | Death* |
| Clifford-Jones et al.[118] | 43/M | ICH, recurrent | Myelopathy | Corticosteroids, surgery (drainage ICH) | ‡Survived |
| Launes et al.[119] (Case 1) | 26/F | ICH | None | Corticosteroids | †Survived |
| Kattah et al.[120] | 64/F | ICH, recurrent | Myelopathy | Corticosteroids, cyclophosphamide | ‡Survived |
| Biller et al[121] (2 cases) | 70/M | ICH | None | Corticosteroids | Death* |
| | 50/F | SAH, possible aneurysms | None | Corticosteroids, cyclophosphamide | †Survived |

Abbreviations: M = male, F = female, VZ = varicella zoster, R = right 2° = secondary.
*Primary CNS vasculitis documented at postmortem examination.
†No pathological documentation of vasculitis (only presumptive diagnosis based on angiographic features).
‡Primary CNS vasculitis documented on surgical biopsy.

similar pattern of sclerotic spinal arteries and heavily inflamed intracranial arteries was observed by Rawlinson and Braun[116] in their patient with long-standing myelopathy and terminal hemispheric ICH. In two patients, the intracranial hemorrhage was preceded by VZ infection. The patient reported by Magidson et al.[114] had VZ infection of the ophthalmic and maxillary divisions of the right trigeminal nerve, and two months later developed left hemiparesis due to a right frontotemporal infarct. Cerebral angiograms showed prominent "beading" of branches of the right ICA, ACA, MCA, PCA, anterior choroidal artery, posterior-inferior cerebellar artery, and the left PCA. In some areas, the "beading" was accompanied by aneurysmal dilatations of arteries, generally at points of bifurcation. The patient developed a large SAH about three months after the onset of the VZ infection, attributed to rupture of an area of aneurysmal dilatation of the right ACA. There was no pathological confirmation of the diagnosis of "granulomatous angiitis of the CNS." The patient reported by De Reuck et al.[117] had VZ infection of the left thigh preceding the onset of a rapidly ascending myelopathy, followed by a fatal right frontal ICH that occurred approximately two-and-a-half months after hospital admission. These observations suggest that viral infection by the VZ agent, and possibly also by others, may be of pathogenic importance in some cases of primary CNS vasculitis, either by causing direct infection of the intracranial vessels or by triggering an immune response leading to prominent inflammatory changes in the CNS vasculature.[117]

## Moyamoya Disease

Moyamoya disease is a disorder characterized by progressive bilateral stenosis and eventual occlusion of the intracranial arteries of the circle of Willis, a process that is accompanied by the development of profuse collaterals through the deep perforating vessels in the basal ganglia region.[122,123] The latter type of collaterals result in a net-like appearance of the deep vasculature on angiography, an aspect that gives the disease its name, which in Japanese means "something hazy like a puff of cigarette smoke drifting in the air."[123] The occlusive process involves initially the intracranial ICA, often ending in occlusion, subsequently also affecting the proximal trunk of the MCA and ACA, with less frequent and prominent involvement of the posterior circulation. In addition to the development of profuse collaterals through the deep perforating arteries of the basal ganglia, collateral flow to the distal intracranial vessels is also provided by transdural anastomoses derived from external carotid artery branches (middle meningeal and superficial temporal arteries), by transethmoidal communications from the ophthalmic artery and the external carotid artery into the basal ganglionic anastomotic channels, and by leptomeningeal collaterals, mainly from the posterior circulation via the PCA[123] (Figure 13.8). The angiographic features of the disorder generally evolve through a number of stages, in which the typical basal ganglionic moyamoya collaterals, which are prominent in the early stages, become less obvious with the passage of time, the main collaterals present in the late stages originating primarily from the external carotid artery.[123]

Moyamoya disease was originally described in Japanese patients and most of the reported cases are from Japan,[122] but the condition occurs worldwide. Most of the cases are due to an idiopathic noninflammatory arteriopathy of the proximal branches of the circle of Willis, but the characteristic angiographic picture is not exclusive to this form, but represents a nonspecific pattern of development of collateral vessels in response to occlusive involvement of these proximal arteries, usually early in life. The moyamoya pattern of circulation has been described with intracranial ICA stenosis or occlusion in patients with tuberculous meningitis,[124] sickle cell disease,[125] neurofibromatosis,[126] atherosclerosis,[127] after radiation therapy to the neck area,[128] and in disorders of connec-

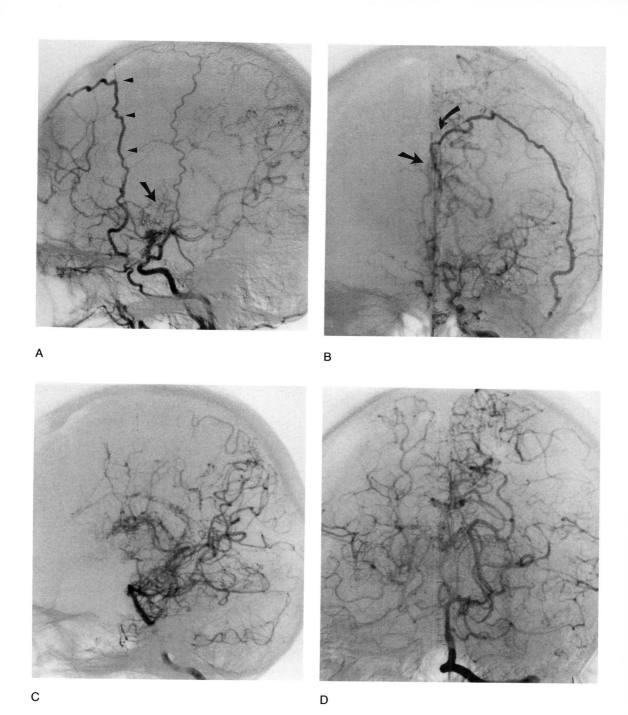

**Figure 13.8.** Angiographic features of moyamoya disease. (A) Lateral carotid angiogram showing occlusion of branches of the intracranial ICA, with deep basal ganglionic collaterals ("puff of cigarette smoke") (arrow), and transdural anatomoses through enlarged meningeal branches (arrowheads). (B) Anteroposterior view, with pale opacification of the MCA, and prominent anastomoses from the middle meningeal artery into the ACA territory (arrows). (C) Lateral view of posterior circulation injection showing prominent leptomeningeal collaterals from the PCA into the MCA and ACA territories. (D) Anteroposterior view of extensive anastomoses between the PCA and the MCA and ACA bilaterally (Courtesy of Dr. Takenori Yamaguchi, National Cardiovascular Center, Osaka, Japan.)

tive tissue.[129] This has led to the idea that moyamoya should be considered as a clinico-radiological syndrome of various possible causes, rather than a specific disease.[130]

The pathology of moyamoya disease is restricted to the cerebral vasculature. It is characterized by thickening of the intima by fibrous tissue, thinning of the media, and prominent infolding, thickening, and fragmentation of the internal elastic lamina of the proximal trunks of the circle of Willis[131,132] (Figure 13.9). The prominent basal collateral channels show intimal thickening, thinning of the media and, at times, discontinuity of the internal elastic lamina and fibrin deposits on the wall.[132] Occasionally, these vessels are the site of microaneurysm formation.[132] Vascular inflammation and necrosis are not features of this disorder.

The clinical presentation of moyamoya disease has a peculiar bimodal distribution. In young patients, with a peak incidence in the first decade, the disorder predominantly presents with cerebral infarction, whereas in adults, with a peak incidence in the fourth decade, it presents most frequently with intracranial hemorrhage (Table 13.6).[122,123] The young patients often develop transient episodes of hemiparesis or other focal neurological deficits, as well as single or multiple episodes of persistent deficits of sudden onset secondary to infarction. This is thought to be the result of the progressive occlusive phenomena taking place in the proximal trunks of the circle of Willis. In the adult, on the other hand, the predominant presentation is with intracranial hemorrhage, including ICH, SAH, and intraventricular hemorrhage.

Intracranial hemorrhage in moyamoya disease has been extensively reported, especially in Japanese populations. Its most common form is probably ICH, which usually occurs in the basal ganglia, thalamus, and deep hemispheric white matter[123,133] (Figure 13.10). ICH has been reported in a variety of forms, with examples of occurrence during pregnancy[134] and as four episodes of recurrent ICH over a period of nine years.[135] The mechanism of these hemorrhages,

which involve deep hemispheric structures close to the midline and with frequent ventricular extension, is thought to be rupture of the abnormal deep anastomotic arteries that are characteristic of the disease.[131,132] These arteries frequently develop microaneurysm formation along with the other features previously described, and their rupture has been documented histologically at sites of ICH or intraventricular hemorrhage.[131,132] In the latter situation of so-called primary intraventricular hemorrhage, it is possible that some of the reported patients actually represent examples of small caudate nucleus parenchymal hemorrhages with prominent ventricular extension.[128,133]

The pathogenesis of the rare examples of pure SAH in moyamoya disease is controversial. There is evidence that pure basal SAH due to rupture of anastomotic channels is either very rare or nonexistent,[133] and the reported examples of SAH have resulted from rupture of an associated saccular aneurysm.[136–138] Approximately half of the reported patients with SAH due to ruptured aneurysm in moyamoya disease have had an aneurysm of the basilar artery.[123,138] This finding has led to the suggestion that compromise of the anterior circulation may alter the circulatory dynamics in the posterior circulation in a way conducive to the development of basilar artery aneurysms,[138] possibly on the basis of a developmental vascular anomaly, which has been suggested by some authors[122] to represent the basic pathogenesis of the disorder. In other instances in which aneurysms occur in the intracranial ICA or in other proximal affected vessels, they are most likely the result of the local arterial pathology, and as such probably represent pseudoaneurysms formed as a result of arterial wall destruction, rather than true aneurysms due to a developmental or degenerative mechanism.[137,139] These observations have led to the recommendation that physicians should search for an associated saccular aneurysm, especially in the posterior circulation, in patients with moyamoya disease who present with pure SAH.[138] The

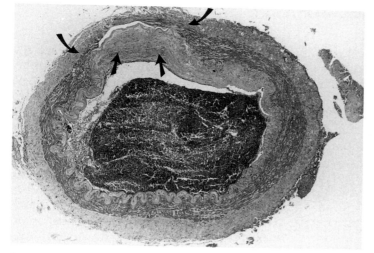

A

**Figure 13.9.** Histological arterial changes in moyamoya disease, MCA trunk. Intimal fibrocellular thickening (A and B, arrows), atrophy of the media (A, curved arrows), and reduplication of elastic lamina (C, arrows). (Elastic-van Gieson, ×30) (Courtesy of Dr. Jun Ogata, National Cardiovascular Center, Osaka, Japan.)

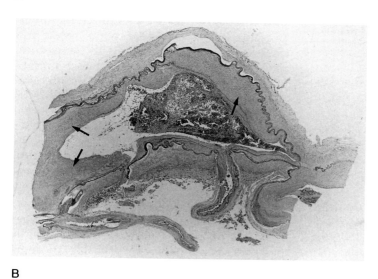

B

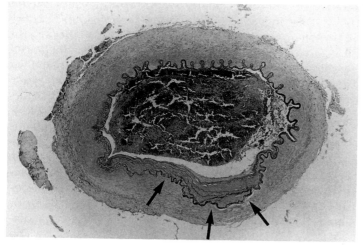

C

**Table 13.6.** Forms of Presentation in Moyamoya Disease, in Relationship to Age

| Symptoms/Signs | Age | |
| --- | --- | --- |
| | Under 15 (73 Pts.) | Above 15 (38 Pts.) |
| Hemiplegia | 38 | 10 |
| Monoplegia | 17 | 0 |
| Seizures | 15 | 2 |
| Headache | 14 | 11 |
| Involuntary movements | 6 | 0 |
| SAH | 3 | 19 |

Abbreviations: Pts. = patients, SAH = subarachnoid hemorrhage.
(Based on data reported by Nishimoto A, Takeuchi S. Moyamoya disease: abnormal cerebrovascular network in the cerebral basal region. In Vinken PJ, Bruyn GW (eds): Handbook of Clinical Neurology, vol. 12, chap. 11. New York: Elsevier Scientific Publishing, 1972, pp. 352–383.)

treatment of such lesions should follow the same criteria used in the treatment of saccular aneurysms in general.[138]

## Arterial Dissection

Arterial dissection is a well recognized cause of stroke, especially in young patients.[140] The process involves dissection of blood from the lumen into the wall of the artery, via an intimal tear. This results in an area of accumulation of blood within the arterial wall, which produces partial or total obliteration of the lumen. The longitudinal extent of the process is variable, and it can involve several-cm-long segments of the artery, or it may be confined to a short segment of a few mm in length.[141,142] In instances of stenosis secondary to dissection, the angiogram shows a characteristic "string sign,"[143] produced by a generally long (several cm), thin layer of contrast within the stenotic lumen, with normal-size lumens proximally and distally to the dissection. On occasions, the area of dissection into the wall opens distally into the lumen, and the arteriogram can show a "double lumen,"[144] due to the circulation of blood through both the "true" stenotic lumen and the "false" lumen created by the circulating blood within the arterial wall.[142]

Pathologically, arterial dissection is characterized by the presence of blood in the arterial wall, with variable degrees of obliteration of the lumen. Blood within the arterial wall accumulates in either the media-subintimal region or, less commonly, in the media-adventitial interface.[145] In the latter situation, the area of dissection can result in a local outpouching of the vessel wall, which is often referred to as a "dissecting aneurysm." There is evidence to suggest that these two patterns of arterial dissection have a certain topographic selectivity in the cerebral vasculature, as well as different clinical presentations. In a report of four cases, and analyses of fifty-one from the literature, O'Connell et al.[146] pointed out that subintimal dissection is more common in intracranial vessels, a condition usually affecting the younger patients (average age 27.4) with dissection. Medial dissection, on the other hand, favors the extracranial vessels, and affects older patients (average age 52.3). In the vertebrobasilar system, the pattern of dissection was found to affect either arterial plane, without specific anatomic predilection.

The pathogenesis of arterial dissection remains unclear. In a number of instances it has been associated with pathological demonstration of preexistent local arterial disease. This has included atherosclerosis,[147] fibromuscular dysplasia,[148] cystic medial necrosis,[149,150] Marfan's syndrome,[151] arteritis,[152] a congenital anomaly of the arterial wall,[153] and migraine.[154] In other instances, however, the condition occurred in the absence of known pre-existent disease, generally as a result of direct trauma, at times trivial, presumably causing an intimal tear followed by dissection. In the case of the vertebral artery, precipitating traumatic events have included extremes of head rotation or extension during normal daily activities or in the practice of sports, and chiropractic manipulations.[141] The actual mechanism of bleeding into the arterial wall in dissection is unclear. In instances of local trauma, an inti-

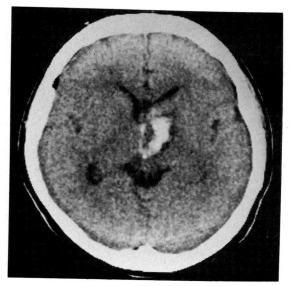

A

**Figure 13.10.** ICH in 40-year-old woman with moyamoya disease (angiogram showed in Figure 13.8). (A) Left thalamic hemorrhage with extension into the third ventricle and slight midline shift. (B) Ventricular extension. (C) T1-weighted MRI on day 57 from onset of ICH, showing residual low signal abnormality in the left thalamus. (Courtesy of Dr. Takenori Yamaguchi, National Cardiovascular Center, Osaka, Japan.)

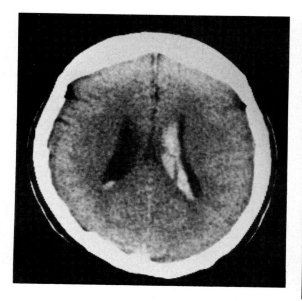

B

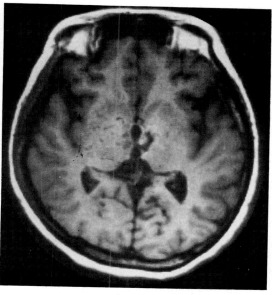

C

mal tear is thought to be responsible for initiating the process of dissection, with blood collecting in the medial-subintimal plane. In those patients in whom blood dissects into the medial-adventitial plane, presumably without intimal involvement, it has been proposed that the mechanism may be rupture of vasa vasorum within the arterial wall.[145] This mechanism is thought to lead to limited areas of dissection, and occurs more often in extracranial than intracranial arteries, since the latter lack vasa vasorum.[145]

The clinical presentation of arterial dissection varies depending on the type and site of artery involved. In the carotid territory, most dissections occur extracranially, usually starting in the ICA about 1.5 to 3.0 cm from its origin.[143] Clinical findings often include prominent ipsilateral hemicranial headache or facial pain, at times with vomiting, along with an ipsilateral Horner's syndrome,[140,142] combined with either transient (TIA, often as "transient monocular blindness"[142]) or permanent ipsilateral ischemic events. The latter are thought to result from distal intracranial embolization from the area of dissection or, less commonly, from distal hypoperfusion.[141,155] Focal cerebral ischemia is the most common neurological consequence of dissections in the carotid territory.[142] Hemorrhagic strokes, on the other hand, are distinctly uncommon. Rare examples of ICH or SAH secondary to MCA, ACA, and intracranial ICA dissection have been reported.[144,147,156,157,157a] Ramsey and Mosquera[156] reported a 47-year-old man who presented with symptoms suggestive of SAH and left hemiplegia, and at postmortem examination had massive SAH due to a ruptured dissecting aneurysm of the MCA, with rupture at a site "30 mm from the circle of Willis," presumably at the distal end of the MCA stem, "in an area near the insula." On microscopic examination, the affected artery was described as showing "marked arteriosclerosis and cystic medial degeneration" at the point of rupture. Kunze and Schiefer[144] reported a 34-year-old alcoholic man who developed a large left basal ganglia ICH due to MCA dissection, which involved pathologically the whole extent of its stem, over a 5-cm segment. Another instance of ICH in a patient with intracranial ICA and MCA dissection was the result of bleeding into an area of hemorrhagic infarction while on anticoagulants, rather than rupture of the dissected vessel.[157] Guridi et al.[157a] recently described the case of a 72-year-old hypertensive woman who developed sudden headache and neck pain, with nuchal rigidity and right hemi-

paresis. CT showed subarachnoid and interhemispheric hematomas, and cerebral angiography was normal. She died suddenly as a result of massive gastrointestinal bleeding, and the brain at autopsy showed a large interhemispheric hemorrhage involving the whole extent of the corpus callosum. The ICH proved to be due to a transmural dissection of the left ACA. The onset of the dissection was thought to be in an area of hemorrhage in an atheromatous plaque ("intraplaque" hemorrhage) with transmural extension of the hematoma into the adventitia, resulting in arterial rupture into the subarachnoid space and corpus callosum. Adams et al.[147] reported a 75-year-old woman who developed SAH due to an angiographically documented dissecting aneurysm of the distal intracranial ICA. Treatment with carotid clamping was followed by signs of left hemispheric infarction, and follow-up angiogram was reported as showing left MCA occlusion, presumably indicating that the dissecting ICA aneurysm had become thrombosed.

Intracranial hemorrhage is a more common occurrence in dissections of the vertebral and basilar arteries. Although ischemic syndromes, especially lateral medullary and cerebellar infarction, are the most common feature in patients with intracranial vertebral artery dissection,[158] this condition has resulted in posterior fossa SAH in a number of occasions (Table 13.7). The clinical presentation is almost uniformly with the sudden onset of SAH, but in rare instances a short preceding period of ipsilateral neck pain[160,162] probably represents the onset of dissection, followed by delayed SAH. This course of vertebral artery dissection is illustrated by the following patient:

A 50-year-old man in previous good health, woke up on 12/16/89 with severe pain on the left side of the neck posteriorly, for which he took ibuprofen, without relief. On the evening of that day, while standing at a store, he suddenly developed severe pain in the trapezius area bilaterally, and immediately collapsed to the ground,

**Table 13.7.** Subarachnoid Hemorrhage Secondary to Vertebral Artery Dissection

| Author | Age/Sex | A-gram/Path Aneurysm | Predisposing Factors | Outcome |
|---|---|---|---|---|
| Yonas et al.[145] | 44/F | R VA | — | Died, 2° GI bleed. |
| Waga et al.[159] | 53/M | R VA | — | Normal |
| Senter and Sarwar[160] | 45/M | L VA | — | Normal |
| Manz and Luessenhop[161] | 57/M | R VA | Hypertension, mucoid subst. in media | Died |
| Farrell et al.[162] | 63/M | R VA | Hypertension | Died |
| Berger and Wilson[163] | 46/M | R VA | — | Postop. stroke |
| (2 cases) | 39/M | L VA | — | Slight deficit |
| Friedman and Drake[164] | 36–63 | R VA (7 pts.) | Hypertension (8 pts.) | Normal |
| (11 cases) | 6M | L VA (2 pts.) | | |
| | 5F | Bilat. (1 pt.) | | |
| | | N/S (1 pt.) | | |
| Caplan et al.[165] | 43/M | Bilateral | ? | Died |
| (3 cases) | 54/M | R VA | Hypertension | Severe deficit |
| | 48/M | L VA | — | Normal |
| Kaplan et al.[165a] | 41/F | L VA, extracranial | ?Trauma (delivery) | Normal, after endovascular balloon occlusion of VA |

Abbreviations: a-gram = angiogram, path = pathology, R = right, L = left, VA = vertebral artery, M = male, F = female, GI = gastrointestinal, postop. = postoperative, bilat. = bilateral, N/S = not stated 2° = secondary to, bleed. = bleeding.
(Modified from Caplan LR, Baquis GD, Pessin MS, et al. Dissection of the intracranial vertebral artery. Neurology 1988;38:868–877.)

without loss of consciousness or seizure activity. On arrival at the hospital minutes later, he had a generalized tonic-clonic seizure. His neurologic examination showed only lethargy, without focal deficits, neck stiffness, or abnormalities in funduscopic examination. Head CT showed extensive subarachnoid bleeding in the posterior fossa (Figure 13.11A), with moderate hydrocephalus. Arteriography on the day of admission revealed an area of suspected dissection of the distal portion of the right intracranial vertebral artery (Figure 13.11B). No aneurysm was identified.

His course was characterized by progressive improvement in the level of consciousness, along with gradual resolution of the posterior fossa SAH, and disappearance of the area of segmental narrowing of the right vertebral artery. This was thought to represent an area of medial-adventitial dissection with rupture, followed by healing.

This patient is an example of SAH secondary to distal vertebral dissection, with prodromal neck pain indicative of the onset of dissection, prior to its rupture.

The most consistent associated condition in patients with posterior fossa SAH due to vertebral artery dissection has been hypertension, present in approximately half of the reported patients (see Table 13.7). These dissecting vertebral aneurysms result from bleeding into the medial-adventitial plane, where the thinness of both layers and the lack of external elastic lamina[145] promote outpouching of the arterial wall and rupture. A fatal outcome occurred in five of the twenty-one (24%) patients reported, while ten of the twenty-one (48%) survived without neurological deficits. In a number of instances the dissecting aneurysms were surgically

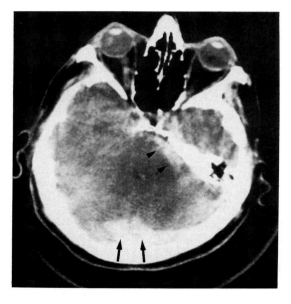

A

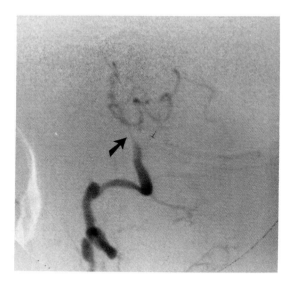

B

**Figure 13.11.** Posterior fossa SAH due to vertebral artery dissection. (A) Acute SAH in the basal cisterns of the posterior fossa, especially in the cisterna magna (arrows) and prepontine cistern (arrowheads). (B) Posterior fossa angiogram showing area of vertebral artery dissection, with "string" of flow in the distal intracranial portion of the artery (arrow).

clipped or ligated, and the patients survived without residual neurologic deficits.

Dissecting aneurysms of the basilar artery are less common than those of the vertebral artery, and they generally present with signs of brainstem ischemia,[166] but examples of SAH have been described as well. These have been reported in six patients,[147,154,162–164] between ages 39 and 69, four in women and two in men; this contrasts with a male predominance of basilar artery dissection in general, with a reported 61% of patients (eight of thirteen reported) being men.[166] The aneurysms have usually been located in the midbasilar region (five patients). Four of these patients died, and the other two survived with slight or moderate neurological deficits. In one instance,[147] a subadventitial dissection was shown to start at the site of an atheromatous plaque, in others it occurred in patients with migraine[154] or who were using oral contraceptives.[163]

## Migraine and Intracerebral Hemorrhage

Stroke during a migrainous attack generally results from cerebral infarction, which predominates in the posterior circulation.[167,168] Its mechanism is felt to be prolonged intense vasoconstriction of intracranial arteries, leading to infarction either directly by severely compromising blood flow or indirectly by promoting vascular thrombosis, presumably facilitated by the platelet activation that accompanies migraine attacks.[168]

A less common occurrence is ICH during an episode of migraine. A possible example of a deep right hemispheric ICH during a migraine attack was reported by Dunning in 1942.[169] The patient was a 35-year-old woman with long-standing history of migraine who developed a sudden left hemiplegia with bloody-xanthochromic CSF. However, further details of the mechanism of the hemorrhage were unavailable, since the patient survived the event, and there was no pathological examination of the cerebral vasculature, in order to rule out an aneurysm or AVM as the cause of the bleeding. In the modern literature, CT-documented instances of ICH during migraine episodes have been reported by Shuaib et al.[170] and by Cole and Aubé.[171] All four patients with this complication were middle-aged women who developed ICH during a particularly long and severe migraine attack. Three of the ICH were lobar,[171] and the other was basal ganglionic.[170] Cerebral angiograms in the three patients reported by Cole and Aubé[171] showed transient spasm of the MCA or the extracranial ICA ipsilateral to the hemorrhage. This finding suggests that the pathogenesis of this type of ICH may involve intracranial migrainous vasoconstriction as the initial event, accompanied by ischemia of intracranial vessel walls, followed by rupture as a result of subsequent reperfusion.[171,172] One of us (LRC) has postulated that this mechanism of ICH, in conjunction with increased cerebral blood flow and transient hypertension, may be the common factor in the pathogenesis of ICH in a number of situations.[172] These include ICH in response to extreme cold, after use of sympathomimetic drugs, during severe pain induced by dental interventions, following carotid endarterectomy, and during migraine attacks.[172] In several of these instances, as well as in idiopathic cases,[173] angiographic studies have revealed transient vasoconstriction of the intracranial vasculature, lending further support to the notion that vasoconstriction may be the initial feature in a chain of events that culminates in vessel rupture upon reperfusion of an ischemic vascular bed.

## Summary

In this chapter we have discussed a wide range of disorders. The common thread is injury to arterial structures leading to *vascular friability and rupture*. Damage to vessel walls can be due to immunogenic mechanisms, infection, or trauma. In moyamoya disease, vascular injury probably derives from overburdening of small arteries with high-

volume flow. A similar mechanism occurs in arteries feeding AVM. At times, the vascular injury leads to aneurysmal outpouchings of the arteries and thinning of the arterial wall. Rupture of the diseased arteries may be precipitated by reperfusion of ischemic zones (as in migraine) and sudden increases in blood pressure and blood flow.

Hemorrhages have usually been due to vascular injury caused by the disease process. However, in patients with vasculitis there is often involvement of other body systems, especially the kidneys and the hematopoietic system. Bleeding tendencies can result from the hematological involvement (e.g., in SLE), and cause ICH. In some patients a concomitant nephropathy leads to hypertension, which causes ICH. In yet other patients with vasculopathies, ICH can be caused by other disorders that have no relation to the primary disease, for example, older patients with bleeding due to cerebral amyloid angiopathy. Concurrent disease should be especially suspected in patients with conditions that rarely cause ICH.

## References

1. Cohen BA, Biller J. Hemorrhagic stroke due to cerebral vasculitis and the role of immunosuppressive therapy. Neurosurg Clin NA 1992;3: 611–624.
2. Moore PM, Cupps TR. Neurological complications of vasculitis. Ann Neurol 1983;14:155–167.
3. Arkin A. A clinical and pathological study of periarteritis nodosa: a report of five cases, one histologically healed. Am J Path 1930;6: 401–426.
4. Griffith GC, Vural IL. Polyarteritis nodosa: a correlation of clinical and postmortem findings in seventeen cases. Circulation 1951;3:481–491.
5. Ford RG, Siekert RG. Central nervous system manifestations of periarteritis nodosa. Neurology 1965;15:114–122.
6. Summers VK. The nervous manifestations of periarteritis nodosa. Lancet 1950;1:1148–1149.
7. Hiller F. Cerebral hemorrhage in hyperergic angiitis. J Neuropath Exp Neurol 1953;12:24–40.

8. Tuhy JE, Maurice GL, Niles NR. Wegener's granulomatosis. Am J Med 1958;25:638–646.

9. Mickle JP, McLennan JE, Chi JG, et al. Cortical vein thrombosis in Wegener's granulomatosis: case report. J Neurosurg 1977;46:248–251.

10. MacFadyen DJ. Wegener's granulomatosis with discrete lung lesions and peripheral neuritis. Can Med Assoc J 1960;83:760–764.

11. Drachman DA. Neurological complications of Wegener's granulomatosis. Arch Neurol 1963; 8:145–155.

12. Nishino H, Rubino FA, DeRemee RA, et al. Neurological involvement in Wegener's granulomatosis: an analysis of 324 consecutive patients at the Mayo Clinic. Ann Neurol 1993;33: 4–9.

13. Johnson RT, Richardson EP. The neurological manifestations of systemic lupus erythematosus: a clinical-pathological study of 24 cases and review of the literature. Medicine 1968;47:337–369.

14. Ellis SG, Verity MA. Central nervous system involvement in systemic lupus erythematosus: a review of neuropathologic findings in 57 cases, 1955–1977. Semin Arthritis Rheum 1979;8:212–221.

15. Harvey AM, Shulman LE, Tumulty PA, et al. Systemic lupus erythematosus: review of the literature and clinical analysis of 138 cases. Medicine 1954;33:291–437.

16. Kelley RE, Stokes N, Reyes P, et al. Cerebral transmural angiitis and ruptured aneurysm: a complication of systemic lupus erythematosus. Arch Neurol 1980;37:526–527.

17. Sakaki T, Morimoto T, Utsumi S. Cerebral transmural angiitis and ruptured cerebral aneurysms in patients with systemic lupus erythematosus. Neurochirurgia 1990;33: 132–135.

18. Steiner JW, Gelbloom AJ. Intracranial manifestations in two cases of systemic rheumatoid disease. Arthritis Rheum 1959;2:537–545.

19. Watson P, Fekete J, Deck J. Central nervous system vasculitis in rheumatoid arthritis. Can J Neurol Sci 1977;4:269–272.

20. Gobernado JM, Leiva C, Ràbano J, et al. Recovery from rheumatoid cerebral vasculitis. J Neurol Neurosurg Psychiat 1984;47:410–413.

21. Delaney P. Neurologic manifestations in sarcoidosis: review of the literature, with a report of 23 cases. Ann Intern Med 1977;87:336–345.

22. Meyer JS, Foley JM, Campagna-Pinto D. Granulomatous angiitis of the meninges in sarcoidosis. Arch Neurol Psychiat 1953;69:587–600.

23. Urich H. Neurosarcoidosis or granulomatous angiitis: a problem of definition. Mt Sinai J Med 1977;44:718–725.

24. Ferrer-Roca O, Coca A. Sarcoidosis with granulomatous angiitis. Hum Pathol 1980;11:302 (letter).

25. Rottino A, Hoffman G. A sarcoid form of encephalitis in a patient with Hodgkin's disease: case report with review of the literature. J Neuropath Exp Neurol 1950;9:103–108.

26. Caplan L, Corbett J, Goodwin J, et al. Neuro-ophthalmologic signs in the angiitic form of neurosarcoidosis. Neurology 1983;33:1130–1135.

27. Kozin F, Haughton V, Bernhard GC. Neuro-Behçet disease: two cases and neuroradiologic findings. Neurology 1977;27:1148–1152.

28. Chajek T, Fainaru M. Behçet's disease: report of 41 cases and a review of the literature. Medicine 1975;54:179–196.

29. O'Duffy JD, Goldstein NP. Neurologic involvement in seven patients with Behçet's disease. Am J Med 1976;61:170–178.

30. Jenkins AM, Macpherson AIS, Nolan B, et al. Peripheral aneurysms in Behçet's disease. Br J Surg 1976;63:199–202.

31. Nagata K. Recurrent intracranial hemorrhage in Behçet disease. J Neurol Neurosurg Psychiat 1985;48:190–192 (letter).

32. Altinörs N, Şenveli E, Arda N, et al. Intracerebral hemorrhage and hematoma in Behçet's disease: case report. Neurosurgery 1987;21: 582–583.

33. Al Kawi MZ, Bohlega S, Banna M. MRI findings in neuro-Behçet's disease. Neurology 1991;41:405–408.

34. Bousser M-G, Chiras J, Bories J, et al. Cerebral venous thrombosis—a review of 38 cases. Stroke 1985;16:199–213.

35. Wechsler B, Vidailhet M, Piette JC, et al. Cerebral venous thrombosis in Behçet's disease: clinical study and long-term follow-up of 25 cases. Neurology 1992;42:614–618.

36. Pankey GA. Subacute bacterial endocarditis at the University of Minnesota Hospital, 1939 through 1959. Ann Intern Med 1961;55: 550–561.

37. Jones HR, Siekert RG, Geraci JE. Neurologic manifestations of bacterial endocarditis. Ann Intern Med 1969;71:21–28.

38. Pruitt AA, Rubin RH, Karchmer AW, et al. Neurologic complications of bacterial endocarditis. Medicine 1978;57:329–343.

39. Jones HR, Siekert RG. Neurological manifestations of infective endocarditis: review of clinical and therapeutic challenges. Brain 1989;112:1295–1315.

40. Le Cam B, Guivarch G, Boles JM, et al. Neurologic complications in a group of 86 bacterial endocarditis. Eur Heart J 1984;5(suppl C):97–100.

41. Keyser DL, Biller J, Coffman TT, et al. Neurologic complications of late prosthetic valve endocarditis. Stroke 1990;21:472–475.

42. Greenlee JE, Mandell GL. Neurological manifestations of infective endocarditis: a review. Stroke 1973;4:958–963.

43. Dreyer NP, Fields BN. Heroin-associated infective endocarditis: a report of 28 cases. Ann Intern Med 1973;78:669–702.

44. Masuda J, Yutani C, Waki R, et al. Histopathological analysis of the mechanisms of intracranial hemorrhage complicating infective endocarditis. Stroke 1992;23:843–850.

45. Ziment I. Nervous system complications in bacterial endocarditis. Am J Med 1969;47:593–607.

46. Hart RG, Kagan-Hallet K, Joerns SE. Mechanisms of intracranial hemorrhage in infective endocarditis. Stroke 1987;18:1048–1056.

47. Lieberman A, Hass WK, Pinto R, et al. Intracranial hemorrhage and infarction in anticoagulated patients with prosthetic valves. Stroke 1978;9:18–24.

48. Salgado AV, Furlan AJ, Keys TF. Mycotic aneurysm, subarachnoid hemorrhage, and indications for cerebral angiography in infective endocarditis. Stroke 1987;18:1057–1060.

49. Frazee JG, Cahan LD, Winter J. Bacterial intracranial aneurysms. J Neurosurg 1980;53:633–641.

50. Roach MR, Drake CG. Ruptured cerebral aneurysms caused by micro-organisms. N Engl J Med 1965;273:240–244.

51. Morawetz RB, Karp RB. Evolution and resolution of intracranial bacterial (mycotic) aneurysms. Neurosurgery 1984;15:43–49.

52. Bohmfalk GL, Story JL, Wissinger JP, et al. Bacterial intracranial aneurysm. J Neurosurg 1978;48:369–382.

52a. Cole DG, Richardson EP. Case records of the Massachusetts General Hospital (case 10-1993). N. Engl J Med 1993;328:717–725.

53. Cantu RC, LeMay M, Wilkinson HA. The importance of repeated angiography in the treatment of mycotic-embolic intracranial aneurysms. J Neurosurg 1966;25:189–193.

54. Moskowitz MA, Rosenbaum AE, Tyler HR. Angiographically monitored resolution of cerebral mycotic aneurysms. Neurology 1974;24:1103–1108.

55. Barrow DL, Prats AR. Infectious intracranial aneurysms: comparison of groups with and without endocarditis. Neurosurgery 1990;27:562–573.

56. Wilson WR, Giuliani ER, Danielson GK, et al. Management of complications of infective endocarditis. Mayo Clin Proc 1982;57:162–170.

57. Simmons KC, Sage MR, Reilly PL. CT of intracerebral hemorrhage due to mycotic aneurysms: case report. Neuroradiology 1980;19:215–217.

58. Siekert RG, Jones HR. Transient cerebral ischemic attacks associated with subacute bacterial endocarditis. Stroke 1970;1:178–183.

59. Takeshita M, Kagawa M, Kubo O, et al. Clinicopathological study of bacterial intracranial aneurysms. Neurol Med Chir 1991;31:508–513.

60. Molinari GF, Smith L, Goldstein MN, et al. Pathogenesis of cerebral mycotic aneurysms. Neurology 1973;23:325–332.

61. Bingham WF. Treatment of mycotic intracranial aneurysms. J Neurosurg 1977;46:428–437.

62. Schold C, Earnest MP. Cerebral hemorrhage from a mycotic aneurysm developing during appropriate antibiotic therapy. Stroke 1978;9:267–268.

63. Venger BH, Aldama AE. Mycotic vasculitis with repeated intracranial aneursymal hemorrhage: case report. J Neurosurg 1988;69:775–779.

64. Richardson JV, Karp RB, Kirklin JW, et al. Treatment of infective endocarditis: a 10-year comparative analysis. Circulation 1978;58:589–597.

65. Ojemann RG, New PFJ, Fleming TC. Intracranial aneurysms associated with bacterial meningitis. Neurology 1966;16:1222–1226.

66. Suwanwela C, Suwanwela N, Charachinda S, et al. Intracranial mycotic aneurysms of extravascular origin. J Neurosurg 1972;36:552–559.

67. Walsh TJ, Hier DB, Caplan LR. Aspergillosis of the central nervous system: clinicopathological analysis of 17 patients. Ann Neurol 1985;18:574–582.

68. Mielke B, Weir B, Oldring D, et al. Fungal aneurysm: case report and review of the literature. Neurosurgery 1981;9:578–582.

69. Komatsu Y, Narushima K, Kobayashi E, et al. Aspergillus mycotic aneurysm: case report. Neurol Med Chir 1991;31:346–350.

70. Kikuchi K, Watanabe K, Sugawara A, et al. Multiple fungal aneurysms: report of a rare case implicating steroid as predisposing factor. Surg Neurol 1985;24:253–259.

71. Hadley MN, Martin NA, Spetzler RF, et al. Multiple intracranial aneurysms due to Coccidioides immitis infection. J Neurosurg 1987;66:453–456.

72. McKee EE. Mycotic infection of brain with arteritis and subarachnoid hemorrhage: report of case. Amer J Clin Path 1950;20:381–384.

73. Corvisier N, Gray F, Gherardi R, et al. Aspergillosis of ethmoid sinus and optic nerve, with arteritis and rupture of the internal carotid artery. Surg Neurol 1987;28:311–315.

74. Lau AHC, Takeshita M, Ishii N. Mycotic (aspergillus) arteritis resulting in fatal subarachnoid hemorrhage: case report. Angiology 1991;42:251–255.

75. Visudhiphan P, Bunyaratavej S, Khantanaphar S. Cerebral aspergillosis: report of three cases. J Neurosurg 1973; 38:472–476.

76. Horten BC, Abbott GF, Porro RS. Fungal aneurysms of intracranial vessels. Arch Neurol 1976;33:577–579.

77. Vu N, Kim RC, Choi BH. Aspergillotic cerebral arterial aneurysm formation complicating hemodialysis. Surg Neurol 1986;25:582–586.

78. Ahuja GK, Jain N, Vijayaraghavan M, et al. Cerebral mycotic aneurysm of fungal origin: case report. J Neurosurg 1978;49:107–110.

79. Iihara K, Makita Y, Nabeshima S, et al. Aspergillosis of the central nervous system causing subarachnoid hemorrhage from mycotic aneurysm of the basilar artery: case report. Neurol Med Chir 1990;30:618–623.

80. Kowall NW, Sobel RA. Case records of the Massachusetts General Hospital (Case 7-1988). N Engl J Med 1988;318:427–440.

81. Davidson P, Robertson DM. A true mycotic (Aspergillus) aneurysm leading to fatal subarachnoid hemorrhage in a patient with hereditary hemorrhagic telangiectasia: case report. J Neurosurg 1971;35:71–76.

82. Fernando SSE, Lauer CS. Aspergillus fumigatus infection of the optic nerve with mycotic arteritis of cerebral vessels. Histopathology 1982;6:227–234.

83. Beal MF, O'Carroll CP, Kleinman GM, et al. Aspergillosis of the nervous system. Neurology 1982;32:473–479.

84. Fukumoto S, Kinjo M, Hokamura K, et al. Subarachnoid hemorrhage and granulomatous angiitis of the basilar artery: demonstration of the varicella-zoster-virus in the basilar artery lesions. Stroke 1986;17:1024–1028.

85. Mizusawa H, Hirano A, Llena JF, et al. Cerebrovascular lesions in acquired immune deficiency syndrome (AIDS). Acta Neuropathol 1988;76:451–457.

86. Gilbert GJ. Herpes zoster ophthalmicus and delayed contralateral hemiparesis: relationship of the syndrome to central nervous system granulomatous angiitis. JAMA 1974;229; 302–304.

87. Doyle PW, Gibson G, Dolman CL. Herpes zoster ophthalmicus with contralateral hemiplegia: identification of cause. Ann Neurol 1983;14:84–85.

88. Linnemann CC, Alvira MM. Pathogenesis of varicella-zoster angiitis in the CNS. Arch Neurol 1980;37:239–240.

89. McArthur JC. Neurologic manifestations of AIDS. Medicine 1987;66:407–437.

90. Snider WD, Simpson DM, Nielsen S, et al. Neurological complications of acquired immune deficiency syndrome: analysis of 50 patients. Ann Neurol 1983;14:403–418.

91. Levy RM, Bredesen DE, Rosenblum ML. Neurological manifestations of the acquired immunodeficiency syndrome (AIDS): experience at UCSF and review of the literature. J Neurosurg 1985;62:475–495.

92. Engstrom JW, Lowenstein DH, Bredesen DE. Cerebral infarctions and transient neurologic deficits associated with acquired immunodeficiency syndrome. Am J Med 1989;86:528–532.

93. Sharer LR, Kapila R. Neuropathologic observations in acquired immunodeficiency syndrome (AIDS). Acta Neuropathol 1985;66: 188–198.

94. Anders KH, Guerra WF, Tomiyasu U, et al. The neuropathology of AIDS: UCLA experience and review. Am J Pathol 1986;124: 537–558.

95. Vinters HV, Tomiyasu U, Anders KH. Neuropathologic complications of infection with the human immunodeficiency virus (HIV). Progr AIDS Pathol 1989;1:101–130.

96. Berger JR, Harris JO, Gregorios J, et al. Cerebrovascular disease in AIDS: a case-control study. AIDS 1990;4:239–244.

97. Yankner BA, Skolnik PR, Shoukimas GM, et al. Cerebral granulomatous angiitis associ-

ated with isolation of human T-lymphotropic virus type III from the central nervous system. Ann Neurol 1986;20:362–364.

98. Schwartz ND, So YT, Hollander H, et al. Eosinophilic vasculitis leading to amaurosis fugax in a patient with acquired immunodeficiency syndrome. Arch Intern Med 1986; 146:2059–2060.

99. Rhodes RH. Histopathology of the central nervous system in the acquired immunodeficiency syndrome. Hum Pathol 1987;18: 636–643.

100. Vinters HV, Guerra WF, Eppolito L, et al. Necrotizing vasculitis of the nervous system in a patient with AIDS-related complex. Neuropathol Appl Neurobiol 1988;14:417–424.

101. Chaudhari AB, Singh A, Jindal S, et al. Haemorrhage in cerebral toxoplasmosis: a report on a patient with the acquired immunodeficiency syndrome. S Afr Med J 1989;76: 272–274.

102. Cupps TR, Moore PM, Fauci AS. Isolated angiitis of the central nervous system: prospective diagnostic and therapeutic experience. Am J Med 1983;74:97–105.

103. Cravioto H, Feigin I. Noninfectious granulomatous angiitis with a predilection for the nervous system. Neurology 1959;9:599–609.

104. Kolodny EH, Rebeiz JJ, Caviness VS, et al. Granulomatous angiitis of the central nervous system. Arch Neurol 1968;19:510–524.

105. Hankey GJ. Isolated angiitis/angiopathy of the central nervous system. Cerebrovasc Dis 1991;1:2–15.

106. Griffin J, Price DL, Davis L, et al. Granulomatous angiitis of the central nervous system with aneurysms on multiple cerebral arteries. Trans Am Neurol Assoc 1973;98:145–148.

107. Rosenblum WI, Hadfield MG. Granulomatous angiitis of the nervous system in cases of herpes zoster and lymphosarcoma. Neurology 1972;22:348–354.

108. Arthur G, Margolis G. Mycoplasma-like structures in granulomatous angiitis of the central nervous system: case reports with light and electron microscopic studies. Arch Pathol Lab Med 1977;101:385–387.

109. Victor M, Taft EB, Richardson EP. Case records of the Massachusetts General Hospital (Case 41152). N Engl J Med 1955;252: 634–641.

110. Koo EH, Massey EW. Granulomatous angiitis of the central nervous system: protean man-

ifestations and response to treatment. J Neurol Neurosurg Psychiat 1988;51:1126–1133.

111. Harrison PE. Granulomatous angiitis of the central nervous system. J Neurol Sci 1976;29: 335–341.

112. Harbitz F. Unknown forms of arteritis, with special reference to their relation to syphilitic arteritis and periarteritis nodosa. Am J Med Sci 1922;163:250–272.

113. Peison B, Padleckas R. Granulomatous angiitis of the central nervous system. Ill Med J 1964;126:330–334.

114. Magidson MA, Rajendran MM, Leutcher WM. Granulomatous angiitis of the central nervous system with an unusual angiographic feature. Surg Neurol 1978;10:355–360.

115. Shuangshoti S. Localized granulomatous (giant cell) angiitis of brain with eosinophil infiltration and saccular aneurysm. J Med Assoc Thai 1979;62:281–288.

116. Rawlinson DG, Braun CW. Granulomatous angiitis of the nervous system first seen as relapsing myelopathy. Arch Neurol 1981;38: 129–131.

117. De Reuck J, Crevits L, Sieben G, et al. Granulomatous angiitis of the nervous system: a clinicopathological study of one case. J Neurol 1982;227:49–53.

118. Clifford-Jones RE, Love S, Gurusinghe N. Granulomatous angiitis of the central nervous system: a case with recurrent intracerebral haemorrhage. J Neurol Neurosurg Psychiat 1985;48:1054–1056.

119. Launes J, Iivanainen M, Erkinjuntti T, et al. Isolated angiitis of the central nervous system. Acta Neurol Scand 1986;74:108–114.

120. Kattah JC, Cupps TR, DiChiro G, et al. An unusual case of central nervous system vasculitis. J Neurol 1987;234:344–347.

121. Biller J, Loftus CM, Moore SA, et al. Isolated central nervous system angiitis first presenting as spontaneous intracranial hemorrhage. Neurosurgery 1987;20:310–315.

122. Nishimoto A, Takeuchi S. Moyamoya disease: abnormal cerebrovascular network in the cerebral basal region. In: Vinken PJ, Bruyn GW, eds. Handbook of Clinical Neurology. Vol. 12. New York: Elsevier, 1972:352–383.

123. Suzuki J, Kodama N. Moyamoya disease: a review. Stroke 1983;14:104–109.

124. Mathew NT, Abraham J, Chandy J. Cerebral angiographic features in tuberculous meningitis. Neurology 1970;20:1015–1023.

125. Stockman JA, Nigro MA, Mishkin MM, et al. Occlusion of large cerebral vessels in sickle-cell anemia. N Engl J Med 1972;287:846–849.

126. Tomsick TA, Lukin RR, Chambers AA, et al. Neurofibromatosis and intracranial arterial occlusive disease. Neuroradiology 1976;11:229–234.

127. Hinshaw DB, Thompson JR, Hasso AN. Adult arteriosclerotic moyamoya. Radiology 1976;118:633–636.

128. Sato M, Kohama A, Fukuda A, et al. Moyamoya-like diseases associated with ventricular hemorrhages: report of three cases. Neurosurgery 1985;17:260–266.

129. Richman DP, Watts HG, Parsons D, et al. Familial moyamoya associated with biochemical abnormalities of connective tissue. Neurology 1977;27:382 (abstract).

130. Caplan LR. Stroke, A Clinical Approach. Second edition, Stoneham, MA: Butterworth-Heinemann, 1993.

131. Oka K, Yamashita M, Sadoshima S, et al. Cerebral haemorrhage in moyamoya disease at autopsy. Virchows Arch (Pathol Anat) 1981;392:247–261.

132. Yamashita M, Oka K, Tanaka K. Histopathology of the brain vascular network in moyamoya disease. Stroke 1983;14:50–58.

133. Aoki N, Mizutani H. Does moyamoya disease cause subarachnoid hemorrhage? review of 54 cases with intracranial hemorrhage confirmed by computerized tomography. J Neurosurg 1984;60:348–353.

134. Enomoto H, Goto H. Moyamoya disease presenting as intracerebral hemorrhage during pregnancy: case report and review of the literature. Neurosurgery 1987;20:33–35.

135. Kaufman M, Little BW, Berkowitz BW. Recurrent intracranial hemorrhage in an adult with moyamoya disease: case report, radiographic studies and pathology. Can J Neurol Sci 1988;15:430–434.

136. Debrun G, Lacour P. A new case of moyamoya disease associated with several intracavernous aneurysms. Neuroradiology 1974;7:277–282.

137. Kodama N, Suzuki J. Moyamoya disease associated with aneurysm. J Neurosurg 1978;48:565–569.

138. Adams HP, Kassell NF, Wisoff HS, et al. Intracranial saccular aneurysm and moyamoya disease. Stroke 1979;10:174–179.

139. Yuasa H, Tokito S, Izumi K, et al. Cerebrovascular moyamoya disease associated with an intracranial pseudoaneurysm: case report. J Neurosurg 1982;56:131–134.

140. Fisher CM, Ojemann RG, Roberson GH. Spontaneous dissection of cervico-cerebral arteries. Can J Neurol Sci 1978;5:9–19.

141. Hart RG, Easton JD. Dissections of cervical and cerebral arteries. Neurol Clin 1983;1:155–182.

142. Anson J, Crowell RM. Cervicocranial arterial dissection. Neurosurgery 1991;29:89–96.

143. Ojemann RG, Fisher CM, Rich JC. Spontaneous dissecting aneurysm of the internal carotid artery. Stroke 1972;3:434–440.

144. Kunze S, Schiefer W. Angiographic demonstration of a dissecting aneurysm of the middle cerebral artery. Neuroradiology 1971;2:201–206.

145. Yonas H, Agamanolis D, Takaoka Y, et al. Dissecting intracranial aneurysms. Surg Neurol 1977;8:407–415.

146. O'Connell BK, Towfighi J, Brennan RW, et al. Dissecting aneurysms of head and neck. Neurology 1985;35:993–997.

147. Adams HP, Aschenbrener CA, Kassell NF, et al. Intracranial hemorrhage produced by spontaneous dissecting intracranial aneurysm. Arch Neurol 1982;39:773–776.

148. Ringel SP, Harrison SH, Norenberg MD, et al. Fibromuscular dysplasia: "spontaneous" dissecting aneurysms of the major cervical arteries. Ann Neurol 1977;1:301–304.

149. Thapedi IM, Ashenhurst EM, Rozdilsky B. Spontaneous dissecting aneurysm of the internal carotid artery in the neck: report of a case and review of the literature. Arch Neurol 1970;23:549–554.

150. Wolman L. Cerebral dissecting aneurysms. Brain 1959;82:276–291.

151. Austin MG, Schaefer RF. Marfan's syndrome, with unusual blood vessel manifestations: primary medionecrosis dissection of right innominate, right carotid, and left carotid arteries. Arch Pathol 1957;64:205–209.

152. Chang V, Rewcastle NB, Harwood-Nash DCF, et al. Bilateral dissecting aneurysms of the intracranial internal carotid arteries in an 8-year-old boy. Neurology 1975;25:573–579.

153. Johnson AC, Graves VB, Pfaff JP. Dissecting aneurysm of intracranial arteries. Surg Neurol 1977;7:49–52.

154. Alexander CB, Burger PC, Goree JA. Dissecting aneurysms of the basilar artery in 2 patients. Stroke 1979;10:294–299.

155. Bogousslavsky J, Despland P-A, Regli F. Spontaneous carotid dissection with acute stroke. Arch Neurol 1987;44:137–140.

156. Ramsey TL, Mosquera VT. Dissecting aneurysm of the middle cerebral artery. Ohio State Med J 1948;44:168–170.

157. Hochberg FH, Bean C, Fisher CM, et al. Stroke in a 15-year-old girl secondary to terminal carotid dissection. Neurology 1975;25:725–729.

157a. Guridi J, Gállego J, Monzón F, Aguilera F. Intracerebral hemorrhage caused by transmural dissection of the anterior cerebral artery. Stroke 1993;24:1400–1402.

158. Caplan LR, Zarins CK, Hemmati M. Spontaneous dissection of the extracranial vertebral arteries. Stroke 1985;16:1030–1038.

159. Waga S, Fujimoto K, Morooka Y. Dissecting aneurysm of the vertebral artery. Surg Neurol 1978;10:237–239.

160. Senter HJ, Sarwar M. Nontraumatic dissecting aneurysm of the vertebral artery: case report. J Neurosurg 1982;56:128–130.

161. Manz HJ, Luessenhop AJ. Dissecting aneurysm of intracranial vertebral artery: case report and review of literature. J Neurol 1983;230:25–35.

162. Farrell MA, Gilbert JJ, Kaufmann JCE. Fatal intracranial arterial dissection: clinical pathological correlation. J Neurol Neurosurg Psychiat 1985;48:111–121.

163. Berger MS, Wilson CB. Intracranial dissecting aneurysms of the posterior circulation: report of six cases and review of the literature. J Neurosurg 1984;61:882–894.

164. Friedman AH, Drake CG. Subarachnoid hemorrhage from intracranial dissecting aneurysm. J Neurosurg 1984;60:325–334.

165. Caplan LR, Baquis GD, Pessin MS, et al. Dissection of the intracranial vertebral artery. Neurology 1988;38:868–877.

165a. Kaplan SS, Ogilvy CS, Gonzalez R, Gress D, Pile-Spellman. Extracranial vertebral artery pseudoaneurysm presenting as subarachnoid hemorrhage. Stroke 1993;24:1397–1399.

166. Caplan LR, Tettenborn B. Vertebrobasilar occlusive disease: review of selected aspects. 1. Spontaneous dissection of extracranial and intracranial posterior circulation arteries. Cerebrovasc Dis 1992;2:256–265.

167. Bogousslavsky J, Regli F, Van Melle G, et al. Migraine stroke. Neurology 1988;38:223–227.

168. Caplan LR. Migraine and vertebrobasilar ischemia. Neurology 1991;41:55–61.

169. Dunning HS. Intracranial and extracranial vascular accidents in migraine. Arch Neurol Psychiat 1942;48:396–406.

170. Shuaib A, Metz L, Hing T. Migraine and intracerebral hemorrhage. Cephalalgia 1989;9:59–61.

171. Cole AJ, Aubé M. Migraine with vasospasm and delayed intracerebral hemorrhage. Arch Neurol 1990;47:53–56.

172. Caplan L. Intracerebral hemorrhage revisited. Neurology 1988;38:624–627.

173. Rousseaux P, Scherpereel B, Bernard MH, et al. Angiopathie cérébrale aiguë bénigne: six observations. Presse Med 1983;12:2163–2168.

# PART THREE
# Clinical Features at Different Sites

In Chapter 3 of Part 1 of this book we characterized the general symptoms in patients with intracerebral hemorrhage (ICH). These general symptoms relate to the rapid introduction of blood into the brain with any accompanying increase in local or intracranial pressure. These general symptoms do not depend on the cause or site of the hemorrhage. In the second part of the book, we considered the various causes of ICH and the particular findings in patients with various specific mechanisms. This third portion of the book considers the influence of the location of the hematoma. Symptoms and signs clearly vary with the site. In this section we detail the usual sites of ICH, the accompanying symptoms, signs and radiological features, and the prognosis and management.

Hematomas were one of the first focal brain lesions recognized by physicians. Their rapid onset and high mortality made clinicopathological correlations readily feasible when postmortem examinations were performed. By the late nineteenth century, clinicians were aware of the usual sites of brain hemorrhage in persons with hypertension, and knew the usual symptoms and signs in patients with basal ganglionic and pontine hemorrhages.[1] During the middle years of this century, the clinicopathological studies of Aring and Merritt[2] led to knowledge of the clinical differentiation between hemorrhage and infarction, and the studies of Fisher helped clarify the usual findings in patients with large putaminal, thalamic, pontine, and cerebellar hematomas.[3]

Neurologists and neurosurgeons literally "went to school" on intracerebral hematomas. Hematomas were the prototype of focal brain lesions. Knowledge of the findings in a patient with a thalamic hemorrhage gave general knowledge about the findings in patients with other thalamic lesions, for example, tumors, abscesses, infarcts, and so forth. Since hypertensive damage to penetrating arteries caused vascular changes that could lead to either hemorrhage or ischemia, the locations of hematomas were guideposts for where small deep infarcts were likely to be located. Knowledge of the clinical findings in patients with thalamic, caudate, and lateral pontine tegmental hemorrhages led clinicians to look for and recognize groups of patients with infarcts in these regions.

Initial studies were clinico*pathological* and depended on necropsy localization of hematomas since in life there were no procedures that could accurately define hematoma location. These necropsy series were biased to large fatal hematomas since these were the only kind that led to necropsy. Table III.1 lists those necropsy series of ICH[1–6] that contained more than 100 cases. None recognized caudate hemorrhage as a separate category and most did not separate primary intraventricular bleeding. Tooth[1] and Aring and Merritt[2] did not separate putaminal and thalamic locations. Considering all of these necropsy series, putaminal hemorrhages were by far the most common (cumulative average, 58%) and lobar hemorrhages were relatively rare (13%).

**Table III.1.** Autopsy Series

| Series | N | Lobar | Caudate | Putamen | Thalamus | Pons | Cerebellum | Ventricular |
|---|---|---|---|---|---|---|---|---|
| Tooth[*] | 118 | 9 (8%) | — | 76(65%) | | 19(16%) | 2 (2%) | 12(10%) |
| Aring and Merritt[2] | 108 | 35(32%) | — | 66(61%) | | 3 (3%) | 3 (3%) | 1 (1%) |
| Fisher[3] | 101 | 22(22%) | — | 47(46%) | 13(13%) | 9 (9%) | 9 (9%) | 1 (1%) |
| Mutlu et al.[4] | 135 | 33(26%) | — | 83(61%) | 11 (8%) | 8 (6%) | — | — |
| Freytag[5] | 373 | 38(10%) | — | 165(44%) | 60(16%) | 63(17%) | 47(13%) | — |
| Dinsdale[6] | 511 | 30 (6%) | — | 351(69%) | 48 (9%) | 30 (6%) | 52(10%) | — |
| Total | 1316 | 167(13%) | — | 646(57%) | 132(12%) | 132(10%) | 113 (9%) | — |

*Quoted in reference 1.
Mutlu[4] did not separate caudate from thalamic, but called them mesial.
Tooth and Aring and Merritt[2] did not separate thalamic or caudate from basal ganglionic (putaminal).
Totals in putaminal and thalamic hematoma groups omit Tooth and Aring and Merritt[2]

The advent of CT scanning completely changed clinicians' abilities to document the sizes and locations of hematomas during life. This led to recognition of small hematomas. Table III.2 lists various series[7–19] containing more than 50 cases of ICH studied by *neuroimaging* (mostly CT, some with MRI). The incidence of pontine and cerebellar hemorrhages does not change much from the necropsy series, but lobar, caudate, and thalamic hematomas are more often recognized, and now fewer hematomas are putaminal. The distribution of lobar hematomas in these series is noted in Table III.3. Frontal and temporal hematomas are more common than parietal and occipital lesions.

CT and, later, MRI also allowed more precise localization of small hematomas. The original clinicopathological studies of Fisher and his colleagues defined the clinical findings in patients with prototypic large hematomas. CT now made it clear that there were subtypes of hematomas at each site that had different clinical findings. For example, putaminal hemorrhages could be far anterior, involve the middle portion including the posterior limb of the capsule, or be far posterior and involve the retrolenticular portion of the white matter near the temporal isthmus. The clinical syndromes and prognosis differ in each of these subtypes. Similarly, anterior, ventrolateral, medial, and

**Table III.2.** Imaging Series

| Series | N | Lobar | Caudate | Putamen | Thalamus | Pons | Cerebellum | Ventricular |
|---|---|---|---|---|---|---|---|---|
| Stroke Data Bank[7,8] | 209 | 65(31%) | 10(5%) | 51(24.5%) | 46(22%) | 11(5%) | 26(12.5%) | — |
| Weisberg et al.[9] | 265 | 98(37%) | 10(4%) | 50(19%) | 50(19%) | 21(8%) | 28(10%) | 8 (3%) |
| Schütz[10] | 336 | 132(39%) | 6(2%) | 115(17%) | 57(17%) | 15(4.5%) | 11 (4%) | — |
| Schütz et al.[11] | 100 | 27(27%) | 3(3%) | 31(31%) | 26(26%) | 3(3%) | 7 (7%) | — |
| Lausanne Registry[12] | 109 | 43(40%) | — | 46(42%) | 4 (4%) | 7(6%) | 9 (8%) | — |
| Harvard Registry[13,14] | 60 | 14(23%) | — | 32(53%) | 7(12%) | 1(2%) | 6(10%) | — |
| M. Reese and S. Alabama[15] | 194 | 38(19.5%) | 17(9%) | 63(32.5%) | 43(24%) | 20(1%) | 14 (7%) | |
| Brott et al.[16] | 154 | 73(47%) | — | 36(23%) | 15(10%) | 5(3%) | 11 (7%) | 14(10%) |
| Paillas and Alliez[17*] | 239 | 106(44%) | 21(9%) | 108(45%) | | 1(.5%) | 3(1.5%) | — |
| Giroud et al.[18] | 87 | 16(19%) | — | 36(42%) | 22(26%) | 5(4%) | 8 (9%) | — |
| Fieschi et al.[19] | 103 | 31(30%) | — | 38(37%) | 18(18%) | 6(6%) | 8 (8%) | 2 (2%) |
| Total | 1856 | 643(35%) | 67(4%) | 498(31%) | 288(18%) | 95(5%) | 31 (7%) | 24(1%) |

*Surgical series, arteriograms and surgery used for localization.

**Table III.3.** Lobar Hematomas

| Series | N | Frontal | Parietal | Temporal | Occipital |
|---|---|---|---|---|---|
| Stroke Data Bank[7,8] | 65 | 37% | 24% | 19.5% | 19.5% |
| Weisberg et al.[9] | 98 | 25.5% | 25.5% | 31% | 18% |
| Schütz[10] | 132 | 26% | 17% | 43% | 14% |
| Lausanne Registry[12] | 43 | 47% | (10%) | 33% | (10%) |
| Fieschi et al.[19] | 31 | 23% | 19% | 48% | 10% |
| Mutlu et al.[4] | 33 | 27% | 18% | 19% | 36% |
| Totals | 402 | 29% | 20.5% | 32.4% | 18% |

Figures in parentheses are an even split of the "pariet O = Occipital" location, given a one figure (20%) for the two lobes together.

pulvinar types of thalamic hemorrhage all differ as do large tegmentobasal, lateral tegmental and basal types of pontine hemorrhages. Hematomas (and infarcts) occur in the territories of each of the penetrating artery branches. The chapters on the various sites of ICH review in detail the findings in each subtype of hematoma, knowledge that has been gained from recent neuroimaging-clinical correlations.

# References

1. Wilson SAK, Bruce AN. Neurology. Second edition. London: Butterworth, 1955;1377.
2. Aring CD, Merritt HH. Differential diagnosis between cerebral hemorrhage and cerebral thrombosis: a clinical and pathological study of 245 cases. Arch Int Med 1935;56:435–456
3. Fisher CM. The pathology and pathogenesis of intracerebral hemorrhage. In: Fields WS, ed. Pathogenesis and Treatment of Cerebrovascular Disease. Springfield, IL: Charles C Thomas, 1961; 295–317.
4. Mutlu N, Berry RG, Alpers BJ. Massive cerebral hemorrhage: clinical and pathologic correlations. Arch Neurol 1963;8:644–661.
5. Freytag E. Fatal hypertensive intracerebral haematomas: a survey of the pathological anatomy of 393 cases. J Neurol Neurosurg Psychiat 1968;31:616–620.
6. Dinsdale HB. Spontaneous hemorrhage in the posterior fossa: a study of primary cerebellar and pontine hemorrhages with observations on their pathogenesis. Arch Neurol 1964;10: 200–217.
7. Foulkes MA, Wolf PA, Price TR, et al. The Stroke Data Bank: design, methods, and baseline characteristics. Stroke 1988;19:547–554.
8. Massaro AR, Sacco RL, Mohr JP, et al. Clinical discriminators of lobar and deep hemorrhages: the Stroke Data Bank. Neurology 1991;41:1881–1885.
9. Weisberg LA, Shamsnia M, Elliott D. Seizures caused by nontraumatic parenchymal brain hemorrhages. Neurology 1991;41:1197–1199.
10. Schütz H. Spontane intrazerebrale Hämatome: pathophysiologie, klinik und therapie. Heidelberg: Springer-Verlag, 1988.
11. Schütz H, Bödeker RH, Damian M, et al. Age-related spontaneous intracerebral hematoma in a German community. Stroke 1990;21: 1412–1418.
12. Bogousslavsky J, Van Melle G, Regli F. The Lausanne Stroke Registry: analysis of 1,000 consecutive patients with first stroke. Stroke 1988;19:1083–1092
13. Mohr JP, Caplan LR, Melski JW, et al. The Harvard Cooperative Stroke Registry: a prospective registry. Neurology 1978;28:754–762.
14. Caplan LR, Mohr JP. Intracerebral hemorrhage: an update. Geriatrics 1978;33:42–52.
15. Caplan LR, Stein RW. Stroke: A Clinical Approach. Boston: Butterworth, 1986;267.
16. Brott T, Thalinger K, Hertzberg V. Hypertension as a risk factor for spontaneous intracerebral hemorrhage. Stroke 1986;17:1078–1083
17. Paillas JE, Alliez B. Surgical treatment of spontaneous intracerebral hemorrhage: immediate and long-term results in 250 cases. J Neurosurg 1973;39:145–151.
18. Giroud M, Gras P, Chadan N, et al. Cerebral hemorrhage in a French prospective popula-

tion study. J Neurol Neurosurg Psychiat 1991;54:595–598.

19. Fieschi C, Carolei A, Fiorelli M, et al. Changing prognosis of primary intracerebral hemorrhage: results of a clinical and computed tomographic follow-up study of 104 patients. Stroke 1988;19:192–195.

# Chapter 14
# Putaminal Hemorrhage

## Louis R. Caplan

## Historical Aspects

When ancient physicians wrote of apoplexy, they almost invariably referred to the most obvious extreme manifestation, paralysis of one side of the body, a phenomenon known to Hippocrates before the common era.[1] When hemiplegia was caused by brain hemorrhage, the most likely anatomical site was clearly, in retrospect, the internal capsule and basal ganglionic region deep in the cerebral hemisphere, although this fact was not established until the 19th century. Interest in the morbid anatomy of disease was most stimulated by the appearance of Morgagni's monumental work on the seats and causes of disease *De Sedibus*, in 1761. However, not until the publication of atlases that illustrated the appearance and location of the lesions found in the brain at necropsy was there much interest or knowledge in correlating the pathological anatomy with the clinical manifestations. Hooper included in his atlas on *The Morbid Anatomy of the Human Brain* a lithograph of a specimen showing a putaminal hemorrhage.[2] We have included this figure (see Chapter 1, Figure 1.2) in the discussion of the historical aspects of the general topic of intracerebral hemorrhage (ICH). Charcot, and his protegés Bouchard and Duret, who worked in his pathology laboratory, studied many specimens of brains of patients dying with apoplexy. Brain hemorrhage was often found and Charcot and his followers found that by far the most common location of ICH was the lateral ganglionic region, the corpus striatum.[3,4] Duret was so impressed with the frequency of hemorrhage into this lateral ganglionic region that he called the artery supplying this area, the lateral lenticulostriate artery, "the artery of cerebral hemorrhage."[4]

By the turn of the twentieth century, prominent general texts such as Osler's *The Principles and Practices of Medicine*[5] and Gowers' *A Manual of Diseases of the Nervous System*[6] devoted considerable space to putaminal hemorrhage. Each noted that this was the most common location of ICH and each included discussions on the pathological and clinical features of putaminal hemorrhage. Other necropsy series corroborated the high frequency of striate hemorrhages. In the classic series of Aring and Merritt on differentiating ICH and thrombosis, over half (58 of 101, 57%) of the hemorrhages were "basal ganglionic."[7] Fisher described and analyzed the clinical signs in patients with putaminal hemorrhage in 1961.[8] The advent of computed tomography (CT) and magnetic resonance imaging (MRI) have undoubtedly helped in the separation of putaminal from caudate, lobar, and thalamic sites, and ICH from infarction. Stroke registries and population studies have helped determine the relative frequency of putaminal origin and involvement in series of ICH patients and the incidence of the disorder in the community.

## Anatomy and Physiology

In horizontal brain sections, the putamen has a rather long extent measured in the anterior-posterior dimension. The putamen and its neighbor medially, the internal and external portion of the globus pallidus, form a diamond-shaped zone of grey matter separating the internal and external capsules. The anterior limb of the internal capsule divides the putamen far anteriorly from the medially located caudate nucleus, and more posteriorly, the anterior limb separates the pallidum and putamen from the caudate. The posterior limb of the internal capsule separates the thalamus medially from the pallidum and putamen, and far posteriorly from just the putamen. The pyramidal tract lies within the anterior two thirds of the posterior limb of the internal capsule. Some observers have lumped hematomas originating from the two large medial, paraventricular gray matter structures, the caudate nucleus and the thalamus, together as "medial" ganglionic hematomas as contrasted with "lateral" ganglionic hematomas arising from the putamen. For reasons not well understood, hemorrhages either very seldom arise from the pallidum, or when they do, the site of origin cannot be identified as either pallidal or putaminal. We herein follow common usage and refer to lateral ganglionic hemorrhages as putaminal, recognizing that some in fact may arise from the globus pallidus or from the internal capsule.

The external capsule lies just lateral to the putamen. Then from medial to lateral lie the claustrum, the extreme capsule, and the insula of Reil. The putamen stretches from the most anterior portion of the insula to its most posterior extent. Lateral to the insular cortex lie the infoldings of the Sylvian fissure, the frontal and parietal opercula, and the convexal portions of the frontal, parietal, and temporal lobes. On coronal sections, the putamen also has a long dorsal-ventral dimension. Figure 14.1 depicts the relations of the putamen found in a CT section through the foramen of Monro.

The major afferent projections to the putamen come from the cerebral cortex, substantia nigra, thalamus, and raphe nuclei.[9,10] Though virtually all major cortical areas project to both the caudate nucleus and the putamen, the major motor and sensory-motor regions project more to the putamen. These corticostriate projections arise from small pyramidal cells restricted for the most part to the upper half of the fifth cortical lamina.[10] Somatic motor areas 4 and 6 project laterally to a large anteroposterior division of the putamen primarily in its more lateral portion.[11,12,13] This motor projection is somatotopically organized. Fibers from the lower limb regions project to the rostral dorsal putamen and the face region projects more caudoventrally. The contralateral projections cross in the midline in the corpus callosum and enter the putamen through the external capsule. Fibers from somatosensory areas 1, 2, and 3 project only ipsilaterally but the somatotopic distribution is very similar to that arising from area 4.[12] Though the motor and sensory areas project to nearly the entire anteroposterior extent of the putamen, these critical regions have only minor projections to the caudate nucleus. Next to the cerebral cortex, the substantia nigra is the major source of afferent input to the striatum. The striatal projection comes mostly from the *pars compacta* but the *pars reticulata* and paranigral cell groups also project to the striate nuclei. The nigrostriatal projection is, of course, dopaminergic while most of the corticostriate projection involves glutamate as the neurotransmitter. There are also important thalamostriate projections emanating mostly from the intralaminar thalamic nuclei and the center medianum.[9,10] Projections from the dorsal raphe nuclei to the striatum are serotonergic.

Efferents from the putamen project primarily to the globus pallidus (internal and external segments) and the substantia nigra.

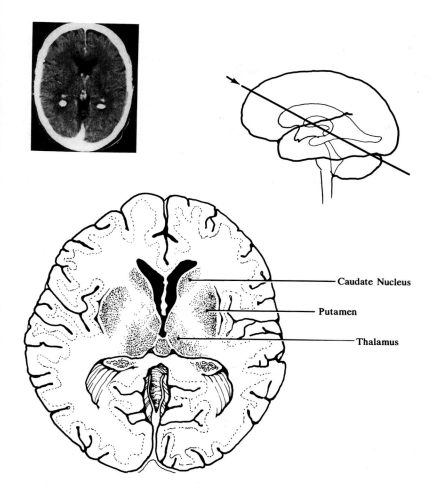

**Figure 14.1.** Anatomy of the basal ganglia on CT. Upper left is an axial CT section taken through a plane shown in the figure on the upper right. Lower figure shows the location of anatomical structures in this section. (Drawn by Harriet Greenfield.)

The striatofugal fibers are mostly thin and poorly myelinated. The fibers travel in small bundles that converge medially upon the pallidum passing through and around its borders. In transverse sections, these fibers pass through the lightly stained putamen and are directed ventromedially toward the pallidum. These fibers are most prominent in the medial part of the putamen. Further caudally, the striatofugal fibers pass to the substantia nigra traversing the cerebral peduncle. The striatonigral and nigrostriatal fibers are topographically and reciprocally organized.

Putaminal hemorrhage often involves the adjacent lateral segment of the globus pallidus. This region has been shown to project to the dorsolateral portion of the subthalamic nucleus.[14] The subthalamic nucleus has strong projections to both the internal and external segments of the globus pallidus and to the substantia nigra, *pars reticulata*.[14,15]

The functions of the lateral basal gangli- onic structures have been studied mostly in primates. The putamen seems to participate in a critical basal ganglionic-thalamic-cortical loop that has predominantly motor func- tions. This "motor loop" receives input mostly from premotor and secondary-motor cortex and directs its influences to specific premotor areas.[16] The study of neural activity during various controlled movements shows putaminal discharge during slow and rapid movements and during isometric contrac- tions, and during both voluntary spontaneous movements and those triggered by sensory stimuli.[17] The putamen is also undoubtedly involved in the preparation for movement as well as in its execution.[18,19] Marsden concluded that "the basal ganglia are responsible for the automatic execution of learned motor plans."[19] Abnormalities of tone and posture, and abnormal movements such as tremors and chorea, are also often found in humans and animals with lesions in the putamen and lateral pallidum. Injections of gamma-aminobutyric acid (GABA) antagonists into the lentiform nucleus complex can produce chorea in the contralateral limbs of monkeys.[14] The putaminal region probably also participates in eye as well as limb movements.[20]

The blood supply of the putamen is derived predominantly from penetrating branches of the middle cerebral artery. However, the most anterior portion of the putamen is supplied in part by branches of the recurrent arteries of Heubner.[21] These penetrators sweep from the anterior perforated substance to enter the anteromedial putamen from its medial aspect. The medial lenticulostriate branches usually arise at the very medial origin of the middle cerebral artery and penetrate the anterior perforated substance just lateral to the penetrating anterior cerebral artery branches.[22–24] The medial lenticulostriates supply predominantly the globus pallidus. The lateral lenticulostriate arteries are a series of vessels that originate most often from the mainstem middle cerebral artery to supply the lateral third of the globus pallidus and most of the putamen and internal capsule. In almost one-fourth of patients, the lateral lenticulostriates arise from the middle cerebral artery bifurcation and in 20% of specimens, the vessels originate from the superior division branch of the middle cerebral artery.[22–25] Slanting first laterally, the fan of three to six lateral lenticulostriate arteries arc through and around the putamen and then course medially toward the superior portion of the internal capsule. Figure 14.2 depicts diagrammatically the blood supply of the lateral ganglionic region.

### Pathology

Lateral ganglionic hemorrhages can be tiny and round, globoid, or linear in shape. As the hematoma expands, it often dissects along white matter pathways, most often along the anterior-posterior dimension.[26]

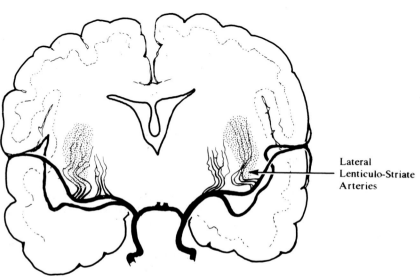

Lateral
Lenticulo-Striate
Arteries

Figure 14.2. Artist's diagram of the lateral lenticulostriate arteries which supply the putamen. The medial lenticulostriate artery branches of the middle cerebral artery are just medial to the lateral lenticulostriate arteries. (Drawn by Harriet Greenfield.)

Larger lesions exert pressure and often push the medially related structures, the pallidus, internal capsule, and caudate nucleus, in a more medial direction, sometimes across the midline. The laterally located structures are similarly pushed more laterally so that the external and extreme capsules, the claustrum and insular and opercular cortex, lie closer to the skull surface. Hemorrhages may dissect medially draining into the lateral ventricles or laterally toward the subarachnoid surface within or adjacent to the sylvian fissure. In the past, drainage into the ventricular system was considered a disastrous complication usually leading to coma and death. Actually, ventricular or subarachnoid drainage helps to decompress the enlarging hematoma. The alternative to this drainage is further bleeding into the brain parenchyma. Studies have shown that patients with putaminal hemorrhages that drain into the ventricles have a poorer prognosis for survival and recovery than those without such drainage, but the poor outcome is entirely accounted for by the size of the hematomas.[27–29] Only large hematomas that have dissected across the internal capsule drain into the medially located lateral ventricles. At times, putaminal hemorrhages spread posteriorly into the thalamus. These lesions are probably best referred to as putaminal-thalamic hemorrhages since it is often difficult to know where the bleeding originated.

Large hematomas, especially those that develop quickly, often cause secondary pressure-related changes. Pressure on the medial structures often shifts the midline, putting pressure on the contralateral paramedian structures. Distortion of the ventricular system can cause obstruction at the foramen of Monro with dilatation of the contralateral lateral ventricle. Sometimes, posteriorly located putaminal hemorrhages can compress the ipsilateral atrial region leading to trapping and dilatation of the ipsilateral temporal horn. A pressure cone can develop causing ipsilateral uncal herniation in which the posterior cerebral artery is compressed at the uncal notch. This vascular pressure causes

infarction of the medial temporal lobe and occipital lobe supplied by this artery, the infarct causing further brain swelling and mass effect. The most severe pressure effects are due to compression of the brainstem. Both "central herniation" with downward symmetrical compression of the diencephalon and unilateral lateral compression of the midbrain have been noted in large putaminal hemorrhages. The distortion of the brainstem often leads to secondary Duret hemorrhages. Figures 14.3, 14.4, and 14.5 shows necropsy specimens of large sized lateral ganglionic hemorrhages. Figure 14.6 illustrates two different pressure effects caused by a large putaminal hematoma. Compression of the foramen of Monro leads to dilatation of the contralateral lateral ventricle, and compression at the tentorial notch leads to infarction of the temporal lobe supplied by the compressed posterior cerebral artery. Figures 14.7 and 14.8 show Duret hemorrhages found at necropsy in patients with large fatal putaminal hematomas. Figures 14.9 and 14.10 show CT scans of large putaminal hemorrhages and Figure 14.11 a small lesion.

A morphological study in which putaminal hemorrhage cavities were tagged with radiopaque material at the time of surgical drainage serves as the best source of data about the frequency of various localizations of lesions within the lateral ganglionic region.[30] Most often hematomas are found in the *middle* part of the putamen as viewed in horizontal brain sections. This portion of the putamen lies just lateral to the corticospinal (pyramidal) tract fibers that traverse the posterior limb of the internal capsule. In this location, the thalamus is located medial to the internal capsule and the hematoma. The next most common location is the *posterior* type in which the hematoma occupies the most posterior portion of the putamen and internal capsule often spreading to the retrolenticular regions of the white matter behind the capsule. Some of these posteriorly situated lesions dissect along white matter pathways and turn laterally to produce a hockey-stick-like configuration turning laterally into the

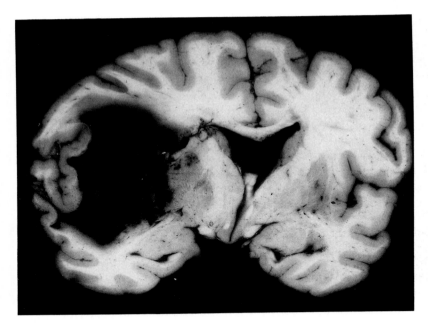

**Figure 14.3.** Necropsy specimen showing a very large putaminal hematoma. The hemorrhage has tracked medially draining into the lateral ventricles. The pallidum and other medial structures are displaced medially with considerable midline shift. The insula and cortical structures lateral to the hematoma are compressed.

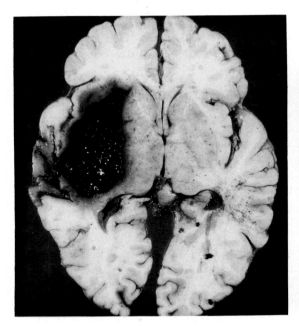

**Figure 14.4.** Necropsy specimen showing large putaminal hemorrhage in axial section comparable to CT. This hematoma has dissected laterally emptying onto the surface.

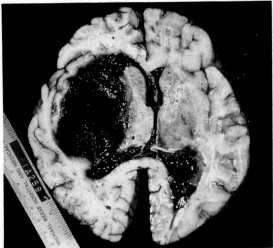

**Figure 14.5.** Necropsy specimen showing large putaminal hematoma in axial section. Drainage into the ventricular system, and medial and lateral displacement of normal brain tissues are shown.

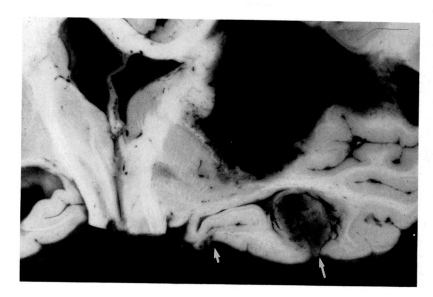

**Figure 14.6.** Necropsy specimen showing large putaminal hematoma with shift of midline structures. The medial inferior temporal lobe has been compressed against the tentorial notch (short white arrow) causing compression of the temporal branch of the posterior cerebral artery and infarction in the medial temporal lobe (long white arrow).

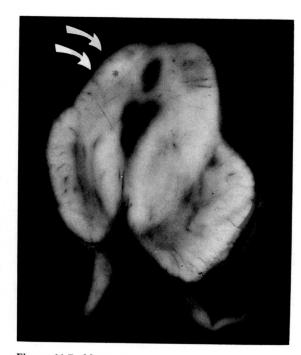

**Figure 14.7.** Necropsy specimen of midbrain in a patient with a large putaminal hemorrhage. Pressure from above and from the right side has compressed the left midbrain against the tentorial edge (arrows). Duret hemorrhages are seen in the midline which is shifted from right to left.

white matter of the temporal isthmus leading into the temporal lobe (Figure 14.12). Least often, hematomas are found in the *anterior* segment of the putamen adjacent to the anterior limb of the internal capsule. In these lesions, the head of the caudate nucleus is situated medial to the lesions. Figure 14.13 diagrammatically shows the location of the anterior, middle, and posterior groups of putaminal hemorrhages. It is usually possible using modern neuroimaging tests to determine to which location or group of putaminal hemorrhages the patient belongs. To a great extent, the anterior-posterior location of the lesion and its size and spread determine the physical findings and prognosis of the hemorrhage. With time, the cavity of the hematoma collapses leaving a "slit" (Figure 14.14).

The lateral ganglionic region is the most common location of deep hypertensive ICH. In the introduction to this section, we have reviewed the frequency of putaminal hemorrhages in various large series.[31-39] Various studies described the lesions differently, for example, basal ganglionic, capsular, lateral ganglionic, and so forth. Some did not distinguish between the deep structures and called the hematomas putaminothalamic. Probably about one-third of all spontaneous ICH are

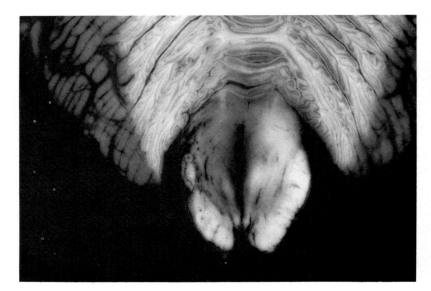

**Figure 14.8.** Necropsy specimen of midbrain in a patient with a large putaminal hematoma. The midbrain is elongated, the tegmentum is diffusely swollen and necrotic, and there is a midline Duret hemorrhage.

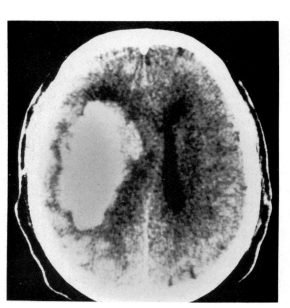

**Figure 14.9.** CT showing very large putaminal hematoma with compression of the ipsilateral adjacent lateral ventricle.

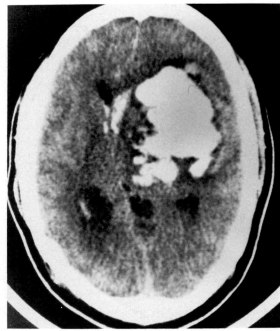

**Figure 14.10.** CT showing large putaminal hematoma with drainage into the ventricular system and massive midline shift.

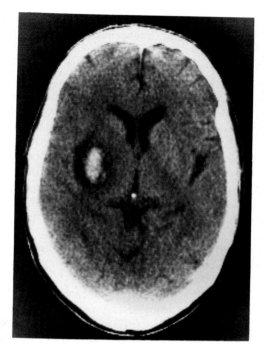

**Figure 14.11.** CT showing rather small putaminal hematoma with surrounding edema.

pia, conjugate deviation of the eyes toward the side of the lesion, decreased level of alertness, and aphasia in left-sided lesions and neglect of the left side of space in right-sided hematomas.[5,6] The syndrome was developed from the study of patients who came to postmortem with putaminal hemorrhages, since in the pre-CT era there was no other way to accurately localize the lesions. We now know that the findings in patients with putaminal hemorrhage are very variable. Signs and symptoms depend on a number of factors including:

1. The location of the hematoma within the putamen especially whether the lesion occupies the middle, anterior, or posterior segments (see Figure 14.13).
2. The size of the lesion and its spread to adjacent regions, especially the internal capsule and thalamus.
3. The presence and distribution of surrounding edema and pressure exerted on

putaminal in location. A great proportion of hematomas found in the putaminal region are hypertensive, or at least not due to other known causes such as trauma, amyloid angiopathy, aneurysms, and bleeding diatheses. Weisberg[35] analyzed a large series of ganglionic-thalamic hematomas shown by CT according to mechanism. Only ten among 232 (4%) were of defined nonhypertensive cause (two angiomas, two aneurysms, five coagulopathy, one tumor) and 187 (81%) were considered hypertensive.[35] When a typically located putaminal hemorrhage is found on CT in a patient with high blood pressure, a search for a nonhypertensive cause is almost always fruitless.

## Symptoms and Signs

Early writings emphasized the uniformity of findings in putaminal hemorrhage patients. The "syndrome" included a contralateral hemiplegia, hemisensory loss, and hemiano-

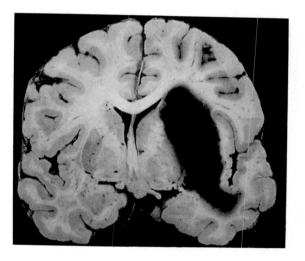

**Figure 14.12.** Large left putaminal hemorrhage dissecting along white matter tracts into the temporal lobe, adopting a hockey-stick-like configuration. (From Kase CS, Mohr JP, Caplan LR. Intracerebral hemorrhage. In Barnett HJM, et al., eds. Stroke: pathophysiology, diagnosis, and management. Second edition. New York: Churchill Livingstone, 1992;561–616. Reprinted with permission).

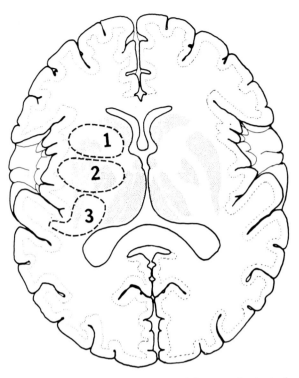

**Figure 14.13.** Artist's diagram of three major loci of putaminal hematomas. (1) is anterior type, (2) is middle type, (3) is posterior. As shown, the posterior type often dissects into the temporal lobe. (Drawn by Harriet Greenfield.)

adjacent structures. The presence of pressure shifts or herniation is especially important.

4. Disconnection of brain regions. The long linear lesions often interrupt wiring connecting the overlying cerebral cortex with the deep basal gray nuclei, and connecting different cortical regions with each other. As has been emphasized in the pathology section, the medially located structures are pushed further medially toward the ventricle, and the laterally situated cortex and external and extreme capsules are pushed further laterally. Though distorted and compressed, these regions may retain their viability but their fiber interconnections are irreparably interrupted.

5. Metabolic effects on the cerebral cortex. Metabolic studies using positron emmision tomography (PET) scan technology and fluorodeoxyglucose show that putaminal hemorrhages often are accompanied by significant and persistent depression of glucose metabolism in zones of overlying, anatomically preserved, cerebral cortex.[40] In anteriorly placed lesions, the metabolic depression is predominantly in the frontal lobe ipsilateral to the hemor-

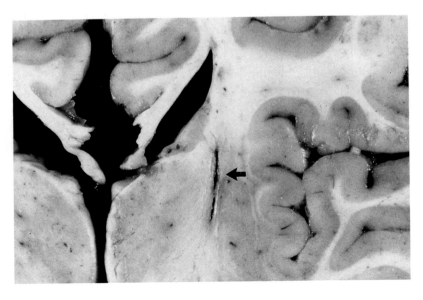

**Figure 14.14.** Necropsy specimen showing slit cavity (arrow) representing an old putaminal hemorrhage. The tear in the corpus collosum is artifactual.

rhage.[40] Posteriorly located lesions cause metabolic depression in the cortex of the temporal and parietal lobes. Small hematomas cause less effects on cortical metabolism.

Disconnection and metabolic effects probably account for the very high frequency of higher cortical function abnormalities in patients with putaminal hemorrhages. The vast majority of patients with left putaminal hematomas have some abnormalities of language function, while neglect of contralateral space, poor drawing and copying, dysprosody, anosognosia, and motor impersistence are commonly found in patients with right putaminal lesions.

The single most important and most frequent findings are *abnormalities of the motor system.*[26,30,36,41] Weakness or paralysis usually involves the contralateral face, arm, and leg and is almost invariably accompanied by hyperreflexia and a Babinski sign. The hyperreflexia is noted very early in the course of the illness and is nearly always present on the initial neurological examination. When the hematoma occupies the middle part of the putamen and spreads medially to the adjacent internal capsule, the paralysis is usually severe and persistent and does not recover well.[30,41–43] Some patients with small hematomas located predominantly at the genu or within the posterior limb of the internal capsule present with a syndrome closely mimicking pure motor hemiparesis due to lacunar infarction.[44,45] Hematomas limited to the middle putamen have also caused a pure motor hemiparesis usually with excellent resolution.[46] At times, capsular involvement results from spread of small hematomas arising in the pallidum and dissecting medially.[45]

Most often, there are at least slight subjective *sensory symptoms* in the weak limbs, even in patients with small hematomas. Patients describe the weak limbs as feeling funny, heavy, or numb even when there are no objective sensory abnormalities.[41] Hematomas in the posterior portion of the putamen and

posterior capsule are often associated with a predominantly *ataxic syndrome* in which limb incoordination and ataxia are the major abnormalities in the arm and leg contralateral to the hemorrhage.[45,47] In these patients, the gait may also be slightly ataxic, usually the patient veering toward the side of the affected limbs. Rarely the predominant motor abnormality is a *hemichorea*. Jones et al. reported a single patient with a right putaminal hemorrhage of moderate size who suddenly developed continuous purposeless choreic movements of the left arm and leg.[48] When extended, the left hand maintained a "dystonic striatal posture" and the left limbs were hyperreflexic and a left Babinski sign was present.

Some patients with putaminal hemorrhage have *ipsilateral abnormal arm movements.* These movements are noted at the onset of symptoms by the patient, a spouse, or other observers who describe a tremor or shaking of the ipsilateral arm. Some patients with right putaminal lesions and left neglect and anosognosia will report only the right limb shaking and will be unaware and unconcerned with their hemiplegia. When examined, the ipsilateral arm is restless and incoordinated without weakness, ataxia, or hyperreflexia. The abnormal movements are probably best explained by ipsilateral descending projections from the basal ganglia. The ipsilateral adventitious movements in our experience do not persist once the contralateral hemiplegia becomes established.

In patients with large hemorrhages and shift of midline structures, ipsilateral weakness and pyramidal dysfunction develop as the patient is clinically worsening. Most often when a history is available, the patient or observers report first a hemiplegia contralateral to the hemorrhage and then the onset of bilateral weakness. Some patients with larger hemorrhages when first examined have bilateral paralysis, hyperreflexia, and Babinski signs closely mimicking pontine hemorrhage. The bilateral motor signs relate to compression of the contralateral cerebral peduncle or upper brainstem. These patients with bilateral motor signs also invariably have other signs of increased pressure, such as decreased alertness, bilateral conjugate gaze paresis, and abnormal pupils.

*Sensory abnormalities* are also very common, although most patients with hemiplegia do not complain of paresthesias. Numbness, or dead anesthesic feelings are most often described. On examination, almost invariably there is a decrease in touch and pin perception in the weak limbs.[26] When the hematoma is large or involves the middle or posterior segments of the putamen there is also diminished ability to discern position sense in the involved limbs. Localization of tactile stimuli may be preserved. Rarely in patients with far posteriorly placed hematomas that affect the posterior limb of the capsule, there may be a predominantly sensory syndrome with only very minor weakness.[49]

Hemianopia and neglect of the left side of visual space are common findings in patients with large putaminal hemorrhages.[26] The predominant abnormality is visual neglect. Most patients do not have a persistent hemianopia after recovery since seldom is the lesion posterior enough to interrupt the geniculocalcarine tract. Asking the patient to read a newspaper or magazine page, or to describe a scene outside of a window are the best ways to detect the visual neglect abnormality. Usually patients will read or describe only those stimuli on the side of the hemorrhage and will ignore those in the opposite visual field. Neglect is more predominant in right lateral ganglionic hemorrhages but is occasionally found in left-sided lesions. Some posterior hematomas that dissect near the atrium or temporal horn of the lateral ventricle can interrupt the temporal visual radiation causing an upper *quadrantanopia*.

Extraocular movement abnormalities are very important diagnostic features in patients with lateral ganglionic hemorrhages. The most common finding is a conjugate gaze paresis.[8,26,38] The eyes are both deviated conjugately at rest to the side of the hematoma. Patients have a delay or inability to generate saccades voluntarily to the opposite

side and often do not visually follow objects moving into the contralateral visual field. Optokinetic responses are also abnormal. Conjugate eye deviation at rest is invariably present in patients with large hematomas, especially those that are located in the anterior and middle segments of the putamen and internal capsule. In contrast, conjugate eye deviation is virtually never found in patients with pure motor hemiparesis due to capsular lacunar infarction. In posteriorly placed putaminal hemorrhages, patients may have difficulty following objects into the opposite visual field but the eyes are not deviated at rest. Oculocephalic and oculovestibular stimuli induce full horizontal eye movements but in the early period after the stroke, reflex conjugate movements to the contralateral side may be difficult to elicit. Sometimes both ice water caloric and doll's eye maneuvers must be used simultaneously to obtain full conjugate movement to the contralateral side.

In large hematomas, pressure shifts can lead to additional oculomotor abnormalities. Compression of fibers in the opposite hemisphere may lead to defective eye movements to the ipsilateral side. The eyes, originally deviated ipsilaterally, are now midline and there is bilateral horizontal conjugate gaze paresis. Pressure on the rostral brainstem can cause a vertical gaze palsy or elements of an ipsilateral third nerve palsy. Even sixth nerve palsies have been described and are presumably related to the increased intracranial pressure.[26] The development of any oculomotor abnormality other than a unilateral conjugate gaze palsy is a very poor prognostic sign since it signifies important changes in intracranial pressure and contents.

The *pupils* are normal in the vast majority of patients with putaminal hemorrhages. Usually they are of normal size and react normally to light. Exceptions include patients with hematomas that dissect far ventrally and medially affecting the hypothalamus and upper diencephalon. However, when hematomas are very large and pressure on the upper brainstem develops, the ipsilateral pupil may change. At first pressure causes ipsilateral pupillary constriction. Later, the ipsilateral pupil dilates. When the upper brainstem is severely compromised, both pupils become abnormal. When the pressure cone is far lateral, uncal herniation can cause an ipsilateral third nerve palsy with a dilated pupil without a preliminary period of pupillary constriction. Any pupillary abnormality that develops in a patient with putaminal hemorrhage adversely affects the prognosis for survival and recovery.[38,41]

*Higher cortical function* abnormalities are very common in patients with putaminal hemorrhages. Large and medium left putaminal hematomas are usually accompanied by some degree of aphasia. Most often the language abnormality is a global aphasia affecting production, repetition, and comprehension of spoken and written language. In hematomas within the anterior segment, the major finding is often decreased output of speech. Speech is sparse and often poorly articulated.[38,50] Posterior temporal hematomas cause a Wernicke-type aphasia. Posterior lesions that spread to the temporal isthmus are especially hard to diagnose clinically as putaminal hemorrhages by the unwary since motor signs may be minimal; the findings include a hemisensory loss, slight limb weakness, an upper quadrantanopia, and a fluent aphasia with paraphasic errors. The syndrome mimics the findings in patients with embolic infarction in the distribution of the inferior division of the left middle cerebral artery. Writing is particularly affected and usually to a severe degree.[50] Curiously and diagnostically, in patients with global aphasia, speech repetition and echoing of words returns early in the course so that the aphasic syndrome resembles a transcortical aphasia. The preservation of speech repetition despite the presence of a deep lesion that interrupts the arcuate fasciculus, a white matter fiber tract connecting frontal and temporal lobes, provides strong argument against the interpretation that the arcuate fasciculus is important in the production of conduction aphasia. The aphasia syndromes that accompany putaminal hemor-

rhages are more transient that the language abnormality seen in patients with extensive middle cerebral artery cortical infarcts.[50] Neglect and inattention toward left-sided stimuli accompany right putaminal hemorrhages of appreciable size. Other so-called right hemisphere behavior abnormalities, such as poor drawing and copying, speech dysprosody, anosognosia, abulia, and motor impersistence are frequently found in patients with right-sided hematomas[51,52] and may cause persistent problems in recovery.[53]

Putting together the various signs and symptoms yields useful prototypic syndromes in patients with putaminal hemorrhages located at the common sites. In *anteriorly placed lesions,* the syndrome is primarily motor and there are few, if any, sensory or visual abnormalities. The eyes are conjugately deviated to the side of the lesion. Abulia and a transcortical motor aphasia are the commonest behavioral abnormalities. Although moderately severe, the hemiparesis is usually temporary and reversible. Patients with anterior lesions usually make good recoveries. Hemorrhages in the *middle part of the putamen* usually cause the most severe deficits and recover least well. Visual, sensory, and behavioral abnormalities accompany the severe hemiplegia, and conjugate eye deviation is invariably present. *Posteriorly situated lesions* have the least prominent motor abnormalities and sensory, visual, ataxic, or behavioral deficits may predominate. The eyes are usually not conjugately deviated at rest. Table 14.1 lists the most common features found in patients with putaminal hemorrhages at the various sites.

The onset of symptoms is usually abrupt and the deficit accumulates during a period of fifteen minutes to several hours. Most often, the progression of the neurological deficit is halted by the time the patient is examined in the emergency room.[26,38] In one large series of patients with putaminal hemorrhage, among twenty-one patients seen within six hours of the onset of symptoms, the neurological deficits had stabilized in fifteen patients by the time of the examina-

**Table 14.1.** Clinical Findings in Putaminal Hemorrhages at Various Sites

| Type | Contralateral | | | | Cognitive and Behavioral | |
|---|---|---|---|---|---|---|
| | Motor | Sensory | Visual | Oculomotor | Left Lesions | Right Lesions |
| Anterior | moderate, often temporary hemiparesis; Babinski sign | subjective numbness | | conjugate deviation to side of lesion; conjugate voluntary gaze palsy to opposite side | abulia, non-fluent aphasia, preserved repetition; poor writing | abulia, motor impersistence; temporary L neglect |
| Middle | severe persistent hemiplegia, hyper-reflexia, Babinski sign | decreased pin, touch, position sense | visual neglect | conjugate deviation to side of lesion; horizontal conjugate gaze palsy to opposite side | global aphasia with relatively preserved repetition; poor writing | anosognosia, left neglect |
| Posterior | Slight hemiparesis; ataxia; hyperreflexia; Babinski sign | paresthesias, decreased pin, touch, position sense | prominent neglect, occasional severe hemianopia or quadrantanopia | decreased visual pursuit towards contralateral visual field | fluent aphasia; poor reading and writing; paraphasic errors | L neglect, poor drawing and copying |
| Small Capsular | Hemiparesis, usually moderate but temporary; hyperreflexia; Babinski sign | slight subjective | | | | |

tion.[26] Some patients, however, do progress. During the acute phase worsening can sometimes be shown to be caused by persistent bleeding which can continue for minutes and hours after onset.[54,55] Later, edema develops and increases local and generalized mass effect. Worsening may be manifested solely by a worsening of the neurological signs already present, for example, development of a more severe hemiplegia or more severe aphasia. More ominous is the development of signs that indicate compression of the contralateral hemisphere or brainstem. Patients with significant shifts of the midline become less alert. Stupor and coma may ensue. Development of an ipsilateral extensor plantar reflex and hyperreflexia in the limbs on the same side as the hematoma are the earliest signs of dysfunction of the contralateral hemisphere. Paratonic stiffness and weakness of the ipsilateral limbs denote more severe compromise and by now the patient is stuporous and quadraparetic. The development of pupillary changes and bilateral horizontal gaze palsies or vertical gaze abnormalities means pressure on the upper brainstem. In hypertensive putaminal hemorrhages, worsening usually develops within the first seventy-two hours or not at all.

## Prognosis

The outlook for recovery in patients with putaminal hemorrhage depends on a number of clinical and neuroimaging findings. The data to judge prognosis are available during the first day of admission and usually within a few hours. Demographic features do not seem to correlate with outcome. We might have predicted that older patients would do less well but statistical analysis does not bear this out.[56,57] In fact, in one study, younger patients, mostly black men, did less well than older black and white patients.[56] Perhaps the atrophy that comes with age provides reserve room inside the cranium for ICH with a resulting decreased frequency of herniation. Blood pressure in

one study correlated with the size of hemorrhage[27] but did not in another.[26] The Pilot Stroke Data Bank analysis showed that pulse pressure was one of the three strongest predictors of poor outcome, the others being size of hemorrhage and Glasgow coma score.[57] Tuhrim et al. hypothesized that increased intracranial pressure (ICP) had led to a higher systolic and lower diastolic pressure and that pulse pressure might have been a "surrogate" for intracranial pressure which was usually not formally measured and so was not analyzed.[57]

Physical signs are helpful predictors. All studies have found that coma carries a dire prognosis in patients with putaminal hemorrhage.[8,28,31,36,41,56,57] Any lessening of alertness adversely affects prognosis. The severity of the hemiplegia always is related to survival since putaminal hemorrhage patients with little or no weakness usually have smaller hematomas.[57] The Pilot Stroke Data Bank found that horizontal conjugate gaze paresis also correlated with poor outcome,[57] probably for the same reason as severity of hemiplegia. Vertical gaze palsy and other abnormalities of brainstem function, not surprisingly, also predict poor outcome since they indicate compression of the rostral brainstem by mass effect or spread of the putaminal hematoma.[57] Worsening of the clinical deficit while the patient is under clinical observation is also an adverse prognostic sign.[8,26,36,57]

In all series, the size of the hematoma predicts outcome. The larger the hematoma the less the chance for survival and the poorer the outlook for recovery of function.[27,28,29,32,35,56,57] Hier et al. found that patients with putaminal hematomas larger than 140 $mm^2$ (as measured by cross-sectional area at the slice with the most blood) did poorly.[26] The Pilot Stroke Data Bank investigators found that size was one of the most important predictors of outcome.[57] They subdivided lesions by estimating whether the hematomas were small (less than half of a lobe), moderate (between one-half to one lobe), or large (greater than one lobe). Among forty patients with large hematomas, seventeen (42.5%) died, while only four of thirty-two (12.5%) patients with small hematomas died.[57] Young et al. studied the effect of the size of hematomas and the presence and amount of ventricular blood on prognosis.[29] The volume of parenchymal and ventricular blood were calculated by computer read-out after the edges of the hematoma were marked, and the data were digitalized and stored. In this study, among 20 putaminal hemorrhage patients, the average volume of parenchymal blood was 33.7 cm[3] and the average volume of ventricular blood was 6.6 cm[3]. Outcome was highly correlated with parenchymal and parenchymal plus ventricle volume of blood, but the volume of ventricular blood was less significant.[29] Patients with more than 20 cm[3] of ventricular blood did poorly but also invariably had large intracerebral hematomas. Similarly, Stein et al. found that patients with ventricular blood did poorly but also invariably had large intracerebral hematomas. The presence of ventricular blood was also a poor prognostic sign in patients with putaminal hemorrhage.[27] We believe that hemorrhages that dissect from the putamen far medially to the ventricle are invariably large, and ventricular spread in itself does not cause major

problems unless the volume is large. Ventricular blood does not correlate with outcome in caudate hematoma.[27] The Pilot Stroke Data Bank analysis also found hydrocephalus to be an adverse prognostic factor.[57] Ropper and Gress analyzed CT findings in comatose patients with large hematomas (greater than 55 cm[3], range 55 to 161 cm[3]).[58] Coma could be attributed to 8 mm or greater horizontal shift of the midline at the pineal region or diencephalic spread.

The location of the putaminal hematoma is important in gauging the likelihood of recovery from hemiplegia. Persistent hemiplegia is usually due to destruction of the posterior limb of the internal capsule when the hematoma spreads medially from the putamen. The location of the hematoma on various imaging and radiographic studies can help predict involvement of this capsular region. Mizukami et al. studied the prognosis for recovery of hemiplegia in a large series of patients with putaminal hemorrhage.[42] The outcome correlated best with the presence or absence of blood on a CT section through the bodies of the lateral ventricles. When blood was found at this level, usually the posterior limb of the capsule contained hematoma and hemiplegia would persist (Figure 14.15). Earlier, Mizukami had correlated the angio-

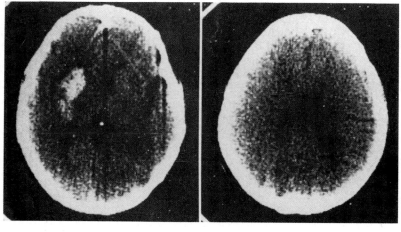

A          B

**Figure 14.15.** CT scans in a patient with anterior type of putaminal hematoma. Scan at level of the foramen of Monro (A) shows the hematoma, but no hematoma is seen at the level of the bodies of the lateral ventricle (B), indicating that the posterior limb of the capsule is not involved. (From Mizukami M, Nishijima M, Kin H. Computed tomographic findings of good prognosis for hemiplegia in hypertensive putaminal hemorrhage. Stroke 1981;12:648–652, with permission.)

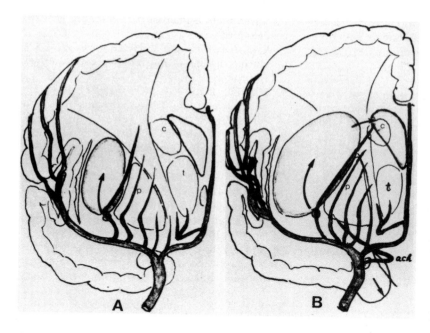

**Figure 14.16.** Schematic drawing of angiographic changes in putaminal hematomas. (A) The hematoma displaces the lateral lenticulostriate branch medially but does not affect its distal portion which courses through the posterior limb of the capsule. (B) The distal portion of this artery is displaced medially by a larger hematoma that extends into the posterior limb of the internal capsule. (From Mizukami M, Araki G, Mihara H. Angiographic sign of good prognosis for hemiplegia in hypertensive intracerebral hemorrhage. Neurology 1974;24:120–126, with permission.)

graphic appearance of the lenticulostriate artery with recovery from hemiplegia.[43] Putaminal hemorrhages usually cause the proximal portion of the lentriculostriate artery to deviate medially. When the posterior limb of the capsule is involved, the distal portion of the artery is also deviated medially. When the posterior limb is spared, the terminal portion of the artery retains its natural course[43] (Figure 14.16).

The discussion on prognosis considered mostly conservatively treated patients. Treatment of all hematomas will be considered in Chapter 22. The advent of CT- and MRI-guided stereotactic surgery has recently allowed percutaneous drainage of hematomas providing a new treatment to be evaluated.[59]

## References

1. Adams F. The Genuine Works of Hipocrates: translated from the Greek. Baltimore: Williams & Wilkins, 1939.
2. Hooper R. The Morbid Anatomy of the Human Brain. Illustrated by Coloured Engravings of the most frequent and important Organic Diseases to which that viscus is subject. London: Longman, Ries, Orme, Brown and Green, 1828.
3. Charcot JM, Bouchard C. Nouvelles recherches sur la pathogénie de l'hémorrhagie cérébrale. Arch Physiol Norm Path 1868;1:110–127, 643–665, 725–734.
4. McHenry LC. Garrison's History of Neurology, revised and enlarged. Springfield, IL: Charles C Thomas, 1969.
5. Osler W. The Principles and Practice of Medicine. Fifth Edition. New York: D. Appleton, 1903;997–1008.
6. Gowers WR. A Manual of Diseases of the Nervous System. London: Churchill, 1893;384–413.
7. Aring CD, Merritt HH. Differential diagnosis between cerebral hemorrhage and cerebral thrombosis: a clinical and pathologic study of 245 cases. Arch Intern Med 1935;56:435–456.
8. Fisher CM. Clinical syndromes in cerebral hemorrhage. In: Fields WS, ed. Pathogenesis and Treatment of Cerebrovascular Disease. Springfield, IL: Charles C Thomas, 1961; 318–342.
9. Brodal A. Neurological Anatomy in Relation to Clinical Medicine. Third Edition. Oxford: Oxford University Press, 1981;211–226.
10. Carpenter MB, Sutin J. Human Neuroanatomy. Eight Edition. Baltimore: Williams & Wilkins, 1983;579–591.

11. Künzle H. Bilateral projections from precentral motor cortex to the putamen and other parts of the basal ganglia. Brain Res 1975;88: 195–210.

12. Jones EG, Coulter JD, Burton H, et al. Cells of origin and terminal distribution of corticostriatal fibers arising in the sensory-motor cortex of monkeys. J Comp Neurol 1977;173:53–80.

13. Denny-Brown D. The basal ganglia and their relation to disorders of movement. London: Oxford University Press, 1962.

14. Mitchell IJ, Jackson A, Sambrook MA, et al. The Role of the Subthalamic Nucleus in Experimental Chorea. Brain 1989;112:1533–1548.

15. Nauta HJW, Cole M. Efferent projections of the subthalamic nucleus: an autoradiographic study in monkey and cat. J Comp Neurol 1978;180:1–16.

16. DeLong MR, Alexander GE. Organization of basal ganglia. In Asbury AK, et al., eds. Diseases of the Nervous System: Neurobiology. Philadelphia: Ardmore Medical Books, 1986; 379–393.

17. DeLong MR, Georgopoulos AP. Motor functions of the basal ganglia. In: Brookhart JM, et al., eds. Handbook of Physiology, The Nervous System. Bethesda: American Physiological Society, 1981;1017–1061.

18. Alexander GE. Instruction-dependent neuronal activity in primate putamen. Soc Neurosci Abstr 1984;10:515.

19. Marsden CD. The mysterious motor function of the basal ganglia: The Robert Wartenberg Lecture. Neurology 1982;32:514–539.

20. Alexander GE, DeLong MR, Strick PL. Parallel organization of functionally segregated circuits linking basal ganglia and cortex. Annu Rev Neurosci. 1986; 9:357–381.

21. Gorczyca W, Mohr G. Microvascular anatomy of Heubner's recurrent artery. Neurol Res 1987;9:259–264.

22. Kaplan HA. Anatomy and embryology of the arterial system of the forebrain. In Vinken PJ, Bruyn GW, eds. Vascular disease of the nervous system, Part I. Handbook of Clinical Neurology. Amsterdam: North Holland, 1972; 1–23.

23. Herman LH, Ostrowski AZ, Gurdjian ES. Perforating branches of the middle cerebral artery. Arch Neurol 1963;8:32–34.

24. Marinković SV, Kovačević MS, Marinković JM. Perforating branches of the middle cerebral artery: microsurgical anatomy of their extracerebral segments. J Neurosurg 1985;63: 266–271.

25. Caplan L, Babikian V, Helgason C, et al. Occlusive disease of the middle cerebral artery. Neurology 1985;35:975–982.

26. Hier DB, Davis KR, Richardson EP, et al. Hypertensive putaminal hemorrhage. Ann Neurol 1977;1:152–159.

27. Stein RW, Caplan LR, Hier DB. Outcome of intracranial hemorrhage: role of blood pressure and location and size of lesions. Ann Neurol 1983;14:132–133 (abstract).

28. Helweg-Larsen S, Sommer W, Strange P, et al. Prognosis for patients treated conservatively for spontaneous intracerebral hematomas. Stroke 1984;15:1045–1048.

29. Young WB, Lee KP, Pessin MS, et al. Prognostic significance of ventricular blood in supratentorial hemorrhage: a volumetric study. Neurology 1990;40:616–619.

30. Koba T, Yokoyama T, Kaneko M. Correlation between the location of hematoma and its clinical symptoms in the lateral type of hypertensive intracerebral hemorrhage: observations on pantopaque radiography of the hematoma cavity in cases of early surgical treatment. Stroke 1977;8:676–680.

31. Wilson SAK, Bruce AN. Neurology. Second Edition. London: Butterworth, 1955;1377.

32. Fisher CM. The pathology and pathogenesis of intracerebral hemorrhage. In: Fields WS, ed. Pathogenesis and Treatment of Cerebrovascular Disease. Springfield, IL: Charles C Thomas, 1961;295–317.

33. Mutlu N, Berry RG, Alpers BJ. Massive cerebral hemorrhage: clinical and pathological correlations. Arch Neurol 1963;8:644–661.

34. Freytag E. Fatal hypertensive intracerebral haematomas: a survey of the pathological anatomy of 393 cases. J Neurol Neurosurg Psychiat 1968;31:616–620.

35. Weisberg LA. Computerized tomography in intracerebral hemorrhage. Arch Neurol 1979;36:422–426.

36. Mohr JP, Caplan LR, Melski JW, et al. The Harvard Cooperative Stroke Registry: a prospective registry. Neurology 1978;28:754–762.

37. Bogousslavsky J, Van Melle G, Regli F. The Lausanne Stroke Registry: analysis of 1,000 consecutive patients with first stroke. Stroke 1988;19:1083–1092.

38. Caplan LR, Stein RW. Stroke: Clinical Approach. Boston: Butterworth, 1986;267.

39. Foulkes MA, Wolf PA, Price TR, et al. The Stroke Data Bank: design, methods and baseline characteristics. Stroke 1988;19:547–554.

40. Metter EJ, Jackson C, Kempler D, et al. Left hemisphere intracerebral hemorrhages studied by (F-18)-fluorodeoxyglucose PET. Neurology 1986;36:1155–1162.

41. Caplan LR, Mohr JP. Intracerebral hemorrhage: an update. Geriatrics 1978;33:42–52.

42. Mizukami M, Nishijima M, Kin H. Computed tomographic findings of good prognosis for hemiplegia in hypertensive putaminal hemorrhage. Stroke 1981;12:648–652.

43. Mizukami M, Araki G, Mihara H. Angiographic sign of good prognosis for hemiplegia in hypertensive intracerebral hemorrhage. Neurology 1974;24:120–126.

44. Weisberg LA, Wall M. Small capsular hemorrhages: clinical-computed tomographic correlations. Arch Neurol 1984;41:1255–1257.

45. Mori E, Tabuchi M, Yamadori A. Lacunar syndrome due to intracerebral hemorrhage. Stroke 1985;16:454–459.

46. Tapia J, Kase CS, Sawyer RH, et al. Hypertensive putaminal hemorrhage presenting as pure motor hemiparesis. Stroke 1983;14:505–506.

47. Mori E, Yamadori A, Kudo Y, et al. Ataxic hemiparesis from small capsular hemorrhage: computed tomography and somatosensory evoked potentials. Arch Neurol 1984;41:1050–1053.

48. Jones HR, Baker RA, Kott HS. Hypertensive putaminal hemorrhage presenting with hemichorea. Stroke 1985;16:130–131.

49. Groothuis DR, Duncan GW, Fisher CM. The human thalamocortical sensory path in the internal capsule: evidence from a small capsular hemorrhage causing a pure capsular sensory stroke. Ann Neurol 1977;2:328–331.

50. Alexander MP, LoVerme SR. Aphasia after left hemispheric intracerebral hemorrhage. Neurology 1980;30:1193–1202.

51. Hier DB, Stein R, Caplan LR. Cognitive and behavioral deficits after right hemisphere stroke. Current Concepts of Cerebrovascular Disease (Stroke) 1985;20:1–5.

52. Hier DB, Mondlock J, Caplan LR. Behavior abnormalities after right hemisphere stroke. Neurology 1983;33:337–344.

53. Hier DB, Mondlock J, Caplan LR. Recovery of behavioral abnormalities after right hemisphere stroke. Neurology 1983;33:345–350.

54. Broderick JP, Brott TG, Tomsick T, et al. Ultra-early evaluation of intracerebral hemorrhage. J Neurosurg 1990;72:195–199.

55. Kelley RE, Berger JR, Scheinberg P, et al. Active bleeding in hypertensive intracerebral hemorrhage: computed tomography. Neurology 1982;32:852–856.

56. Douglas MA, Haerer AF. Long-term prognosis of hypertensive intracerebral hemorrhage. Stroke 1982;13:488–491.

57. Tuhrim S, Dambrosia JM, Price TR, et al. Prediction of intracerebral hemorrhage survival. Ann Neurol 1988;24:258–263.

58. Ropper A, Gress DR. Anatomical causes of coma in large cerebral hemorrhage. Ann Neurol 1989;26:161 (abstract).

59. Niizuma H, Shimizu Y, Yonemitsu T, et al. Results of stereotactic aspiration in 175 cases of putaminal hemorrhage. Neurosurgery 1989;24:814–819.

# Chapter 15
# Caudate Hemorrhage

Louis R. Caplan

## Historical Aspects

Among all the common sites of intracerebral hemorrhage (ICH), caudate nucleus hemorrhages are the subject of the fewest reports and studies. In the pre-CT era, deep hemispheric hematomas were often referred to as "ganglionic" referring to the general location of the basal gray nuclei including the thalamus, pallidum, caudate, and putamen. Some spoke of medial ganglionic hemorrhages referring to caudate and thalamic hematomas, and lateral ganglionic lesions meaning putaminal hemorrhages. Clinicopathological correlations in patients with brain hematomas came only from analysis of fatal cases. One plausible reason why caudate hematomas were ignored or at least not recognized in early writings on brain hemorrhage was that patients with hemorrhages limited to the caudate nucleus and adjacent ventricular system generally had a favorable prognosis for recovery. Only those with large hemorrhages extending into the thalamus or lateral ganglionic regions expired, and in these larger hematomas, the prosector likely could not identify the origin of the bleeding. Few necropsy specimens of hematomas limited to the caudate nucleus and ventricular system were available for study. To this date we know of only one such specimen and that (Figure 15.1) was in a young patient who, while recovering, had a fatal massive pulmonary embolism.[1]

Osler makes probably the first reference to caudate hemorrhage. In his textbook of medicine, in the discussion on ventricular hemorrhage, he states, "In the cases which I have seen in adults, it (ventricular bleeding) has almost always been caused by rupture of a vessel in the neighborhood of the caudate nucleus."[2] Gowers also was aware of caudate hemorrhages and included them in his anterior group of hemorrhages in the corpus striatum but did not distinguish the findings in patients with caudate hematomas from those at other sites.[3] Fisher later noted, in a presentation to the Houston Neurological Society in 1959, "Occasionally hemorrhages occur into the head of the caudate nucleus with prompt rupture into the ventricular system producing the picture of subarachnoid hemorrhage without focal signs."[4] In discussing Fisher's paper, Dr. Robert Siekert showed a slide of a patient in whom a caudate hemorrhage was found at autopsy with only minimal clinical findings.[4] In their collection of massive hemorrhages, Mutlu et al. diagrammed the location of their mesial hemorrhages, illustrating caudate and thalamic locations (Figure 15.2).[5]

Computed tomography (CT) made it possible to distinguish hematomas arising in the head of the caudate nucleus from thalamic hematomas arising more posteriorly and

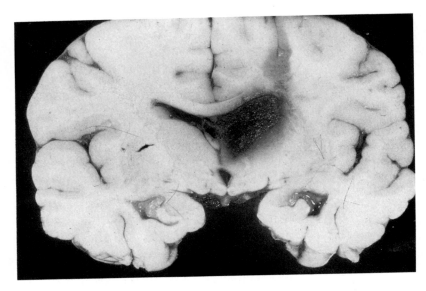

**Figure 15.1.** Necropsy specimen, coronal section. Hematoma is limited to the right caudate nucleus and adjacent lateral ventricle. The brownish stain above the ventricle is artifactual. (From Stein RW, Kase CS, Hier DB, et al. Caudate hemorrhage. Neurology 1984;34:1549–1554, with permission.)

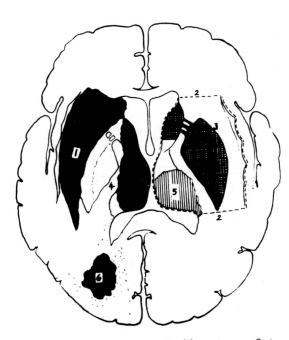

**Figure 15.2.** 1 refers to putaminal hematomas; 2, to hematomas involving the quadrilateral space; 3, are small putaminal hematomas; 5, are thalamic hematomas; 4 refers to medial hematomas; including the caudate nucleus and thalamus. (From Mutlu N, Berry R(G), Alpers B(J). Massive cerebral hemorrhage: clinical and pathological correlations. Arch Neurol 1963;8:644–661, with permission.)

putaminal hemorrhages arising more laterally. Yet at this writing, clinicoradiological studies of caudate hemorrhages are still rare. We could locate only four series of patients with spontaneous caudate nucleus hemorrhages.[1,6,7,8] These reports contain a total of thirty-four patients with hypertensive caudate hemorrhages, four with arteriovenous malformation (AVM) related hemorrhages, and four with ruptured basal aneurysms that bled into the caudate nucleus and adjacent structures. Other reports were usually isolated case reports that discussed a particular neurobehavioral phenomenon in a patient with caudate hemorrhage.[9–11] In these early reports of the findings in patients with caudate hematomas, it was always difficult to separate those findings due to involvement of the caudate nucleus and its connections, from those related to subarachnoid and intraventricular bleeding and changes in intracranial pressure. The restless agitation and confusion often found in patients with caudate hemorrhages were very similar to the findings in patients with subarachnoid hemorrhage due to aneurysmal rupture who had no bleeding in the brain parenchyma. Identification of patients with infarction within the caudate nucleus and its adjacent structures helped solve the puzzle.[12–15] In patients with caudate infarcts, changes in intracranial pressure and subarachnoid bleeding are not present so that the findings must be due only to dysfunction of the infarcted tissues and their connections.

## Anatomy

The caudate nuclei are paired robust ovoid deep gray matter structures that jut into the lateral ventricles. Throughout their course, the caudate nuclei are adjacent to the lateral ventricles, separated from the ventricles medially only by a thin layer of ependyma. Vascular malformations commonly arise from this subependymal region. The caudate nuclei first appear in coronal sections of the brain quite anteriorly and remain related to the anterior horn of the lateral ventricles so that they are generally considered as components of the deep portion of the *frontal lobes*. Laterally and ventrally the caudate nuclei are bordered by the obliquely oriented anterior limb of the internal capsule. Inferiorly are located the gray nuclei near the orbital surface of the frontal lobe including the basal nuclei of Meynert and the *substantia innominata*. This region is often called the anterior perforated substance because the deep medial branches of the anterior portion of the circle of Willis penetrate into the brain in this orbital frontal region. In more posterior coronal sections, the hypothalami appear medial and inferior to the caudate nuclei. The bulk of the caudate nucleus diminishes greatly at the genu of the internal capsule at which anteroposterior level the anterior portions of the thalami appear. More posteriorly, the body of the caudate nucleus is much less prominent and the nucleus curves with the lateral ventricle so that the tails of the caudate nuclei are very small structures related closely to the temporal horns of the lateral ventricles. Figure 15.3 illustrates the major anatomical relations of the caudate nuclei found on a CT slice through the frontal region.

The caudate nuclei are surrounded by white matter pathways that connect the caudate nucleus to the cerebral cortex, and with the putamen, pallidum, substantia nigra, and thalamus. The largest pathway is the anterior limb of the internal capsule which lies adjacent and ventral to the head of the caudate nucleus throughout its course. Anatomical and physiological studies mostly in primates have defined a number of complex circuits involving the caudate nuclei.[16–20] These circuits include elements usually considered functionally to be part of the motor, oculomotor, cognitive and behavioral, and limbic systems, and share a common general theme of organization. Regions of the cerebral cortex project to the striatum (sometimes predominantly caudate, sometimes mostly putaminal) and then projections go successively to the globus pallidus or substantia nigra, or both, then to specific thalamic relay nuclei, then projections return to the originating regions of the cerebral cortex. For example, in the monkey, the primary motor, primary sensory-motor and supplementary motor regions of the cortex all project to the striatum and then, via pallidonigral pathways, to the ventrolateral thalamus and back to the cortex in a so-called motor circuit.[16,17] Other circuits include cortex usually considered associative. The ventrolateral caudate nucleus receives projections from orbitofrontal and temporal lobe visual and auditory association cortical regions and then projects to the globus pallidus, rostromedial substantia nigra, ventral anterior and dorsomedial thalamic nuclei, and then back to the originating cortical areas. The dorsolateral caudate nucleus receives fibers projecting from the prefrontal convexal cortical surface and then projects to the dorsomedial globus pallidus, rostral substantia nigra, and then to the ventral anterior and medial dorsal thalamic nuclei and then back to the cortex. A "limbic circuit" includes projections from the anterior cingulum, orbitofrontal region, hippocampi, amygdala, entorhinal and perirhinal cortex to the ventral striatum which then in turn projects to the ventral pallidum and substantia nigra and then to the mediodorsal thalamic nuclei back to the originating cortical regions. Projections from these striatal

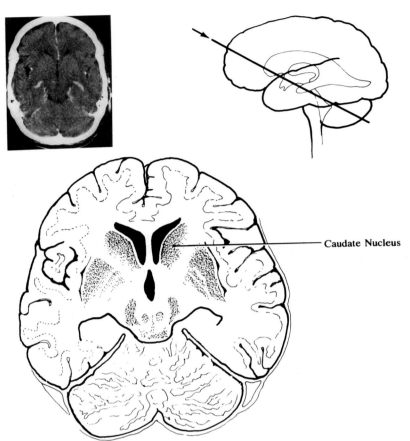

Caudate Nucleus

circuits can be interrupted by lesions involving the caudate nucleus or by lesions involving the anterior limb of the internal capsule undercutting caudate projections. The striatum receives input from all major sensory, motor, limbic, and multimodal sensory association regions of the cerebral cortex. The cortical projections are very highly patterned and specific; cortical areas that are reciprocally connected by corticocortical connections project in turn to similar regions within the caudate nucleus.[20] Radionuclide studies of patients with caudate nucleus hemorrhages have shown depression of large areas of the cerebral cortex during the acute phase.[21]

The caudate nuclei receive their blood supply from four main sources: Heubner's arteries, arteries that penetrate directly from the most proximal portions of the anterior ce-

rebral arteries, and both medial and lateral lenticulostriate branches arising from the proximal middle cerebral arteries. The *recurrent artery of Heubner* most often originates from the beginning of the $A_2$ segment of the anterior cerebral artery near the junction of the anterior cerebral and anterior communicating arteries.[22–24] The artery then loops and courses posteriorly travelling parallel to the $A_1$ segment of the anterior cerebral artery. Initially considered to be a single artery, we now know that the vessel is single in only approximately one-fourth of patients.[22] More often, on each side there are two, three, and even four or more parallel arteries. The multiplicity of parallel arteries supplying deep gray structures is similar to the pattern of penetrating arteries in the lenticulostriate and thalamogeniculate artery systems supplying the lateral basal ganglia and thalami, respectively. Heubner's arteries supply the anterior limb of the internal capsule but give little supply to structures posterior to the anterior commissure. The most *medially located lenticulostriate arteries* arising from the proximal portion of the mainstem of the middle cerebral artery (MCA) supply the anterior limb of the internal capsule and a small portion of the most lateral border of the caudate nuclei.[25-27] The *lateral lenticulostriate arteries* branch from the mainstem MCA or superior division to supply the major portion of the head of the caudate nucleus as well as the adjacent internal capsule. Anastomoses are often present between these medial and lateral striate branches and Heubner's arteries.[22] Observers have also identified arteries that *penetrate directly from the proximal main trunk of the anterior cerebral artery* that course through the anterior perforated substance to supply the deep medial structures of the frontal lobe. One of these arteries, the short central artery, is more consistently present than others and sometimes supplies a portion of the caudate nucleus and the anterior limb of the internal capsule.[28] All of the arteries that supply the caudate nuclei and adjacent structures are short, penetrating arteries similar morphologically to the penetrating lenticulostriate artery branches of the middle cerebral artery, the thalamogeniculate artery branches of the posterior cerebral artery, and the medial brainstem penetrators from the basilar and vertebral arteries. Figure 15.4 depicts diagrammatically the blood supply of the caudate nucleus and adjacent structures.

## Pathology

Some hemorrhages originating in the main region of the caudate remain small and are entirely confined to the caudate nucleus itself. Most however dissect into adjacent structures. There are two main patterns of spread of larger hemorrhages—medially into the ventricular system, or into adjacent brain tissue away from the ventricular system.

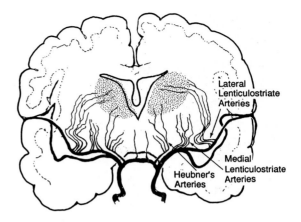

**Figure 15.4.** Artist's diagram of arterial supply of the caudate nucleus from Heubner's arteries and the medial and lateral lenticulostriate arteries. Although Heubner's arteries are drawn as originating from the A, segment of the anterior cerebral artery, their actual site of origin is from the $A_2$ portion of that artery, near the junction with the anterior communicating artery. (Drawn by Harriet Greenfield.)

Since these patterns of dissection determine the clinical symptoms and signs, it is useful to divide caudate hemorrhages into Group I cases in which spread is predominantly into the ventricular system and Group II in which spread is into the nearby white and grey matter structures.

In Group I hematomas, blood dissects medially emptying into the anterior horns of the lateral ventricles. The presence and degree of ventricular drainage probably depends on the size, direction, rapidity, and pressure of the bleeding. Once blood drains into the ipsilateral ventricle, it quickly disseminates within the ventricular system and spreads to the exit foramina of the fourth ventricle to empty into the subarachnoid space. Rarely, the force of blood is so great that the septum is broken and the lateral ventricles form a single clot-filled ventricle. When the bleeding originates from near the subependymal surface, as it often does in children with vascular malformations, the bulk of the bleeding is intraventricular and only a tiny amount of blood is found within the parenchyma of the caudate nucleus. Intraventricular bleeding

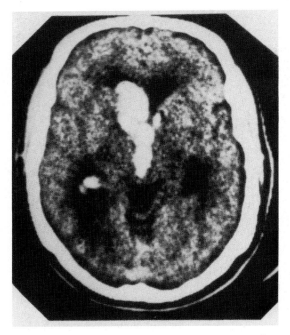

**Figure 15.5.** CT of caudate origin hematoma with spread to adjacent lateral ventricle and IIIrd ventricle medially. (From Stein RW, Kase CS, Hier DB, et al. Caudate hemorrhage. Neurology 1984;34:1549–1554, with permission.)

cleus and dissect away from the ventricular system. As in hematomas in other sites, dissection usually follows white matter pathways. Lateral or posterolaterally dissecting hemorrhages involve the anterior or posterior, or both, limbs of the internal capsule and sometimes the putamen. Sometimes it is difficult to tell if the hematoma originated in the putamen and spread medially towards the caudate nucleus, or began in the caudate and dissected laterally to the putamen. This uncertainty is best handled by referring to these large hemorrhages as caudatoputaminal. Some caudate hemorrhages dissect predominantly posteriorly into the thalamus or inferiorly into the hypothalamus. These posterior or posterior-inferior dissecting lesions can also enter the ventricular system after their spread to the diencephalon, emptying into the third ventricle. Occasionally, lesions beginning in the lateral portion of the caudate may spread inferiorly to the subfrontal and medial frontal surfaces of the brain and empty into the subarachnoid space without entering the lateral ventricle. These latter le-

was once believed to be a cataclysmic, usually fatal event that invariably led to high fever, rigidity, coma, and death. Actually ventricular dissection may lead to effective drainage of the enlarging clot. The alternative to spread to the ventricular system is spread into brain tissue with brain destruction. Spread to the ventricular system has sometimes been described using the term "rupture", a word that implies rather forceful release of contents. In most cases, the ventricular spread is probably more like a slow leak allowing egress of hematoma contents and alleviation of building pressure. Figures 15.5, 15.6 and 15.7 show examples of Group I caudate hemorrhages. On CT scans, it may be difficult to separate the intraparenchymatous component of the hemorrhage from that within the lateral ventricular system.

Group II hematomas usually originate in the more lateral or inferior portions of the nu-

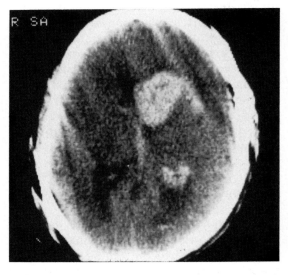

**Figure 15.6.** CT of somewhat larger hematoma. Most of the spread is medial and into the ventricle. (From Stein RW, Kase CS, Hier DB, et al. Caudate hemorrhage. Neurology 1984;34:1549–1554, with permission.)

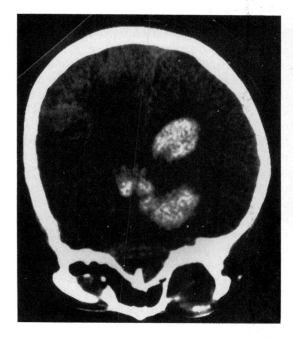

Figure 15.7. CT, Caudate hematoma with a great deal of ventricular blood.

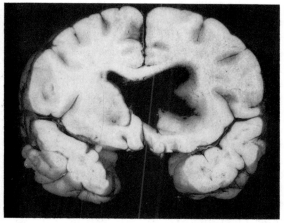

Figure 15.8. Caudate hematoma at necropsy. Lesion has dissected laterally across the internal capsule into the anterior putamen.

sions remain anterior to the hypothalamus. Since some thalamic hemorrhages spread dorsally towards the caudate, very large hematomas involving the thalamus and caudate should be referred to as caudatothalamic indicating the uncertainty of the origin of the lesions. Figures 15.8 and 15.9 show examples of Group II caudate hemorrhages.

In adults, the most common cause of caudate hemorrhages, by far, is hypertension. In neonates, hemorrhages arise from the germinal matrix just under the ependyma of the lateral ventricles and spread to the caudate nucleus, internal capsule, and other deep structures. This subependymal site is also a favorite place for small AVMs, which are the second most common cause of caudate hemorrhages. Since most series of patients with ICH do not separate caudate from putaminal hemorrhage, precise statistics concerning the frequency of hypertensive caudate hemorrhages have been difficult to obtain. Using our own figures from the Michael Reese Hospital, University

of South Alabama, and the Stroke Data Bank, we estimate that approximately 7% of hypertensive hemorrhages are caudate hematomas. This figure may be even higher in Japan where they seem to have a disproportionately higher incidence of medial (cau-

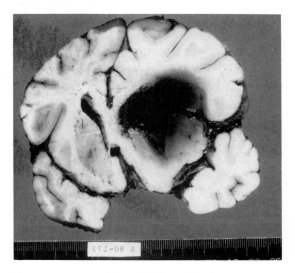

Figure 15.9. Very large, fatal caudate hematoma with considerable spread laterally, ventrally, and medially into the ventricle. Massive shift of the midline.

date and thalamic) ganglionic hypertensive hemorrhages.

The two lesions that can closely mimic caudate hemorrhages are rupture of anterior communicating artery aneurysms and head trauma. Traumatic lesions often emphasize paramedian structures especially the dorsolateral brainstem tegmentum and the corpus callosum. The septum pellucidum may also be torn. Contusions or small hematomas may affect the caudate nuclei as well as the more commonly involved orbital frontal brain surface. Traumatic caudate hematomas also are accompanied by some degree of subarachnoid bleeding. Aneurysms arising directly from the internal carotid artery or at the anterior cerebral-anterior communicating artery junction can bleed into the inferior frontal region and dissect into the caudate nucleus. These aneurysms usually also bleed into the subarachnoid space causing true meningocerebral hemorrhages. Aneurysmal rupture breaks the pial surface of the orbital frontal lobe and the jet of blood involves the subfrontal region, septum pellucidum, lateral ventricles, and often the corpus callosum as well as the caudate nucleus. On CT scan it may be difficult to separate an aneurysmal caudate-subfrontal hematoma from a caudate hemorrhage that dissected inferiorly or posteroinferiorly.[2] However when caudate hemorrhages are confined to the nucleus, or spread medially or laterally, the subfrontal region between the orbital brain surface and the caudate nucleus is free of blood. An aneurysmal hemorrhage involving the caudate nucleus always must affect the subfrontal region first. The amount and distribution of the subarachnoid blood also helps differentiate caudate ICH from aneurysmal bleeding.[29,30] In some cases, angiography may be needed to exclude an aneurysm or AVM from other primary spontaneous caudate hemorrhages.

## Symptoms and Signs

The clinical findings depend on the size of the hematoma, the rapidity and extent of the ventricular drainage, and dissection of the hematoma into adjacent lateral, inferior, and posterior brain structures. Stein et al. in their original description of twelve patients with hypertensive caudate hemorrhages divided the series into two groups of patients.[1] Their Group I patients had symptoms of subarachnoid bleeding and behavioral changes but no focal neurological signs, while Group II patients did have abnormal focal signs. These clinical groups conform to the groups separated pathologically by their pattern of spread. Stein et al.'s Group I patients conform to our pathologically characterized Group I in whom the hemorrhages are confined to the caudate nucleus and adjacent ventricular system. Their clinical Group II patients all had extensive hematomas spreading laterally, posteriorly or inferiorly, thus making them identical pathologically with our Group II.

In Group I patients the most frequent and important symptoms are headache, drowsiness, vomiting, and altered mental state and behavior. When examined early in their course, neck stiffness is usually found. The level of consciousness is usually decreased, especially in large hemorrhages. Restlessness, agitation, and drowsiness predominate. Some patients are also confused and may be disoriented. Restless patients often move incessantly in bed making it nearly impossible to obtain a coherent account of their symptoms or to properly examine them. Poor recall of recent events[1] and abnormal mental function[2,6–10] have also been noted in this group of patients. One patient, a practicing physician, was discovered confused in his automobile. When he had not returned home for twenty-four hours, his wife initiated a search for him.[1] When found, he could give no coherent account of where he had been or what he had been doing during this twenty-four-hour period and he could make no new memories when tested. Even after recovery, he remained amnesic for the original lost day.

The mechanism of symptoms in these patients relates to the presence of ventricular and subarachnoid bleeding and to disruption of cognitive and behavior functions mediated by the caudate nuclei and their connections. The onset of symptoms is usually abrupt and the common symptom complex of headache, vomiting, altered alertness, and neck stiffness are also the usual findings in patients with primary subarachnoid hemorrhage. CT in this patient group nearly always shows blood in the ventricular system. The ipsilateral lateral ventricle may also be dilated. Lumbar puncture usually shows blood-tinged fluid under higher than normal pressure. Most often obtundation or stupor is temporary, usually resolving within forty-eight hours. In Group I patients with large hematomas, decreased level of consciousness may last up to a week. When these patients with Group I large caudate hemorrhages become more alert and can be tested more completely, confusion, agitation, restlessness, decreased spontaneity, slow responses, apathy, and poor memory are often noted. These abnormalities may take time to recover.

At times, the behavioral and cognitive abnormalities are the predominant features. One woman, described as intermittently confused and disoriented after a right caudate hemorrhage, had vivid visual and auditory hallucinations of an alligator that made unpleasant noises with its teeth.[10] This illusion was so vivid that she was able to draw a likeness of the alligator from her recall. Another patient with a left caudate hemorrhage of medium size with slight extension into the adjacent white matter had prominent aphasic abnormalities.[9] Though there was no hemiparesis or limb weakness, she named poorly, perseverated ideas, and made semantic errors in her spoken and written language production. Another patient with a small hemorrhage limited to the left caudate nucleus and adjacent lateral ventricle, was disoriented to time and place and had impaired short-term memory during the acute stroke.[21] When tested three years later he still had slight abnormalities of verbal comprehension and verbal memory. One patient, sixteen months after a bilateral caudate hemorrhage remained persistently abulic.[21] He showed

no interest in the results of his tests and had less spontaneous conversation than before his stroke. His mood and affect were flat. Single-photon-emission computed tomography (SPECT) scans in these latter two patients with persistent cognitive and behavioral abnormalities showed decreased radionuclide activity in the left cerebral hemisphere, especially in the left frontal lobe.

The mental state abnormalities described are more prominent and persistent than those found in patients with uncomplicated subarachnoid bleeding. Similar abnormalities have also been found in patients with infarction in the caudate nucleus, in whom there are no pressure effects and no subarachnoid or ventricular blood. In a series of eighteen patients with infarction limited to the caudate nucleus and adjacent white matter, the major abnormalities were in the sphere of the mental state.[13] The two most common abnormalities related to the *amount* and *speed* of behavior. Ten of the eighteen patients were abulic, that is, they had reduced spontaneity and activity and were slow in their speech and actions. These patients were described as apathetic, mentally slow, poorly attentive, and easily distracted. When given sufficient time and prodding, their answers and intellect were normal. The second most common abnormality was the presence of an agitated, restless, hyperactive state. These patients were described as anxious, talkative, and easily distracted. Their conversations flitted from one topic to another. At times they became excited and aggressive and shouted aloud. Restraints and sedation were often needed. These two abnormalities, abulia and restless agitation, almost mirror-opposite patterns of behavior, were also prominent findings in another series of patients with behavioral abnormalities after caudate infarction.[12] Abulia has been described in patients with frontal lobe lesions, and restlessness and agitation are common after limbic lobe lesions. Presumably interruption of the extensive corticostriate-thalamic-cortical circuits described in the anatomy section of this chapter is responsible for the behavioral abnormalities. Less often, there are cognitive abnormalities related to left or right cerebral hemisphere dysfunction. Aphasia, dysnomia, left-sided neglect or extinction of double simultaneous stimuli, dysarthria, poor drawing and copying, and anosognosia have all been described in patients with caudate hemorrhages or infarcts.

Group II patients, in whom hemorrhage has extended laterally, posteriorly, or inferiorly, also usually present with headache, vomiting, and decreased alertness. But in addition, they also have limb weakness or hemiparesis, hemisensory symptoms, oculomotor abnormalities, and oculosympathetic (Horner's syndrome) dysfunction. Hemiparesis usually occurs only when there has been dissection of the hematoma laterally toward and across the internal capsule. Most often, the motor weakness affects face, arm, and leg, but occasionally only the face and arm are involved. Most often the weakness is slight or at most moderate and is often quite transient. By the time of discharge from the hospital, weakness nearly always has cleared or is minimal. Seldom is hemiplegia persistent or disabling. In the series of Stein et al., only one patient had a persistent hemiparesis and that patient had developed a basal ganglionic infarct on the same side as the caudate hemorrhage during recovery.[1] The motor abnormalities are caused by interruption of frontopontine fibers coursing in the anterior limb of the internal capsule. Loss of these fibers causes some changes in tone and agility but seldom produces persistent paralysis. A single patient reported by Valenstein and Heilman with a large right caudate hemorrhage had a contralateral motor deficit that the authors characterized as "unilateral hypokinesia."[11] They interpreted the patient's motor abnormality as a decrease in the "intention" to act with the left arm. This patient had decreased spontaneous movement of the left arm and a very prolonged reaction time limited only to the left upper extremity. When asked to hold up his arms, he would raise the right arm and only after several seconds would slowly raise the left arm. When

asked to raise the arm touched by the examiner, he raised only the right arm after bilateral tactile stimuli but said that he felt both the right and left touch.

Hemisensory symptoms or findings are much more unusual than motor abnormalities. When present, the abnormalities are often a description that the limbs do not feel "the same" as the other side. Paresthesias are less common. Sensory symptoms are usually transient and not accompanied by objective sensory loss to touch, position sense, or pain or temperature perception. Persistent sensory signs are found only when the hemorrhage dissects extensively in a posterior or posterolateral direction involving the posterior limb of the capsule and the thalamus.

The most frequent oculomotor abnormality is deviation of the eyes conjugately to the side of the hemorrhage. Defective voluntary conjugate gaze to the opposite side is also present but oculocephalic and oculovestibular responses are normal. Hemiparesis, to some degree, nearly always accompanies the conjugate gaze palsy. The fibers from the "frontal eye center" course deeply within the internal capsule and must be affected by the hemorrhage. Less often, some patients with large hemorrhages have bilateral conjugate gaze paresis with defective horizontal eye movements in either direction. These patients usually have extensive intraventricular blood and raised intracranial pressure. Bilateral conjugate gaze paresis is also found in patients with primary intraventricular hemorrhages and so could be caused by either massive ventricular drainage of blood or brainstem dysfunction due to the increased intracranial pressure. Rarely, some patients with caudate hemorrhage have had transient paralysis of vertical gaze.[1] Vertical gaze paresis results from spread of the hematoma to the thalamus or is explained by a central herniation effect with compression of the upper brainstem.

Some Group II patients have elements of a Horner's syndrome especially an ipsilaterally small pupil.[1] Spread of the hemorrhage

**Table 15.1.** Clinical Findings Among Three Series (25 Patients) with Hypertensive Caudate Hemorrhages[1,2,4]

| | | |
|---|---|---|
| Headache | 22/25 | (88%) |
| Stiff neck | 21/25 | (84%) |
| Decreased level of consciousness | 18/25 | (72%) |
| Abnormal mental state | 16/25 | (64%) |
| Vomiting | 15/25 | (60%) |
| Hemiparesis | 13/25 | (52%) |
| Memory abnormality | 7/25 | (28%) |
| Contralateral gaze paresis* | 3/12 | (25%) |
| Hemisensory findings | 5/25 | (20%) |
| Vertical gaze paresis* | 2/12 | (16%) |
| Abulia* | 2/12 | (16%) |
| "Right hemisphere" behavioral abnormalities* | 1/12 | (8%) |
| Bilateral horizontal gaze paresis* | 1/12 | (8%) |
| Aphasia | 1/25 | (4%) |

*Commented on only in one series, reference 1.

ventrally toward the orbital surface causes involvement of the descending sympathetic fibers in the hypothalamus and rostral diencephalon. A full Horner's syndrome (ptosis, miosis, and anhydrosis) or just miosis may be found. The oculosympathetic abnormalities are on the side ipsilateral to the hemorrhage and may be only temporary. The cognitive and behavioral abnormalities found in Group I caudate hemorrhage patients are also prominent in Group II hemorrhage patients indicating that the necessary feature is involvement of the caudate nucleus and its connections, *not* the ventricular spread of blood.

Table 15.1 lists the clinical findings in twenty-five patients with hypertensive caudate hemorrhage.

## Prognosis

Hypertensive caudate hemorrhages have a relatively good prognosis.[1,2–11] Among forty reported cases only five (12%) died during the acute hospitalization. While recovering well, one of these patients died suddenly and another died of a confirmed pulmonary embolus.[1] Another patient who died had meningitis, pneumonia, and disseminated intravascular coagulation.[8] Only two patients, each with large hematomas, died of the direct intracranial effects of the hemorrhage, and each died during ninety-six hours after onset.[6] Prognosis for recovery of the clinical deficits was also good. Among thirty patients who survived the acute hemorrhage, and in whom follow-up data were available, twenty-four (80%) were characterized as "normal," "excellent," "good," or "returned to normal activity and work." Among the six patients with significant residual deficits, two had other vascular lesions that contributed to their disability. Only four had important residual disability solely attributable to their caudate hemorrhages. In these series of patients with caudate hemorrhages, few patients had extensive neuropsychological testing after recovery. It is our feeling that the mood and behavioral abnormalities found usually recover within six months of the stroke and that persistent mental state changes are unusual in patients with unilateral caudate hemorrhages.

The prognosis for recovery from caudate hemorrhages due to rupture of an AVM is also good, though of course the lesions may later rebleed. In the cases reported in the literature, the malformations were often detected only at necropsy. This means that the sample of cases reported was biased toward the larger fatal hemorrhages. Caudate AVMs detected during life by angiography have often been removed surgically so that postoperative disability contributes to the residual deficits.[8] Caudate AVMs are often not detected by angiography and are presumed to have often "destroyed themselves" during the initial hemorrhage. Their presence is presumed if the patient is young, normotensive, and has no other cause for bleeding.

## References

1. Stein RW, Kase CS, Hier DB, et al. Caudate hemorrhage. Neurology 1984;34: 1549–1554.

2. Osler W. The principles and practices of medicine. Fifth Edition. New York: D. Apleton, 1903;999–1000.

3. Gowers WR. A Manual of Diseases of the Nervous System. London: J and A Churchhill, 1893;384–413.

4. Fisher CM. Clinical syndromes in cerebral hemorrhage. In: Fields WS, ed. Pathogenesis and Treatment of Cerebrovascular Disease. Springfield, IL: Charles C Thomas, 1961; 318–342.

5. Mutlu N, Berry RG, Alpers BJ. Massive cerebral hemorrhage: clinical and pathological correlations. Arch Neurol 1963;8:644–661.

6. Weisberg LA. Caudate hemorrhage. Arch Neurol 1984;41:971–974.

7. Tsubokawa T, Shinozaki H, Nishimoto H, et al. Hypertensive caudate hemorrhage: its classification and treatment. Surg Cerebr Stroke (Sendai, Japanese Society for Surgery of Cerebral Strokes) 1978;3:85–89.

8. Waga S, Fujimoto K, Okada M, et al. Caudate hemorrhage. Neurosurgery 1986;18:445–450.

9. Cambier J, Elghozi D, Strube E. Hémorragie de la tête du noyau caudé gauche: désorganisation du discours et de l'expression graphique, perturbations des séries gestuelles. Rev Neurol 1979;135:763–774.

10. Pardal MMF, Micheli F, Asconapé J, et al. Neurobehavioral symptoms in caudate hemorrhage: two cases. Neurology 1985;35:1806–1807 (letter).

11. Valenstein E, Heilman KM. Unilateral hypokinesia and motor extinction. Neurology 1981;31: 445–448.

12. Mendez MF, Adams NL, Lewandowski KS. Neurobehavioral changes associated with caudate lesions. Neurology 1989;39:349–354.

13. Caplan LR, Schmahmann JD, Kase CS, et al. Caudate infarcts. Arch Neurol 1990, 47, 133–143.

14. Richfield EK, Twyman R, Berent S. Neurological syndrome following bilateral damage to the head of the caudate nuclei. Ann Neurol 1987;22:768–771.

15. Kawamura M, Takahashi N, Hirayama K. Hemichorea and its denial in a case of caudate infarction diagnosed by magnetic resonance imaging. J Neurol Neurosurg Psychiat 1988; 51:590–591 (letter).

16. Selemon LD, Goldman-Rakic PS. Longitudinal topography and interdigitation of corticostriatal projections in the rhesus monkey. J Neurosci 1985;5:776–794.

17. Alexander GE, DeLong MR, Strick PL. Parallel organization of functionally segregated circuits linking basal ganglia and cortex. Annu Rev Neurosci 1986;9:357–381.

18. Alexander GE, DeLong MR. Microstimulation of the primate neostriatum. I. Physiological properties of striatal microexcitable zones. J Neurophysiol 1985;53:1401–1416.

19. Goldman PS, Nauta WJH. An intricately patterned prefronto-caudate projection in the rhesus monkey. J Comp Neurol 1977;171: 369–386.

20. Yeterian EH, Van Hoesen GW. Cortico-striate projections in the rhesus monkey: the organization of certain cortico-caudate connections. Brain Res 1978;139:43–63.

21. Pozzilli C, Passafiume D, Bastianello S, et al. Remote effects of caudate hemorrhage: a clinical and functional study. Cortex 1987;23: 341–349.

22. Gorczyca W, Mohr G. Microvascular anatomy of Heubner's recurrent artery. Neurol Res 1987;9:259–264.

23. Dunker RO, Harris AB. Surgical anatomy of the proximal anterior cerebral artery. J Neurosurg 1976;44:359–367.

24. Gomes F, Dujovny M, Umansky F, et al. Microsurgical anatomy of the recurrent artery of Heubner. J Neurosurg 1984;60:130–139.

25. Jain KK. Some observations on the anatomy of the middle cerebral artery. Can J Surg 1964;7:134–139.

26. Herman LH, Ostrowski AZ, Gurdjian ES. Perforating branches of the middle cerebral artery. Arch Neurol 1963;8:32–34.

27. Caplan LR, Babikian V, Helgason C, et al. Occlusive disease of the middle cerebral artery. Neurology 1985;35:975–982.

28. Selman J, Dujovny M, Vazquez M, et al. Microanatomical basis for lenticulostriate surgery. In: Microsurgery for Cerebral Ischemia, Ninth International Symposium. Vienna: Springer-Verlag, 1990.

29. Weisberg LA. Computed tomography in aneurysmal subarachnoid hemorrhage. Neurology 1979;29:802–808.

30. Caplan LR. Computed tomography and stroke. In: McDowell FH, Caplan LR, eds. Cerebrovascular Survey Report, for the National Institute of Neurological and Communicative Disorders and Stroke, 1985. Washington: 1985;61–74.

# Chapter 16
# Thalamic Hemorrhage

## Louis R. Caplan

## Historical Aspects

Early authors did not consider thalamic he-matomas as a separate category but usually lumped them together with caudate and putaminal hemorrhages in the general category of basal ganglionic hemorrhages. Miller Fisher deserves credit for emphasizing the frequency of thalamic intracerebral hemor-rhage (ICH) and for describing the usual clin-ical features. His first report was a brief description of the pathological and clinical aspects of thalamic hemorrhage presented at a meeting of the American Neurological Association in 1959.[1] Several years later he fur-ther elaborated on the syndrome of thalamic ICH.[2,3] Among his own necropsy series of 102 hemorrhages, Fisher found that thalamic hemorrhages accounted for thirteen, or 13% of the total.[1] Commenting on the paper, Dr. Zimmerman studied the results of Dr. Hirano who found 12.5% of his specimens of ICH had a thalamic location.[1] Since then, most necropsy series have found that 10% to 15% of hematomas are thalamic while computed tomography (CT) studies yield a somewhat higher figure.

Fisher summarized the cardinal clinical features as: "(1) predominance of sensory deficit over motor, (2) ocular motor distur-bances, especially impairment of vertical gaze with lesions medially placed, and (3) dysphasia when the dominant hemisphere is involved."[1] Probably Fisher's major contribu-tion was an analysis of the characteristic eye signs: "vertical gaze upwards and down-wards may be in abeyance; or gaze upwards is absent, while gaze downwards is only im-paired. The eyes may be tonically deviated downwards, seeming to peer at the tip of the nose. The pupils may be small and fixed to light . . . the pupil on the side of the lesion is slightly small and may be combined with a mild ptosis. Skew deviation of the eyes is common. Conjugate horizontal gaze may be impaired on voluntary effort mimicking palsy of the lateral rectus or even a conjugate gaze disturbance and irregular nystagmoid jerks are seen as well."[1] Most of Fisher's fatal cases were large hematomas occupying much of the thalamus, but he recognized that most thalamic hemorrhages lay in the poste-rior thalamus and that medial thalamic he-matomas most often had abnormal eye signs while posterior-lateral lesions had more sen-sory and motor abnormalities.

Fisher's initial observations on thalamic hemorrhage, of course, preceded CT. When CT became available, smaller hematomas could be diagnosed and separated from inf-arcts, and the anatomical details could be readily defined. In the late 1970s, several authors[4-7] analyzed the clinical-CT features of thalamic hemorrhage. When CT became available, it became clear that some of the "Parinaud syndrome" features were probably due to increased intracranial pressure and hydrocephalus.[8,9] The fact that patients with thalamic lesions were often aphasic stimulated analysis of the speech disturbance, since before Fisher's time, aphasia was generally thought to result only from cortical and subcortical white matter lesions near the sylvian fissure. Aphasiologists were fascinated by the unusual aspects of "thalamic aphasia."[10–16] More recently, authors have begun to describe clinical subtypes of thalamic hemorrhage recognized by careful MRI- and CT-clinical correlations of patients with small thalamic hematomas.[17–20]

## Anatomy

Space will not allow a detailed analysis of the anatomy of the human thalamus. We will merely outline the key features that are needed to understand anatomoclinical correlations in patients with small thalamic hemorrhages. The diencephalon probably makes up only about 2% of the neuraxis by volume but its extensive afferent and efferent connections and its central location make it almost a microcosm of the cerebral cortex. It can be considered the gateway to the cortex. The thalamus extends from the foramen of Monro rostrally to the posterior commissure caudally. It is bounded medially by the third ventricle and laterally by the posterior limb of the internal capsule and far posteriorly by the retrolenticular capsular fibers. Figure 16.1 shows the anatomical relations of the thalamus as found on a CT section taken near the foramen of Monro.

### Divisions of the Thalamus

Various schemes have been used to describe the divisions of the thalamus, including purely anatomical or functional classifications. Herein, we will divide the nuclear groups into anterior, medial, ventral lateral, and posterior (dorsal) portions of the thalamus, following Carpenter[21] and Kawahara et al.[19] Figure 16.2 is a diagram showing the various nuclear groups.

**Anterior Group.** This group lies within the most rostral portion of the thalamus where it projects forward as the anterior tubercle. The major nucleus is the *anteroventral* (AV) while the *anterodorsal* (AD) and *anteromedial* (AM) nuclei are smaller. These nuclei receive projections from the mamillary bodies through the mamillothalamic tract and also receive projections from the fornix. These anterior nuclei project to the cingulum through the posterior portion of the anterior limb of the internal capsule.

**Medial Group.** We include within the medial nuclei those usually classified as intralaminar nuclei that lie just lateral to the dorsomedial nucleus. This group lies posteromedially extending from just behind the anterior group to the pulvinar. The *dorsomedial* (DM) nucleus is the largest structure within this group. This nucleus has extensive connections with other thalamic nuclei, especially the intralaminar and posterior nuclei. It receives input from the amygdala, temporal lobe neocortex, and the orbital frontal cortex. A large projection goes to the prefrontal cortex. The midline nuclei (paratenial, paraventricular, reunines nuclei) lie medial to parts of DM and connect with the hypothalamus. The intralaminar nuclei lie within the internal medullary lamina which divides the medial and lateral thalamus. The largest intralaminar nucleus is the *centromedian nucleus* (CM), which is located between DM and the ventral posterior nucleus. The other prominent intralaminar nucleus is the *parafascicular nucleus* (PF). The intralaminar nuclei receive input mostly from the brainstem reticular formation and project to the putamen and caudate nuclei.

**Ventral Lateral Group.** This group is composed of the *ventral anterior nucleus* (VA) rostrally, and the *ventral lateral* (VL) and *ventral posterior nuclei* (VP) more caudally. The VA receives input from the medial portion of the

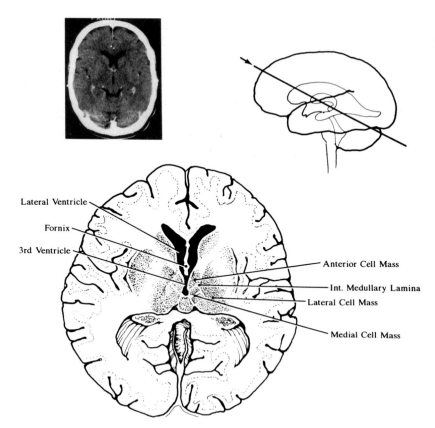

**Figure 16.1.** Section of brain cut in CT plane through the foramen of Monro. Upper right figure shows plane of section. Upper left is a CT at this level. Lower picture is artist's drawing of thalamus and other brain structures at this level. (Drawn by Harriet Greenfield.)

Lateral Ventricle
Fornix
3rd Ventricle
Anterior Cell Mass
Int. Medullary Lamina
Lateral Cell Mass
Medial Cell Mass

globus pallidus and the *pars reticulata* of the substantia nigra. There are connections with intralaminar and midline thalamic nuclei and projections to orbital frontal cortex. The *ventral lateral nucleus* (VL) receives major input from the globus pallidus, substantia nigra, contralateral cerebellum (via the brachium conjunctivum), and from the precentral cortex. Projections are primarily to the precentral motor cortex. The *ventral posterior nucleus* is divided into ventral posteromedial (VPM) and ventral posterolateral (VPL) subdivisions. This nucleus receives projections from the sensory relay tracts, the medial lemniscus, and the spinothalamic tracts, and subserves primarily somatosensory functions. VPM contains fibers related to sensory functions in the face and mouth while VPL receives fibers relaying somatosensory information from the trunk and limbs.

**Posterior (Dorsal) Group.** These nuclei lie dorsolaterally and caudally in the thalamus. Carpenter classifies them as the lateral group,[21] but clinical classification usually refers to them as posterior or dorsal. Included are the *lateral dorsal nucleus* (LD), the *lateral posterior nucleus* (LP) and the *pulvinar* (P). The pulvinar is one of the largest nuclear structures within the thalamus. It receives afferent input mostly from other thalamic nuclei including the medial and lateral geniculate bodies. Projections from the pulvinar go to the posterior parietal lobe, the posterior temporal lobe, and the visual cortex surrounding area 17.

The *medial* and *lateral geniculate bodies*, the auditory and visual relay nuclei, lie far posteriorly. Inferior to the main body of the thalamus are the subthalamus and hypothalamus. Hematomas can also extend caudally

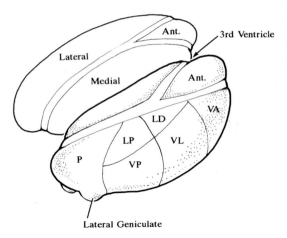

**Figure 16.2.** Diagram showing various thalamic regions. On the left at the top are the anterior, medial, and lateral portions of the thalamus. On the right are shown the locations of some of the thalamic nuclei. Ant = anterior; VA = ventral anterior; LD = lateral dorsal; VL = ventral lateral; LP = lateral posterior; VP = ventral posterior; P = pulvinar. (Drawn by Harriet Greenfield.)

to the diencephalic-midbrain junction and even into the midbrain. The thalamic projections reciprocally connect the cerebral cortex and the thalamus. They consist of an *anterior projection* to the frontal lobe which travels lateral to the caudate nucleus within the anterior limb of the internal capsule, a *superior thalamic radiation* which connects the perirolandic and adjacent frontal and parietal cortex with the ventral lateral thalamic nuclei, and a *posterior radiation* to the posterior parietal and occipital cerebral cortex. The latter includes the retrolenticular portion of the capsule including the geniculocalcarine optic radiation.

In perhaps a very oversimplified view, the anterior thalamic nuclear group can be thought of as primarily subserving memory and emotional behavioral functions.[22] The connections are mostly with the mamillary bodies, fornices, and cinguli. The medial group can be thought of as relating to memory and behavior, especially those functions usually classified as "frontal," because they are defective in patients with large prefrontal

cortical lesions. DM projects heavily to prefrontal cortex. Also, the intralaminar nuclei relate to the brainstem reticular formation and state of alertness and consciousness. The ventral lateral group has mostly somatosensory and motor functions. VPM and VPL are the principal somatosensory relay nuclei. VL and to a lesser extent VA, receive inputs from cerebellar and basal ganglionic structures and project to motor cortex. The posterior (dorsal) group probably has the most poorly characterized functional status. This group projects mostly to association cortex in the posterior parietal, temporal, and occipital lobes. It probably relays complex multimodal sensory data (auditory, visual, somatosensory) to the posterior hemisphere and might be related to some visual-spatial and language functions.

### Arterial Supply

The arterial supply to these thalamic regions derives mostly from arteries that branch from the parent basilar, posterior communicating, and posterior cerebral arteries near the region of the apex of the basilar artery. In general, there are two categories of arteries: thalamoperforating arteries, which supply the medial thalamic structures, and thalamogeniculate and circumferential arteries, which supply more lateral and posterior thalamic structures.[23–27] The two major groups of thalamoperforating arteries are the more anterior tuberothalamic artery (polar artery) and the more posterior thalamic-subthalamic paramedian artery. The *tuberothalamic artery* has been referred to as the polar artery by Percheron,[24] and the premamillary pedicle by Foix and Hillemand.[23] This artery usually arises from the middle third of the posterior communicating artery but may be absent in 30–40% of cases.[28] When the polar artery is absent, the anterior and anterolateral thalamic territory is supplied by the thalamic-subthalamic paramedian artery.[23,28] The tuberothalamic artery supplies the reticular nucleus, the mamillothalamic tract, and parts of the ventrolateral and dorsomedial nuclei, and the lateral aspect of the anterior thalamic pole.[24,28] Hemorrhage from this artery accounts for anterior and anterolateral thalamic hemorrhages.

The *thalamic-subthalamic paramedian arteries* supply the medial thalamus more posteriorly. These vessels are also referred to as the deep interpeduncular profunda arteries, the paramedian thalamic arteries by Percheron,[25] and the thalamoperforating pedicle by Foix and Hillemand.[23] Sometimes the arteries to both sides arise from a single artery or from a pedicle of vessels.[25,29] These arteries arise from the very proximal portion of the posterior cerebral arteries, from a segment also referred to as the basilar communicating or mesencephalic artery. They supply the intralaminar nuclei, dorsomedial nucleus, part of the ventral posterior nucleus, the subthalamus, and the centromedian nucleus.[23,28,29] Bleeding from these arteries cause medial (posteromedial) thalamic hematomas.

The *thalamogeniculate arteries* arise as a group of parallel arteries from the posterior cerebral arteries after the level of the posterior communicating artery branches. These arteries penetrate the thalamus between the medial and lateral geniculate bodies and then arc anteriorly to supply the posterior half of the lateral thalamus. The anterior half is supplied by the polar artery. The nuclei supplied include the medial geniculate body, the medial half of the lateral geniculate body, the ventral posterior and ventral lateral nuclei, parts of the centromedian and intralaminar nuclei, and the ventral lateral portion of the pulvinar.[28] Hemorrhages from these arteries cause posterior lateral hematomas. These hematomas are the most frequent and largest of the thalamic hemorrhages.

The *posterior choroidal arteries* supply the posterior, dorsal region of the thalamus. The lateral posterior choroidal arteries arise from the posterior cerebral artery after that vessel has passed around a portion of the midbrain. There are usually two or three lateral posterior choroidal arteries.[30] The medial posterior choroidal arteries also originate from the P2 ambient segment of the posterior cerebral arteries just after the thalamogeniculate artery branches. Branches from the posterior choroidal arteries supply most of the dorsal medial nucleus and the pulvinar, and then course forward to supply the anterior nuclei. Hemorrhages from the posterior choroidal arteries probably explain far posterior, dorsal hematomas, especially those limited to the pulvinar. Figures 16.3 and 16.4 show the arterial supply of the thalamus.

## Pathology

As with hematomas at other sites, bleeding may be very restricted and remain less than 2 cm in maximal diameter or may be massive and affect nearly the entire thalamus and adjacent structures. Small hematomas are most often located in the ventrolateral region in the territory fed by the thalamogeniculate arteries (Figure 16.5). These vessels are larger than the thalamoperforating medial branches and the posterior choroidal arteries. Some small hematomas are situated more medially (Figure 16.6). In the series of small restricted thalamic hematomas reported by Kawahara and colleagues, twenty-eight of thirty-seven were located posterolaterally in the ventrolateral region.[19] A much smaller percentage are situated anterolaterally, dorsally, and medially. Larger lesions often dissect medially into the third ventricle. The thalamic hematoma and clot within the third ventricle often shift the midline impinging on the contralateral thalamus (Figures 16.7 and 16.8). Blood can also extend into the atrium of the lateral ventricle. Lateral spread of thalamic hemorrhages into the globus pallidus and internal capsule, and even putamen, is relatively common. At times, the lateral extension is so prominent that the hematomas are designated putaminothalamic because it is impossible to tell the site of origin. Thalamic hematomas may also extend caudally into the midbrain. The expanding thalamic mass often compresses the diencephalic-midbrain region near the posterior commis-

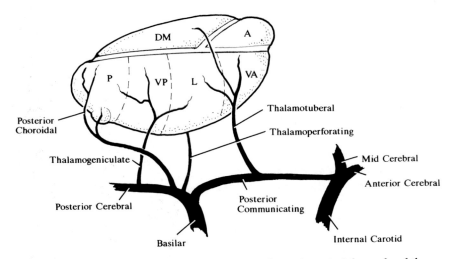

**Figure 16.3.** Drawing of a lateral view showing the major arterial supply of the thalamus. Nuclei are A = anterior; VA = ventral anterior; DM = dorsomedial; L = lateral; VP = ventral posterior; P = pulvinar. (Drawn by Harriet Greenfield.)

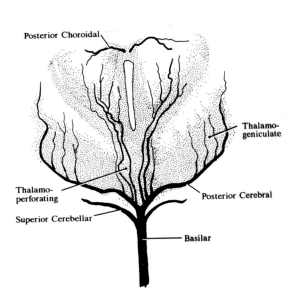

**Figure 16.4.** Anteroposterior view of the thalamic arterial supply schematically drawn by artist. (Drawn by Harriet Greenfield.)

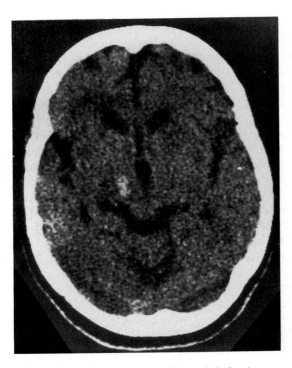

**Figure 16.5.** CT showing small lateral thalamic hematoma.

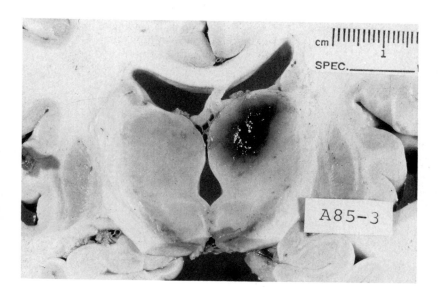

**Figure 16.6.** Necropsy specimen of small to moderate, medial thalamic hemorrhage. Note pressure directed mostly toward ipsilateral lateral ventricle distorting fornix.

sure and exerts pressure on the quadrigeminal plate region or extends into the midbrain (Figure 16.9). The aqueduct or third ventricle can be blocked leading to hydrocephalus (Figures 16.8 and 16.10). MRI, especially using sagittal sections, can show the posterior location of thalamic hematomas (Figure 16.11).

## Clinical Findings

We will begin by analyzing the clinical phenomenology that has been described and personally observed in patients with thalamic hematomas. In many patients, the hemorrhages were large and occupied most of the thalamus, or their anatomy within the

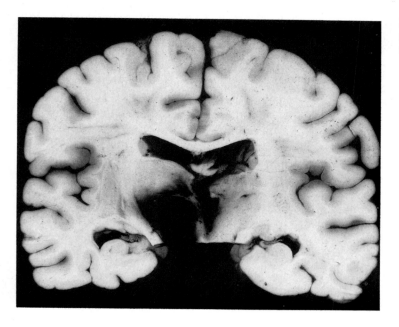

**Figure 16.7.** Large thalamic hemorrhage. Note dissection into third ventricle and midline shift.

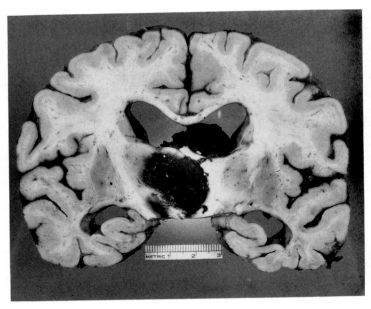

**Figure 16.8.** Large thalamic hematoma spreading to opposite side. The third ventricle is compressed and hydrocephalus is present. Clot is also seen in the lateral ventricles.

region was not defined further by neuroimaging tests or necropsy. In general, the signs and symptoms are nearly identical to those found in patients with rostral basilar artery occlusion[31–35] and in those with thalamic infarction.[23,28,29,36,37,38] After describing the general findings, we will then attempt to correlate the findings with regions of the thalamus from the few available clinicopathological-imaging studies of patients with small, well localized hemorrhages within the thalamus.

### State of Consciousness and Awareness

Fisher commented in his initial report on thalamic hemorrhage that "if the hemorrhage is massive, consciousness is promptly lost."[1] In a single case report that appeared in 1970, Ingvar and Sourander described in detail the case of a barber who suddenly became ill after a visit to the washroom and developed confusion, headache, and loss of consciousness.[39] He remained in coma for thirty-five months until his death. At necropsy, he had a very large thalamic hemorrhage cavity that extended into the third ventricle and sylvian

aqueduct, and into the contralateral medial thalamus and the ipsilateral midbrain tegmentum. During life, EEG showed severe depression of activity with continuous delta slowing that was not influenced by sensory stimulation.[39] The authors believed that the long-term coma was due to a lesion of the rostral brainstem reticular activating system (RAS) with loss of "the *activating* effects upon the cortex from the brainstem."[39] Previously, two reports of patients with bilateral paramedian thalamic and rostral midbrain tegmental infarcts had described a state of prolonged *hypersomnolence* before death.[40,41] In our experience, excessive sleepiness is much more common than coma after thalamic bleeding. Patients go from an awake state into rather deep sleep from which they can only be aroused with difficulty. Many sleep much of the time but when aroused they become quite alert and interactive. Another altered state of behavior has been called "akinetic mutism," after Segarra, who described severe apathy, inertia, and decreased motor activity and speech after rostral brainstem infarction in the territory of the proximal posterior cerebral artery (mesencephalic artery).[42] We prefer the term *abulia*, after

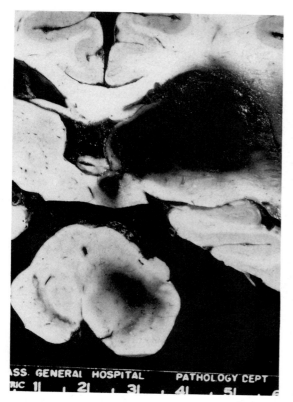

**Figure 16.9.** Very large thalamic hemorrhage seen in top section. Blood has dissected into the adjacent midbrain. At bottom, the hemorrhage can be seen in the midbrain laterally on the same side as the thalamic hematoma.

pontine levels causes stupor and coma. The mechanism of abulia is likely different. As noted previously in this chapter in the section on anatomy, the anterior and medial thalamic nuclei have extensive prefrontal projections. Abulia is often seen after frontal lobe lesions.[43] Interruption of the thalamic-prefrontal pathways could mimic frontal lobe disease. Unilateral lesions might produce temporary abulia as has been described in patients with occlusion of the tuberothalamic artery unilaterally.[28,34]

### Motor and Sensory Signs

Fisher, in his original note, emphasized that in thalamic hemorrhage, there is "predominence of sensory deficit over motor."[1] He went on to say that hemiparesis or hemiplegia occur because of involvement of the adjacent internal capsule and that when motor

Fisher, for the findings of decreased spontaneity, prolonged latency, and difficulty persevering with tasks.[43]

Prolonged stupor, coma, and hypersomnolence probably require bilateral involvement of the brainstem RAS. This occurs when the hematoma dissects into the opposite thalamus, when pressure effects compress the contralateral thalamus or rostral mesencephalon, and when the hematoma dissects into the third ventricle, aqueduct, or upper brainstem bilaterally. It is possible (but not well studied or proven) that diencephalic involvement of the RAS leads to hypersomnolence with arousability, while involvement of the RAS at midbrain and

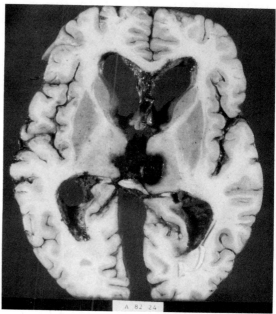

**Figure 16.10.** Horizontal section. Thalamic hemorrhage with clot in the third ventricle causing acute hydrocephalus. The walls of the lateral ventricles are blood stained.

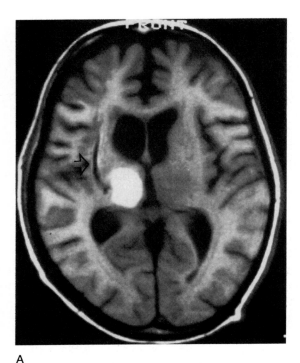

A

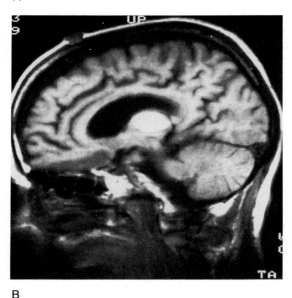

B

**Figure 16.11.** MRI showing posteriorly placed thalamic hematoma. (A) Horizontal section showing large thalamic hemorrhage (bright). A linear dark cavity (open arrow) is the result of an older healed putaminal "slit" hemorrhage. (B) Sagittal view. The hematoma is located posteriorly in the pulvinar region.

signs are present, "a sensory deficit of relatively greater severity affecting all modalities will be found due to involvement of the posteroventral nucleus."[1] Often, the earliest symptoms described in patients who are alert at the onset of their hemorrhage relate to the somatosensory system. Paresthesias, numbness, and dysesthesias are common and are usually hemicorporeal but can be in isolated body parts. In some of these patients, there is a profound sensory loss to all modalities, but others have very trivial objective threshold increase in touch, temperature, and pain perception. We now know from studies of patients with "pure sensory strokes" that infarction of the VPL nuclei can occur with little objective sensory loss.[44,45] On the other hand, involvement of the thalamoparietal radiations in the internal capsule[46] or thalamoparietal pedicle in the deep white matter or temporal isthmus can lead to more obvious objective sensory loss.[36] Mistakenly, students have been taught that all or most of the somatosensory projections in the spinothalamic and medial lemniscal tracts end in the VPL and VPM nuclei. Actually, many fibers branch off in the brainstem to travel medially with the RAS where they probably serve to help activate the brain after noxious somatosensory stimuli. Only when the fibers from both the medial and lateral thalamus (either because of a large thalamic lesion or involvement of the fibers in the thalamoparietal radiations from thalamus to Sensory I and Sensory II cortical zones) are affected does much of a sensory loss develop. Of course, after thalamic hemorrhage, so-called thalamic pain may develop and be very disturbing to the patient. Pain is seldom a problem acutely.

Although the thalamus is often thought of as a sensory relay station, there are also ample motor system connections. Nearly all patients with thalamic hemorrhages that involve the lateral thalamic region have some motor abnormalities. Severe hemiplegia, however, is only found when the hematoma spreads laterally to involve the posterior limb of the internal capsule, in which case the hemiplegia may persist. When thalamic hematomas are located anteriorly or anterolaterally, there is often slight hemiparesis and hemisensory loss that rapidly improve.[19] These lesions are confined to the anterior half of the posterior limb of the capsule or dissect into the posterior portion of the anterior limb. When the hematomas involve the ventral lateral portion, by far the most common site of bleeding, and the bleeding is confined to the thalamus, there is usually some weakness, clumsiness and incoordination of the contralateral limbs but not a severe hemiparesis. The most common motor abnormality in our experience is clumsiness with some features of cerebellar type incoordination. Rapid alternating movements are done poorly. A side-to-side displacement and overshoot of the target occur on finger-to-nose or toe-to-object testing. If the patient is asked to abruptly lower the arm but to brake it quickly before stopping, there is often some rebound. Often, there is some accompanying gait ataxia. In some patients, the ataxia is very prominent and mimics closely the ataxic hemiparesis syndrome found in patients with lacunar infarcts in the posterior limb of the capsule or the pons.[47] Occasionally, patients with lateral thalamic hematomas develop a severe tremor, usually after recovery from hemiparesis. Schlitt et al. described a young woman who developed an acute hemiparesis and hemisensory loss in relation to a posterolateral right thalamic hemorrhage that probably involved a part of the posterior limb of the internal capsule.[48] Four months later as her weakness improved, she developed severe shaking in her left arm and leg. Movements produced a coarse amplitude tremor involving the shoulder, arm and forearm. The tremor was reduced after a stereotaxic cryothalamotomy lesion. The cerebellar type symptoms surely relate to involvement of cerebellofugal fibers which synapse in the lateral thalamus before influencing the cortex. The brachium conjunctivum contains fibers projecting from the dentate nucleus which course through the midbrain and synapse mostly in the ventral lateral and, to

a lesser extent, in the ventral anterior thalamic nuclei.

In patients with ventral lateral thalamic hematomas, there are also often some abnormal so-called "extrapyramidal" features. The arm and hand contralateral to the hemorrhage may move spontaneously less than the opposite arm. Choreic or irregular athetoid-like movements of the hand and arm occur and are best observed by watching the patient walk. Dystonic postures are common. The wrist may be hyperpronated. The fingers are commonly flexed in a fist posture with the thumb trapped in the palm. Some patients tend to keep their hand in the pocket, especially a back pocket, when they walk to avoid adventitious motions of the arm. Prominent choreoathetosis has also been described.[49] Resistance to passive movement is also increased in the limbs contralateral to the hematoma. The extrapyramidal dysfunction partially relates to interruption of striatofugal fibers that course in the ansa lenticularis and other tracts that will synapse in the VL and VA nuclei, or to involvement of these nuclei directly. Occasionally, patients with thalamic hemorrhage have unilateral asterixis on the side opposite the hemorrhage.[50]

### Speech Abnormalities

Altered voice, speech, and language functions have been noted in patients with thalamic hemorrhage.[10–16] The language abnormalities have varied. Often there has been decreased spontaneity and a reduced amount of speech.[10,13,15] Other patients have been described as fluent, meaning that the amount of speech output was considered normal or even that the patients were loquacious.[14,16] Speech content often shows some paraphasic word errors. The unusual feature of the patients' spontaneous speech output has been the variability. The patient of Mohr et al. had periods of near normal speech, then lapsed into gross jargon with many paraphasic errors, especially when fatigued.[11] In one patient, the variability of speech seemed to relate to the topic of discussion.[16] When that patient discussed familiar topics such as personal history, paraphasias were unusual and word-finding difficulties were relatively minor. However, when the patient discussed unfamiliar subjects, paraphasias were so frequent and word-finding deficits so severe that speech deteriorated into irrelevant jargon.[16]

Occasionally the rhythm, loudness, and articulatory aspects of speech have been noted to be abnormal. Reduced speech volume, dysarthria, and changed speech rhythms have been described, but usually are transient and not severe. Reduced voice volume has also been described in the immediate postoperative period in patients with surgery on the thalamus.[15] Altered amount, rhythm, and pronunciation also occur after thalamic stimulation,[51,52] and after thalamotomy for treatment of Parkinson's and other diseases.

A relatively uniform feature of aphasia in patients with thalamic hemorrhage has been preservation of the ability to repeat spoken language.[10,11,13,15] Even patients with many paraphasic errors and jargon output seem to repeat very well. This feature separates "thalamic aphasia" from Wernicke aphasia due to temporal lobe disease. Wernicke aphasia patients and patients with conduction aphasia have severe deficits in speech repetition. Preserved repetition is the hallmark of the so-called transcortical aphasias.

Comprehension of spoken language has been variable. In some patients, comprehension has been well preserved and in others, obviously impaired. Perseveration and echolalia are other features often commented upon.[10,11,13] Some patients seem to duplicate and repeat the last letters of words they say or write. Defective writing is also a very common feature, at times being involved out of proportion to other language functions.[10,13,15] Reading and naming abilities are also quite variable.

To summarize, the aphasia in patients with thalamic hemorrhage is a relatively unique syndrome, probably best classified as an unusual type of transcortical sensory aphasia or mixed transcortical motor and sensory aphasia. The language abnormality is characterized by preserved repetition, variable fluency, word errors that vary with the discussion topic and degree of alertness, poor writing, and perseverations. Transcortical sensory aphasia is the predominant speech syndrome in patients with infarction in the posterior cerebral artery territory.[53] Of course, the thalamus and its posterior white matter connections are supplied almost entirely by the posterior cerebral arteries. Aphasia has also been noted in patients with thalamic tumors,[51] during thalamic stimulation,[52] and in patients with thalamic infarcts.[23,54–57]

The anatomical aspects of thalamic hemorrhage aphasia are complex. Most often, aphasia has followed left thalamic hemorrhage but there are two cases of aphasia after right-sided thalamic bleeding.[14,15] One patient was left-handed and the other, although right-handed at the time of the stroke, had been shifted as a boy from his left-handed status. Often, the thalamic hemorrhages causing aphasia have been large and involve most of the thalamus.[10] Cappa et al. in their review cited the observation that most thalamic lesions causing aphasia were anterolateral or ventrolateral in location.[54] Medial lesions seemed not to cause aphasia. On the other hand, Crosson et al. marshall arguments favoring the anterior superior lateral part of the pulvinar as the crucial region for production of thalamic aphasia.[16] This portion of the dorsal-lateral thalamus was involved in their case[16] and that of others.[10,11] In addition, retrograde degeneration has been found in this portion of the pulvinar in patients with cortical aphasia.[16,58] Also important is the observation that some patients with left thalamic hemorrhage, especially in the posterior portions, do not have aphasia.[53]

Rousseaux et al. recently studied blood flow asymmetries in twenty patients with aphasia and left thalamic or "capsulothalamic" hemorrhage.[59] They used $Xe^{133}$ inhalation and a single-photon-emission computed tomography (SPECT) technique to analyze asymmetries in blood flow in various cortical and subcortical regions of interest. Reduced verbal fluency correlated with reduced frontal lobe activity, whereas abnormalities of verbal comprehension, naming, and paraphasic errors correlated with reduced flow in the putamen, insular region, and temporal and posterior cortex.[59] The anatomy and clinical features of thalamic hemorrhage aphasia are complex, and relate to involvement of various thalamic nuclei which project to different subcortical and cortical areas in basal ganglionic-thalamic-cortical circuits.

### Other Cognitive and Behavioral Abnormalities

Nearly all abnormalities described in patients with right cerebral infarcts and hemorrhages have also been noted in patients with right thalamic hematomas. *Unilateral spatial neglect* is a prominent feature in patients with large right thalamic hemorrhages. Watson and Heilman in 1979 reported three patients with right thalamic hematomas and left spatial neglect and inattention.[60] They emphasized that lesions anywhere in a reticular-limbic-cortical loop could lead to neglect. Cambier et al. a year later, described two patients with right thalamic hemorrhage and one with a right thalamic infarct who had left neglect.[61] These authors suggested that the posterior portion of the thalamus, especially the medial pulvinar, was probably the critical region for the direction of attention to the contralateral extrapersonal space.[61] Motomura et al. studied the incidence and anatomy of unilateral spatial neglect more formally and prospectively.[62] They investigated thirty-three patients with thalamic hemorrhage irrespective of the side of the lesion. Testing for spatial neglect involved bisecting lines, canceling out lines on a paper, and drawing and copying tasks. Unilateral spatial neglect was found in eleven patients

(33%) and all had right thalamic hematomas. Most of the hemorrhages causing neglect were large or posteriorly located. The authors analyzed the anatomical regions involved and suggested that medial or posterior thalamic structures were critical for attention to contralateral space. Waxman et al. also reported a single case of right thalamic hemorrhage with prominent left spatial neglect.[63] Their patient had "contralateral motor neglect" also called limb "akinesia" or "hypokinesia." The so-called motor neglect is a concept popularized by Heilman et al.[64,65] The affected limbs had decreased spontaneous movements and decreased arousability or reaction to stimuli but moved well to command. Waxman et al. described the left motor neglect as follows: "the patient tended to move the left side much less than the right. Even in responding to noxious stimuli on the left side of the body, he tended to use the right hand. However, with urging he could move the left side with as much facility as the right and exhibited full strength."[63] Mesulam, in reviewing the concept of attention and hemi-inattention, has cited the role of the various anatomical sites that affect attention including the RAS, limbic, motor, and trimodal sensory (vision, hearing, somatosensory) systems.[66]

*Auditory neglect* or extinction often accompany the hemi-inattention when tested. The standard tests for inattention are visual—drawing, copying, or heeding bilateral stimuli. When Motomura et al. looked for auditory extinction, they found that eight of their thirty-three patients with thalamic hematomas had spatial neglect.[62] Auditory neglect may take the form of simply failing to turn toward or heed sound or word input from the left. Other patients have a failure of localization of auditory input from the left and they look to the right for the stimulus. Some observers have even misinterpreted the pattern as left ear deafness.

*Constructional dyspraxia* (abnormal drawing and copying) also frequently accompanies unilateral spatial neglect, but neglect and constructional dyspraxia are not synonymous. Unilateral spatial neglect in drawing refers to omission of one side (nearly always the left) of figures drawn or copied.[67] Constructional dyspraxia, in contrast, refers to defects in formulation or reconstruction of the entire figure. The size, angles, proportions and conceptualization of the object are globally defective, not just on one side of the figure. Though not identical, constructional dyspraxia and unilateral spatial neglect often coexist in patients with right cerebral infarcts and hematomas.[67] In the series of Motomura et al. ten of the thirty-three patients with thalamic hemorrhage had constructional disturbances, all had right thalamic hematomas, and nine of the ten also had unilateral spatial neglect.[62]

*Anosognosia*, a lack of awareness of abnormalities, is also very common in patients with right thalamic hemorrhage, just as it is in right frontal and parietal cerebral infarcts.[67] Patients with right thalamic hemorrhage also may fail to recognize their left limbs or believe that the limbs are distorted, absent, or distant. Some patients speak of a dead fish or body toward their left. This type of deficit, wrongly called *hemi-asomatognosia* is also common in patients with right parietal lobe lesions.

*Disorientation to place* can also occur in patients with right thalamic hematomas. This can take the form of reduplication of place. One striking example was a patient from Argentina who had a right thalamic hemorrhage and insisted his home and the clinic were, on various days, in Finland, Chile, Spain, and anywhere other than Buenos Aires.[68] Fisher has described this type of abnormality in patients with right posterior hemisphere lesions.[69]

Generalized behavioral disturbances have also been often described in patients with thalamic hemorrhages. The most common disturbances involve the amount of activity. Some patients have markedly decreased activity (*abulia*) while others are restless, agitated, loquacious, and overactive. Abulia is a term popularized by Fisher.[43] Abulia is defined by three characteristics: decreased spontaneity of speech and body movement, prolonged latency in responding to verbal and other stimuli (often the patient fails to respond or responds slowly), and difficulty persevering with tasks. Verbal responses are usually short, terse, and incomplete, and much prodding is needed to continue with tasks such as counting backwards from twenty to zero or crossing off all the "b's" on a page. Slowing of behavior is prominent. In our experience, abulia is a common finding in patients with thalamic hemorrhage. Waxman et al. detailed a prototypic example: "the patient was awake but markedly apathetic and indifferent. He expressed no concern when he was told that he had suffered a stroke. There was a paucity of spontaneous movements and of facial expression. The patient was markedly hypokinetic and would sit without any movements except blinking for periods of minutes. During these periods, the patient's eyes were open, and he would follow the examiner around the room with his gaze. These periods of immobility were punctuated by very slow (30 seconds to shift position) changes in posture after which the patient would sit, statue-like, without moving. The patient moved very slowly in response to vigorous commands, taking 30 seconds for example, to rise from a chair and 3–4 minutes to write a sentence."[63] The anatomy of abulia has not been well defined. Waxman et al. equated the global apathy with motor neglect but we believe they are different phenomena and often do not coexist.[63] Abulic patients may have no motor or lateralized signs. Apathy, indifference, and abulia occur in both right and left thalamic lesions. Studies are insufficient at present to know whether there is a predominance of either side.

*Agitation and delirium* are also commonly seen in patients with thalamic hemorrhage, sometimes only during the acute phase of the illness. Hyperactivity can take the form of restless moving, yelling, agitation, or pressured loquacious speech. Many patients flit from one conversational topic to another. Usually accompanying agitation is an inability to sustain attention to any task. At times, both abulia and agitation are seen in the same patient and the two opposite states may even alternate. Guard et al. described a striking example of a 68-year-old man with a right thalamic hematoma located in the pulvinar and dorsomedial nucleus who was at times apathetic, inert, sleepy, and indifferent, but had frequent agitated spells in which he had stereotypic gestures and soliloquies.[70] Similarly, caudate nucleus lesions can also cause abulia, agitated delirium, or a combination of the two disorders.[71] There are extensive reciprocal relations between the caudate nucleus and the thalamus.

Hallucinations have also been described in patients with thalamic hemorrhages. Fisher, in his 1959 paper, noted that five of his patients with thalamic hematomas had hallucinations.[1] Fisher referred to the hallucinations as "peduncular" after the original French literature description of L'Hermitte and Van Bogaert.[1,31] "Pedonculaire" referred to the midbrain but it is now well known that hallucinations arise also from lesions of the thalamus. The hallucinations are often vivid and include bright colorful objects, animals, and flowers. Often there are auditory components also. The hallucinations occur when the patient is very alert and awake but usually develop in the evening or at night. The peduncular hallucinations often begin during the early part of the illness but can persist for days and even weeks. These types of hallucinations have also been described in patients with thalamic infarcts.[72]

*Altered memory function* has been described in patients with thalamic lesions and undoubtedly can complicate thalamic hemorrhage. Unfortunately, there are very few well studied cases of amnesia from thalamic hemorrhage that would allow precise anatomoclinical correlation. Waxman et al.'s patient with a right thalamic hemorrhage and left neglect also had severely impaired memory.[63] That patient's thalamic hemorrhage occurred in the postoperative period after a left carotid endarterectomy, and hydrocephalus is evident from the published CT scans. Choi et al.

described three patients with thalamic hemorrhage and amnesia.[73] Two of these patients had caudatothalamic lesions, and memory disorders can occur in lesions of the caudate nucleus.[73] The third patient had a recent right thalamic hematoma but had previously had a left thalamic hemorrhage. Hankey and Stewart-Wynne described a single patient with confusion and memory loss and a left anteromedial thalamic hemorrhage.[74] That patient also had an ependymitis and meningitis with thrombosed cortical veins and sagittal sinus, making it difficult to correlate the cognitive deficits with only the thalamic lesion. Memory loss is well known after bilateral thalamic infarction,[75,76] bilateral thalamic tumors, and in Wernicke-Korsakoff syndrome with involvement of the medial dorsal thalami and mamillary bodies bilaterally.[77] Memory loss also may occur after unilateral thalamic lesions, most often infarctions. In most such cases, however, the thalamic infarct has not been an isolated finding. The medial thalamus, which contains the dorsomedial nuclei, the mamillary bodies, and the mamillothalamic tracts, is the expected location in which hemorrhage would cause memory deficits.

### Eye Signs

Most of the oculomotor abnormalities found in patients with thalamic hemorrhage were described in Fisher's original communication[1] or in a subsequent article on neuroophthalmological signs.[78] Fisher noted that the *pupils were usually small and reacted poorly to light*. The lesion affects the most rostral sympathetic system accounting for the small size of the pupils and also interrupts the pupillary reflex arc of fibers going from the optic tract towards the third nerve nuclei in the midbrain. At times, both pupils are miotic but the ipsilateral pupil is smaller. Rarer is unilateral miosis with a normal contralateral pupil. When the hematoma dissects into the midbrain or compresses the midbrain, the pupils may become midposition (neither dilated nor constricted), or oval,[79] or eccentrically placed (corectopia).[80] The eyelid ipsilateral to the hematomas may droop. Occasionally, one or both of the upper lids are retracted (so-called Collier's sign).[81]

The most diagnostic and characteristic oculomotor findings relate to *abnormalities of vertical gaze.* Fisher pointed out that the eyes often were deviated downward (and inward) seeming to peer at the nose.[1] Usually, both upward and downward gaze are abnormal but upward gaze is usually more severely involved. Often the vertical axis is not parallel, but the eyes are skewed with one remaining above the other in all planes of gaze. Gilner and Avin showed that in their patient with a right thalamic hemorrhage, the vertical gaze abnormality related to intraventricular and intracranial pressure.[8] The patient's eyes were deviated downward and medially but immediately after an intraventricular catheter was placed, the eyes assumed a normal vertical position but were directed to the right. Intraventricular pressure was monitored. When the pressure rose steeply to two to three times the baseline value, the eyes would deviate downward and medially.[8] Waga et al. similarly showed that in their patient with a left thalamic hemorrhage and a dilated third ventricle, drainage of the ventricle caused an upgaze palsy to disappear.[9] Vertical gaze palsies are also commonly found in patients with embolism to the rostral basilar artery and with infarcts in the territory of the thalamic-hypothalamic arteries in the posteromedial thalamus.[31,33] The crucial structures for vertical gaze are probably located in the pretectal region at the diencephalic-midbrain junction and include the rostral interstitial nucleus of the medial longitudinal fasciculus (MLF) and the posterior commissure.

*Abnormalities of horizontal conjugate gaze* are also common. Most often the eyes are deviated toward the side of the hemorrhage similar to the conjugate deviation found in putaminal and lobar hematomas. Occasionally, the eyes deviate to the "wrong side" and rest contralateral to the side of the hematoma.[78] Brigell et al. studied horizontal eye movements in detail in their patient with a right thalamic hemorrhage.[82] At first, the eyes rested to the right and spontaneous eye movements occurred mainly in the right hemifield of gaze. Later, when the gaze preference had improved, saccades were hypometric when directed away from the side of the lesion, and pursuit was low in gain with many interposed saccades when gaze was deviated ipsilateraly. This type of saccade and eye movement pattern is similar to patients with decorticating lesions.[83] Similarly, Hirose et al. found in their six patients with posteriorly located thalamic hematomas, there was hypometria away from the lesion and defective pursuit toward the lesion.[17] The horizontal gaze abnormality in thalamic hemorrhage probably relates to interruption of efferent fibers from the cerebral zones mediating saccadic and smooth-pursuit eye movements. When the horizontal gaze deviation is to the contralateral side, there is always spread of the hematoma to the third ventricle, or compression of the third ventricle and contralateral thalamus by the mass of the hematoma.[78]

Keane described a different type of horizontal eye movement abnormality in three patients with right thalamic hemorrhages. Each developed continual, predominantly horizontal binocular saccades lasting less than eighteen hours on the second or third day after their hemorrhages.[84] Sometimes the abnormality began with a burst of saccades. Keane called this abnormality *transient opsoclonus* although the movements were less chaotic and irregular than usually thought of as opsoclonus.[84]

Horizontal eye movements are not always conjugate in patients with thalamic hemorrhage. Fisher described a phenomenon that he referred to as a *pseudo–sixth nerve palsy.*[1] By this, he referred to a failure of monocular abduction not due to injury to the abducens nerve. In this condition, one or both eyes are deviated medially. The medial deviation is more pronounced in the eye ipsilateral to the hemorrhage. In looking to the opposite hemifield, the adducting eye remains deviated medially and the abducting eye fails to look far laterally. Gaze is thus dysconjugate in lateral gaze giving the appearance of a sixth nerve palsy. However, in contrast to a sixth nerve palsy, the abducting eye usually can deviate well past the midline. When the adducting eye is covered, the abducting eye can deviate further laterally. Also, if the abducting eye is watched carefully, there will often be inward jerks that interrupt gaze laterally. Necropsy in patients with this pseudo–sixth palsy shows that the pons and sixth nerve fibers are intact. We believe that two factors account for the failure of abduction and for the medial deviation of the eyes. These are *hyperconvergence tendencies* and *monocular fixation with the adducting eye. Hyperconvergence, convergence spasms*, and *convergence nystagmus* are well known after thalamic hemorrhages and infarcts.[31,33] Hyperconvergence probably accounts for the tendency of the eyes to deviate inward. Convergence nystagmus can be elicited by asking the patient to view an optokinetic drum or tape that moves upward. The inward directed jerks of the abducting eye on lateral gaze probably represent convergence vectors. Thus, on lateral gaze the convergence vectors balance and neutralize lateral gaze and limit abduction. Also, because the adducting eye is hyperconverged, gaze becomes dysconjugate. Closing or covering the adducting eye is usually followed by improved ability to abduct the contralateral eye, showing that the fixating eye was most likely the adducting one. Gomez et al. reported three patients with unilateral thalamic infarcts and acute esotropia of the contralateral eye, which remained hyperadducted.[85] Subcomponents of the oculomotor complex relate to tonic activities.[86] Hyperconvergence might be caused by a lesion of the corticooculomotor pathways that cross the thalamus.[85]

Oculomotor abnormalities are present in virtually all patients with large thalamic hemorrhages. Among the eighteen patients studied by Walshe et al., all but the one with the smallest hemorrhage had oculomotor signs.[4] Vertical gaze abnormalities were present in seventeen patients. In ten patients, the eyes rested downwards by 1 to 3 mm and, in the remainder, gaze upwards or downwards was impaired either on pursuit or as a reflex response to vertical head movements. In nine there was horizontal gaze deviation, three ipsilaterally and six contralaterally.[4]

Hemianopia is found transiently in many patients with thalamic hemorrhage but rarely persists. Usually the abnormality is severe visual neglect rather than interruption of the geniculocalcarine pathway. The lateral geniculate body lies far posteriorly and is usually spared, although thalamic hematomas may dissect laterally across the retrolenticular part of the internal capsule to affect the visual radiations. Aoki and Fujino reported two patients with an isolated hemianopia from thalamic hemorrhages located far posteriorly and laterally.[87]

### Correlations in Patients with Smaller Hematomas

The advent of CT and later MRI has allowed detection of small hematomas that previously would have gone undetected. Patients with hematomas less than 2 cm in maximal diameter nearly always survive. The most common location of these small hematomas is in the posterolateral thalamus in the territory of supply of the thalamogeniculate arteries. In one large series of small thalamic hematomas, among thirty-seven lesions, twenty-nine (76%) were posterolateral.[19] The other sites, anterolateral, medial, and posterior (dorsal) probably each account for 8% of small hematomas.

*Anterior and anterolateral lesions* affect nuclei that project to the frontal lobe. The hematomas also often reach the ventral lateral nucleus, which is a motor relay structure. Anterolateral thalamic hematomas often spill out of the boundaries of the thalamus laterally to involve the far anterior portion of the posterior limb of the internal capsule. The major clinical findings are a slight sensory and motor "hemiparesis," and behavior and cognitive abnormalities. The sensory-motor limb abnormalities are often slight and reversible. The behavioral syndrome is characterized by abulia with decreased spontaneity, apathy, and indifference to the environment. Memory dysfunction may also be present and often persists.[18,19] The behavioral syndrome is very similar to that found in patients with occlusion of the tuberothalamic (polar) artery.[23,28,38] Usually patients remain alert. Oculomotor signs are usually not present.

The *posterolateral* site is by far the most frequent location for small and large thalamic hematomas.[4,5,19] These lesions arise from thalamogeniculate branches. These hematomas often dissect out of the thalamus laterally and involve the posterior limb of the internal capsule. Figure 16.12 shows a CT scan of a typical lateral thalamic hematoma. Alertness is usually maintained in the small hematomas. Severe sensory-motor deficits are found because of the involvement of the thalamic somatosensory relay nuclei (VPM and VPL) and the pyramidal tract fibers in the internal capsule. Hemiplegia usually persists when the hematoma affects the internal capsule. Ataxia can also often be found in the weak limbs as can dystonic and choreic movements. Behavioral abnormalities are not prominent. When present, they usually are characterized by aphasia in dominant hemisphere hematomas, and left-sided neglect and poor drawing and copying in right posterolateral thalamic hematomas.[17] Neuroophthalmological findings are an ipsilateral small pupil and ptosis, and abnormalities of conjugate lateral gaze. Hypometric saccades are found in gaze to the contralateral side and there are abnormalities of pursuit to the side of the lesion with so-called "catch up" saccades.[17,82] Occasionally, a persistent hemianopia occurs. Disturbances of alertness and consciousness, memory loss, and abnormalities of vertical gaze or convergence are not found, unless the posterolateral hematomas

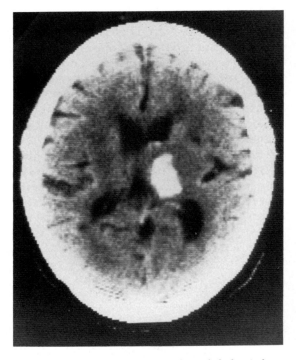

**Figure 16.12.** CT showing large lateral thalamic hematoma. Note pressure on ipsilateral lateral ventricle.

are large and spread medially and posteriorly towards the diencephalic-midbrain junction.

*Medial hematomas* usually involve the dorsomedial and centromedian nuclei. Sensory-motor abnormalities are usually absent or minor and transient. The major abnormalities are reduced alertness and cognitive and behavioral abnormalities.[19,73,74] Lethargy and even stupor in larger medial lesions are due to involvement of the RAS near the third ventricle. Early in the course, these patients are often described as confused. Later, they are abulic and have difficulty making new memories. The amnesia may be severe and persistent after recovery from the stroke.[73,74] Oculomotor abnormalities are not present in the small medial lesions.

The *far posterior-dorsal lesions* are probably the least common of all the small thalamic hematomas. These lesions predominantly involve the pulvinar and are in the distribution of the posterior choroidal arteries. Slight sensory-motor signs may be present but are usually transient. The most important problem in left pulvinar hematomas is aphasia. The first few sentences may be normal except for minor paraphasic errors. As patients continue to talk, they lapse into jargon aphasia. Repetition of spoken language is good but writing is poor. Patients with right pulvinar and posterior hematomas may have constructional apraxia, abnormal topographic memory, and disorientation to place.[17,68]

## Prognosis

The two most consistent features that correlate with prognosis are the size of the hematoma and the state of alertness of the patient. All studies have found that patients with larger hematomas have a higher fatality rate. In Weisberg's series, the patients with thalamic hematomas larger than 3 cm in greatest diameter died.[5] Kwak et al. also showed that patients with hematomas over 2.5 cm in greatest diameter had a worse outlook for survival than those with hematomas less than 2 cm.[88] These authors also measured hematoma volume. When the volume was less than 10 ml, the outlook was good for recovery. Penetration of the hematoma into the third ventricle probably does not greatly affect survival,[87,88] but midline shifts and generalized ventricular enlargement due to compression of the aqueduct or third ventricle are correlated with poor recovery and higher mortality.[88]

All studies have shown that coma, especially when prolonged, is a poor prognostic sign.[4,7,88,89] In one series, four of the five patients admitted in coma died, as did three of six who were stuporous and two of six who were obtunded.[4] In another series, only one patient admitted in coma with thalamic hemorrhage survived.[7] Progression from alertness to coma is a particularly bad sign.

## References

1. Fisher CM. The pathologic and clinical aspects of thalamic hemorrhage. Tr Am Neurol Assoc 1959;84:56–59.
2. Fisher CM. The pathology and pathogenesis of intracerebral hemorrhage. In Fields WS [Ed.] Pathogenesis and treatment of cerebrovascular disease. Springfield, IL: Charles C Thomas, 1961;295–317.
3. Fisher CM. Clinical syndromes in cerebral hemorrhage. In: Fields WS, ed. Pathogenesis and treatment of cerebrovascular disease. Springfield IL: Charles C Thomas, 1961:318–342.
4. Walshe TM, Davis KR, Fisher CM. Thalamic hemorrhage: a computed tomographic-clinical correlation. Neurology 1977;27:217–222.
5. Weisberg LA. Computed tomography in intracranial hemorrhage. Arch Neurol 1979;36:422–426.
6. Scott WR, New PFJ, Davis KR, et al. Computerized axial tomography of intracerebral and intraventricular hemorrhage. Radiology 1974;112:73–80.
7. Barraquer-Bordas L, Illa I, Escartin A, et al. Thalamic hemorrhage: a study of 23 patients with diagnosis by computed tomography. Stroke 1981;12:524–527.
8. Gilner LI, Avin B. A reversible ocular manifestation of thalamic hemorrhage: a case report. Arch Neurol 1977;34:715–716.
9. Waga S, Okada M, Yamamoto Y. Reversibility of Parinaud syndrome in thalamic hemorrhage. Neurology 1979;29:407–409.
10. Ciemins VA. Localized thalamic hemorrhage: a cause of aphasia. Neurology 1970;20:776–782.
11. Mohr JP, Watters WC, Duncan GW. Thalamic hemorrhage and aphasia. Brain Lang 1975;2:3–17.
12. Samarel A, Wright TL, Sergay S, et al. Thalamic hemorrhage with speech disorder. Tr Am Neurol Assoc 1976;101:283–285.
13. Cappa SF, Vignolo LA. "Transcortical" features of aphasia following left thalamic hemorrhage. Cortex 1979;15:121–130.
14. Kirshner HS, Kistler KH. Aphasia after right thalamic hemorrhage. Arch Neurol 1982;39:667–669.
15. Chesson AL. Aphasia following a right thalamic hemorrhage. Brain Lang 1983;19:306–316.

16. Crosson B, Parker JC, Kim AK, et al. A case of thalamic aphasia with postmortem verification. Brain Lang 1986;29:301–314.

17. Hirose G, Kosoegawa H, Saeki M, et al. The syndrome of posterior thalamic hemorrhage. Neurology 1985;35:998–1002.

18. Ikeda K, Yamashima T, Uno E, et al. Clinical manifestation of small thalamic hemorrhage. Brain Nerv 1985;37:173–179.

19. Kawahara N, Sato K, Muraki M, et al. CT classification of small thalamic hemorrhages and their clinical implications. Neurology 1986;36:165–172.

20. Weisberg LA. Thalamic hemorrhage: clinical-CT correlations. Neurology 1986;36:1382–1386.

21. Carpenter MB. Core text of Neuroanatomy. Second Edition. Baltimore: Williams & Wilkins, 1978.

22. Afifi AK, Bergman RA. Basic neuroscience. A structural and functional approach. Baltimore: Urban and Schwarzenberg, 1986.

23. Graff-Radford NR, Damasio H, Yamada T, et al. Nonhaemorrhagic thalamic infarction: clinical, neuropsychological and electrophysiological findings in four anatomical groups defined by computerized tomography. Brain 1985;108:485–516.

24. Percheron G. Les artères du thalamus humain I. Artère et territoire thalamiques polaires de l'artère communicante postérieure. Rev Neurol 1976;132:297–307.

25. Percheron G. Les artères du thalamus humain II. Artères et territoires thalamiques paramédians de l'artère basilaire communicante. Rev Neurol 1976;132:309–324.

26. Takahashi S, Goto K, Fukasawa H, et al. Computed tomography of cerebral infarctions along the distribution of the basal perforating arteries: Part II: Thalamic arterial group. Radiology 1985;155:119–130.

27. Lazorthes G, Salamon G. The arteries of the thalamus: an anatomical and radiological study. J Neurosurg 1971;34:23–26.

28. Bogousslavsky J, Regli F, Assal G. The syndrome of unilateral tuberothalamic artery territory infarction. Stroke 1986;17:434–441.

29. Castaigne P, Lhermitte F, Buge A, et al. Paramedian thalamic and midbrain infarcts: clinical and neuropathological study. Ann Neurol 1981;10:127–148.

30. Stephens RB, Stilwell D. Arteries and veins of the human brain. Springfield, IL: Charles C Thomas, 1969.

31. Caplan LR. "Top of the basilar syndrome." Neurology 1980;30:72–79.

32. Mehler MF. The rostral basilar artery syndrome: diagnosis, etiology, prognosis. Neurology 1989;39:9–16.

33. Mehler MF. The neuro-ophthalmologic spectrum of the rostral basilar artery syndrome. Arch Neurol 1988;45:966–971.

34. Caplan LR. Vertebrobasilar occlusive disease. In: Barnett HJM, et al., eds. Stroke: Pathophysiology, Diagnosis, and Management. New York: Churchill-Livingstone, 1986;549–619.

35. Caplan LR. Vertebrobasilar system syndromes. In: Vinken P, et al., eds. Handbook of clinical Neurology (Revised). Vol. 53. Vascular Disease Part I. Amsterdam: North Holland, 1988;371–408.

36. Caplan LR, DeWitt LD, Pessin MS, et al. Lateral thalamic infarcts. Arch Neurol 1988;45:959–964.

37. Dejerine J, Roussy G. Le syndrome thalamique. Rev Neurol 1906;14:521–532.

38. Bogousslavsky J, Regli F, Uske A. Thalamic infarcts: clinical syndromes, etiology and prognosis. Neurology 1988;38:837–848.

39. Ingvar DH, Sourander P. Destruction of the reticular core of the brainstem: a patho-anatomical follow-up of a case of coma of three years' duration. Arch Neurol 1970;23:1–8.

40. Façon E, Steriade M, Wertheim N. Hypersomnie prolongée engendrée par des lésions bilatérales du système activateur médial: le syndrome thrombotique de la bifurcation du tronc basilaire. Rev Neurol 1958;98:117–133.

41. Castaigne P, Buge A, Escourolle R, et al. Ramollissement pédonculaire médian, tegmento-thalamique avec ophtalmoplégie et hypersomnie (étude anatomo-clinique). Rev Neurol 1962;106:357–367.

42. Segarra JM. Cerebral vascular disease and behavior: I. the syndrome of the mesencephalic artery (basilar artery bifurcation). Arch Neurol 1970;22:408–418.

43. Fisher CM. Abulia minor vs. agitated behavior. Clin Neurosurg 1983;31:9–31.

44. Fisher CM. Pure sensory stroke involving face, arm and leg. Neurology 1965;15:76–80.

45. Fisher CM. Pure sensory stroke and allied conditions. Stroke 1982;13:434–447.

46. Groothuis DR, Duncan GW, Fisher CM. The human thalamocortical sensory path in the internal capsule: evidence from a small capsular

hemorrhage causing a pure sensory stroke. Ann Neurol 1977;2:328–331.

47. Verma AK, Maheshwari MC. Hypestheticataxic-hemiparesis in thalamic hemorrhage. Stroke 1986;17:49–51.

48. Schlitt M, Brown JW, Zeiger HE, et al. Appendicular tremor as a late complication of intracerebral hemorrhage. Surg Neurol 1986;25: 181–184.

49. Freilich RJ, Chambers BR. Choreoathetosis and thalamic hemorrhage. Clin Exper Neurol 1980;25:115–120.

50. Donat JR. Unilateral asterixis due to thalamic hemorrhage. Neurology 1980;30:83–84.

51. Hermann K, Turner JW, Gillingham FJ, et al. The effects of destructive lesions and stimulation of the basal ganglia on speech mechanisms. Confin Neurol 1966;27:197–207.

52. Ojemann GA, Ward AA. Speech representation in ventrolateral thalamus. Brain 1971;94: 669–680.

53. Kertesz A, Sheppard A, MacKenzie R. Localization in transcortical sensory aphasia. Arch Neurol 1982;39:475–478.

54. Cappa SF, Papagno C, Vallar G, et al. Aphasia does not always follow left thalamic hemorrhage: a study of five negative cases. Cortex 1986;22:639–647.

55. Archer CR, Ilinsky IA, Goldfader PR, et al. Aphasia in thalamic stroke: CT/stereotactic localization. J Comput Assist Tomogr 1981;5: 427–432.

56. Davous P, Bianco C, Duval-Lota AM, et al. Aphasie par infarctus thalamique paramédian gauche: observation anatomo-clinique. Rev Neurol 1984;140:711–719.

57. Gorelick PB, Hier DB, Benevento L, et al. Aphasia after left thalamic infarction. Arch Neurol 1984;41:1296–1298.

58. Van Buren JM. The question of thalamic participation in speech mechanisms. Brain Lang 1975;2:31–44.

59. Rousseaux M, Steinling M, Griffié G, et al. Corrélations de l'aphasie thalamique avec le débit sanguin cérébral. Rev Neurol 1990;146: 345–353.

60. Watson RT, Heilman KM. Thalamic neglect. Neurology 1979;29:690–694.

61. Cambier J, Elghozi D, Strube E. Lésions du thalamus droit avec syndrome de l'hémisphère mineur: discussion du concept de négligence thalamique. Rev Neurol 1980;136: 105–116.

62. Motomura N, Yamadori A, Mori E, et al. Unilateral spatial neglect due to hemorrhage in the thalamic region. Acta Neurol Scand 1986;74:190–194.

63. Waxman SG, Ricaurte GA, Tucker SB. Thalamic hemorrhage with neglect and memory disorder. J Neurol Sci 1986;75:105–112.

64. Heilman KM, Valenstein E. Frontal lobe neglect in man. Neurology 1972;22:660–664.

65. Heilman KM, Schwartz HD, Watson RT. Hypoarousal in patients with the neglect syndrome and emotional indifference. Neurology 1978;28:229–232.

66. Mesulam M-M. A cortical network for directed attention and unilateral neglect. Ann Neurol 1981;10:309–325.

67. Hier DB, Mondlock J, Caplan LR. Behavioral abnormalities after right hemisphere stroke. Neurology 1983;33:337–344.

68. Leiguarda RC. Environmental reduplication associated with a right thalamic haemorrhage. J Neurol Neurosurg Psychiat 1983;46: 1154 (letter).

69. Fisher CM. Disorientation for place. Arch Neurol 1982;39:33–36.

70. Guard O, Bellis F, Mabille JP, et al. Démence thalamique après lésion hémorragique unilatérale du pulvinar droit. Rev Neurol 1986;142: 759–765.

71. Caplan LR, Schmahmann JD, Kase CS, et al. Caudate infarcts. Arch Neurol 1990;47: 133–143.

72. Feinberg WM, Rapcsak SZ. 'Peduncular hallucinosis' following paramedian thalamic infarction. Neurology 1989;39:1535–1536.

73. Choi D, Sudarsky L, Schachter S, et al. Medial thalamic hemorrhage with amnesia. Arch Neurol 1983;40:611–613.

74. Hankey GJ, Stewart-Wynne EG. Amnesia following thalamic hemorrhage. Stroke 1988;19: 776–778.

75. von Cramon DY, Hebel N, Schuri U. A contribution to the anatomical basis of thalamic amnesia. Brain 1985;108:993–1008.

76. Winocur G, Oxbury S, Roberts R, et al. Amnesia in a patient with bilateral lesions to the thalamus. Neuropsychologia 1984;22:123–143.

77. Victor M, Adams RD, Collins GH. The Wernicke-Korsakoff syndrome. Philadelphia: F.A. Davis, 1971.

78. Fisher CM. Some neuro-ophthalmological observations. J Neurol Neurosurg Psychiat 1967;30:383–392.

79. Fisher CM. Oval pupils. Arch Neurol 1980;37:502–503.

80. Selhorst JB, Hoyt WF, Feinsod M, et al. Midbrain corectopia. Arch Neurol 1976;33:193–195.

81. Collier J. Nuclear ophthalmoplegia, with special reference to retraction of lid and ptosis and to lesions of the posterior commissure. Brain 1927;50:488–498.

82. Brigell M, Babikian V, Goodwin JA. Hypometric saccades and low-gain pursuit resulting from a thalamic hemorrhage. Ann Neurol 1984;15:374–378.

83. Sharpe JA, Lo AW, Rabinovitch HE. Control of the saccadic and smooth pursuit systems after cerebral hemidecortication. Brain 1979;102:387–403.

84. Keane JR. Transient opsoclonus with thalamic hemorrhage. Arch Neurol 1980;37:423–424.

85. Gomez CR, Gomez SM, Selhorst JB. Acute thalamic esotropia. Neurology 1988;38:1759–1762.

86. Büttner-Ennever JA, Akert K. Medial rectus subgroups of the oculomotor nucleus and their abducens internuclear input in the monkey. J Comp Neurol 1981;197:17–27.

87. Aoki N, Fujino T. Hypertensive basal ganglionic hemorrhage with a single manifestation of isolated homonymous hemianopia: report of two cases. Brain Nerve 1983;35:1141–1144.

88. Kwak R, Kadoya S, Suzuki T. Factors affecting the prognosis in thalamic hemorrhage. Stroke 1983;14:493–500.

89. Young WB, Lee KP, Pessin MS, et al. Prognostic significance of ventricular blood in supratentorial hemorrhage: a volumetric study. Neurology 1990;40:616–619.

# Chapter 17
# Lobar Hemorrhage

## Carlos S. Kase

Lobar intracerebral hemorrhage (ICH) occurs in the white matter of the cerebral lobes. Its site of origin is frequently at the cortical-subcortical grey-white matter junction, from where it extends for variable degrees into the adjacent white matter (Figure 17.1). After the acute event has passed and the hemorrhage has been slowly absorbed, the residual from it after months from the onset appears macroscopically as a "slit" with orange-stained margins. This represents the collapsed cavity of the original hematoma along with collections of ochre hemosiderin-laden macrophages at its periphery, resulting from phagocytosis of blood products from the original hematoma. This form of ICH has distinctive clinical features, mechanisms, and prognosis, which separate it from the basal ganglionic and thalamic forms of ICH.

### General Features

#### Frequency

Lobar ICH is reported to account for between 23% and 46% of the cases of ICH in clinical series.[1–6] A lower relative frequency, between 8% and 37.5%, has been documented in autopsy series.[7–10] Lobar ICH has been associated with a generally lower mortality rate than that of other locations of hematomas.[1]

In clinical series, lobar ICH is only second to putaminal ICH in frequency,[1,4] being as common or more common than thalamic hemorrhage (Table 17.1). In some series[5,10a] lobar

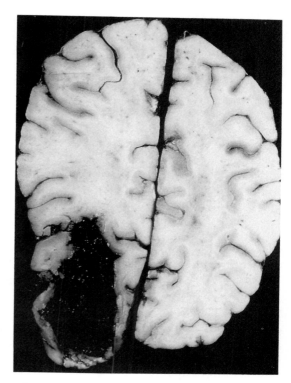

**Figure 17.1.** Pathology specimen of large left occipital white matter hemorrhage.

**Table 17.1.** Distribution by Site of Ninety-three Cases of ICH

| Type of ICH | No. of Cases | % of Total |
|---|---|---|
| Putaminal | 31 | 33 |
| Lobar | 22 | 23 |
| Thalamic | 19 | 20 |
| Cerebellar | 7 | 8 |
| Pontine | 6 | 7 |
| Miscellaneous | 8 | 9 |
| Total | 93 | 100 |

(From Kase CS, Williams JP, Wyatt DA, Mohr JP. Lobar intracerebral hematomas: Clinical and CT analysis of 22 cases. Neurology 1982;32:1146–1150, with permission.)

ICH is reported with the highest frequency (34% and 33%, respectively) among spontaneous ICH, even surpassing the putaminal location (23% and 18%, respectively). The frequency of the lobar type among patients with ICH is even higher when one considers the group of patients younger than age 45. Toffol et al.[11] studied seventy-two patients with nontraumatic ICH between ages 15 and 45 and found a lobar location in forty (55%), representing by far the highest frequency site, followed by only eleven patients with putaminal and four with thalamic ICH. Similarly, Gras et al.[12] reported thirty-three patients with ICH between ages 9 and 44, twenty-one (64%) of them having lobar ICH, in contrast to only eleven (33%) with "deep" and one (3%) with infratentorial ICH. Despite this, lobar ICH has received relatively little attention in the literature, until the late

1970s to early 1980s, when several publications addressed its clinical and computed tomography (CT) features.[1,13,14]

*Mechanisms*

Lobar ICH is thought to be less commonly due to hypertension than any of the other varieties of ICH. In five large series from the literature, the cause of lobar ICH was thought to be hypertension in 20% to 47.5% of the patients (Table 17.2). This compares with figures of 67% for putaminal,[16] 57% for thalamic,[17] 86% to 97% for pontine,[18,19] and 52% to 75% for cerebellar[20–22] hemorrhage. One possible explanation for these differences is that the arterial lesions thought to cause ICH in hypertensive individuals, lipohyalinosis[23] and microaneurysms,[24] tend to be located in the deep portions of the cerebral hemispheres, brainstem, and cerebellum, with relative sparing of vessels in the corticosubcortical junction.[24] Secondly, nonhypertensive mechanisms of ICH, including cerebral amyloid angiopathy (CAA), vascular malformations, sympathomimetic drugs, and bleeding disorders (especially use of fibrinolytic agents for the treatment of myocardial infarction), all have a tendency to produce predominantly subcortical lobar ICH, with a lower frequency of deep hemispheric and brainstem hemorrhages. Depending on the age group under consideration, certain nonhypertensive mechanisms of lobar ICH are characteristic: CAA in the elderly,[25] vascular

**Table 17.2.** Causes of Lobar ICH in Series from the Literature

| Cause | Kase et al.[1] (N = 22) N (%) | Weisberg et al.[2] (N = 25) N (%) | Schütz[5] (N = 98) N (%) | Ropper and Davis[14] (N = 26) N (%) | Lipton et al.[15] (N = 42) N (%) |
|---|---|---|---|---|---|
| Hypertension | 10 (45) | 5 (20) | 36 (37.0) | 8 (30.5) | 20 (47.5) |
| Bleeding diathesis | 1 (5) | 2 (8) | 14 (14.0) | 2 (8.0) | 8 (19.0) |
| Neoplasms | 3 (14) | 1 (4) | 4 (4.0) | 1 (3.5) | — |
| Vasc. malf., aneurysm | 2 (9) | 8 (32) | 24 (24.5) | 2 (8.0) | 4 (9.5) |
| Other | — | — | — | 3 (11.5) | 10 (24.0) |
| Unknown | 6 (27) | 9 (36) | 20 (20.5) | 10 (38.5) | — |

Abbreviations: N = number of patients, vasc. malf. = vascular malformation.

malformations,[11] aneurysms,[26,27] and sympathomimetic drugs[28,29] in the young, and neoplasms[1] and bleeding disorders, in particular ICH from fibrinolytic agent use[30] in the intermediate age groups.

Despite these various reasons to explain a predominance of nonhypertensive mechanisms in lobar ICH, Broderick at al.[30a] have recently provided evidence for a substantial contribution of hypertension to its pathogenesis. They found hypertension as the mechanism in 67% of 66 patients with lobar ICH, a figure that was not significantly different from that of 77 patients with deep hemispheric (73%), eleven with cerebellar (73%), and nine with pontine (78%) hemorrhage. Furthermore, the frequency of hypertension as the mechanism of ICH remained virtually unchanged with advancing age, suggesting that the impact of hypertension does not decline in the elderly as a consequence of the relative increase of other nonhypertensive causes of ICH, such as CAA. These data led the authors to conclude that hypertension is at least as important as CAA in the pathogenesis of lobar ICH.

Other causes of lobar ICH are well documented. Small, "occult" (i.e., not visible angiographically) *vascular malformations* in surgical specimens from patients with predominantly lobar ICH have been reported on several occasions. VanderArk and Kahn[31] operated on thirty patients with predominantly lobar hematomas of unknown cause, and found small vascular malformations on histological examination in eight patients (27%). Similarly, Krayenbühl and Siebenmann[32] reported seven patients with ICH due to histologically proven vascular malformations, six of whom presented with lobar hematomas. Recently, Wakai et al.[33] reported the operative results in twenty-nine patients with lobar ICH and negative angiography, and found nine with vascular malformations (six arteriovenous malformations [AVM], three cavernous angiomas) and eleven with microaneurysms, for a total of twenty of twenty-nine patients, or 69%, with these vascular lesions. Five of the eleven patients with

microaneurysms had no evidence of hypertension. There were six patients with CAA, and two with brain tumors; only one of the twenty-nine had no diagnosis after histological examination of the hematoma and its wall. These data confirmed their previous observation of the frequent finding of microaneurysms by performing serial histological sections of surgical samples in patients with lobar ICH.[34] In that study, six patients with surgically-drained lobar ICH had no diagnosis made by routine histological study of biopsy materials but, after serial histological sections were performed, all cases were found to have microaneurysms. Only two of the six patients had evidence of hypertension. The lesions were labeled as microaneurysms if they corresponded to either true microaneurysms[24] or "bleeding globes,"[23] as the authors considered both lesions related to the pathogenesis of ICH.

Other less common causes of lobar ICH include: (1) *Cerebral tumors*, which are for the most part malignant, more often metastatic than primary.[1,14] The lobar location of these ICH follows the predilection of hematogenous deposits for the grey/white junction of the cerebral hemispheres. The presence of an underlying tumor is a consideration in patients presenting with lobar ICH that has a disproportionate amount of surrounding edema and mass effect, as well as postcontrast enhancement of nodules at the periphery of the acute ICH.[34a] (2) The use of *anticoagulant and fibrinolytic agents*, when complicated by ICH, frequently results in hemorrhages of lobar location. Those due to the use of warfarin are generally large and of poor prognosis, with a mortality in the 55% to 70% range. The use of the fibrinolytic agents streptokinase and tissue plasminogen activator (tPA) for the treatment of acute myocardial infarction has resulted in ICH in 0.5% to 5% of patients.[30,34b] The majority of the ICHs are lobar, and a role for CAA in their causation has been suggested.[34c,34d] (3) *Sympathomimetic drugs*, including amphetamines, phenylpropanolamine, and cocaine, have been implicated in numerous instances of ICH, which have been predominantly lobar in location.[29,34e] The hemorrhages generally occur minutes or hours after drug use, and acute hypertension has been present in approximately 50% of the patients. These agents are associated with a vasculopathy on cerebral angiography characterized by alternating areas of focal constriction and dilatation ("beading"), thought to represent vasculitis. However, such pathology has only rarely been confirmed histologically.[34f,34g] (4) *Cerebral amyloid angiopathy*, which involves the small and medium-size arteries and veins of the cerebral cortex and leptomeninges,[25] often leads to lobar ICH. The angiopathy is strongly age-related, and is thus responsible for ICH in the elderly. Additional features include a recurrent character and, occasionally, the occurrence of several simultaneous lobar ICHs.[34h] (5) *Vasculitis* is an uncommon cause of ICH, as the main effect of the angiopathy is cerebral infarction. On rare occasions, "granulomatous angiitis of the nervous system" has resulted in ICH, which has been predominantly lobar.[34i,35]

Finally, a host of less common disorders such as dural vein thrombosis,[9,27] hemodialysis,[36] and lumbar metrizamide myelography[37] have been reported in association with lobar ICH. Despite the documentation of these multiple causes of lobar ICH, a substantial proportion (20% to over 40%) of the cases are of unknown mechanism (see Table 17.2).[38,39]

## Clinical Features

These will be discussed in two parts, first referring to the *general* clinical features of lobar ICH, irrespective of its location, and secondly to the specific neurological manifestations in the *various anatomical sites* of lobar ICH.

### General Clinical Features

Lobar ICH is frequently described as having a *sudden onset* during activity, like ICH at other sites, with no cases reported as having an onset during sleep.[1,14] Progression of neurological deficits over minutes to hours is commonly observed, and has been reported in 22%[40] and 54%[14] of patients in two large series. The most common symptom at onset is *headache*, either alone or accompanying other symptoms, a feature that characterizes the onset in 60% to 70% of the patients.[1,14,40,41] The specific characteristics of the headache depend on the anatomical location of the ICH, and they are discussed in the next section. Associated *vomiting* has been reported in over one-third of the patients (30% to 45%)[1,14,40,41] a feature that tends to occur early after the onset of ICH, usually in the first hours of illness.

The occurrence of *seizures* at the onset of lobar ICH has been repeatedly documented.[1,3,4,15,40–43] Seizures probably occur more frequently in lobar ICH than in other locations of brain hemorrhage.[1] In large series in the literature, seizures at onset of lobar ICH have been reported in 16.3%,[41] 21%,[15] 23%,[1] 28%,[4,40] 29%,[3] and 36%[43] of the patients. In virtually all instances, seizures occur at the time of onset of the ICH.[44] Sung and Chu[43] reported the highest frequency (36%) of seizures at onset of lobar ICH, and over half of their patients presented in status epilepticus. Berger et al.[44] reported a 17% frequency of seizures in 112 patients with supratentorial ICH, including patients with lobar and deep hemispheric hemorrhages. The most significant feature associated with the occurrence of seizures was the presence of blood extending into the cerebral cortex: seizures occurred in seventeen of sixty-five (26%) patients with cortical involvement by the ICH, whereas only one of thirty-three (3%) patients without cortical extension of the hemorrhage had seizures. The seizure type in lobar ICH was described as generalized in thirteen of nineteen (68%) patients and focal in six of nineteen (32%) patients in the series of Berger et al.[44] However, a predominance of focal seizures in patients with lobar hemorrhage has been more often reported in the literature.[1,40–43] The propensity of subcortical hemorrhages to cause seizures has been attributed to either sudden interruption of blood flow to the sensorimotor cortex[45] or isolation of a segment of cerebral cortex by the subcortical hematoma,[1] the latter presumably resulting in the generation of paroxysmal electrical activity from the isolated segment of cortex.[46]

The following case description illustrates the presentation of temporal ICH with focal motor "status epilepticus"[47]:

> A 45-year-old hypertensive woman collapsed to the ground while eating breakfast, and had focal motor convulsions involving the face and arm on the left. Shortly thereafter she vomited. On admission her blood pressure was 260/130. Rhythmic clonic jerking of the left limbs and face continued after two 5-mg intravenous doses of diazepam, and 750 mg of intravenous diphenylhydantoin were required to control the seizure activity. In the postictal period she was stuporous, with left hemiplegia and conjugate ocular deviation to the right, with midline crossing with the doll's head maneuver. The pupils were 3 mm, reactive to light.
>
> A CT scan showed a subcortical hematoma in the midportion of the right temporal lobe (Figure 17.2). No mass effect or ventricular extension were present.
>
> After a 24-hour seizure-free period she was alert and oriented, the left limbs were slightly paretic, and she had full eye movements. On day 4, she had regained full strength in the left leg, the arm was slightly weak distally, and no facial asymmetry was present. No abnormalities were detected in sensory or visual field testing. An angiogram on day 11 revealed slight signs of right midtemporal mass effect, without a vascular malformation or tumor stain.

This patient presented in focal motor "status epilepticus" at onset of a small temporal hemorrhage. The admission left hemiplegia was a manifestation of postictal (Todd's) paralysis, as it improved after hours from the onset with later return of motor strength to normal.

The occurrence of *coma* at presentation has been reported in small proportions of patients with lobar ICH: 19% in the Stroke Data

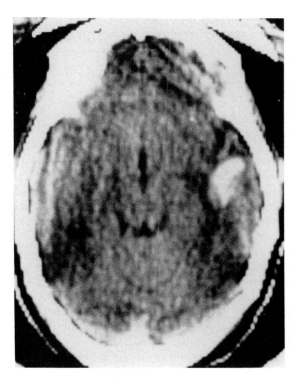

**Figure 17.2.** CT of small right subcortical temporal hematoma (From Kase CS, Mohr JP. Supratentorial intracerebral hemorrhage. In Barnett HJM, Mohr JP, Stein BM, Yatsu FM, eds. Stroke: Pathophysiology, Diagnosis, and Management. New York: Churchill Livingstone, 1986; 525–547, with permission.)

Bank,[41] 18% in the series of Kase et al.,[1] 5% in that of Schütz,[5] and 0.4% by Ropper and Davis.[14] This relatively low frequency of coma at onset has been interpreted as reflecting the peripheral location of the lobar hemorrhages, with a lesser likelihood of distorting midline structures,[1,14] in comparison with hematomas of putaminal and thalamic locations.

These various features of presentation of lobar ICH have been thought to be different from those of the deep hemispheric varieties[1] (Table 17.3). In particular, higher frequency of headache and seizures at onset, lower frequency of coma, and lower frequency of hypertension as its cause have been noted. A relatively higher frequency of headache may

**Table 17.3.** Comparison of Clinical Features of Lobar ICH with all Forms of ICH

| Feature | All Forms of ICH (%) | | Lobar ICH (%) | | | |
|---|---|---|---|---|---|---|
| | HSR[4] | Lausanne[6] | Kase et al.[1] | Ropper and Davis[14] | Weisberg[40] | SDB[41]* |
| Hypertension | | | | | | |
| History | 72 | 55[†] | 22 | 31 | 30 | 55 |
| On admission | 91 | | 66 | 46 | 56 | ? |
| Headache | 33 | 40 | 61 | 46 | 72 | 60 |
| Vomiting | 51 | ? | 33 | 61 | 32 | 29 |
| Seizures | 6 | 7 | 33 | 0 | 28 | 16 |
| Coma | 24 | 22 | 18 | 0.4 | ? | 19 |

Abbreviations: HSR = Harvard Stroke Registry, SDB = Stroke Data Bank, ? = information not provided.
*Percentages rounded to the closest whole number (decimals from the original omitted).
[†]Not specified whether hypertension was diagnosed by history or at entry examination.

simply reflect the lower likelihood of coma at presentation, thus allowing for a higher probability of reporting of the symptom.[1] However, other series[15,41] have not found a significant difference between lobar and deep hemorrhages in their frequency of coma at onset. In a comparison of forty-two patients with lobar ICH with seventy patients with deep (putaminal and thalamic) hemispheric hemorrhages, Lipton et al.[15] reported different results. They only documented the lower frequency (48%) of the hypertensive mechanism in lobar ICH as compared with the deep (67%) varieties, but failed to show significant differences in the frequency of headache (52% lobar, 41% deep ICH), seizures (21% lobar, 14% deep ICH), and coma at presentation (36% lobar, 53% deep ICH). The latter figure on frequency of coma at onset of lobar ICH is so discrepant with that from the literature[1,4,14] that one wonders about their data representing a collection of unusually severe forms of lobar ICH, possibly having significantly larger hematoma sizes than those from other studies. Since the methods of hematoma measurement have not been uniform across studies, some using either a computation of maximal longitudinal and transverse axis[15] or mean diameter in the horizontal plane only,[14] others reporting volumetric measurements,[1] comparisons of hematoma size among series are not possible. The unusually high frequency (19%) of lobar hematomas due to bleeding disorders in the series of Lipton et al.[15] may have been one factor responsible for suspected larger hematoma sizes, since ICH in patients receiving anticoagulants tend to be larger than those in patients not receiving anticoagulants.[48,49] Another feature suggestive of larger hematomas in their series is the high frequency (40%) of ventricular extension of the hemorrhage (in comparison with a figure of 24.6% reported in the Stroke Data Bank[41]), a feature that correlates with lobar hematoma size[1,41] and its closely related clinical effect, the degree of compromise of consciousness. Large hematomas with ventricular extension have consistently been associated with severely depressed level of consciousness and increased mortality.[50,51] Similarly, Massaro et al.,[41] in reporting the NINDS Stroke Data Bank experience in patients with lobar and deep hemispheric hemorrhages, found coma at onset in 19% of patients with lobar ICH, and in 20.2% of those with deep ICH. A possible explanation for this finding is their reporting a significantly larger mean volume of hematomas in the lobar (49 cm³) than in the deep (29 cm³) hemorrhage patients.

### Clinical Features by Anatomical Site

Lobar ICH occurs in the various cerebral lobes with different frequencies, most often favoring the posterior (parietal, occipital) areas of the brain[1,4,5,14,39] although some series[27,40] have documented a high proportion of patients (27% and 22%, respectively) with frontal hemorrhages. Multiple lobar ICH occasionally occur,[52] a feature found in three of the sixty-seven (4.5%) patients reported by Loes et al.[27] The various locations of lobar ICH determine distinct clinical presentations, which have been analyzed in detail by Ropper and Davis[14] and by Weisberg et al.[2,40,53–56]

*Frontal Hematomas*

Frontal hemorrhages are characterized by prominent limb paresis and headache at onset. The headache is generally described as bifrontal,[14,40] at times predominating on the side of the hemorrhage.[14] The pattern of motor weakness has differed among series, probably reflecting differences in hematoma location within the frontal lobe. Ropper and Davis,[14] based on their four patients with frontal hemorrhages, described contralateral arm weakness as the leading symptom, in two patients corresponding to isolated arm monoplegia. Leg and face weakness were slight, and gaze preference toward the side of the hematoma was present in two of their four patients.

The series of patients with frontal ICH reported by Weisberg[40] and Weisberg and Stazio[53] included hematomas in various portions of the frontal lobe. The authors established some clinical-radiological correlations that related to the topography of the lobar hematomas within the frontal lobe. In patients with hemorrhages located *superiorly* (Figure 17.3), above the frontal horns of the lateral ventricle, hematomas of 1.7 to 2.1 cm caused frontal headache and contralateral leg weakness. These were generally round or oval hemorrhages of moderate size. Larger hematomas in that location generally presented with leg monoparesis that rapidly progressed to hemiparesis. In contrast, patients with *inferior frontal hemorrhages*, located below the frontal horn of the lateral ventricle, generally

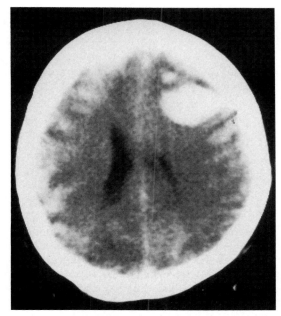

**Figure 17.3.** Superior frontal hematoma, with mass effect on the frontal horn of the lateral ventricle.

had larger hematomas, 3.8 to 5.4 cm in diameter, triangular or wedge-shaped, and with the apex pointing toward the frontal horn. These patients had a more dramatic clinical presentation, with impaired consciousness, hemiparesis, hemisensory loss, and horizontal gaze palsy toward the side of the hemiparesis. Other anatomical forms of frontal hemorrhage reported by these authors[40,53] included examples of unilateral or bilateral hematomas in basal portions of the frontal lobe, at times with blood in the interhemispheric fissure or the sylvian subarachnoid space. These were generally the result of ruptured anterior communicating-anterior cerebral artery aneurysms or local AVM, rarely occurring within a glioblastoma multiforme.

On occasion, frontal hematomas in anterior locations can present without focal motor deficits or aphasia, but rather with an acute change in mental status. This behavioral change most often takes the form of apathy or abulia, with a general decline in spontaneous motor or verbal behavior, along with slowness in responding to questions and commands, the latter being typically followed after an abnormally long latency. The following patient is an example of this presentation of an anterior frontal lobe hematoma:

> An 82-year-old hypertensive man was noted by relatives to become "confused and forgetful," with instability of gait, but without weakness or incoordination of the limbs. On examination he was oriented to time and person, but not to place. His speech was fluent but laconic, and he had no language abnormality. He had severe motor impersistence, prominent bilateral grasp reflexes, and positive snout reflex. He was abulic, with lack of spontaneity in language and movement, and showed great delays in following commands. Motor strength, tendon reflexes, coordination, and sensory examination were all normal, as was cranial nerve function. His gait was unstable, with increased base and poor balance, and he was unable to perform tandem walking.
>
> CT showed a large right frontal lobar ICH, with surrounding edema and local mass effect (Figure 17.4). The suspected cause of the ICH was CAA, but the diagnosis was not confirmed pathologically.
>
> He remained essentially unchanged throughout the hospital stay, despite gradual resolution of the mass effect from the hematoma, and he was discharged to a rehabilitation facility after 14 days from onset.

This patient is an example of a common presentation of anterior frontal lobar hematomas, which spare the motor tracts but produce prominent mental status changes accompanied by "frontal release signs."

The general clinical features of the twenty-five patients with frontal hemorrhages reported by Weisberg and Stazio[53] included a high frequency of headache (80%), vomiting (80%), and seizures (32%). An abnormal level of consciousness was a feature in 52% of their patients, all twenty-five of them had a contralateral hemisensory syndrome, and 40% had gaze preference. The cause of the hemorrhage was hypertension in 20%, ruptured

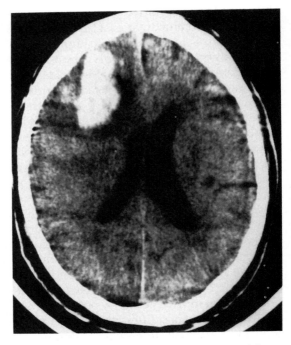

**Figure 17.4.** Right anterior (polar) parasagittal frontal hemorrhage, with low-density edema and mass effect with effacement of the frontal horn of the lateral ventricle.

aneurysm or AVM in 32%, brain tumor, anticoagulant treatment, or coagulopathy in 4% each, while 36% of the patients had no known mechanism for the hemorrhage, even after twenty-four of the twenty-five had undergone cerebral angiography.

*Temporal Hematomas*

Temporal hematomas present with distinct syndromes depending on their laterality as well as their location within that lobe. Hematomas occurred on the left side in seven of eight patients in the series of Ropper and Davis.[14] Headache was a common symptom, and the pain usually was centered in front of the ear or around the eye. The dominant hemisphere hematomas generally produced a fluent aphasia with poor comprehension, abundant paraphasias, and marked anomia.[14,40] An accompanying right-sided visual field defect, either a hemianopia or a superior quadrantanopia is the rule, although anterior hematomas have presented without it. Hemiparesis is uncommon, being present in only one of the seven patients reported by Ropper and Davis,[14] and in three of the eight patients in Weisberg's series.[40] A hemisensory syndrome with decreased sensation to pinprick in the limbs was reported in only two of the seven patients of Ropper and Davis.[14]

A more extensive series of thirty patients with temporal lobe hematomas was analyzed by Weisberg et al.[54] The hemorrhage was purely temporal in only twelve patients (posterior in five and inferior-basal in seven). The remainder had temporal hematomas that extended into either the frontal lobe (four patients), parietal lobe (eight patients), or basal ganglia (six patients). Seven patients (23%) had seizures on presentation. In five patients with *posterior* temporal hematomas, retroauricular headache at onset was common, and those with left-sided lesions presented with Wernicke aphasia and right homonymous hemianopia, while right-sided hemorrhages produced "confusion without focal neurological signs."[54] The "confusion" showed rapid resolution, within four to seven days after onset, whereas the Wernicke aphasia of the dominant-side hematomas took longer to improve, usually after about three weeks from onset. A sometimes early and dramatic improvement of Wernicke aphasia has been reported in patients with dominant temporal lobe hematomas.[57] This course was followed by two of three patients with small temporal hematomas in the series of Kase et al.[1] The features of Wernicke aphasia cleared after four and ten days from onset, respectively. The third patient, who had a large temporoparietal hemorrhage (75 cm$^3$), remained aphasic after surgical drainage of the hematoma. These anecdotal data suggest that small temporal hematomas may at times be associated with a surprisingly rapid improvement of Wernicke aphasia. The following patient is an example of such a situation:

A 72-year-old hypertensive woman developed focal seizures in the right arm and right side of the face, without loss of consciousness or generalized convulsions. Shortly after admission, the seizure activity was controlled with intravenous diazepam, followed by a loading dose of 1000 mg of intravenous phenytoin. On examination she was awake and alert, able to follow some simple commands by using visual cues, but unable to follow auditory commands, name objects, or read aloud. She had fluent speech output that was virtually jargon because of abundant paraphasias. She had full and symmetric limb strength, with flexor plantar reflexes. Her response to visual threat suggested a right visual field defect.

CT showed a small posterior left temporal hematoma with minimal effacement of the Sylvian fissure, without ventricular extension (Figure 17.5).

Her course was characterized by rapid amelioration of her Wernicke aphasia. She started to follow some auditory commands on hospital day 2, and to name objects on hospital day 3, along with a marked reduction in her paraphasias, her speech contact becoming clear. By day 4, she had rare paraphasias on naming and reading aloud, but the rest of her language functions were preserved. At the time of discharge on day 10, she had intact language functions, and her visual field defect was limited to extinction to double simultaneous stimulation in the right upper quadrants. At no time during her course was there evidence of paroxysmal discharges on EEG, which only showed focal theta slowing in the left temporal region.

This patient illustrates the rapid resolution of Wernicke aphasia in a patient with a small posterior temporal hematoma. Although the possibility of the deficit clearing as a result of the control of the focal temporal lobe seizures cannot be excluded, the persistence of aphasic disturbances into day 4, when no focal seizure activity was detected clinically or on EEG, suggests that other mechanisms may account for this unusual phenomenon. This

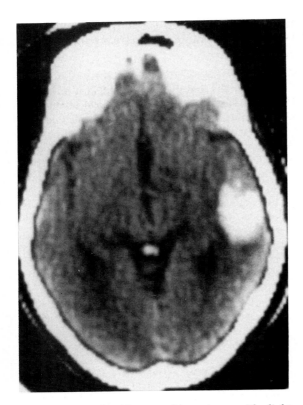

**Figure 17.5.** Left midtemporal hematoma with slight mass effect (effacement of the sylvian fissure).

is further supported by the lack of seizure activity, clinically and electrically, in a patient who had resolution of Wernicke aphasia after four days from onset of a left temporoparietal ICH.[1]

Among several patients with *inferior-basal* temporal hematomas, five had blood in the basal cisterns or cortical sulci on CT in the series of Weisberg et al.[54] Three of these patients had middle cerebral artery (MCA) aneurysms, and two had AVMs documented by angiography. The cause of the ICH remained undetermined in only two of the seven patients after cerebral angiography. These findings stress the high probability of the bleeding being secondary to MCA aneurysm or AVM in inferiorly located hematomas of the temporal lobe. Large temporal hematomas with *extension to adjacent lobes* produce less well defined clinical syndromes.

Hemorrhages that extend medially into the basal ganglia area acquire large sizes and frequently reach the ventricular system.[54] This is accompanied by marked focal neurological deficits, including hemiplegia, hemisensory defects, aphasia, hemianopia, and paresis of horizontal gaze. The clinical deficit in these patients is indistinguishable from large, primary putaminal ICH.[16] Right temporal hematomas that extend superiorly into the parietal lobe can produce prominent syndromes of left-sided hemineglect.[1]

On rare occasions, temporal hematomas have presented with purely cognitive and behavioral abnormalities, without deficits on elementary neurological examination. Cohen et al.[58] recently reported the remarkable case of a 30-year-old man who abruptly developed the visual hallucination of a friend's face in association with a large right temporal ICH. The hallucination lasted for about thirty seconds, and the patient described the face as being of normal size and color, without specific emotional expression, comparable to a passport photograph. On examination he showed no abnormalities in mental status testing, and had no focal neurological deficits. Head magnetic resonance imaging (MRI) documented an acute ICH that involved most of the anterior two-thirds of the right temporal lobe. No cause for the hemorrhage was found after cerebral angiography and subsequent pathological examination of brain tissue. The latter was obtained at the time of surgical hematoma evacuation that followed hemorrhage recurrence one month after the original ICH. The authors interpreted this short, elaborate, visual hallucination as possibly resulting from a right temporal seizure discharge at the time of ICH onset, based on the suggestion that the nondominant temporooccipital areas are essential for the processing of face recognition.[59]

*Parietal Hematomas*

Parietal hematomas frequently present with prominent unilateral headache,[14,55] usually localized around the temple region.[14] Hemisensory syndromes are often severe, at times involving the limbs and trunk,[14] with deficits in superficial and deep sensation,[1] in all with associated hemiparesis.[1,14,40] Seizures at onset were reported in seven (28%) of the twenty-five patients reported by Weisberg and Stazio.[55] These authors analyzed the clinical features of their twenty-five patients in relation to the location of the hematomas within the parietal lobe. In six patients with *anterior-lateral* hemorrhages, all of whom were normotensive, motor and sensory deficits were always present, in three with an associated homonymous hemianopia. Aphasia or hemi-inattention was present depending on the laterality of the ICH. The cause of these hematomas could not be determined. Prognosis was good, as all patients survived the acute event, four of them becoming functionally independent. In six patients with *anterior-medial* parietal hematomas, the clinical syndromes were similar to those of patients with lateral hemorrhages, except for the more common finding of altered consciousness in those with medial hematomas. These ICH were of similar size in comparison with the lateral ones, and were described on CT as extending into the thalamic area, presumably distorting midline structures and causing impaired consciousness. A causal mechanism could not be defined in these patients, four of whom were hypertensive and two normotensive. The latter two patients, ages 70 and 72, were demented and their hemorrhage was suspected to be due to CAA, but neither had pathological confirmation of the diagnosis. All three patients with *posterior* parietal hematomas had seizures at onset, and their clinical features included constructional apraxia, dressing apraxia, and hemi-inattention syndromes. They had relatively small hematomas (1.0 to 1.8 cm in diameter), and they all survived the event, followed by good functional recovery. In instances of *extension* into the frontal, temporal, or occipital lobes, the hematomas reach larger sizes than those confined to only the parietal lobe, and their clinical syndromes reflect the expected combination of clinical features from the various lobes involved.[1,55] The larger size of these hemorrhages is also responsible for the high frequency of altered level of consciousness at presentation, found in four of the eight (50%) patients with hematomas with frontal and temporal extension in the series of Weisberg and Stazio.[55] Smaller hematomas of parietal-occipital location were associated with less severe neurological deficits and improved outcome.[55]

The following patient presented initially with a small parasagittal parietal hematoma that evolved into a severe neurological deficit as a result of extension of the hemorrhage:

An 84-year-old man suddenly slumped over at the dinner table and was unable to get up, despite being awake and conversant, complaining of a diffuse headache. On examination he was oriented to place and person, could answer simple questions appropriately with fluent and slightly dysarthric speech, and was able to follow simple commands. He had a left hemiparesis of proximal predominance in the arm, with paretic leg, but without facial involvement. Sensation to pin-prick was markedly decreased in the left limbs and left side of the face, and joint position sense was decreased in the left toes. He had a left homonymous visual field defect that included an inferior quadrantanopia and extinction to double simultaneous stimulation in the superior quadrants.

CT on 7/11/91 showed a small, high convexity right parasagittal parietal lobar hematoma (Figure 17.6A). He remained stable until four days later, when he became lethargic, with left leg paralysis, and developed hemi-inattention for the left side of space. A CT (7/15/91) showed enlargement of the original parietal hematoma (Figure 17.6B), as well as a new area of acute hemorrhage along the falx, anteriorly in the frontoparietal area (Figure 17.6C). Further deterioration to stupor with arm and leg paralysis, facial weakness, and ocular deviation to the right were associated with the demonstration on CT (7/18/91) of a new large area of hemorrhage in the lateral parietal convexity (Figure 17.6D, E). He remained stuporous, only responsive to deep pain, with left hemiplegia, hemisensory loss, and hemianopia, until discharge to a chronic care facility after 13 days in the hospital.

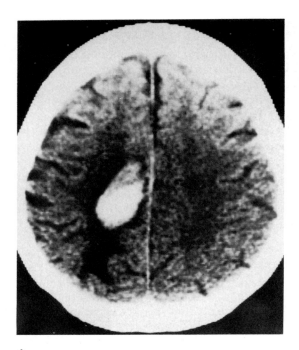

A

**Figure 17.6.** (A) Small right parasagittal parietal hemorrhage. (B) Enlarged right parietal hemorrhage. (C) New focus of hemorrhage in the frontoparietal area, adjacent to the falx. (D and E) New area of hemorrhage in the lateral parietal convexity, with adjacent white matter edema.

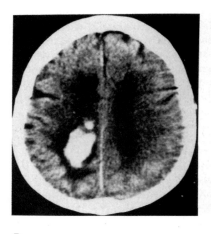

B

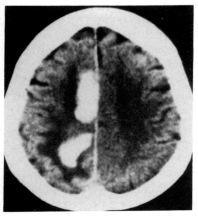

C

This patient initially had the characteristic features of a parasagittal parietal hematoma, with subsequent gradual worsening as a result of repeated episodes of bleeding near the initial hemorrhage. The cause was suspected to be CAA, but no histological demonstration of it was possible, as the family declined consent for surgical drainage of the enlarging hematomas.

*Occipital Hematomas*

Occipital hemorrhages caused severe headache, usually in or around the ipsilateral eye,

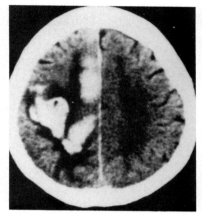
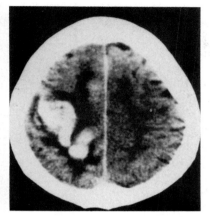

D                                          E

in seven of eleven patients reported by Ropper and Davis.[14] Nine of these patients were acutely aware of a visual disturbance at the onset of the ICH. This correlated with the finding of a contralateral homonymous hemianopia in all eleven patients. Motor weakness was not present, but three patients had contralateral extinction with double simultaneous touch stimulation, and two had dysgraphia and dyslexia. The syndrome of "alexia without agraphia" was reported in two patients with lobar hematomas by Weisberg and Wall.[60] Their Case 1 had a small left posterior-inferior temporal hematoma, and Case 3 had a larger hyperdense left parietal-occipital lesion. The authors were uncertain whether the latter lesion represented a primary ICH or a hemorrhagic infarction. Neither patient had CT evidence of involvement of the splenium of the corpus callosum by the vascular lesion.

Weisberg and Stazio[56] analyzed eighteen consecutive patients with occipital hemorrhages. The hematoma was of *medial* occipital location in six patients, all of whom presented with headache and "visual blurring." The latter description was also given by two of nine patients reported by Ropper and Davis,[14] whereas the remainder described either unilateral homonymous visual loss (four

patients) or a tendency to "bump into things" (three patients). All six patients with medial occipital hematomas in the series of Weisberg and Stazio[56] had homonymous hemianopia, without motor or memory deficits, and with fully preserved mental alertness. They all survived, and were described as not having "functional neurological impairment." One of two patients with a dense homonymous hemianopia from an occipital hematoma reported by Kase et al.[1] improved to a superior homonymous quadrantanopia that was persistent. In three patients with *lateral* occipital hematomas, Weisberg and Stazio[56] reported headache at onset, but without neurological abnormalities on examination, including visual field defects, motor-sensory deficits, or behavioral abnormalities. Among nine patients with occipital hematomas with parietal or temporal *extension*, which were of larger diameter than those confined to the occipital lobe, six had "visual blurring," and four had an acute mental change labeled as "confusion." One of the latter, a 47-year-old man on anticoagulant treatment, developed agitation and visual hallucinations (not further described), confusion, left-sided inattention, and left homonymous hemianopia, with a large right occipitoparietal ICH with ventricular extension. All nine of these patients had a cause for the ICH documented: excessive anticoagulation for thrombophlebitis (two), blood dyscrasias (three), systemic lupus erythematosus (three, but only one with laboratory evidence of abnormal coagulation, and none with abnormalities on cerebral angiography), and bacterial endocarditis (one, although no mycotic aneurysm or other vascular lesions were detected on cerebral angiography).

The following patient illustrates most of the characteristic features of occipital lobar hemorrhage:

A 71-year-old hypertensive man on treatment with atenolol and amiloride hydrochloride, was noted to "bump" into a fire extinguisher and into a cement column, both located on his left side, during the three days that preceded admission. He did not volunteer any complaints about visual dysfunction, but reported having a persistent headache in the right temporo-occipital area, which was made worse by coughing or bending. On examination he had an intact mental status, with preserved orientation, topographic sense, and face recognition. There were no motor or sensory deficits in the limbs or face. He had a congruous left homonymous hemianopia, with more severe involvement of the inferior than the superior quadrants, and with preservation of optokinetic nystagmus in both directions.

CT showed a moderate size right occipital hemorrhage located between the medial and lateral portions of that lobe, with extension to the superficial occipital cortex, but without subarachnoid or intraventricular extension (Figure 17.7).

His course was uncomplicated, and a posterior circulation angiogram showed only an avascular mass in the area of the hemorrhage, without local vascular or tumoral lesions. On day 5 after admission, the left homonymous hemianopia had improved into an inferior quadrantanopia, which persisted at the time of discharge and on subsequent follow-up.

This patient presented with an occipital hemorrhage in the nondominat hemisphere, characterized by a dense homonymous hemianopia and anosognosia, with subsequent

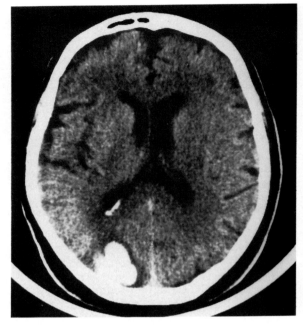

**Figure 17.7.** Right occipital hematoma, with extension to the cortical surface, without mass effect.

shrinking of the visual field deficit to an inferior quadrantanopia, which correlated with a predominantly superior extension of the hemorrhage.

## Outcome

The mortality and morbidity of lobar ICH have been thought to be less than in deep hemispheric (putaminal, thalamic) and posterior fossa hemorrhages[1,10,14,38] *Mortality rates* of 11.5%,[14] 13%,[61] 14%,[62] 20%,[13] 28%,[63] and 32%[1] have been reported for lobar hemorrhage, whereas figures between 37% for putaminal[16] and 97% for pontine ICH[19] have been quoted. Steiner et al.[62] found a mortality of 13% (three of twenty-three patients) for lobar ICH, compared to 42% (five of twelve patients) for basal ganglionic and thalamic ICH, and 43% (three of seven patients) for posterior fossa hemorrhages. However, in larger series of patients with ICH diagnosed by CT, when lobar and "deep" forms of ICH were compared, no significant differences in mortality were found. Massaro et al.[41] reported a thirty-day fatality rate of 27.7% for patients with lobar hemorrhage, and 31.8% for those with deep hemorrhages. Similarly, nonsignificant differences in one-year survival rates of 51.1% and 60.9%, respectively, were found in their NINDS Stroke Data Bank series of sixty-five patients with lobar and 107 patients with deep ICH.

It is possible that differences in mortality among series of lobar and deep ICH are more a reflection of hematoma size variation than of their location. The most important determinants of survival in ICH are hematoma size and its closely related clinical sign, reduction in the level of consciousness during the acute stage of the stroke.[15,38,50,51,63] Intraventricular extension of the hemorrhage usually, but not always, correlates with hematoma size, and as such represents an additional poor prognostic factor.[15,38] This is particularly the case for basal ganglionic and thalamic hemorrhage,[38,64] in which ventricular extension is common in large hemorrhages at these sites. In other instances, ventricular extension is a reflection of the proximity of the parenchymal ICH to the ventricular system, the hemorrhage being mostly intraventricular, with only a small component of parenchymal bleeding. This is the case in caudate hemorrhage, which almost invariably communicates with the ventricular system,[65] but this feature does not have an adverse effect on outcome.[64] However, the importance of intraventricular extension of the hemorrhage in relationship to the prognosis of ICH has not been fully elucidated. Young et al.[66] have recently reported a correlation between volume of intraventricular blood and outcome, irrespective of the location of the parenchymal component of the hemorrhage. Finally, a role for hematoma location in the frequency of coma in large cerebral hemorrhages has been suggested.[67] In addition to hematoma size, a major determinant of coma or lethargy in ICH is the amount of displacement of midline structures, measured on CT by the shift of the calcified pineal gland. This phenomenon is more likely to occur in deep hemispheric hemorrhages that are adjacent to midline structures, than in the more peripherally-located lobar hemorrhages.[67] Furthermore, large temporal lobar hematomas are more likely than similar size hematomas in the frontal or occipital lobes to produce brainstem compression, as a reflection of more prominent displacement of midline structures.[68]

In conclusion, although not all series agree, it appears that mortality in lobar ICH may be lower than in deep hemispheric hemorrhages. However, differences in mortality rates between these two types of ICH may reflect other parameters that are important for survival, such as hematoma size, displacement of midline structures, and ventricular extension, rather than just the location of the hematoma.

The *functional outcome* in lobar ICH has also been reported as better than in the deep varieties of ICH[1,14,38,61,62] (Table 17.4). How-

**Table 17.4.** Outcome in Lobar and Deep Hemorrhages

| | Type of ICH | | | | | |
| | LOBAR | | | DEEP | | |
| Author | Mortality | Good Outcome | Poor Outcome | Mortality | Good Outcome | Poor Outcome |
|---|---|---|---|---|---|---|
| Richardson[61] | 14% | 85% | 1% | 32% | 54% | 14% |
| Steiner et al.[62] | 13% | 57% | 30% | 42% | 16% | 42% |
| Helweg-Larsen et al.[38] | 24% | 65%* | 11%* | 26% | 40%* | 34%* |

*Values are calculated approximations from the authors'[38] Figure 1, since follow-up did not include all the survivors.

ever, these data are likely to be at least partially biased by patient selection. In some series,[14] a very low frequency of coma at onset (0.4%) suggests that patients with large hematomas may have been excluded from referral to the institution, because of severe neurological signs at onset, early mortality, or poor surgical risk. In other instances[38] elderly patients with severe neurological deficits may have been excluded from the study group.

Other large series[15,41,50] have found no differences in functional outcome between lobar and deep hemorrhages. In the series of Portenoy et al.,[50] nineteen of forty-two patients (45%) with lobar ICH and twenty-six of seventy patients (37%) with deep ICH had a favorable outcome. When outcome was related to four quartiles of hematoma size, those with the largest hematomas fared poorly and those with the smallest hematomas did well, irrespective of hematoma location. However, in the middle two quartiles of hematoma size, a good outcome occurred in lobar hematomas (46%) more often than in deep ones (21%).

These series, albeit subjected to variability in their results due to biases in patient selection, suggest a better functional prognosis in lobar than in deep hemispheric hemorrhages. In addition to ICH location, hematoma size, level of consciousness at onset, and ventricular extension, Weisberg[40] suggested that a hypertensive cause of lobar ICH entails a worse prognosis than in normotensive patients. Among eighteen hypertensive patients with lobar ICH, five (28%) died and ten of the thirteen survivors (77%) had residual disability, mainly hemiparesis or aphasia; only three patients (23%) had good functional recovery. In contrast, all thirty-two normotensive patients with lobar hematomas survived, and only eleven of them (34%) showed residual deficits, the remaining twenty-one (66%) had almost complete recovery or slight residual deficits. These striking differences between hypertensive and normotensive patients were related to significantly larger hematomas in hypertensive patients. The va-

lidity of these observations needs to be tested in future series of patients with ICH at various locations, in which hypertensive status and hematoma size, the latter measured in a standardized and reproducible fashion, are related to survival rates and functional outcome measures.

## Management

The choice of treatment in lobar ICH, either conservative or surgical, has been controversial. On the basis of their findings of low mortality and good functional outcome in patients not undergoing surgery, Ropper and Davis[14] and Iwasaki and Kinoshita[39] concluded that surgical treatment is not indicated in lobar hemorrhage. However, other series have suggested an improved outcome in a subgroup of patients with lobar ICH subjected to operative treatment.[1, 33, 40, 69] This controversy was highlighted in the report of Masdeu and Rubino,[70] who distributed two case histories of patients with a left parietal ICH among eighty-eight neurologists and 114 neurosurgeons, and requested their opinion regarding medical or surgical treatment. The responses were quite discrepant within each group of specialists, as well as between neurologists and neurosurgeons, the latter group opting for surgical clot removal more often than the group of neurologists: 52% of the neurologists and 28% of the neurosurgeons would have referred neither patient for surgery, while both patients would have been referred for surgery by 24% of the neurologists and 47% of the neurosurgeons.

Although no study has prospectively and randomly assigned patients with CT-proven lobar ICH to medical or surgical therapy, in order to properly compare the two, uncontrolled data suggest a better outcome in surgically-treated patients with medium-sized hematomas. Kase et al.[1] analyzed outcome in twenty-two patients with lobar ICH in relation to form of therapy and hematoma volume on CT. All patients with small ICH (less than 20 cm$^3$) improved without surgical treatment, whereas those with large hematomas (greater than 40 cm³) did poorly, without clear differences between medical and surgical therapy. In the intermediate group of patients, with hematoma volumes between 20 and 40 cm³, outcome was better following surgical hematoma drainage. In a group of patients with basal ganglionic and lobar hemorrhages analyzed together, Volpin et al.[69] reached similar conclusions. All patients with hematoma volumes below 26 cm³ survived and did not require surgical therapy, while all patients with hematomas larger than 85 cm³ died, irrespective of the form of therapy used. In the intermediate group of patients, with hematoma volumes between 26 and 85 cm³, the surgical group fared better than the nonsurgical group, but only with statistical significance in the patients with hematoma volumes between 66 and 85 cm³. Finally, in the nonsurgical series of fifty-three patients reported by Helweg-Larsen et al.,[38] twenty-nine of whom had lobar ICH, a hematoma volume below 50 cm³ resulted in good prognosis (mortality of 10%), while poor prognosis (mortality of 90%) was the rule in patients with hematoma volumes larger than 50 cm³. The data in the series of Gårde et al.[63] also suggest that surgical treatment is of no value in the small (5 to 30 cm³) or in the very large (70 to 80 cm³) hematomas, but in those of intermediate size (30 to 80 cm³), surgery improves survival rates in those patients who are not deeply comatose preoperatively.

In view of the above uncontrolled data, it is our policy to treat conservatively patients with small (up to 20 to 30 cm³ volume) lobar hematomas who are alert or drowsy, and clinically stable during hospital observation. We only provide supportive measures for those patients in the poor prognostic group of large (greater than 80 cm³) hematomas, especially if they are comatose and have CT features of marked mass effect and midline shift on hospital presentation. For patients with intermediate size hematomas (30 to 80 cm³), who are obtunded or lethargic at presentation with midline shift on CT, we

recommend surgical evacuation of the hematoma. If such patients are alert or drowsy at presentation, any further decline in the level of consciousness or increase in mass effect on CT after hospital admission are indications for emergency surgical treatment.

In addition to its possible value in improving vital prognosis, surgical treatment of lobar ICH has been recommended for the purpose of resection of lesions with potential for recurrent bleeding. Wakai et al.,[33] in reporting their experience with twenty-nine patients with lobar ICH and negative angiography who underwent surgical treatment, emphasized the finding of vascular lesions in twenty patients (AVM in six, cavernous angioma in three, and microaneurysm in eleven). The diagnosis of these lesions with potential for rebleeding was only possible after histological examination of surgical biopsy materials. Good outcome was reported in twenty-four of the twenty-nine patients (83%), the best results being in the group with vascular malformations or microaneurysms, whereas only 50% of patients with CAA as the cause of the ICH had a good outcome.

The decision regarding therapy in lobar ICH continues to be based on the specific features of the individual patient, including level of consciousness at presentation, cause of ICH, site and size of the hematoma, associated mass effect, and ease of surgical accessibility by virtue of its proximity to the cortical surface. The relative value of medical and surgical therapy will only be ultimately assessed by a large scale clinical trial involving randomization of comparable groups of patients to one or the other form of treatment.

## References

1. Kase CS, Williams JP, Wyatt DA, et al. Lobar intracerebral hematomas: clinical and CT analysis of 22 cases. Neurology 1982;32:1146–1150.
2. Weisberg LA, Stazio A, Shamsnia M, et al. Nontraumatic parenchymal brain hemorrhages. Medicine 1990;69:277–295.
3. Gras P, Arveux P, Clavier I, et al. Étude rétrospective d'une série hospitalière de 238

hémorragies intracérébrales spontanées. Sem Hôp Paris 1990;66:1677–1683.

4. Mohr JP, Caplan LR, Melski JW, et al. The Harvard Cooperative Stroke Registry: a prospective registry. Neurology 1978;28: 754–762.

5. Schütz H. Spontane intrazerebrale Hämatome: pathophysiologie, klinik und therapie. Heidelberg: Springer-Verlag, 1988.

6. Bogousslavsky J, Van Melle G, Regli F. The Lausanne Stroke Registry: analysis of 1,000 consecutive patients with first stroke. Stroke 1988;19:1083–1092.

7. Mutlu N, Berry RG, Alpers BJ. Massive cerebral hemorrhage: clinical and pathological correlations. Arch Neurol 1963;8:644–661.

8. Freytag E. Fatal hypertensive intracerebral haematomas: a survey of the pathological anatomy of 393 cases. J Neurol Neurosurg Psychiat 1968;31:616–620.

9. McCormick WF, Rosenfield DB. Massive brain hemorrhage: a review of 144 cases and an examination of their causes. Stroke 1973; 4:946–954.

10. Omae T, Ueda K, Ogata J, et al. Parenchymatous hemorrhage; etiology, pathology, and clinical aspects. In: Vinken PJ, et al., eds. Handbook of Clinical Neurology. New York: Elsevier, 1989;287–331.

10a. Boonyakarnkul S, Dennis M, Sandercock P, et al. Primary intracerebral hemorrhage in the Oxfordshire Community Stroke Project: 1. Incidence, clinical features and causes. Cerebrovasc Dis 1993;3:343–349.

11. Toffol GJ, Biller J, Adams HP. Nontraumatic intracerebral hemorrhage in young adults. Arch Neurol 1987;44:483–485.

12. Gras P, Arveux P, Giroud M, et al. Les hémorragies intracérébrales spontanées du sujet jeune: étude de 33 cas. Rev Neurol 1991;147: 653–657.

13. Weisberg LA. Computerized tomography in intracerebral hemorrhage. Arch Neurol 1979;36:422–426.

14. Ropper AH, Davis KR. Lobar cerebral hemorrhages: acute clinical syndromes in 26 cases. Ann Neurol 1980;8:141–147.

15. Lipton RB, Berger AR, Lesser ML, Lantos G, Portenoy RK. Lobar vs thalamic and basal ganglion hemorrhage: clinical and radiographic features. J Neurol 1987;234:86–90.

16. Hier DB, Davis KR, Richardson EP, et al. Hypertensive putaminal hemorrhage. Ann Neurol 1977;1:152–159.

17. Piepgras U, Rieger P. Thalamic bleeding: diagnosis, course and prognosis. Neuroradiology 1981;22:85–91.

18. Okudera T, Uemura K, Nakajima K, et al. Primary pontine hemorrhage: correlations of pathologic features with postmortem microangiographic, and vertebral angiographic studies. Mt Sinai J Med 1978;45:305–321.

19. Dinsdale HB. Spontaneous hemorrhage in the posterior fossa: a study of primary cerebellar and pontine hemorrhages with observations on their pathogenesis. Arch Neurol 1964;10:200–217.

20. Freeman RE, Onofrio BM, Okazaki H, et al. Spontaneous intracerebellar hemorrhage: diagnosis and surgical treatment. Neurology 1973;23:84–90.

21. Ott KH, Kase CS, Ojemann RG, et al. Cerebellar hemorrhage: diagnosis and treatment: a review of 56 cases. Arch Neurol 1974;31: 160–167.

22. Dunne JW, Chakera T, Kermode S. Cerebellar haemorrhage—diagnosis and treatment: a study of 75 consecutive cases. Quart J Med 1987;64:739–754.

23. Fisher CM. Pathological observations in hypertensive cerebral hemorrhage. J Neuropathol Exp Neurol 1971;30:536–550.

24. Cole FM, Yates P. Intracerebral microaneurysms and small cerebrovascular lesions. Brain 1967;90:759–768.

25. Vinters HV. Cerebral amyloid angiopathy: a critical review. Stroke 1987;18:311–324.

26. Toffol GJ, Biller J, Adams HP, et al. The predicted value of arteriography in nontraumatic intracerebral hemorrhage. Stroke 1986; 17:881–883.

27. Loes DJ, Smoker WRK, Biller J, et al. Nontraumatic lobar intracerebral hemorrhage: CT/angiographic correlation. Am J Neuroradiol 1987;8:1027–1030.

28. Nalls G, Disher A, Daryabagi J, et al. Subcortical cerebral hemorrhages associated with cocaine abuse: CT and MR findings. J Comput Assist Tomogr 1989;13:1–5.

29. Kase CS, Foster TE, Reed JE, et al. Intracerebral hemorrhage and phenylpropanolamine use. Neurology 1987;37:399–404.

30. Kase CS, Pessin MS, Zivin JA, et al. Intracranial hemorrhage after coronary thrombolysis with tissue plasminogen activator. Am J Med 1992;92:384–390.

30a. Broderick J, Brott T, Tomsick T, Leach A. Lobar hemorrhage in the elderly: the undiminishing importance of hypertension. Stroke 1993;24:49–51.

31. VanderArk GD, Kahn EA. Spontaneous intracerebral hematoma. J Neurosurg 1968;28: 252–256.

32. Krayenbühl H, Siebenmann R. Small vascular malformations as a cause of primary intracerebral hemorrhage. J Neurosurg 1965; 22:7–20.

33. Wakai S, Kumakura N, Nagai M. Lobar intracerebral hemorrhage: a clinical, radiographic, and pathological study of 29 consecutive operated cases with negative angiography. J Neurosurg 1992;76:231–238.

34. Wakai S, Nagai M. Histological verification of mircoaneurysms as a cause of cerebral haemorrhage in surgical specimens. J Neurol Neurosurg Psychiat 1989;52:595–599.

34a. Kase CS. Intracerebral hemorrhage: nonhypertensive causes. Stroke 1986;17:590–595.

34b. Longstreth WT, Litwin PE, Weaver WD, and the MITI Project Group. Myocardial infarction, thrombolytic therapy, and stroke: a community-based study. Stroke 1993;24: 587–590.

34c. Pendlebury WW, Iole ED, Tracy RP, Dill BA. Intracerebral hemorrhage related to cerebral amyloid angiopathy and t-PA treatment. Ann Neurol 1991;29:210–213.

34d. Wijdicks EFM, Jack CR. Intracerebral hemorrhage after fibrinolytic therapy for acute myocardial infarction. Stroke 1993;24: 554–557.

34e. Levine SR, Brust JCM, Futrell N, et al. Cerebrovascular complications of the use of the "crack" form of alkaloidal cocaine. N Engl J Med 1990;323:699–704.

34f. Glick R, Hoying J, Cerullo L, Perlman S. Phenylpropanolamine: an over-the-counter drug causing central nervous system vasculitis and intracerebral hemorrhage. Neurosurgery 1987;20:969–974.

34g. Tapia JF, Golden JA. Case records of the Massachusetts General Hospital (Case 27-1993). N Engl J Med 1993;329;117–124.

34h. Finelli PF, Kessimian N, Bernstein PW. Cerebral amyloid angiopathy manifesting as recurrent intracerebral hemorrhage. Arch Neurol 1984;41:330–333.

34i. Clifford-Jones RE, Love S, Gurusinghe N. Granulomatous angiitis of the central nervous system: a case with recurrent intracerebral haemorrhage. J Neurol Neurosurg Psychiat 1985;48:1054–1056.

35. Biller J, Loftus CM, Moore SA, Schelper RL, Danks KR, Cornell SH. Isolated central nervous system angiitis first presenting as spontaneous intracranial hemorrhage. Neurosurgery 1987;20:310–315.

36. Onoyama K, Ibayashi S, Nanishi F, et al. Cerebral hemorrhage in patients on maintenance hemodialysis: CT analysis of 25 cases. Eur Neurol 1987;26:171–175.

37. Overbeek HC, Keyser A. Multiple subcortical haemorrhages following lumbar metrizamide myelography. J Neurol 1987;234:177–179.

38. Helweg-Larsen S, Sommer W, Strange P, Lester J, Boysen G. Prognosis for patients treated conservatively for spontaneous intracerebral hematomas. Stroke 1984;15:1045–1048.

39. Iwasaki Y, Kinoshita M. Subcortical lobar hematomas: clinico-computed tomographic correlations. Comput Med Imag Graph 1989; 13:195–198.

40. Weisberg LA. Subcortical lobar intracerebral haemorrhage: clinical-computed tomographic correlations. J Neurol Neurosurg Psychiat 1985;48:1078–1084.

41. Massaro AR, Sacco RL, Mohr JP, et al. Clinical discriminators of lobar and deep hemorrhages: The Stroke Data Bank. Neurology 1991;41:1881–1885.

42. Faught E, Peters D, Bartolucci A, Moore L, Miller PC. Seizures after primary intracerebral hemorrhage. Neurology 1989;39: 1089–1093.

43. Sung C-Y, Chu N-S. Epileptic seizures in intracerebral haemorrhage. J Neurol Neurosurg Psychiat 1989;52:1273–1276.

44. Berger AR, Lipton RB, Lesser ML, et al. Early seizures following intracerebral hemorrhage: implications for therapy. Neurology 1988;38: 1363–1365.

45. Richardson EP, Dodge PR. Epilepsy in cerebral vascular disease: a study of the incidence and nature of seizures in 104 consecutive autopsy-proven cases of cerebral infarction and hemorrhage. Epilepsia 1954;3:49–74.

46. Echlin FA, Arnett V, Zoll J. Paroxysmal high voltage discharges from isolated and partially isolated human and animal cerebral cortex. EEG Clin Neurophysiol 1952;4:147–164.

47. Kase CS, Mohr JP. Supratentorial intracerebral hemorrhage. In: Barnett HJM et al., eds. Stroke: pathophysiology, diagnosis, and management. New York: Churchill Livingstone, 1986;525–547.

48. Kase CS, Robinson RK, Stein RW, et al. Anticoagulant-related intracerebral hemorrhage. Neurology 1985;35:943–948.

49. Rådberg JA, Olsson JE, Rådberg CT. Prognostic parameters in spontaneous intracerebral hematomas with special reference to anticoagulant treatment. Stroke 1991;22:571–576.

50. Portenoy RK, Lipton RB, Berger AR, et al. Intracerebral haemorrhage: a model for the prediction of outcome. J Neurol Neurosurg Psychiat 1987;50:976–979.

51. Tuhrim S, Dambrosia JM, Price TR, et al. Prediction of intracerebral hemorrhage survival. Ann Neurol 1988;24:258–263.

52. Weisberg L. Multiple spontaneous intracerebral hematomas: clinical and computed tomographic correlations. Neurology 1981;31:897–900.

53. Weisberg LA, Stazio A. Nontraumatic frontal lobe hemorrhages: clinical-computed tomographic correlations. Neuroradiology 1988;30:500–505.

54. Weisberg LA, Stazio A, Shamsnia M, et al. Nontraumatic temporal subcortical hemorrhage: clinical computed tomographic analysis. Neuroradiology 1990;32:137–141.

55. Weisberg LA, Stazio A. Nontaumatic parietal subcortical hemorrhage: clinical-computed tomographic correlations. Comput Med Imag Graph 1989;13:355–361.

56. Weisberg LA, Stazio A. Occipital lobe hemorrhages: clinical-computed tomographic correlations. Comput Med Imag Graph 1988;12:353–358.

57. Ojemann RG, Mohr JP. Hypertensive brain hemorrhage. Clin Neurosurg 1976;23:220–244.

58. Cohen L, Verstichel P, Pierrot-Deseilligny C. Hallucinatory vision of a familiar face following right temporal hemorrhage. Neurology 1992;42:2052.

59. Damasio AR, Tranel D, Damasio H. Facial agnosia and the neural substrates of memory. Annu Rev Neurosci 1990;13:89–109.

60. Weisberg LA, Wall M. Alexia without agraphia: clinical-computed tomographic correlations. Neuroradiology 1987;29:283–286.

61. Richardson A. Spontaneous intracerebral and cerebellar haemorrhage. In: Russell RWR, ed., Cerebral arterial disease. New York: Churchill Livingstone, 1976;210–230.

62. Steiner I, Gomori JM, Melamed E. The prognostic value of the CT scan in conservatively treated patients with intracerebral hematoma. Stroke 1984;15:279–282.

63. Gårde A, Böhmer G, Seldén B, et al. 100 cases of spontaneous intracerebral haematoma: diagnosis, treatment and prognosis. Eur Neurol 1983;22:161–172.

64. Stein RW, Caplan LR, Hier DB. Outcome of intracranial hemorrhage: role of blood pressure and location and size of lesions. Ann Neurol 1983;14:132–133 (abstract).

65. Stein RW, Kase CS, Hier DB, et al. Caudate hemorrhage. Neurology 1984;34:1549–1554.

66. Young WB, Lee KP, Pessin MS, et al. Prognostic significance of ventricular blood in supratentorial hemorrhage: a volumetric study. Neurology 1990;40:616–619.

67. Ropper AH, Gress DR. Computerized tomography and clinical features of large cerebral hemorrhages. Cerebrovasc Dis 1991;1:38–42.

68. Andrews BT, Chiles BW, Olsen WL, et al. The effect of intracerebral hematoma location on the risk of brainstem compression and on clinical outcome. J Neurosurg 1988;69:518–522.

69. Volpin L, Cervellini P, Colombo F, et al. Spontaneous intracerebral hematomas: a new proposal about the usefulness and limits of surgical treatment. Neurosurgery 1984;15:663–666.

70. Masdeu JC, Rubino FA. Management of lobar intracerebral hemorrhage: medical or surgical. Neurology 1984;34:381–383.

# Chapter 18
# Primary Intraventricular Hemorrhage

## Louis R. Caplan

In this group of patients, bleeding occurs directly into the ventricular system rather than into the brain parenchyma. Computed tomography (CT) and magnetic resonance imaging (MRI) show a local hematoma limited to one of the ventricles, or blood disseminated within the ventricular system and often also in the basal cisterns, without a parenchymatous lesion. When patients with intraventricular hemorrhage come to necropsy, some have had bleeding limited entirely to the ventricular spaces, while others have small foci of bleeding adjacent to the ependymal surfaces that had dissected into one of the ventricles but the parenchymatous component was not detectable during life. In one large stroke registry, intraventricular hemorrhage accounted for about 3% of all intracerebral hemorrhages (ICH).[1] In this chapter we consider only primary intraventricular hemorrhage (PIVH) in adults.

## Historical Aspects

Sanders, in 1881, clearly separated intracranial hemorrhage into useful subgroups.[2] "Extraencephalic" forms involved the cranial cavity but were meningeal or external to the brain proper, and "encephalic" forms which either involved the brain substance or were "intra-ventricular encephalic, that in which blood is poured out into one or several of the ventricles of the brain."[2] Sanders further separated the ventricular form into a primary or immediate direct form "occurring without previous laceration of the ventricular parietes" and a secondary or indirect form that "follows laceration or influx of blood from some other part, the primary seat of the hem orrhage being external to these cavities."[2] Sanders thoroughly reviewed prior reports of primary direct intraventricular hemorrhages and added ninety-four cases that he was able to collect from his own experience and the literature. His review remains to date the largest and most detailed report on PIVH.

Prior to Sanders, Wepfer[3] and Morgagni[4] had each commented that cerebral hemorrhage or apoplexy was often due to rupture of one of the vessels of the choroid plexus, the seat of the extravasation lying within the lateral ventricles. Duret noted that he had met with cases in which clots of blood or fluid blood filled ventricular cavities. Sanders quotes Duret: "We saw one small clot which closed the aqueduct of Sylvius. . . . Such clots are the result of ruptures of arteries or the veins of the choroid plexus as we have several times shown, or they arise from small hemorrhagic foci on the floor of the fourth ventricle."[2] Hughlings Jackson in his experience found that ventricular blood usually came from bleeding in the thalamus or striatum, but he had "twice known blood ef-

383

fussed into the ventricles without injury of the ganglia on its floor."[2]

Sanders carefully analyzed ninety-four cases.[2] Sixty-nine occurred in one or the other of the lateral ventricles and eleven involved either the third or fourth ventricle. The age distribution was different from that of primary intraparenchymatous hemorrhage since the very young and very old seemed to be preferentially involved. Pathology was carefully studied. Sanders listed the following potential sources of the ventricular bleeding: (1) vessels of the choroid plexus, (2) vessels of the tela choroidea, (3) arteries ramifying in ventricular walls, (4) veins, especially striate and thalamic veins and the vein of Galen, (5) aneurysms, (6) intraventricular tumors and angiomas, and (7) inflammatory conditions of ventricular walls. This list remains relatively complete even today. Causes recognized and reported in detail included bleeding diatheses (leukemia, scurvy, purpura), large aneurysms rupturing into the ventricles, and miliary aneurysms (Charcot-Bouchard type). Sanders attributed some cases to "increased vascular tension."

As far as clinical features, the description by Sanders might serve as a model of obfuscation. "Usually, without the previous existence of premonitory symptoms, while at rest or moving about, generally suddenly but sometimes with more or less degree of slowness, the attack shows itself. It may be ush-ered in by symptoms of apparent slight import, or they may be so violent and overwhelming as to terminate rapidly or perhaps almost instantaneously in death."[2] He was, however, very emphatic that "extravasation of blood into the ventricles was uniformly and rapidly fatal." However, Sanders was aware that necropsy studies of the choroid plexus sometimes revealed lesions that seemed to indicate past bleeding. Table 18.1 from Sanders compares features of primary intraventricular bleeding with intraparenchymatous hemorrhage.[2]

By the turn of the twentieth century, Sanders and others had delineated the major epidemiologic and pathologic features of PIVH but the clinical features that might have allowed diagnosis were vague. Gordon in 1916 collected 12 cases of intraventricular bleeding, and reported in detail the 5 patients with PIVH.[5] Gordon believed the clinical features formed a distinct syndrome. Bleeding emanated from one lateral ventricle in all cases of PIVH. In three cases the hemorrhage "besides destroying the surrounding brain tissue and pushing outward the remaining cortical substance, exercised also considerable pressure on the opposite hemisphere and disfigured it."[5] In two cases, bleeding came from ruptured vessels in the choroid plexus and in these specimens, rounded yellow masses were found in the plexi that were interpreted as "the remains of

**Table 18.1.** Comparison of Features of Ventricular and Cerebral Hemorrhage

| Ventricular Hemorrhage | Cerebral Hemorrhage |
| --- | --- |
| Common in the very young and in the old | Most frequent during middle life |
| Onset very rapid and violent | Onset slower and less violent |
| Coma usually most profound from the very beginning | Coma generally not so profound |
| Convulsions common | Convulsions rare |
| Paralysis frequently absent | Paralysis the rule, generally hemiplegic |
| Transient improvement or remission of symptoms not uncommon | Transient improvement far less frequent |
| Seldom ends in recovery | Often ends in recovery |
| Death rapid, frequently within a few hours | When fatal, life is usually prolonged for several days |

(Modified from Sanders E. A study of primary, immediate, or direct hemorrhage into the ventricles of the brain. Amer J Med Sci 1881;82:85–128.)

former blood effusions." In two other patients, bleeding came from erosions of the ventricular walls; in one the bleeding site was related to miliary aneurysms near the ependyma. Gordon was impressed that four clinical features were uniformly present in the five patients with PIVH: sudden onset, profound coma from onset, convulsions more marked in limbs opposite the side of original bleeding, and the absence of marked limb paralysis. Gordon emphasized the asymmetry of bleeding: "a rapid glance at the brains in the five cases of primary ventricular hemorrhage shows displacement of the brain tissue to the side opposite the blood in three cases, and consequently the possibility of the comatose state as due to undue pressure on the normal side of the brain appears plausible." In one patient, decompressive surgery seemed to increase survival (twenty-four days versus less than one, six, seven, and twelve days) and led to transient improvement in respiration and responsiveness. Gordon favored surgical decompression. "Unfortunately, the operation was consented to only on the 5th day after the apoplectic seizure, vis., after five days of a comatose state. Efforts were made to operate in the other four cases, but permission could not be obtained."[5]

Gordon retained a lifelong interest in PIVH and in 1938, twenty-two years after the original report, he added three new cases and again reaffirmed the uniqueness of the clinical findings.[6] In all cases, hemorrhage emanated from the choroid plexus and miliary aneurysms were identified in fine blood vessels of the plexus. In one of the cases, Gordon again found "displacement and deviation of the cerebral tissue to the side opposite that of the hemorrhage."[6] Again, Gordon suggested surgery in all patients, but his luck had not changed. "Efforts were made to operate on the three cases of the present series, but permission could not be obtained."[6]

Although previous authors had alluded to the possibility of PIVH with recovery, Scully in 1937 reported a single patient with multiple incidents of intraventricular bleeding.[7] A 60-year-old woman suddenly dropped unconscious while sewing, was comatose for fifteen minutes and then had headache and vomiting. After considerable improvement, two weeks later she convulsed and was again stuporous. Cerebrospinal fluid (CSF) was bloody and under high pressure. After again improving, four weeks later she had a severe convulsive attack, became comatose and died. Necropsy showed a spongy mass of clot $4 \times 2$ cm in the anterior horn of the right lateral ventricle emanating from abnormally dilated vessels in the choroid plexus. All the ventricles were filled with blood and blood extended out from the fourth ventricle to the base. All of the ventricles were considerably dilated. Scully emphasized the possibility of repeated bleeding and absorption of blood, and that hydrocephalus could result from PIVH.

In all cases published prior to 1950, the diagnosis of PIVH was made at necropsy. In the early 1960s, angiography and pneumoencephalography led to occasional antemortem recognition of PIVH. Important observations again came from case reports. McDonald, in 1962, described two patients with blood clots in the third ventricle that led to obstructive hydrocephalus.[8] Bleeding was gradual, simulating a tumor. Diagnosis was made by ventriculography and each patient had decompression of the clot and ventricular shunting, but neither patient survived. Paterson and McKissock, in a review of their own experience with intracranial angiomas, included two patients with episodes of minor bleeding from angiomas in one lateral ventricle.[9] The clinical picture was similar to subarachnoid hemorrhage. Avol and Vogel reported two patients in whom ventriculography had shown large intraventricular masses in one lateral ventricle, which on surgery proved to be blood clots.[10] Ojemann and New reported a young man with "cerebral palsy" in whom angiography showed an arteriovenous malformation (AVM) arising from the left posterior cerebral artery, and pneumoencephalography showed a large irregular intraventricular mass extending from the frontal to the occipital horn.[11] After recovery, repeat pneumoencephalography showed spontaneous disappearance of the mass. Butler et al. also reported three patients with relatively minor bleeding episodes into one lateral ventricle.[12] All had vascular malformations fed by either the anterior choroidal or posterior choroidal arteries. Even before the advent of CT, it was known that PIVH often emanated from one lateral ventricle, often came from AVM fed by the choroidal arteries, and included benign as well as severe and fatal forms.

CT, however, clearly was a major advance in diagnosis. The presence and distribution of blood within the ventricular system could readily be seen and undoubtedly many more "benign" instances of PIVH were recognized. Large series of patients whose intraventricular hemorrhages were diagnosed by CT began to appear in the late 1970s and 1980s.[1,13–15] MRI, by allowing easier recognition of AVM and cavernous angiomas, will probably lead to further advances in diagnosis of the cause of many cases of PIVH.

## Anatomy and Pathology

The gross anatomical relationships of the ventricular system are well known to neurologists and neurosurgeons, so that herein we will discuss mostly the choroid plexus and its blood supply.

The two large lateral ventricles connect to the third ventricle through the foramen of Monro, which is situated between the columns of the fornix and the anterior pole of the thalamus. Fluid circulates through the third ventricle, aqueduct of Sylvius, and fourth ventricle. Fluid can escape from the system through the three foramina in the roof of the fourth ventricle, the median foramen of Magendie and the paired lateral foramina of Luschka which are located at the lateral extension of the lateral recess of the fourth ventricle.

The *choroid plexus* of the lateral ventricles extends from the foramen of Monro where it is continuous with the third ventricle choroid plexus to the rostral end of the temporal horn. The plexus does not extend into the anterior or posterior horns. The lateral ventricular portion projects into the lateral wall from under the lateral edge of the fornix as an extension of the tela choroidea of the third ventricle[16] (Figures 18.1 and 18.2). The cleft through which the plexus extends is called the choroidal fissure. The portion of the plexus in the temporal horn lies in the concavity of the hippocampus (Figure 18.3). The choroid plexus of the fourth ventricle protrudes into the ventricle from its roof (Figure 18.4). The plexus extends laterally on each side somewhat beyond the lateral recess of the fourth ventricle.

The choroid plexuses are made up of minute villous processes or tufts of blood vessels brought into the tela choroidea from the pia mater. The tufts are covered by a layer of epithelial cells derived from the ependyma. The blood supply of the choroid plexus of the lateral and third ventricles comes from the choroidal arteries.

The *anterior choroidal artery* (AChA) arises from the intracranial carotid artery posteriorly between the origin of the posterior communicating artery and the bifurcation of the carotid artery into its main middle cerebral and anterior cerebral artery branches.[17,18] Occasionally, the AChA arises from the middle cerebral artery or from the posterior communicating artery. The AChA courses along the optic tract with the temporal lobe laterally and the thalamus and midbrain situated medially. The AChA gives branches to these structures and to the deep basal gray and posterior limb of the internal capsule.[17–19] The AChA ends with distal branches to the lateral geniculate body and the choroid plexus. The terminal plexus arteries enter the choroid plexus at the genu of the temporal horn and turn along its medial border to supply the plexus in the body of the lateral ventricle, the temporal horn, and up to the foramen of Monro.[17]

The *lateral posterior choroidal arteries*, usually two or three in number,[17] originate from the posterior cerebral artery after that vessel

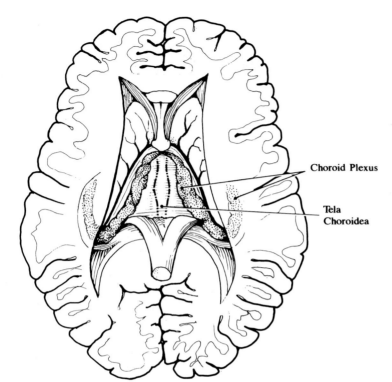

**Figure 18.1.** Artist's drawing of horizontal cut through brain showing choroid plexus of the lateral ventricle and relationship to the tela choroidea of the third ventricle. (Drawn by Harriet Greenfield.)

Choroid Plexus

Tela
Choroidea

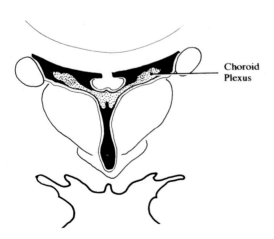

Choroid
Plexus

**Figure 18.2.** Artist's drawing of a coronal section showing the choroid plexus and its relation to the tela choroidea at the roof of the third ventricle. (Drawn by Harriet Greenfield.)

has passed more than halfway around the midbrain. The more anterior of the posterior choroidal arteries enters the temporal horn through the choroidal fissure to supply the choroid plexus of the temporal horn together with the AChA. The more posterior arteries give rise to medial and lateral branches; the lateral branch runs laterally following the choroid plexus around the thalamus into the body of the lateral ventricle, while the medial branch courses above the thalamus medially and joins the choroid plexus under the fornix supplying the medial portion of the plexus.[17]

The choroid plexus of the fourth ventricle is supplied by branches of both the posterior inferior cerebellar artery (PICA) and the anterior inferior cerebellar artery (AICA). The terminal medial branch of PICA courses rostrally and supplies the inferior portion of the vermis giving branches to the choroid plexus of the fourth ventricle. A useful anatomical landmark is the so-called choroidal point of PICA where the vessel lies under the fas-

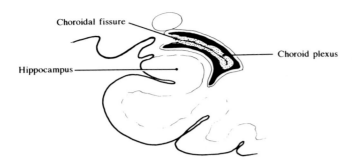

Choroidal fissure

Choroid plexus

Hippocampus

**Figure 18.3.** Artist's drawing of the relation of the choroid plexus within the temporal horn to the hippocampus. (Drawn by Harriet Greenfield.)

tigium of the fourth ventricle. On reaching the cerebellum, AICA branches supply the portion of the choroid plexus of the fourth ventricle near the lateral recess of the foramen of Luschka. The major portion of the choroid plexus of the fourth ventricle is supplied medially from the PICA while a smaller lateral portion gains supply from the AICA. The superior cerebellar artery does not contribute to the supply of the plexus.

The subependymal regions of the lateral ventricles also have a rich arterial supply. The regions around the anterior horn and the central portions of the lateral ventricles are supplied by branches of the striate arteries. Heubner's arteries branching from the proximal anterior cerebral arteries supply the most anterior portion of the caudate nucleus and surrounding white matter. The medial and lateral striate branches of the middle cerebral artery course around the caudate nucleus to reach the external ventricular border; they then send terminal branches running centrifugally back toward the white matter. Van den Bergh studied in detail the supply of the deep periventricular white matter.[20] There is a dual supply with some arteries coursing from the surface centripetally while others course centrifugally from the ventricular surface. This concept is diagramed in Figure 18.5 from Van den Bergh.

The venous system is also very important but quite complex. The anatomy of the veins draining the lateral ventricles are discussed well elsewhere.[16,17] Venous drainage is primarily into the great cerebral vein of Galen which drains the deep internal structures. The major inflow to the vein of Galen comes from the internal cerebral vein and the basal vein of Rosenthal. The major tributaries of the great vein drain both the surface vessels and the ventricular and subependymal veins. The vein of Galen joins the inferior sagittal sinus at the meeting of falx and tentorium forming the straight sinus.

Padget has pointed out that anastomoses between the superior and inferior choroidal veins are present in the fetus and often continue in adults.[21] Also during embryological life, crossing of the larger arterial and venous endothelial tubes is most conspicuous near the relatively enormous choroid plexus. Abnormally dilated capillary nets could lead to arteriovenous communications. Padget considered fistulas between diencephalic arteries that are embryologically choroidal and ve-

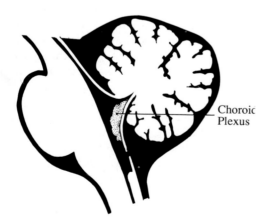

Choroid Plexus

**Figure 18.4.** Artist's drawing of location of choroid plexus in the fourth ventricle. (Drawn by Harriet Greenfield.)

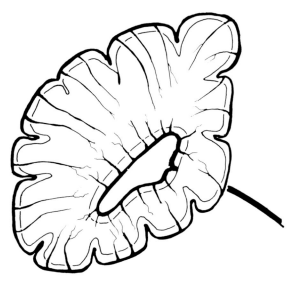

**Figure 18.5.** Artist's drawing of figure from Van den Bergh[20] showing arterial orientation. Arteries emerging near the ventricle have a centrifugal course while surface arteries are centripetal. (Drawn by Harriet Greenfield.)

nous structures of the Galenic system to be very common.[21]

At necropsy, in patients dying of PIVH, the lateral ventricles are usually distended with blood clot which also extends into the third ventricle and aqueduct of Sylvius. The lateral ventricles are usually dilated. Figure 18.6 shows a fatal PIVH. Blood also often extends into the fourth ventricle and through the exit foramina to the basal meninges. Often the massive supratentorial bleeding provides a pressure cone for compression of the midbrain centrally. Duret hemorrhages are sometimes found in the brainstem due to the increased pressure. The tissues around the ventricle are often blood stained and soft, and are damaged by the pressure effects in the expanded ventricles. Less commonly, most of the blood remains confined to one lateral ventricle with considerable shift and compression of the opposite ventricle and hemisphere and the rostral brainstem. Rarely, hemorrhages can be confined almost entirely to the third ventricle, causing acute

obstructive hydrocephalus.[8] In all forms of PIVH, death is invariably due to brainstem compression.

## Clinical Features

The clinical signs and course of illness depend on the cause of the bleeding and the rapidity, symmetry, and volume of the hemorrhage. Patients with PIVH can be conveniently divided into two large groups characterized by either an acute or a more subacute-chronic presentation.[13] Probably about three-fourths of patients with PIVH have the acute form.

### Acute Form

In patients with the acute form of PIVH, the onset is abrupt and the state of consciousness is quickly affected. Stupor or coma are invariably present. Headache and vomiting often precede or accompany the stupor. If the patient is standing at the time of onset, loss of postural tone is frequent and the patient falls or slumps to the floor. Some observers have noted the frequency of seizures during the early course.[1,2,5,6,13] Convulsions may begin focally most often in the limbs opposite the ventricle harboring the initial hematoma, but invariably they become generalized. Sometimes seizures are generalized from the onset or multifocal. Some patients have abnormal movements characterized by shivering, rigidity, and decorticate and decerebrate movements that may be confused with seizures. Similar motor phenomena are frequent in patients with pontine hemorrhage.

On examination, the patient is usually stuporous or may be in frank coma. Blood pressure is often high and the pulse may be slowed. Abnormal respiration is also common. Rapid deep ventilation, Cheyne-Stokes respirations, and ataxic breathing are the most common abnormal respiratory patterns.[13] Meningismus is also very common in patients with the acute form of PIVH and is presumably due to rapid spread of blood into

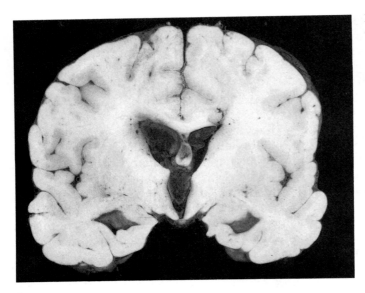

A

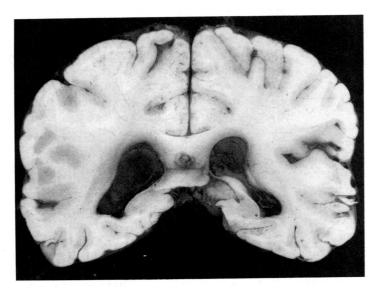

B

**Figure 18.6.** Necropsy brain specimen of fatal PIVH. (A) Cast of blood in the third and lateral ventricles. (B) A more posterior section showing blood in the atria of the lateral ventricles.

the basal meninges and subarachnoid space. Bilateral hyperreflexia and extensor plantar reflexes are often found.

The neuro-ophthalmological signs are very variable. Roving eye movements with preserved oculocephalic and oculovestibular reflex responses are the most common oculomotor findings and are due to bihemispheral loss of supranuclear control. Some patients have eye findings closely mimicking thalamic hemorrhage.[1] In these cases, the eyes are deviated down, or down and in, or remain in midposition. Vertical oculocephalic reflexes may be lost, or only upward movement may be absent. Pupils may be small and poorly reactive. Unilateral or bilateral third nerve palsies are occasionally present. The pupil may be eccentric or oval. Dilatation of the third ventricle with blood or compression or secondary hemorrhage into the brainstem by the sudden increase in supratentorial pressure probably explain the diencephalic dysfunction. Papilledema may develop quickly, especially in younger patients. Subhyaloid hemorrhage are often found in the optic fundus.

In other patients with acute PIVH, the lower brainstem seems to be more involved. Decerebrate movements, shivering, opisthotonic postures, and rigidity are found. Nystagmus and absent horizontal gaze are also described. Apnea may develop as well as chaotic or apneustic breathing. The lower brainstem is affected when the bleeding is infratentorial and the fourth ventricle is acutely dilated. The pons can also be compromised in patients with supratentorial PIVH by increased intracranial pressure with herniation. Duret hemorrhages are often found in these patients in the median and paramedian pons at necropsy.

At times, the motor and oculomotor signs are asymmetric. The frequency of asymmetries is difficult to determine from a review of prior cases since many authors include in their series of patients with intraventricular bleeding patients with parenchymatous lesions that spread to the ventricle. Sanders[2] and Gordon[5,6] described the clinical presentation as that of a unilateral hemispheral-ventricular mass. The patient of Ojemann and New with a mass confined to one ventricle, however, had no focal weakness.[11] Frank hemiplegia must be very rare in PIVH, but minor asymmetries are probably common since bleeding usually originates in one lateral ventricle. In one series of patients with intraventricular hemorrhage and no parenchymatous component by CT, five of eight patients had some focal features.[1] Slight

hemiparesis, asymmetric hyperreflexia or hypotonia or Babinski signs, and asymmetric or unilateral horizontal nystagmus are the most frequent "focal signs." Focality is explained by either a clinically unrecognized parenchymatous component or asymmetrical distension of the ventricles.

### Subacute or Chronic Form

In about 25% of patients, the onset is less sudden. Confusion and headache are the predominant features. Headache, confusion, and gait ataxia may develop gradually during hours or may seem to develop insidiously during weeks to months. At times, the symptoms are recurrent, the patient reporting headache and difficulty concentrating months before with subsequent redevelopment of the same symptom complex after initial improvement. In the subacute form, bleeding probably develops more slowly or intermittently, and the volume of blood is probably less than in the acute form.

Examination usually shows some drowsiness or slight decrease in the level of alertness. Disorientation, restlessness, and decreased ability to concentrate or perform complex cognitive tasks are common. Higher cortical function testing may show poor memory or even isolated deficits in verbal or visual spatial learning function.[1,15,22] Aphasia is unusual. Hyperreflexia and extensor plantar reflexes are often present. Some patients have a slow-stepped shuffling, "marche a petits pas" gait caused by hydrocephalus. Others have lurching and veering with truncal titubation indicative of a vestibulocerebellar abnormality. Asymmetric findings are less common than in the acute form. Papilledema may develop. Eye movements may be normal, but nystagmus may be present.

A recent case will serve to illustrate the subacute presentation. A 23-year-old woman presented in January 1988 because of headache and unusual behavior. She had a long history of headaches. These occurred about once a month, were pounding and throbbing, frequently accompanied by nausea and vomiting, and often occurred during her menstrual periods. Three months before presentation she had been involved in a motor vehicle accident. She was a passenger in the car and briefly lost consciousness after the impact. Headaches had increased in severity and frequency since the injury. During the months before admission, the headaches were particularly severe but resembled qualitatively her usual headaches. Friends said she was more irritable and "not herself" during this period. During the week before admission, headaches were frontal and nearly continuous. She vomited often.

She had no important known past illnesses. She regularly took oral contraceptive pills. She recently had been under some stress because she had two jobs, one as a clerk, the other as a waitress. On the day before hospitalization, she slept all day and was difficult to arouse. On the day of admission, she was very somnolent and disoriented. She walked into a closet and then went into the wrong room to use the toilet. She told her roommates that she had worked the previous day but they knew she had not. She also erroneously reported to them that she had visited the hospital each day of the past week. She spoke of neck and low back pains and was unsteady when she walked. They brought her to the Emergency Room.

On examination, she was sleepy and difficult to interview. She was uncomfortable and complained often of headache and neck discomfort. She was restless and inattentive. She knew she was in Boston at a hospital, but she gave the wrong hospital name. She missed the date by more than a month. She could recall two of three objects after five minutes, but only after prompting. Written and spoken language use and comprehension were normal. She drew and copied simple diagrams adequately. She could not sustain attention long enough to read or interpret a full paragraph. Her neck was stiff. The disc margins of her optic nerves were

blurred and slightly elevated. Strength, reflexes, and sensation were normal. She walked unsteadily holding her head but did not veer, and could walk tandem.

CT scans (Figure 18.7) showed blood in the lateral ventricles and in the third and fourth ventricles. There was no parenchymatous element present. Lumbar puncture showed bloody spinal fluid (270,000 RBC/cc, 40 WBC/cc) under an opening pressure of 280 mm of water. She became more drowsy and confused. Angiography showed a large left cerebellar AVM which clearly communicated directly with the fourth ventricle (Figure 18.8).

Later CT showed increasing hydrocephalus and a ventricular drain was placed in the right lateral ventricle. The clinical course was complicated by thrombophlebitis of the left calf shown by venography to be caused by clot in the deep veins. Three weeks after admission her posterior fossa AVM was removed. She made a gradual but excellent recovery.

## Clinical Course

The course of illness varies greatly depending on the cause, location, and severity of the initial bleeding. Patients with the acute form who have the abrupt onset of deep coma usually do not survive, especially if signs of brainstem dysfunction are present on the initial examination. In patients with stupor, the decreased level of consciousness usually gradually improves. Restlessness, agitation and confusion are present during the recovery period. Examination often shows poor concentration, memory, and ability to retain new information. Gait ataxia is also common just as in the subacute presentation. Generally, if rebleeding does not occur, recovery is very gradual during weeks to months rather than hours or days. Rebleeding may occur during apparent recovery. The natural history of PIVH is now difficult to determine in the CT era since most patients with hydrocephalus have at least temporary ventricular drainage procedures performed after the CT findings are discovered.

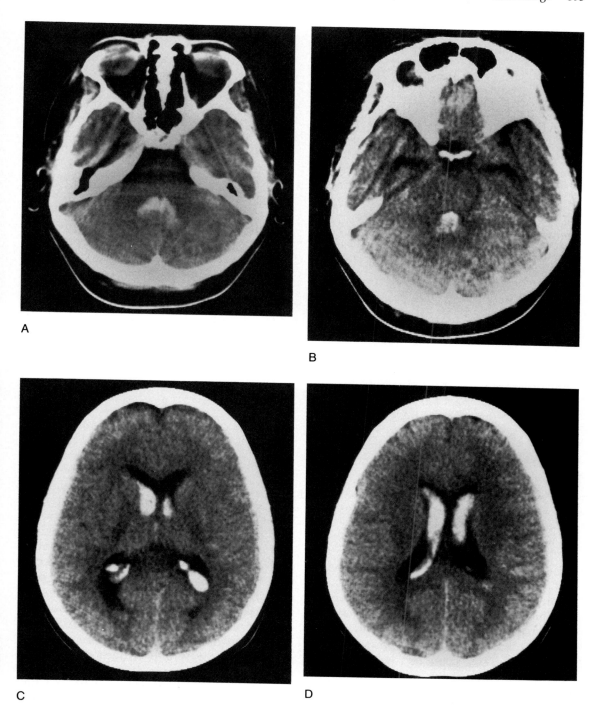

**Figure 18.7.** CT scans showing blood limited to the ventricular system. (A and B) Blood in the fourth ventricle. (C and D) Lateral ventricular blood. There is early hydrocephalus.

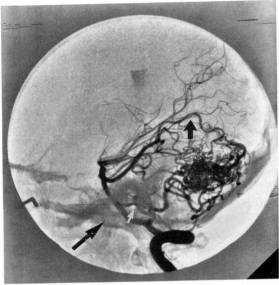

B

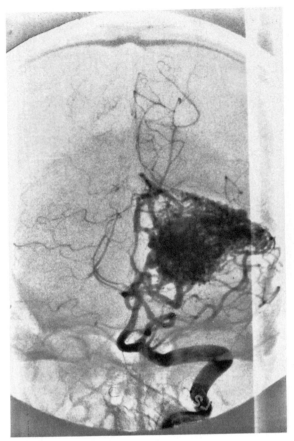

A

**Figure 18.8.** Angiography in the anteroposterior (A) and lateral (B) views showing very large AVM fed primarily by the anterior inferior cerebellar artery (white arrow) and the superior cerebellar artery (upper black arrow). The lower long black arrow points to the basilar artery.

## Laboratory Findings and Investigations

Undoubtedly, to date, the single most important investigation in patients with intraventricular bleeding has been CT scanning. The introduction of CT into clinical practice in the 1970s dramatically changed the clinician's ability to separate PIVH from parenchymatous hemorrhage with or without ventricular extension and from aneurysmal meningocerebral hemorrhages. Blood is found in the lateral ventricles and usually also in the third and fourth ventricles as well as the basal cisterns. At times, bleeding is predominantly in

one or both lateral ventricles, usually in the latter situation with blood also in the third ventricle. Graeb et al. devised a scoring system to quantitate intraventricular hemorrhage.[14] They graded and evaluated each lateral ventricle separately. A score of 1 was given if there was only a trace of blood or slight bleeding. A score of 2 meant that less than half of the ventricle was filled with blood, and a score of 3 was used when the ventricle was more than half blood-filled. A score of 4 was reserved for complete filling and expansion of the ventricle. The third and fourth ventricles were also scored using the same numbers. In some series of patients with intraventricular bleeding, CT has also shown a small hematoma in the caudate nucleus, thalamus, or other periventricular zones.[13,14] In our opinion, the findings of a parenchymatous component should disqualify the patient for the diagnosis of PIVH, but others have included these patients if the predominant clinical findings were related to the ventricular blood. Occasionally, aneurysms or AVMs are seen on contrast-enhanced CT scans. Prognosis usually does not correlate well with the degree of ventricular bleeding, but shifts of brain contents and evidence of transtentorial herniation carry a poor prognosis.

To date, there have not been extensive studies of the utility of MRI in patients with intraventricular bleeding. Possibly, small intraparenchymatous components, especially in the basal frontal or temporal lobes or posterior fossa, would be more readily seen on MRI than CT. Certainly, MRI is more effective at imaging AVMs and cavernous angiomas than CT.

When performed during the first week of bleeding, lumbar puncture usually shows blood-tinged xanthochromic fluid under increased pressure.[13] Spectrophotometry can show increased levels of hemoglobin and bilirubin depending on the length of time after the most recent bleeding. Some patients with intraventricular bleeding have a bleeding diathesis that can be detected by tests of coagulation functions.

Angiography has been a very critical evaluation tool for diagnosing aneurysms and AVMs that cause PIVH. Angiography is indicated in all patients with PIVH in whom the cause remains uncertain after preliminary neuroimaging and blood tests. In the future, MR angiography might also be helpful.

## Cause

The frequency of various causes in series of patients with PIVH depends on: (1) whether patients with some parenchymatous compo-

nent were included, (2) whether the patient was studied on a neurological or neurosurgical service, and (3) the extent of investigations. In contrast to other forms of ICH, the differential diagnosis is much broader and none of the individual causes dominates the list of probabilities.

### Hypertensive Parenchymatous or Choroid Plexus Hemorrhage

Some hypertensive hemorrhages originate in tissues very close to the ventricular system. Hematomas originating in the caudate nucleus may quickly dissect into the adjacent lateral ventricle; the clinical findings and CT might mimic closely PIVH.[23] Similarly, some lesions in the thalamus medially may quickly spread to the third ventricle and hypertensive hematomas arising in the cerebellar vermis might dissect into the fourth ventricle. In all these patients, the parenchymatous component might be so small that it might not be evident on CT.

Early studies found miliary (Charcot-Bouchard) aneurysms within the choroid plexi.[2,5,6] The authors speculated that hypertensive hemorrhages directly into a choroid plexus might occur. In the series of Little et al., hypertensive ICH was diagnosed in twenty-four of fifty-four patients with intraventricular bleeding, making it the single most common cause of IVH in this series.[13]

### Longstanding Cerebrovascular Occlusive Disease and Moya-Moya

In patients with so-called moyamoya occlusive disease, a pattern of dilated arteries develops in the region of the basal ganglia and thalamus. The lenticulostriate and thalamoperforating and thalamogeniculate arteries are often massively dilated.[24] In fact, the term moyamoya, a cloud or puff of smoke, derives from the mass of dilated deep collateral arteries that develop in response to occlusions of the basal arteries usually at the intracranial bifurcations of the carotid arteries. Small microaneurysms form in the dilated deep arteries. Increased flow leads to degenerative changes in the perforating arteries and an increased tendency to bleeding. Increased collateral circulation has also been described in patients with longstanding carotid artery occlusion.[25] There is also a higher instance of intracranial aneurysms in patients with chronic occlusive disease and the moyamoya syndrome.[26–29] In children, moyamoya syndrome patients usually present with seizures or episodes of brain ischemia but in adults, presentation with intracranial hemorrhage is common.[24] At times, the intracranial bleeding is intraventricular. The presumed mechanism of intraventricular hemorrhage in moyamoya syndrome and other extensive occlusive lesions is direct leakage of blood into the ventricle from a periventricular hemorrhage or hemorrhagic infarct, or rupture of small aneurysms into the ventricular system. Gates et al. reported a series of five patients who presented in adult life with PIVH related to severe extensive occlusive disease.[30] Three of these patients had bilateral occlusions of the internal carotid arteries (ICA) at their origins in the neck; one had a unilateral ICA origin occlusion and severe stenosis of the contralateral ICA in the siphon, and one patient had a unilateral middle cerebral artery occlusion.[30] None of these patients had prominent focal clinical signs, but two of the five patients had intraventricular bleeding limited to one lateral ventricle. One patient in the Australian series of patients with PIVH also had moyamoya syndrome.[1] She was a 30-year-old woman with a subependymal hematoma that lay at the external angle of the body of the lateral ventricle at a location where collaterals off the branches of the anterior and posterior choroidal arteries connect the anterior and posterior circulations.

### Arteriovenous Malformations

Small occult aneurysms and AVMs are usually considered to be the most frequent cause of PIVH, especially in young, nonhypertensive individuals. Padget has theorized that the embryological pattern of the arterial and venous choroidal circulation might lead to a high number of choroidal vascular anomalies and malformations.[21] In the series of Darby et al., AVMs accounted for eight of the sixteen instances of PIVH.[1] The AVM are often located in the medial basal ganglia region, for example in the subependymal zone under the head of the caudate nucleus. Some aneurysms lie within the choroid plexus or jut into the lateral ventricle from the periventricular white matter. In most such patients, the lesions are visualized by angiography. At times, cavernous angiomas may primarily be in an intraventricular location. Figure 18.9 is an MRI showing such a lesion. AVMs may cause repeated episodes of slight bleeding or oozing into the ventricular system. AVMs are probably responsible for most examples of subacute or chronic presentations of PIVH. The true incidence of AVMs in patients with PIVH is unknown since some may destroy themselves when they bleed. Others do not opacify on angiography. An occult AVM is usually blamed for PIVH when no other cause is found and the patient is not hypertensive. An illustrative example of a patient with a large cerebellar AVM and subacute PIVH was described earlier in this chapter.

### Systemic Bleeding Disorders

Most series of patients with PIVH contain a few patients with hemorrhage related to a systemic disorder causing a bleeding diathesis. Sanders, in his original monograph on PIVH in 1881, included several such patients.[2] Case 2 of Sanders was a 13-year-old boy with "leukocythemia who had large ecchymoses on the malleoli, purpuric spots on the chest and epistaxis, who developed headache and coma and died of PIVH." An older man with clinical scurvy, a young boy with purpura, and another patient who had a profuse hemorrhage from the gums a few days before, were all described in Sanders report.[2] In the series of Little et al., two patients had a coagu-

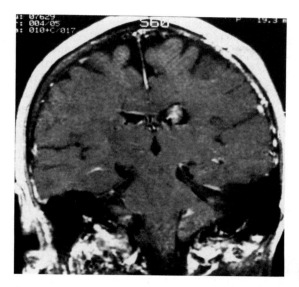

A

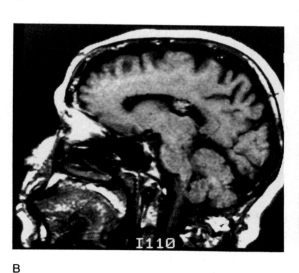

B

**Figure 18.9.** MRI of small AVM in a lateral ventricle. (A) Coronal section. (B) Sagittal section. (C) Transaxial horizontal section. The AVM appears bright on these T-2 weighted images.

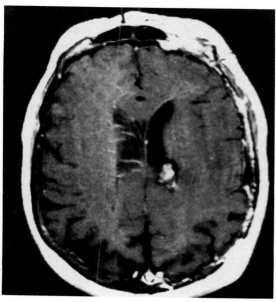

C

lopathy;[13] one patient was receiving heparin and warfarin and had a prolonged partial thromboplastin time, and the other patient had severe liver disease and a prolonged prothrombin time.[13] In the series of Graeb et al., three patients with PIVH had coagulopathy; two had prolonged prothrombin time because of excessive anticoagulation, and the other patient had severe thrombocytopenia due to chemotherapy for leukemia.[14] Platelet

counts, prothrombin and activated thromboplastin times, and studies of bleeding and coagulation should be performed in all patients with PIVH.

### Aneurysms

In surgical series, aneurysms account for a relatively high proportion of cases of PIVH.

The most frequent site of aneurysms causing intraventricular hemorrhage is the anterior cerebral-anterior communicating artery complex.[13,14] These patients also have subfrontal bleeding. Occasionally, aneurysms causing PIVH are located in azygous arteries, pericallosal and callosomarginal branches of the anterior cerebral arteries, and at the ICA-posterior communicating artery junction. Posterior circulation aneurysms, especially those arising from the PICA, have been reported to cause PIVH.[14,31,32] In one such patient, the aneurysm arose from an extracranial lateral medullary branch of the PICA at C1 below the foramen magnum.[31] Sometimes the aneurysms that cause PIVH are located within the lateral ventricles, especially in the terminal branches of the choroidal arteries. Mycotic aneurysms in peripheral periventricular branches of the anterior and middle cerebral arteries have also been reported to cause PIVH.[13] Sanders included in his series of cases several patients with giant aneurysms that caused fatal ICH.[2] Most had preceding symptoms of prior bleeding or mass effect.

CT often yields clues that the bleeding is aneurysmal. Cisternal collections of blood and subarachnoid bleeding are more prominent than in nonaneurysmal PIVH. Anterior communicating artery aneurysms jet blood from the base, usually presenting a characteristic pattern of subfrontal and intraventricular bleeding. In some cases, contrast enhancement will opacify the aneurysms on CT. Large flow voids on MRI are sometimes seen at sites of aneurysmal dilatation. In the future, MR angiography will likely allow detection of most large aneurysms.

## Trauma

Head injury can cause bleeding into the ventricular system as part of the extensive intracranial injury. Sanders quotes Hewett: "a laceration of the floor of the lateral ventricle, even when slight, may give rise to an exten-sive extravasation of blood into the cavity, should it so happen that the injury corresponds to the situation of one of the large veins in this region."[2] Duret, in his experiments with head trauma, had several times found clots of blood in the ventricles of dogs following powerful blows to the head.[2] Traumatic intraventricular bleeding seldom poses a diagnostic problem. Most patients will have a history of recent head injury, outward signs of trauma, or other diagnostic features, such as subdural hematomas, skull fractures, or basal frontal or temporal contusions. In the series of Graeb et al., seventeen of the sixty-eight patients (25%) had traumatic causation.[14] Among these patients, thirteen had swelling or bleeding in the extracranial soft tissues and twelve had additional parenchymatous hemorrhages. Acute subdural hematomas, cerebral contusions, skull fractures, and intracranial air were common CT findings.[14] In contrast, Little et al. found intraventricular bleeding unusual in head injury.[13] They found intraventricular hemorrhage in only one of 196 cases of cerebral trauma, a 40-year-old man who died quickly after a severe motor vehicle accident.[13] The Australian series included only patients with nontraumatic intraventricular hemorrhage.[1] Clearly, trauma occasionally causes massive intraventricular bleeding due to tearing of deep or subependymal veins that empty blood directly into the lateral ventricles. This probably happens only very rarely without other obvious evidence of traumatic brain and skull injury. Traumatic cases seldom qualify strictly as examples of PIVH.

### Other Miscellaneous Causes

Other causes of PIVH are much less common. Tumors, especially intraventricular meningiomas and gliomas have been known to cause intraventricular and subarachnoid bleeding.[2,13,14] Even metastatic lesions, especially those from hypernephroma, choriocarcinoma, and melanoma that often become hemorrhagic, are a known but rare cause of PIVH.[14] In most such cases the diagnosis of metastatic tumor is known before development of the brain hemorrhage. In the series of Little et al., two patients had tumors causing PIVH, a frontal lobe glioblastoma and a hypothalamic oligodendroglioma.[13] Hamartomas[1] and choroid plexus papillomas[33] also are known to cause intraventricular bleeding. Pituitary apoplexy usually causes bleeding into the sella turcica or subarachnoid space but can cause intraventricular bleeding.[34] Occasionally, infectious processes, especially cysticercosis with its predilection for ventricular localization, can cause intraventricular hemorrhage. In all these conditions, CT or MRI should confirm or suggest the diagnosis.

Occasionally, patients with congenital hydrocephalus, for example, related to stenosis of the aqueduct of Sylvius, can have episodes of intraventricular bleeding. Bleeding might be due in these patients to spontaneous tearing of stretched subependymal veins or minor head trauma. Subarachnoid bleeding also occurs in patients with hydrocephalus. Occlusion of the deep draining veins or the vein of Galen can lead to intraventricular bleeding as well as involvement of the diencephalon and deep hemispheric structures. Occasionally, a vein of Galen aneurysm causes PIVH. Surgical cannulation of a ventricle can, of course, be complicated by intraventricular bleeding.

In many patients, the causes of PIVH remains obscure, even after investigations including angiography. In twelve of sixty-eight patients (18%) in the series of Graeb et al., there was no established cause while in the series of Little et al., only two of fifty-four were indeterminate.[13] The majority of these patients are thought to have small cryptic angiomas that are too small to opacify or that destroy themselves when they bleed. Patients who have no demonstrable cause of PIVH, even after angiography, seem to have a better prognosis than those with a documented mechanism of hemorrhage.[14]

## Prognosis

The prognosis depends predominantly on two features: the level of consciousness on admission, and the cause of the intraventricular hemorrhage. Acute onset with coma carries a bad prognosis, especially when there are signs of brainstem dysfunction when the patient is initially evaluated.[13] The sudden increase in intraventricular and intracranial pressure causes immediate damage to the rostral brainstem. Coma in these patients is probably caused by dysfunction of the reticular activating system in the periventricular regions of the diencephalon and/or dysfunction of the paramedian midbrain or pontine tegmentum. Sudden intracranial pressure changes and herniation often provoke subhyaloid retinal hemorrhages and Duret-type brainstem hemorrhages. In these severely affected individuals, the ventricular system is invariably dilated and filled with blood, and blood has escaped into the basal cisterns and subarachnoid space.[2,13] Drainage of the ventricular space by placing a catheter or drain into a lateral ventricle is seldom successful in these patients with extensive bleeding and rapid onset coma.[13] Drainage of clotted blood is technically unsatisfactory. Even when drainage can be accomplished, the patients usually do not survive.

In patients who have a subacute or chronic onset and less severe bleeding, the outlook is better. Jayakumar et al. pointed out that this group had a bimodal outcome—death or survival with little or no deficit.[15] In surviving patients, it takes about ten to seventeen days for blood to be absorbed from the lateral ventricles on CT.[13] Hydrocephalus often develops during the first week but usually is minor.[14] Increase in ventricular size correlates well with the presence and amount of cisternal and subarachnoid blood.[14] This means that in most patients, ventricular enlargement is due to poor absorption of CSF by the basal meninges. Patients with hydrocephalus have a worse outlook for recovery.[15] Occasional patients have obstructive hydrocephalus due to blood in the third ventricle or sylvian aqueduct.[8]

Recently, Darby et al. subjected their patients who recovered from PIVH to a battery of higher cortical function neuropsychological tests.[1] Poor memory and a decline from premorbid levels of intellectual function were common. Some patients could not return to their former work and home activities. Recovery was often slow and incomplete. Other authors have not reported the results of cognitive and behavioral testing.

## References

1. Darby DG, Donnan GA, Saling MA, et al. Primary intraventricular hemorrhage: clinical and neuropsychological findings in a prospective stroke series. Neurology 1988;38:68–75.
2. Sanders E. A study of primary, immediate, or direct hemorrhage into the ventricles of the brain. Amer J Med Sci 1881;82:85–128.
3. Wepfer JJ. Observationes Anatomicae ex cadaveribus eorum, quos sustulit apoplexia cum exercitatione de ejus loco affecto. Schaffhausen, John Caspari, Suteri, 1658.
4. Morgagni GB. The seats and causes of diseases investigated by Anatomy. Translated by B. Alexander. London: Miller and Cadell, 1769 (Birmingham Classics of Medicine Library 1983).
5. Gordon A. Ventricular hemorrhage: a symptom-group. Arch Int Med 1916;17:343–353.
6. Gordon A. Primary ventricular hemorrhage: further contribution to a characteristic symptom group. Arch Neurol Psychiat 1938;39:1272–1276.
7. Scully FJ. Internal hydrocephalus following repeated intraventricular hemorrhages. Ann Int Med 1937;11:684–686.
8. McDonald JV. Midline hematoma simulating tumors of the third ventricle. Neurology 1962;12:805–809.
9. Paterson JH, McKissock W. A clinical survey of intracranial angiomas with special reference to their mode of progression and surgical treatment: a report of 110 cases. Brain 1956;79:233–266.
10. Avol M, Vogel PJ. Circumscribed intraventricular hematoma simulating an encapsulated neoplasm. Bull Los Angeles Neurol Soc 1955;20:25–29.
11. Ojemann RG, New PFJ. Spontaneous resolution of an intraventricular hematoma: report of a case with recovery. J Neurosurg 1963;20:899–902.
12. Butler AB, Partain RA, Netsky MG. Primary intraventricular hemorrhage: a mild and remedial form. Neurology 1972;22:675–687.
13. Little JR, Blomquist GA, Ethier R. Intraventricular hemorrhage in adults. Surg Neurol 1977;8:143–149.
14. Graeb DA, Robertson WD, Lapointe JS, et al. Computed tomographic diagnosis of intraventricular hemorrhage: etiology and prognosis. Radiology 1982;143:91–96.
15. Jayakumar PN, Taly AB, Bhavani UR, et al. Prognosis in solitary intraventricular haemorrhage: clinical and computed tomographic observations. Acta Neurol Scand 1989;80:1–5.
16. Sabotta J, Uhlenhuth E. Atlas of descriptive human anatomy. Vol. III. Blood vessels—nervous system—sense organs, integument and lymphatics. Sixth English edition. New York: Hafner, 1956.
17. Stephens RB, Stilwell DL. Arteries and veins of the human brain. Springfield, IL: Charles C Thomas, 1969.
18. Rhoton AL, Kiyotaka F, Fradd B. Microsurgical anatomy of the anterior choroidal artery. Surg Neurol 1979;12:171–187.
19. Helgason C, Caplan LR, Goodwin J, et al. Anterior choroidal artery-territory infarction: report of cases and review. Arch Neurol 1986;43:681–686.
20. Van den Bergh R. The periventricular intracerebral blood supply. In: Meyer JS, et al. eds. Research on the cerebral circulation. Springfield, IL: Charles C Thomas, 1969;52–63.
21. Padget DH. The cranial venous system in man in reference to development, adult configuration, and relation to the arteries. Amer J Anat 1956;98:307–355.
22. Asín FM, Millán LFP, Miguel EM. Primary intraventricular hemorrhage. Neurology 1989;39:310(letter).
23. Stein RW, Kase CS, Hier DB, et al. Caudate Hemorrhage. Neurology 1984;34:1549–1554.
24. Suzuki J. Moya-Moya disease. Springer-Verlag: Heidelberg, 1986.
25. Fisher CM. Early-life carotid-artery occlusion associated with late intracranial hemorrhage: observations on the ischemic pathogenesis of mantle sclerosis. Lab Invest 1959;8:680–700.

26. Adams HP, Kassell NF, Wisoff HS, et al. Intracranial saccular aneurysm and Moyamoya disease. Stroke 1979;10:174–179.

27. Servo A. Agenesis of the left internal carotid artery associated with an aneurysm on the right carotid siphon: case report. J Neurosurg 1977;46:677–680.

28. Tasker RR. Ruptured berry aneurysm of the anterior ethmoidal artery associated with bilateral spontaneous internal carotid artery occlusion in the neck: case report. J Neurosurg 1983;59:687–691.

29. Hassler O. Experimental carotid ligation followed by aneurysmal formation and other morphological changes in the Circle of Willis. J Neurosurg 1963;20:1–7.

30. Gates PC, Barnett HJM, Vinters HV, et al. Primary intraventricular hemorrhage in adults. Stroke 1986;17:872–877.

31. Ruelle A, Cavazzani P, Andrioli G. Extracranial posterior inferior cerebellar artery aneurysm causing isolated intraventricular hemorrhage: a case report. Neurosurgery 1988;23:774–777.

32. Yeh H-S, Tomsick TA, Tew JM. Intraventricular hemorrhage due to aneurysms of the distal posterior inferior cerebellar artery: report of three cases. J Neurosurg 1985;62:772–775.

33. Ernsting J. Choroid plexus papilloma causing spontaneous subarachnoid haemorrhage. J Neurol Neurosurg Psychiat 1955;18:134–136.

34. Challa VR. Intraventricular hemorrhage from pituitary apoplexy. Arch Neurol 1986;43:544 (letter).

# Chapter 19
# Pontine Hemorrhage

## Louis R. Caplan

## Historical Aspects

Although they account for only 8% to 10% of all intraparenchymal hemorrhages, pontine hematomas have always attracted a disproportionate interest for clinicians and researchers alike. Long before the advent of modern neuroimaging techniques, the distinctive clinical findings in patients with pontine hemorrhage allowed separation from supratentorial location hemorrhages. The major findings in patients with large medial tegmental-basal pontine hemorrhages were known at the turn of the twentieth century, and during the first three-quarters of this century, pontine hematomas were generally considered to be universally fatal. Like hematomas at other loci, the syndrome was considered uniform and homogeneous. More recently, computed tomography (CT) and magnetic resonance imaging (MRI) have allowed the detection of smaller lesions and we now know that the spectrum of clinical findings and outcomes is rather broad and definitely not homogeneous. We will begin the discussion of pontine hemorrhage by reviewing the evolution of information about this disorder. The newer data are best understood against the background of prior knowledge.

Cheyne is generally given credit for the first descriptions of necropsy-verified pontine hemorrhage. The cases were included in his monograph on apoplexy published in 1812.[1] We have already described one of his cases in the opening chapter on the general history of intracerebral hemorrhage (ICH). That patient (Cheyne's case IX) had headache, vomiting, and became "quite insensible." A ragged blood-filled cavity was found in the middle of the pons that communicated with the fourth ventricle. The second patient (Cheyne's case X) was more complex. She was "a corpulent woman, fifty years of age, of sanguine temperament, florid complexion and a spirit drinker." After "falling in a fit" she was confused, then developed a right hemiplegia and later "complete paraplegia," and soon death. At necropsy, Cheyne found "a little mass of clotted blood, not more than would have filled a teaspoon" within the corpus striatum on both sides. In addition, there was a large clot of blood in the pons that communicated with the fourth ventricle.[1,2] Using hog bristles and camel-hair pencils, Cheyne found the vessels leading to the hemorrhages. Perhaps this patient had a bleeding disorder due to her injudicious use of alcohol. Neither of Cheyne's cases had a clinical syndrome that later clinicians could identify as pontine hemorrhage.

Shortly after Cheyne's treatise, Burdach and Serres each reported single cases of pontine bleeding.[3] During the nineteenth century there were a number of scattered case reports, some by names readily recognizable even today—Bright, Abercrombe, Romberg.[3]

There were four relatively large series of cases: Josias (1851, fourteen cases), Larcher (1868), Bode (1877, sixty-seven cases), and Luce (1899, eighteen cases).[3] In 1903, Charles Dana, then professor of Neurology at Cornell University, reviewed the prior cases and his own experience and wrote a classic paper on pontine hemorrhages and softenings.[3] Dana first reviewed the vascular and brain anatomy of the region; these concise descriptions and diagrams would be valid today with only slight changes. He reviewed the frequency of pontine bleeding among large necropsy series. Among a total of 2288 hemorrhages found at necropsy, 205 (9%) were pontine.[3] This figures differs little from modern experience. Pontine hemorrhages occurred most often in persons between ages 30 and 50, and men predominated (95/60) in a ratio close to 3:2. During Dana's time, blood pressure measurements were not in clinical use but the most common associated conditions were nephritis, cardiac hypertrophy, and arterial sclerosis that now would surely be attributed to hypertensive vascular disease. Dana described the prototypic attack:

> The patient has some prodromal headaches and malaise for a few days, with vertigo and sometimes vomiting. Then he falls suddenly, as if by a lightening stroke, into a coma, usually very profound. There are twitching of the face or of the limbs or both, but rarely any general convulsion . . . the respiration is slow, 4 or 6 per minute, or more often irregular, and of Cheyne-Stokes type. The pupils are contracted to a pinpoint and do not respond to light, but may be uneven. There is convergent strabismus or conjugate deviation of the eyes. The limbs are at first stiff, but may be relaxed later and the reflexes increased. The patient can not be aroused but can be made to vomit. A few hours later, the temperature rises, sometimes very high—106 to 108—but usually not . . . the patient dies in six to twenty hours, usually with evidence of paralysis of respiration.[3]

Dana listed the symptoms of "the syndrome of pons lesions" which is quoted in Table 19.1. The twitching, fever, and respiratory

**Table 19.1.** Syndrome of Pontine Hemorrhage

1. Headache, malaise, vomiting.
2. Sudden and profound coma.
3. Twitching of the face and limbs, or both.
4. Miosis and convergent strabismus or conjugate deviation (away from the side of the lesion).
5. Slow, irregular breathing.
6. Irregular pulse.
7. Dysphagia.
8. Paralysis of limbs or crossed paralysis or exaggerated reflexes.
9. Gradual rise of temperature, sometimes to high point.
10. Death inside of twenty-four hours.

(From Dana CL. Acute bulbar paralysis due to hemorrhage and softening of the pons and medulla: with reports of cases and autopsies. Med Rec 1903;64:361–374. With permission.)

changes might not have been readily predicted from knowledge of the anatomy of the region, and attracted great interest during the next half-century. Dana did not describe the necropsy findings but a few years earlier, Gowers[4] had included in his neurology text a rather clear description. The lesions occurred at the tegmentobasal junction toward the rostral end of the pons. They often spread rostrally but rarely spread caudally to the medulla. The hematomas often dissected into the fourth ventricle. Figure 19.1 is an artist's copy of a figure from Gowers' text depicting the usual pontine hematoma.

Oppenheim, in 1905, in his neurological text, reviewed published cases and elaborated on the clinical features of patients with pontine hemorrhages.[5] He also emphasized the sudden onset of coma. Occasionally a hemiplegia or asymmetric bulbar palsy was present, but more commonly there was bilateral limb weakness, and bilateral weakness of the mouth, palate, pharynx, and larynx. Pupils were small, almost pinpoint, but could be dilated. Oppenheim pointed out that eye movements were often lost. Trismus, convulsions and high fever were frequent findings. Oppenheim also emphasized that the lesion

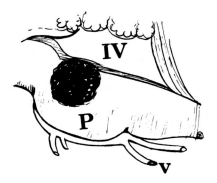

**Figure 19.1.** Artist's drawing of picture from Gowers' textbook of neurology[4] showing location of pontine hemorrhage. P = pons; IV = fourth ventricle; V = vertebral artery. (Drawn by Harriet Greenfield. Modified from Gowers WR. A Manual of Diseases of the Nervous System, 2nd Edition, Vol. 2. London: JA Churchill, 1893.)

was invariably fatal, although, occasionally patients were awake and alert at onset.[5]

Dana, Oppenheim, Gowers and their predecessors, had described patients with hematomas limited to the pons. During the nineteenth century, clinicians and pathologists had become aware that some patients with head trauma and other brain lesions had hematomas within the midbrain and pons at necropsy. In 1878, Henri Duret, working in the laboratory of Jean Martin Charcot, was able to produce brainstem hemorrhages in experimental animals by injecting fluid into the supratentorial tissues of dogs.[2,6] Duret later studied traumatic hemorrhages in humans and pointed out the frequency of hematomas in the pons and midbrain in patients dying of head injury.[7] It was Attwater, however, who in 1911 separated primary pontine hemorrhages from secondary brainstem hematomas.[8] Attwater analyzed seventy-seven examples of pontine hemorrhage found at necropsy at Guy's Hospital in London. Some patients had hemorrhages limited to the center of the pons. Others, especially those whose hemorrhages were caused by trauma, had supratentorial hematomas as well as pontine bleeding. Attwater postulated that some pontine hemor-

rhages could be due to "an increase in intracranial tension produced by the rapid entry of blood into the closed cranial cavity."[8] Subsequent research by Duret[7] and by Dill and Isenhour[9] established that the secondary hemorrhages in the pons, now usually referred to as Duret hemorrhages, were caused by sudden pressure changes that distorted and compressed the brainstem. These secondary hemorrhages clearly had a different cause than the solitary, primary pontine hematomas.

In the second half of the twentieth century, clinicians studied in more detail the clinical phenomena described by Dana and Oppenheim. There were a number of reports of series of patients studied clinically and at necropsy. Steegmann, in 1951, reported seventeen cases of primary pontine hemorrhage, excluding Duret hemorrhages secondary to other intracranial lesions.[10] The hematomas involved the center of the pons and in ten the lesions ruptured into the fourth ventricle. Two patients had hemiplegia (one with crossed facial and limb weakness) and three patients had asymmetrical lesions located more on one side of the tegmentum and basis pontis. Steegmann discussed the irregular abnormal limb movements present in many of the patients. He attributed the shaking, twisting, trembling, and shivering to abnormal motor phenomena and was one of the first to conclude that they were not convulsive in nature.[10] He also described the frequency of "respiratory failure;" four patients had slow, labored breathing and some patients had shallow gasping or irregular respirations.[10] Death was not instantaneous; no patient died in less than twenty-two hours but all lesions were fatal.

Though most authors continued to emphasize the abrupt onset of paralysis and coma, Kornyey, in a striking single case report, described the gradual evolution of symptoms in a man whose hemorrhage developed while under observation.[11] The patient was a 39-year-old printer who was sent to Kornyey's hospital in Szeged, Hungary, for treatment of "malignant hypertension."

While his history was being taken, he reported numbness and tingling of his hands. He became restless and then described difficulty in hearing and swallowing. Blood pressure was 245/170 mm Hg. "Under the eyes of several examiners, complete bilateral palsy of the sixth nerve developed; both pupils dilated and the corneal reflex disappeared. The patient was still able to talk but with a typical bulbar speech and seemed almost totally deaf. The left leg now became paretic, rapid clonic movements being observed. Babinski sign was present bilaterally." Within fifteen minutes he was stuporous and quadriplegic and the pupils were miotic but reacted to light. Kornyey commented "this rapidly progressive chain of events was most unpleasant to witness and produced a depressive effect on the nurses and physicians."[11] The patient died two hours after his presentation to the clinic. At necropsy he had a massive hemorrhage in the pontine tegmentum and small hematomas in the pontine base. The patient had developed "tonic and clonic convulsive" movements of all extremities and Kornyey commented on convulsions in pontine lesions. The patient was quite hypoxic before convulsions commenced, but the author attributed the seizures to the pontine process.

Later, several authors reported their findings in patients with pontine hematomas from large necropsy series. Fang and Foley[12] and later Dinsdale[13] reviewed autopsy studies from the Boston City Hospital—the source of the original Aring and Merritt data. Among 19,093 necropsies, there were 511 intraparenchymatous hematomas among which thirty (6%) were pontine.[13] Two-thirds of the patients with pontine hematomas were comatose when first examined and three-fourths were dead within forty-eight hours. The longest survivor (twenty-three days) had a small hematoma in the pontine tegmentum on one side. All the remainder of the hemorrhages were very large hematomas, usually centered at the junction of the tegmentum and basis pontis. The bleeding usually spread into the fourth ventricle.

Fisher probably best summarized the state of clinical knowledge about pontine hematomas in the preceding era.[14] He summarized the findings: coma usually comes quickly, bilateral pyramidal signs are present and reflex conjugate lateral eye movements are impaired, pupils are small and unreactive, and attacks of tonic bilateral extensor posture are common early. "A sign of some help in diagnosis is the occurrence of an irregular and intermittent, very quick, downward movement of both eyes at intervals of seconds to minutes. This bobbing or dipping movement ("ocular dance") reflects severe damage to the pons with sparing of the midbrain." When evolution of hemorrhage is gradual, a hemiplegia can occur before quadriplegia. Fisher concluded by noting: "the abundance of adventitious movements and rigidities which these patients show . . . unilateral and bilateral decerebrate and decorticate postures, marked rigidity of all limbs, extensor posturing involving these limbs, monospasms—in flexion, frank focal cerebral seizures, or continued focal epilepsy, fine tremblings of the muscles in one or more limbs, moderate tremors of the upper extremities, or rhythmic flexion-extension of the toes or ankles."[14]

As with hematomas at other sites, the advent of CT and MRI allowed better clinicopathological correlations of pontine hematomas and allowed recognition of previously uncharacterized subtypes. In 1982, Caplan and Goodwin[15] reported three patients and reviewed prior reports[13,16–20] of hemorrhages confined to the lateral tegmental region in the distribution of horizontally oriented penetrating branches of the lateral circumferential cerebellar arteries that circle around the pons. This syndrome was quite distinct and involved primarily sensory, cerebellar, and oculomotor signs without stupor or prominent limb paralysis. Subsequent reports noted partial tegmental syndromes, such as pure sensory deficits in the limbs or face.[21–24] During the 1980s clinicians also recognized from neuroimaging tests that some hematomas were confined to the paramedian pontine base, or tegmentum and base. These hematomas caused clinical syndromes identical to those described as lacunar syndromes of pure motor hemiparesis,[25,26] ataxic hemiparesis,[27-29] and the dysarthria–clumsy hand syndrome.[30] The presence of these lesions could have been predicted from a knowledge of the penetrating artery branches to the pons, but these lesions had not been discovered before the modern neuroimaging era.

## Anatomy

Space will not allow a full consideration of the anatomy of the pons. Here we will emphasize those anatomical structures that are important to understand the clinical findings in patients with pontine hemorrhages. Figure 19.2 depicts diagrammatically the major, clinically important, structures.

### Motor Tracts

The descending long motor tracts are located in the ventral pons within the basis pontis. The corticospinal tract fibers are located ventrally and will form compact bundles to make up the medullary pyramids below. The other major components of the basis pontis are corticopontine fibers, which arise primarily from frontal, parietal, and temporal cortex, traverse mainly the anterior limb of the internal capsule and descend in the basis pon-

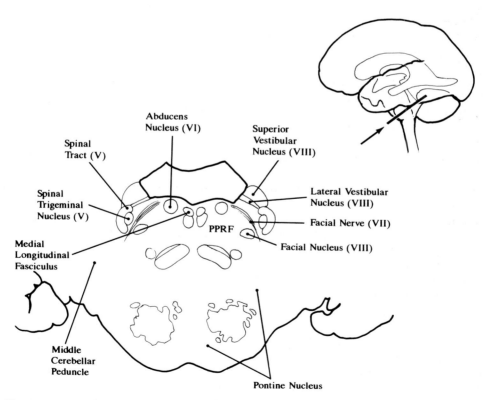

**Figure 19.2.** Artist's drawing of section through pons. The top insert indicates plane and location of the section. Major clinically important structures are labeled. PPRF = Paramedian pontine reticular formation. (Drawn by Harriet Greenfield.)

tis to terminate in the pontine nuclei. The pontine nuclei surround fibers of the corticospinal tracts and are especially numerous medial and lateral to it.[31] The pontine nuclei give rise to fibers that run transversely in the pons, cross the midline, and then course to the cerebellum through the middle cerebellar peduncle. The basis pontis thus contains mostly motor fibers descending towards the spinal cord and toward the contralateral cerebellum. Lesions produce paralysis, "pyramidal signs," and sometimes ataxia if paralysis is not severe.

### Extraocular Movement—Related Structures

Lesions of the pontine tegmentum frequently cause nuclear palsies, conjugate gaze abnormalities, and internuclear ophthalmoplegia. A knowledge of the location and function of the nuclei and tracts of the oculomotor system is necessary to understand the localization of lesions within the tegmentum. The major structures that contribute to the vestibulo-ocular reflex and toward conjugate horizontal gaze are the vestibular nuclei, the paramedian pontine reticular formation (PPRF), the abducens nuclei, and the medial longitudinal fasciculi (MLF). The locations of these structures are depicted on Figure 19.2. Corticofugal fibers mediating conjugate horizontal saccadic and pursuit eye movements descend to the PPRF just ventral to the MLF. Excitatory projections go to the ipsilateral abducens nuclei and through the contralateral MLF to the medial rectus neurons of the opposite side.[32] Lesions of the PPRF cause tonic conjugate contralateral eye deviation and loss of conjugate gaze to the ipsilateral side. Reflex eye movements are preserved. Lesions that include the abducens nucleus cause an ipsilateral gaze palsy and loss of ipsilateral reflex eye movements.[33] When the lesion just involves the intraaxial sixth nerve fibers, then there is intortion of the eye and weakness of ocular abduction. Lesions of the MLF cause the syndrome of internuclear ophthalmoplegia, that is, loss of adduction of the

ipsilateral eye on gaze to the contralateral side and nystagmus of the abducting eye. When the PPRF and MLF are involved on the same side, then a "one-and-a-half syndrome" develops.[32,33,34] In this entity, the only preserved motion is abduction of the contralateral eye.

### Sensory Nuclei and Tracts

The important somatosensory structures are the principal sensory nucleus of V, the spinal tract of V with its nucleus, the lateral spinothalamic tract, and the medial lemniscus. The relative positions of each are shown on Figure 19.2. The principal sensory nucleus of V lies lateral to the entering trigeminal root fibers in the upper pons and mediates tactile and pressure sensation on the face. The spinal tract of V and its nucleus are located laterally in the pontine tegmentum and carry pain and temperature information. The lateral spinothalamic tract is located in the lateral and ventral portion of the tegmentum. As sections proceed more rostrally, the spinothalamic tract courses a bit more medially and joins the medial lemniscus in the far rostral pons–lower midbrain region. The medial lemniscus is located more medially in the ventral pontine tegmentum. Fibers from the descending tract of V synapse in the nucleus of the tract of V; axons from the spinal trigeminal nucleus then project ventromedially, cross the median raphe, and become associated with the contralateral medial lemniscus and spinothalamic tracts and ultimately ascend to the ventral posteromedial nucleus of the thalamus.[31] Lesions of the ventrolateral pontine tegmentum causally cause loss of pain and temperature sensation in the ipsilateral face and contralateral body and limbs. Lesions in the very rostral pons in the ventrolateral tegmentum cause a contralateral loss of sensibility in the face, arm, leg and trunk for all sensory modalities. The location of the facial nuclei, vestibular nuclei, and cerebellar peduncles are also noted in Figure 19.2.

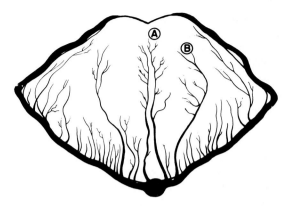

**Figure 19.3.** Artist's drawing of injected arteries from Stephens and Stillwell. (A) Paramedian penetrating arteries. (B) Penetrators from short circumferential arteries. (Drawn by Harriet Greenfield. From Stephens R, Stillwell D. Arteries and veins of the human brain. Springfield, IL: Charles C. Thomas, 1969. With permission.)

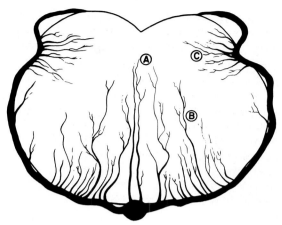

**Figure 19.4.** Artist's drawing from Stephens and Stillwell. (A) Paramedian penetrators. (B) Short circumferential arteries. (C) Penetrators from long circumferential arteries. (Drawn by Harriet Greenfield. From Stephens R, Stillwell D. Arteries and veins of the human brain. Springfield, IL: Charles C Thomas, 1969. With permission.)

The anatomical distribution of the major pontine arteries was worked out by Duret[35] and later, by Foix[36–38] and Stopford.[39–40] The distribution of the arteries is very well shown in the atlas of Stephens and Stillwell.[41] Paramedian branches (labeled A on Figure 19.3 and 19.4) penetrate directly from the basilar artery and are larger than the other penetrating vessels. Short penetrators course more laterally (marked B on Figures 19.3 and 19.4) and run parallel to the median arteries. Lateral penetrating arteries (C in Figure 19.4) arise from the long circumferential arteries, such as the anterior inferior cerebellar artery (AICA), and supply the lateral tegmentum in the midpons. These vessels run perpendicular to the median penetrators. All of these penetrating arteries are susceptible to damage by hypertension. Hemorrhages occur in the distribution of these arteries and are shown diagrammatically on Figure 19.5.

## Pathology

The only pontine hematomas that have been extensively studied are the larger lesions in the middle of the pons. These lesions derive from the large paramedian penetrating arteries, which are probably at least twice the diameter of lateral and dorsal penetrating branches. Clearly, we have more anatomical data on this group because of their tendency to cause a fatal outcome. Figures 19.6 to 19.9 demonstrate examples of such large hemato-

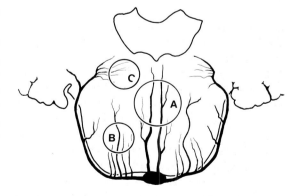

**Figure 19.5.** Artist's drawing of location of pontine hemorrhages. (A) Large central circle is paramedian hematoma. (B) Lateral basal hematoma. (C) Lateral tegmental hematoma. (Drawn by Harriet Greenfield.)

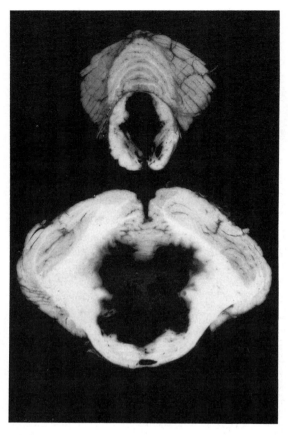

**Figure 19.6.** Massive pontine hematoma (bottom section) with spread to midbrain (upper section). Note lesion partially spares the base of the pons and dissects into IVth ventricle. The tegmentum is destroyed.

mas. Nakajima described the necropsy findings in thirty-eight patients with fatal pontine hemorrhages.[42] Figure 19.10 is from this report and diagrams the location and size of the hemorrhage in twenty-four cases.[42] The hematomas were located mostly in the mid-portion of the pons and virtually always involved the tegmentum bilaterally. The base was also frequently involved but no case involved only the base without tegmental spread. Often, the lesion was asymmetrical, affecting one side more than the other. Many of the lesions (twenty-one of twenty-four) broke into the fourth ventricle, but rupture through the pial surface at the base with spread to the clivus was less common (four of twenty-four). Spread rostrally to the midbrain was found in about half the patients, while downward dissection to the medulla occurred in only one patient. In other large series, the necropsy findings have been identical to those described by Nakajima.[10,12,13,17] In one autopsy series of fatal medial hematomas, the volume of the hematomas varied between 2.4 and 97 ml, with an average of 28.1 ml.[43]

There have been very few autopsies on patients with lateral tegmental hemorrhages. In a case discussed in the clinicopathological conferences of the Massachusetts General Hospital, the patient had a hemorrhage in

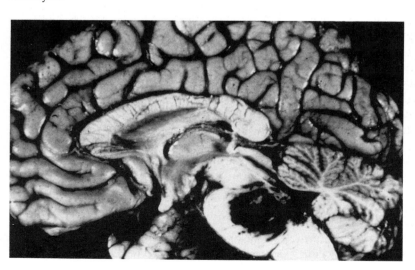

**Figure 19.7.** Large pontine hemorrhage. Sagittal section shows lesion involves the tegmentobasal junction and dissects into the fourth ventricle. Lesion similar to that depicted by Gowers (Figure 19.1) but more caudally placed in the pons.

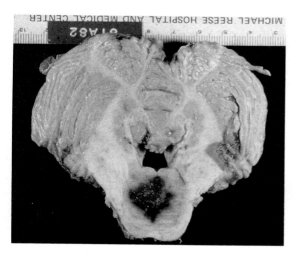

**Figure 19.8.** Paramedian pontine hematoma. Lesion is smaller than that shown in Figures 19.6 and 19.7. No dissection into the fourth ventricle is present.

the right pontine tegmentum that extended over the entire length of the pons for a distance of about 3 cm.[16] The lesion crossed the midline to destroy the left MLF. The lesion was slit-like anteriorly, but enlarged posteriorly and, at the level of the facial nerve, it involved the entire right tegmentum and extended partially into the base. Similar specimens have been briefly noted in the series of Dinsdale[13] and Silverstein.[17] A patient reported by Caplan and Goodwin[15] (Figure 19.11) had a large lesion that was almost entirely limited to the right pontine and mesencephalic tegmental regions. The lesion was predominantly lateral but approached the midline. The hematoma extended into the brachium pontis where it had a shape resembling a bat with wings spread.

Large unilateral paramedian pontine hemorrhages that involve the base and tegmentum have occasionally been reported,[17,43,44] but most case reports of asymmetrical basal or tegmentobasal lesions causing hemiparesis or unilateral motor signs have had only clinical-neuroimaging verification. Figure 19.5 is an artist's diagram showing the location of the most common loci for pontine hemorrhages. Figure 19.12, from Kushner and

Bressman's series, shows the location of their ten hematomas diagnosed by CT.[45] Cases 5 to 10 are large medial tegmentobasal lesions, case 4 is a paramedian tegmentobasal hemorrhage, and cases 1 to 3 are lateral tegmental hematomas.

## Clinical Features

Because of the disparity of symptoms and signs in hematomas at different pontine sites, we will review the clinical findings by location of bleeding.

### Large Middle-of-the-Pons Hematomas

These lesions are the best known and most commonly reported variety. In the large he-

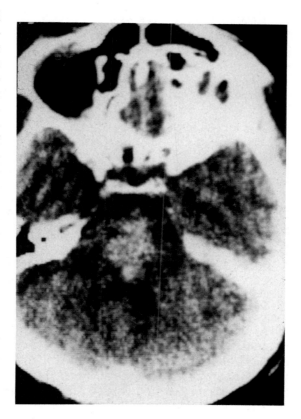

**Figure 19.9.** CT showing massive pontine hematoma with spread to the fourth ventricle.

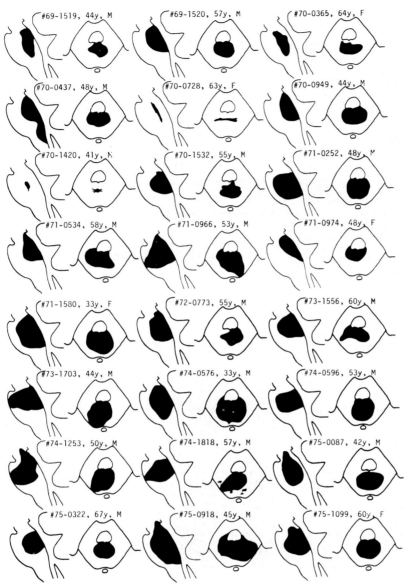

**Figure 19.10.** The size and extension of twenty-four autopsied cases of pontine hematomas (From Nakajima K. Clinicopathological study of pontine hemorrhage. Stroke 1983;14:485–493. With permission.)

matomas, *decrease in the level of alertness* is almost always found. In autopsy series the frequency of *coma* is very high. In one series of eighteen fatal hematomas, four patients were stuporous and fourteen were comatose.[43] In the series from which CT lesions are depicted in Figure 19.12, all six patients with large tegmentobasal medial hematomas (cases 5 to 10) were comatose.[45] Coma sometimes developed after presentation. Nakajima mentioned two patients in whom coma developed three hours after onset and in two the coma developed between three and twenty-four hours.[42] Coma is a very bad prognostic sign. In most series, all comatose patients die or are left very severely disabled.

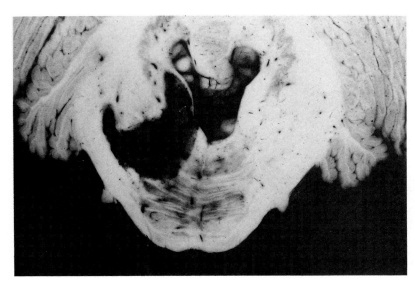

A

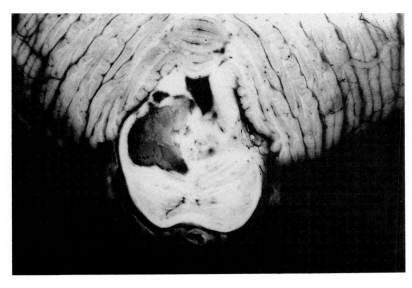

B

**Figure 19.11.** Lateral tegmental pontine hematoma (A) The most caudal section shows hematoma spreading in a scythe shape into the brachium pontis. Some lateral pressure on fourth ventricle. (B) Lesion in more rostral pons. (C) Lesion at midbrain level. Note only most dorsal part of the basis pontis is involved in A and B sections. (From Caplan LR, Goodwin JA. Lateral tegmental brainstem hemorrhages. Neurology 1982;32:252–260, with permission.)

Occasionally, patients remain alert despite severe eye movement abnormalities and imaging tests that indicate bilateral tegmental hemorrhage. One reported patient had bilateral horizontal and vertical gaze palsies but retained alertness.[46] One of us (LRC) has seen another patient with pontine hemorrhage who was alert, but had bilateral horizontal gaze paresis.

*Motor Abnormalities*

Virtually all patients with large tegmentobasal hemorrhages have bilateral abnormal

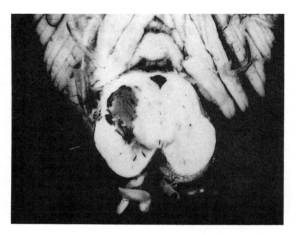

C

**Figure 19.11.** continued

limb motor function. Quadriplegia with stiffness of all limbs is the most common pattern found in large series. A hemiplegic onset has occasionally been described. In the series of Goto et al.[43] four of fifteen patients had hemiplegia but only three of twenty-eight of Silverstein's cases[17] with bilateral hemorrhages had hemiplegia. Even when hemiplegia is present, the limbs on the opposite side have exaggerated reflexes and a Babinski sign. Coma makes assessment of strength difficult; assessment is often based on tone, reflex functions, and the plantar responses. Unusual spontaneous motor movements are

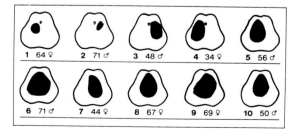

**Figure 19.12.** Diagrammatic figures of the locations of the pontine hematomas in their ten patients. (From Kushner M, Bressman S. The clinical manifestations of pontine hemorrhage. Neurology 1985;35:637–643, with permission.)

common in patients with pontine hematomas. These may take the form of brief shaking tremors, shivering, and dystonic postures. Sudden stiffening may give the false impression of convulsive movement. Decerebrate movements are common and may occur spontaneously or after painful stimuli. Decerebrate posturing was noted in twelve of fifteen patients in the series of Goto et al.[43] Five of the six patients with large tegmentobasal hematomas in the Kushner and Bressman series had "decerebrate and decorticate posturing."[45] The anatomical location of the lesion interrupting pontocerebellar pathways in the basis pontis would predict that limb ataxia might also be present. Ataxia however, has not been described in these patients, because the severity of the paralysis and decreased alertness make the testing of voluntary coordinated movement impossible.

*Cranial Nerve Dysfunction*

Weakness of the face, pharynx, palate, and tongue is nearly invariable in the larger hemorrhages. Even those that remain entirely tegmental destroy the corticobulbar fibers projecting to the bulbar motor cranial nerve nuclei. Formal testing is difficult in comatose patients. Puffing of the cheeks with expiration, decreased eyelid tone, and pooling of secretions in the oropharynx are observed. Patients with asymmetrical hematomas have often had a unilateral facial weakness of the lower motor neuron type, sometimes with a contralateral hemiplegia. Deafness or sudden decrease in hearing, dizziness with vertigo, and numbness of the face are also common symptoms in the early stages of development of the hematoma. Goto et al. studied one patient who complained of taste abnormalities while convalescing from a pontine hemor-rhage.[47] They found there was taste loss on the side of the tongue ipsilateral to the hemorrhage, and at necropsy the neurons and fibers in the solitary tract were decreased in number on the side of the lesion.[47] The tractus solitarius projects rostrally in pathways that course through the pontine tegmental region, possibly near the medial lemniscus.

### Ocular and Eye Movement Abnormalities

All authors have emphasized the presence of bilateral small, sometimes pinpoint pupils that react to light. Anisocoria is sometimes found and was present in thirteen of forty-four (30%) of the fatal cases described by Nakajima.[42] The eyes are most often midline and conjugate at rest but can be deviated inward. Skewing is sometimes seen in asymmetric hemorrhage. Bilateral horizontal conjugate gaze paresis is most often present because of involvement of the PPRF, the so-called pontine lateral gaze center, on each side. Usually both voluntary and reflex horizontal eye movements are lost. Neither ice water nor oculocephalic stimuli produce horizontal movement but can induce vertical movement or bobbing. In some patients in whom the lesion is predominantly in the basis pontis, reflex eye movements are preserved.[44] Patients with asymmetric tegmental hemorrhages may have a unilateral conjugate gaze paresis, usually to the side of the lesion, or more often have a "one-and-a-half syndrome"[34] also called "paralytic pontine exotropia."[32] These terms are used to describe an ipsilateral conjugate gaze palsy plus an abnormality of adduction when the patient looks to the opposite side, often with nystagmus of the abducting eye. One eye deviates only laterally while the other eye can not move either horizontally to the right or to the left. "Ocular bobbing" is another phenomenon often seen in patients with pontine hemorrhage. Bobbing is a term introduced by Fisher to describe sudden, brisk, conjugate ocular depression followed after a few seconds by a slower return to a midposition.[48] Bobbing can be asymmetric and even unilateral, being present on the side of the more severe paralysis of the abducting eye. Sometimes the downward eye movement is slower, and so it has been called dipping. Bobbing or dipping are probably explained by preserva-

tion of vertical gaze centers in the rostral midbrain and diencephalon while horizontal gaze centers (PPRF, sixth nerve nuclei, MLF) are damaged. Downward movement occurs when horizontal movement is lost.

### Respiratory Abnormalities

Early writers described frequent abnormalities of respiration in patients with large pontine hematomas. Steegmann described inspiratory gasps of apneustic respiration, Cheyne-Stokes patterns, slow and labored respirations, gasping, and apnea.[10] Two-thirds of his seventeen patients had apnea or another severe respiratory abnormality. Among Nakajima's forty-three fatal pontine hematomas, 86% had respiratory abnormalities on admission.[42] Respirations are often irregular.

### Hallucinations

Hallucinations were not mentioned prominently by early writers but have been reported in more recent series of hematomas involving the tegmentum. In Nakajima's series, eight patients had visual hallucinations.[42] Often the descriptions were colorful and vivid and included a green coat, colored kettle and bucket, two white dogs, and the landscape of the neighborhood.[42] Other patients have bizarre illusions, such as "a white and black serpent moving on the wall of the building" and a "woman in a black dress standing on a grave." Patients with involvement of the reticular activating system in the midbrain and thalamus have had similar hallucinations, often referred to as peduncular hallucinations.[49,50] The mechanism of the hallucinatory experience probably relates to dysfunction of the reticular formation in the pontine tegmentum.

### Abnormal Sweating

Abnormal sweating (decreased sweating or anhydrosis, or increased sweating) has also been described.[42] *Hyperthermia* sometimes over 40°C is common terminally in fatal cases, but is unusual in patients who are not comatose.

### Gastrointestinal Bleeding

Nakajima also commented on the unusual frequency of gastrointestinal bleeding.[42] Nine of his patients had gastrointestinal hemorrhages during the first week, three during the second week, and two later.[42]

### Survival Time

Massive pontine hematomas are always fatal but death does not come instantly. Steegmann had no deaths in less than two hours among his seventeen patients.[10] Death usually occurred between twenty-four and forty-eight hours in older series.[44] But now, longer survival is common and depends on the vigor of nursing and supportive care, the early use of respiratory assistance, and the presence of complications. Longer survival is especially common in patients with pontine vascular malformations who have had intermittent bleeding. Some of these patients have had surgical drainage.[51–53] CT shows large hemorrhages in the brainstem often spreading to the fourth ventricle (see Figure 19.9).

### Unilateral Basal or Tegmentobasal Paramedian Hemorrhages

Unilateral hematomas remain exclusively or predominantly to one side of the midline. The larger hematomas probably also start more to one side, but spread across the midline instead of in a dorsal-ventral direction. In the series of Goto et al., the authors concluded that all tegmental hematomas were "always localized on one side of the tegmentum."[43] Extension then occurred to the opposite side, and sometimes into the fourth ventricle, rostrally towards the midbrain, and occasionally, but not often, to the base or caudally toward the medulla.[43] Small lesions could, of course, remain confined to the paramedian base or tegmentum. There are then three categories of paramedian unilateral lesions: purely basal, entirely tegmental, and tegmentobasal.

The lesions that occupy the base or basotegmental junction closely mimic lacunar syndromes. Fisher wrote that "the conclusion must be drawn that the same type of hypertensive vascular disease, under some circumstances evokes ischemia and under others leads to bleeding."[54] Lipohyalinotic changes in the arteries that penetrate directly paramedially or from short circumferentials cause lacunar infarction. Degenerative changes in these same arteries can lead to hypertensive bleeding. Hemorrhages in these paramedian loci are probably on average larger than the average lacuna, but the clinical picture is nearly identical. Gobernado et al. reported a 45-year-old hypertensive woman who awakened with an occipital headache and a right hemiplegia.[25] The right limbs were flaccid and plegic. The face and speech articulation were normal. CT showed a tiny hematoma in the most anterior left side of the lower pons. The syndrome conformed to pure motor hemiplegia. The only clinical clue that the lesion might not be ischemic was the headache at onset. In a letter to the editor of *Stroke*, Kameyama et al. described two patients with pure motor hemiplegia caused by small basal paramedian pontine hematomas.[26] Both patients had severe hemiplegia. Dysarthria was present in both (but in one had possibly antedated the stroke), but only one had facial weakness on the side of the hemiparesis. Both patients were alert and headache was not mentioned.

Three reports described patients with ataxic hemiparesis due to small unilateral pontine hemorrhages.[27–29] Kobatake and Shinohara described two patients; each had dysarthria, slight weakness of the arm and leg on one side, a unilateral Babinski sign, and ataxia and incoordination of the weak limbs.[27] One of the patients also had "occipital heaviness" and nausea at onset. Each had paramedian small hematomas in the dorsal part of the basis pontis, one in the rostral pons and the other at the junction of the upper and middle part of the pons.[27] Schnapper's patient also had a dull occipital headache at onset; ataxia of the hemiparetic left limbs, Babinski sign, and nystagmus were noted.[28] The responsible lesion was a small hematoma in the midpons in the dorsal part of the basis pontis. Ambrosetto's patient also had sudden onset of an ataxic right hemiparesis following occipital heaviness and nausea.[29] Nystagmus was found on right gaze, dysarthria was present, and the right side of the face was also involved. The additional feature not noted in other ataxic hemiparesis cases was an ipsilateral decrease in sensation on the left side of the face and a diminished left corneal response. The lesion was in the rostral basis pontis.

Although Tuhrim et al. classified their patient's signs as the dysarthria–clumsy hand syndrome, it conforms better to the ataxic hemiparesis category.[30] This patient's symptoms also began with headache. He vomited once. His left arm and leg were slightly weak and dysmetric, and the left plantar response was extensor. CT showed a right-sided small pontine hematoma in the dorsal basis pontis. The only perhaps distinguishing features in these patients with hematomas and "lacunar syndromes" were the presence of occipital headache or "heaviness," and nausea or vomiting. Headache and vomiting are not common in patients with lacunar infarcts.[55]

Hematomas limited to the paramedian tegmentum have only rarely been reported. Graveleau et al. described the case of a 61-year-old hypertensive woman who noted after coition that her right hand and foot felt abnormal.[21] Within minutes, the abnormal sensation spread to the right side of the face and body. There was also a slight ataxia of the right leg and dystonic posturing of the right arm. She had reduced position sense on the right and also had abnormal stereognosis, two-point discrimination, and ability to localize tactile stimuli in her right hand, but temperature sensibility was preserved. MRI showed a very small hematoma in the location of the medial lemniscus in the left paramedian pontine tegmentum near the junction of the basis pontis in the caudal pons.[21] Hitchings et al. reported a single patient with a small hematoma in the left dorsal midpontine tegmentum extending from the midline towards the lateral tegmentum.[56] This patient was hypertensive and sought medical attention for the sudden onset of diplopia. The abnormal findings were limited to a left "one-and-a-half" syndrome[34] with a right exotropia. There were no motor or sensory abnormalities. He recovered completely in two months.

Unilateral tegmentobasal hematomas occur but also have been infrequently reported. Cases 3 and 4 of Kushner and Bressman (see Figure 19.12) had rather large unilateral tegmentobasal lesions that were paramedian but spread to the lateral tegmentum.[45] Case 3 had dysarthria, anisocoria with the right pupil smaller, one-and-a-half syndrome with only left abduction preserved, right facial palsy, decreased right facial sensation, diminished hearing on the right, and a left hemiplegia. Pain sensation was said to be reduced on the right body. Case 4 had her hemorrhage develop when she had malignant hypertension with papilledema and bilateral sixth nerve palsies. She had a right pontine hemorrhage with decreased sensation on the right side of the face, right facial palsy and a left hemiplegia. One of the cases described by Kase et al. under the title "Partial pontine hematomas" was a left tegmentobasal hematoma.[19] That hypertensive man had a one-and-a-half syndrome, occular bobbing, left facial palsy, right hemiplegia, and severe right hemisensory loss. The cardinal clinical signs in patients with unilateral tegmentobasal hematomas are crossed cranial nerve signs and hemiplegia.

### Lateral Pontine Tegmental Hematomas

Lateral pontine tegmental hemorrhages presumably arise from rupture of small arteries that penetrate into the dorsolateral tegmentum from long circumferential arteries. In

1982, Caplan and Goodwin reported three patients with lateral tegmental hemorrhages and reviewed the seven prior reports.[15] The major clinical features of the ten reported patients were enumerated.

*Neurological Signs*

Anisocoria with ipsilateral pupil smaller and bilaterally small reactive pupils were the most common abnormalities. Defects in *ocular motility* included ipsilateral conjugate gaze palsy (eight of ten), internuclear ophthalmoplegia (seven of ten, five of whom also had a conjugate gaze palsy to conform to the one-and-a-half syndrome), ipsilateral sixth nerve palsy (two of ten), defective upward gaze (three of ten), and ocular bobbing (three of ten). In two, the bobbing was limited to the ipsilateral eye on gaze to the ipsilateral side. *Hemiparesis* contralateral to the hemorrhage was usually slight and transient. More prominent was a *severe loss of all sensory modalities in the contralateral side of the face and body*. The lesion nearly always involved the sensory lemniscus in the rostral pons. Some patients had other cranial nerve signs including decreased hearing (three of ten), dysarthria (five of ten), dysphagia (three of ten), and decreased ipsilateral facial sensation or absent corneal reflex (three of ten). Case 2 of Kase et al.,[19] cases 1 and 2 of Kushner and Bressman,[45] and case 1 of Sharpe et al.[32] conform to the clinical syndrome described by Caplan and Goodwin.[15]

More recently there have been occasional case reports of patients with smaller lateral tegmental hematomas, verified by CT or MRI, who have had much more limited sensory syndromes. Veerapen reported the case of a 70-year-old woman, recently hypertensive, who noted suddenly numbness in the right side of the face and an unsteady gait.[24] Examination showed only decrease in light touch and pin perception on the right side of the face, absent right corneal reflex, and cerebellar-type incoordination of the right limbs. On CT, a small hematoma was seen in the lateral pons that extended into the right

trigeminal nerve root. Holtzman et al. described a 45-year-old man who awoke with numbness in his entire right side of the face, scalp, tongue, and a portion of the auricle.[23] Examination was normal except for decreased trigeminal sensation. CT showed bleeding from a small AVM in the right dorsolateral pontine tegmentum near the middle cerebellar peduncle.

Araga et al. also reported two patients with small lateral tegmental hemorrhages with primarily sensory symptoms, in one corresponding to sensory dysesthesias on one side of the body and in the other predominantly in the face.[22] Kim and Jo reported a patient with a very small right pontine lateral tegmental hematoma with a selective loss of touch, vibration sense, and position sense in the left limbs. Clinically, this patient's only symptoms were left paresthesias and left limb ataxia.[57] Limited syndromes, then, of tiny lateral tegmental hemorrhages include trigeminal sensory signs ipsilaterally, contralateral facial and body sensory changes, and ipsilateral ataxia. Each sign can be seen in isolation.

### Secondary Brainstem Hemorrhages

Duret noted during the nineteenth century that many patients dying of head trauma and supratentorial masses had hemorrhages in the middle of the midbrain and pons at necropsy.[6,7] At the time of Duret, clinicians were not aware of the phenomenology of transtentorial herniation and supratentorial lesions. Transtentorial herniation and pressure cones were not discussed in detail until the middle of the twentieth century.[58–60] Fields and Halpert found seventeen pontine hemorrhages among forty-three patients with raised intracranial pressure and concluded that the secondary hemorrhages occurred when there were dynamic changes in intracranial hydrodynamics.[61] Later, most pathologists and investigators believed that actual distortion of the upper brainstem probably caused the secondary hematomas.[2]

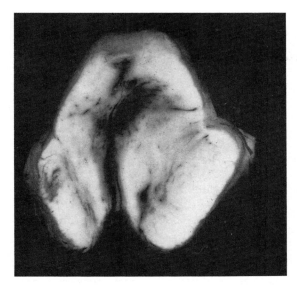

**Figure 19.13.** Duret-type secondary hemorrhage in midbrain. Lower sections also showed pontine hemorrhage.

Midline vessels were stretched or torn when the brainstem was distorted and depressed downward or from the side. Klintworth studied the development of secondary brainstem hematomas in dogs and found that their occurrence depended on the volume and rate of the expansion of the intracranial lesion.[62,63]

Secondary hemorrhages most often involve the midbrain (Figure 19.13). The hemorrhages are generally in the midline and sometimes are periaqueductal affecting the region of the third nerve nuclei. The midbrain is usually elongated and there often is an accompanying Kernohan's notch in the cerebral peduncle, indicating transtentorial pressure cone. Pontine hematomas are usually not found in the absence of midbrain lesions. The pontine lesions are also midline or paramedian and are often linear with larger components in the tegmentum near the floor of the fourth ventricle (Figure 19.14). In all cases, the clinical picture is dominated by the primary lesion. The patients are invariably comatose when the secondary hemorrhages occur. Pupillary dilatation, deeper coma, ophthalmoplegia, and decerebrate rigidity ensues. Herbstein and Schaumburg showed by radionucleide tests that secondary brainstem hemorrhages occurred shortly before death.[64] They labeled red blood cells with Chromium 51, a radionuclide marker, in patients with large hypertensive hematomas. At necropsy, the primary hematomas contained no marker radionuclide, indicating no active bleeding, but the Duret brainstem hemorrhages did contain the radionuclide, indicating that they had bled very recently.[64]

Secondary brainstem and pontine hematomas are probably quite common. Their occurrence was studied in one necropsy series of

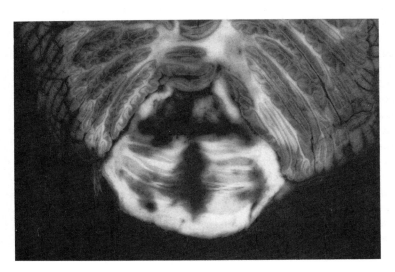

**Figure 19.14.** Duret-type pontine hemorrhages symmetrically placed in the tegmentum and midline of the base in a linear pattern.

435 cases of recent cerebral hemorrhage, brain infarction, or subarachnoid hemorrhage due to aneurysmal rupture.[65] Hemorrhages in the brainstem were most often found in patients with cerebral hemorrhage (45%), compared with aneurysmal rupture (36%) and brain infarcts (15%). Among the patients with ICH, the median survival time was two days and Duret hemorrhages were significantly more frequent during the first forty-eight hours after onset.[65] In an earlier study, Cohen and Aronson had found a frequency of Duret hemorrhages of 57% in fatal supratentorial hemorrhage patients.[66]

### Vascular Malformations

Vascular malformations of all types, arteriovenous malformations (AVM), cavernous angiomas, telangiectasias, and venous angiomas, are common in the pons. The clinical picture is sufficiently different from that found in hypertensive hemorrhages and secondary Duret hemorrhages to warrant separate discussion. Bleeding from pontine vascular malformations occurs most often in childhood.[67–69] There usually is an acute onset, most often with cranial nerve symptoms. Diplopia, ophthalmoplegia, facial weakness, facial pain or numbness, tinnitus, and ataxia are common presenting symptoms. Often there is accompanying headache and a stiff neck. The spinal fluid may or may not be bloody depending on whether the lesion drains into the fourth ventricle. Most often the lesions are tegmental and they are usually asymmetric. CT usually shows some increased density on noncontrast scans. Fresh blood, large well-circumscribed calcifications, or diffuse or punctate calcifications can be seen.[70] MRI better delineates the extent of the lesion and may show flow voids representing draining vessels. The lesions often have mass effect and can bulge into the fourth ventricle. Contrast enhancement on CT is often minimal. The lesions are usually not visualized on angiography and so have been labeled cryptic.[69,70] Capillary telangiec-tasias and cavernous angiomas do not opacify on angiography but the latter can usually be correctly diagnosed by MRI. AVMs do, however, fill and opacify on angiography.[71] In AVMs the bulk of the tangle of vessels can lie in the cisterns around the brainstem or in the cerebellopontine angle,[71] or the majority of the lesion can be embedded in the brainstem with irrigation by small feeding arteries. Often, the detection of unusual draining veins is a major clue to the presence of a vascular malformation.

The course of the lesions is very heterogenous. Many young adults have a fluctuating, relapsing, and remitting course very reminiscent of multiple sclerosis.[70,72,73] In one striking case, the patient had fluctuating signs and symptoms during a period of more than 50 years.[74] This patient's first symptoms were left facial palsy and later left ear hearing loss beginning at about age 20. At age 43 he noted difficulty telling hot and cold on the right side of the body and the right limbs. Later he became ataxic and developed dysarthria. He died of a myocardial infarct at age 77. At necropsy, the vascular malformation involved the left cerebellum and left pons and medulla mostly in the tegmentum. There was abundant evidence of old hemorrhages.[74] At times, the course is gradually progressive closely simulating pontine glioma.[52,68,70,75] Surgical drainage of the lesions is possible and recently, with the diagnostic help of MRI and the use of the dissecting microscope at surgery, operative treatment has become more common.[52,53,71] Cavernous angiomas and telangiectasias can be removed along with drainage of the hematomas. Even large AVMs involving the cisterns of the posterior fossa can be successfully removed.[71]

Curiously, in one reported case[75] and in a personal case of one of the authors (LRC), striking vertical pendular eye movements developed after recovery from a pontine tegmental hemorrhage due to an AVM. The eye movements were continuous and involved large excursion slow vertical movements. In one patient, rhythmic palatal myoclonus was also present and seemed to be synchronous with the eye movements. We have not seen this reported in hematomas not due to vascular malformations.

## Prognosis

The outlook for survival varies greatly with the site and size of the hemorrhage. Bilateral extension into the medial pontine tegmentum is a poor prognostic sign since in this region are the ascending reticular formation fibers that relate to state of consciousness. Bilateral medial tegmental destruction causes coma. Large basotegmental paramedian hematoma patients seldom survive. Occasionally, patients with large median hemorrhages that partially spare the tegmentum on one side will survive with a severe motor handicap. Occasionally, patients with bilateral tegmental disease will survive. Payne et al. presented a patient with complete horizontal ophthalmoplegia and ocular bobbing whose clinical signs and hemorrhage on CT resolved almost completely.[76] That patient remained alert despite the ophthalmoplegia, so that reticular formation fibers must have been spared despite the bilaterality of the lesion. One of the authors (LRC) has encountered a similar patient with alertness despite ophthalmoplegia who survived well. Patients with unilateral hemorrhages in the basis pontis or in the paramedian tegmentum and base frequently survive, often with residual hemiparesis. Patients with unilateral lateral tegmental pontine hematomas generally survive, at times without disabling handicaps. The advent of MRI and stereotactically guided neurosurgery has now made it possible to drain some of the hematomas and this has been done effectively, mostly in patients with AVMs near the fourth ventricle.

## References

1. Cheyne J. Cases of apoplexy and lethargy: with observations upon the comatose diseases. London: T Underwood, 1812.

2. Thompson RK, Salcman M. Brain stem hemorrhage: historical perspective. Neurosurgery 1988;22:623–628.

3. Dana CL. Acute bulbar paralysis due to hemorrhage and softening of the pons and medulla: with reports of cases and autopsies. Med Rec 1903;64:361–374.

4. Gowers WR. A Manual of Diseases of the Nervous System. Second Edition. Vol. II. London: Churchill, 1893;395.

5. Oppenheim H. Trattato della Malattie Nervose. Vol. II. Milan: S.E.I., 1905.

6. Duret H. Études expérimentales et cliniques sur les traumatismes cérébraux in Academie des Sciences. Arts et Belle Lettres de Caën. Paris: Delahage, 1878.

7. Duret H. Traumatismes cranio cérébraux. Paris: Librairie Felix Alcan, 1919.

8. Attwater H. Pontine hemorrhages. Guy's Hosp Rep 1911;65:339–389.

9. Dill LV, Isenhour CE. Etiologic factors in experimentally produced pontile hemorrhages. Arch Neurol Psychiat 1939;41:1146–1152.

10. Steegmann AT. Primary pontine hemorrhage: with particular reference to respiratory failure. J Nerv Ment Dis 1951;114:35–65.

11. Környey S. Rapidly fatal pontile hemorrhage: clinical and anatomic report. Arch Neurol Psychiat 1939;41:793–799.

12. Fang HCH, Foley JM. Hypertensive hemorrhages of the pons and cerebellum. Trans Am Neurol Assoc 1954;79:126–130.

13. Dinsdale HB. Spontaneous hemorrhage in the posterior fossa: a study of primary cerebellar and pontine hemorrhages with observations on their pathogenesis. Arch Neurol 1964;10:200–217.

14. Fisher CM. Clinical syndromes in cerebral hemorrhage. In: Fields WS, ed. Pathogenesis and treatment of cerebrovascular Disease. Springfield, IL: Charles C. Thomas 1961;318–342.

15. Caplan LR, Goodwin JA. Lateral tegmental brainstem hemorrhages. Neurology 1982;32:252–260.

16. Tyler HR, Johnson P. Case records of the Massachusetts General Hospital (Case 36—1972). N Engl J Med 1972;287:506–512.

17. Silverstein A. Primary pontine hemorrhage. In: Vinken PJ, Bruyn GW, eds. Handbook of Clinical Neurology. Vol. 12. Vascular diseases of the nervous system. Part II. Amsterdam: North Holland, 1972;37–53.

18. Müller HR, Wüthrich R, et al. The contribution of computerized axial tomography to the diagnosis of cerebellar and pontine hematomas. Stroke 1975;6:467–475.

19. Kase CS, Maulsby GO, et al. Partial pontine hematomas. Neurology 1980;30:652–655.

20. Freeman W, Ammerman HH, Stanley M. Syndromes of the pontile tegmentum. Foville's syndrome: report of three cases. Arch Neurol Psychiat 1943;50:462–471.

21. Graveleau P, DeCroix JP, Samson Y, et al. Déficit sensitive isolé d'un hemicorps par hématome du pont. Rev Neurol 1986;142:788–790.

22. Araga S, Fukada M, Kagimoto H, et al. Pure sensory stroke due to pontine hemorrhage. J Neurol 1987;235:116–117.

23. Holtzman RNN, Zablozki V, Yang WC, et al. Lateral pontine tegmental hemorrhage presenting as isolated trigeminal sensory neuropathy. Neurology 1987;37:704–706.

24. Veerapen R. Spontaneous lateral pontine hemorrhage with associated trigeminal nerve root hematoma. Neurosurgery 1989;25:451–454.

25. Gobernado JM, Fernández de Molina AR, et al. Pure motor hemiplegia due to hemorrhage in the lower pons. Arch Neurol 1980;37:393.

26. Kameyama S, Tanaka R, Tsuchida T. Pure motor hemiplegia due to pontine hemorrhage. Stroke 1989;20:1288 (letter).

27. Kobatake K, Shinohara Y. Ataxic hemiparesis in patients with primary pontine hemorrhage. Stroke 1983;14:762–764.

28. Schnapper RA. Pontine hemorrhage presenting as ataxic hemiparesis. Stroke 1982;13:518–519.

29. Ambrosetto P. Ataxic hemiparesis with contralateral trigeminal nerve impairment due to pontine hemorrhage. Stroke 1987;18:244–245.

30. Tuhrim S, Yang WC, Rubinowitz H, et al. Primary pontine hemorrhage and the dysarthria-clumsy hand syndrome. Neurology 1982;32:1027–1028.

31. Carpenter M. Core Text of Neuroanatomy. Second Edition. Baltimore: Williams & Wilkins, 1978.

32. Sharpe JA, Rosenberg MA, Hoyt WF, et al. Paralytic pontine exotropia: a sign of acute unilateral pontine gaze palsy and internuclear ophthalmoplegia. Neurology 1974;24:1076–1081.

33. Pierrot-Deseilligny C, Chain F, Serdaru M, et al. The 'one-and-a-half' syndrome: electro-oculographic analyses of five cases with deductions about the physiological mechanisms of lateral gaze. Brain 1981;104:665–699.

34. Fisher C. Some neuro-ophthalmological observations. J Neurol Neurosurg Psychiat 1967;30:383–392.

35. Duret H. Sur la distribution des artères nourricières du bulbe rachidien. Arch Physiol Norm Path 1873;5:97–114.

36. Foix C, Hillemand P. Irrigation du bulbe. CR Soc Biol (Paris) 1925;42:33–35.

37. Foix C, Hillemand P. Les artères de l'axe encéphalique jusqu'au diencéphale inclusivement. Rev Neurol 1925;41:705–739.

38. Caplan LR. Charles Foix—the first modern stroke neurologist. Stroke 1990;21:348–356.

39. Stopford JS. The arteries of the pons and medulla oblongata. Part I. J Anat Physiol 1916;50:130–164.

40. Stopford JS. The arteries of the pons and medulla oblongata. Part II. J Anat Physiol 1916;50:255–280.

41. Stephens R, Stillwell D. Arteries and veins of the human brain. Springfield, IL: Charles C Thomas, 1969.

42. Nakajima K. Clinicopathological study of pontine hemorrhage. Stroke 1983;14:485–493.

43. Goto N, Kaneko M, Hosaka Y, et al. Primary pontine hemorrhage: clinicopathological correlations. Stroke 1980;11:84–90.

44. Kase CS, Caplan LR. Hemorrhage affecting the brainstem and cerebellum. In: Barnett et al., eds. Stroke: Pathophysiology, diagnosis, and management. Vol. I. New York: Churchill-Livingstone 1986;621–641.

45. Kushner MJ, Bressman SB. The clinical manifestations of pontine hemorrhage. Neurology 1985;35:637–643.

46. Dominguez RO, Bronstein AM. Complete gaze palsy in pontine hemorrhage. J Neurol Neurosurg Psychiat 1988;51:150–151 (letter).

47. Goto N, Yamamoto T, Kaneko M, et al. Primary pontine hemorrhage and gustatory disturbance: clinicoanatomic study. Stroke 1983;14:507–511.

48. Fisher CM. Ocular bobbing. Arch Neurol 1964;11:543–546.

49. Lhermitte MJ. Syndrome de la calotte du pédoncule cérébral: les troubles psychosensoriels dans les lésions du mésocéphale. Rev Neurol 1922;38:1359–1365.

50. Caplan LR. "Top of the basilar" syndrome. Neurology 1980;30:72–79.

51. Becker DH, Silverberg GD. Successful evacuation of an acute pontine hematoma. Surg Neurol 1978;10:263–265.

52. Burns J, Lisak R, Schut L, et al. Recovery following brainstem hemorrhage. Ann Neurol 1980;7:183–184.

53. O'Laoire SA, Crockard HA, Thomas DGT, et al. Brain-stem hematoma: a report of six surgically treated cases. J Neurosurg 1982;56:222–227.

54. Fisher CM. Pathological observations in hypertensive cerebral hemorrhage. J Neuropathol Exp Neurol 1971;30:536–550.

55. Mohr JP, Caplan LR, Melski JW, et al. The Harvard Cooperative Stroke Registry: a prospective registry. Neurology 1978;28:754–762.

56. Hitchings L, Crum A, Troost BT. Isolated one-and-one-half syndrome from focal brainstem hypertensive hemorrhage: precise localization with MRI. Neurology 1988;38:1501.

57. Kim JS, Jo KD. Pure lemniscal sensory deficit caused by pontine hemorrhage. Stroke 1992;23:300–30 (letter).

58. Jefferson G. The tentorial pressure cone. Arch Neurol Psychiat 1938;40:857–876.

59. Meyer A. Herniation of the brain. Arch Neurol Psychiat 1920;4:387–400.

60. Finney L, Walker AE. Transtentorial herniation. Springfield, IL: Charles C Thomas, 1962.

61. Fields WS, Halpert B. Pontine hemorrhage in intracranial hypertension. Am J Pathol 1953;29:677–687.

62. Klintworth GK. The pathogenesis of secondary brainstem hemorrhages as studied in an experimental model. Am J Pathol 1965;47:525–536.

63. Klintworth GK. Paratentorial grooving of human brains with particular reference to transtentorial herniation and the pathogenesis of secondary brain-stem hemorrhages. Am J Pathol 1968;53:391–408.

64. Herbstein DJ, Schaumburg HH. Hypertensive intracerebral hematoma: an investigation of the initial hemorrhage and rebleeding using Chromium Cr51-labeled erythrocytes. Arch Neurol 1974;30:412–414.

65. Nedergaard M, Klinken L, Paulson OB. Secondary brain stem hemorrhage in stroke. Stroke 1983;14:501–505.

66. Cohen SI, Aronson SM. Secondary brain stem hemorrhages. Arch Neurol 1968;19:257–263.

67. Teilmann K. Hemangiomas of the pons. Arch Neurol Psychiat 1953;69:208–223.

68. Zeller RS, Chutorian AM. Vascular malformations of the pons in children. Neurology 1975;25:776–780.

69. Yeates A, Enzmann D. Cryptic vascular malformations involving the brainstem. Radiology 1983;146:71–75.

70. Stahl SM, Johnson KP, Malamud N. The clinical and pathological spectrum of brain-stem vascular malformations: long-term course simulates multiple sclerosis. Arch Neurol 1980;37:25–29.

71. Drake CG. Surgical removal of arteriovenous malformations from the brain stem and cerebellopontine angle. J Neurosurg 1975;43:661–670.

72. Britt RH, Connor WS, Enzmann DR. Occult arteriovenous malformation of the brainstem simulating multiple sclerosis. Neurology 1981;31:901–904.

73. Abroms IF, Yessayan L, Shillito J, et al. Spontaneous intracerebral haemorrhage in patients suspected of multiple sclerosis. J Neurol Neurosurg Psychiat 1971;34:157–162.

74. DeJong RN, Hicks SP. Vascular malformation of the brainstem: report of a case with long duration and fluctuating course. Neurology 1980;30:995–997.

75. Lawrence WH, Lightfoote WE. Continuous vertical pendular eye movements after brainstem hemorrhage. Neurology 1975;25:896–898.

76. Payne HA, Maravilla KR, Levinstone A, Heuter J, Tindall RSA. Recovery from primary pontine hemorrhage. Ann Neurol 1978;4:557–558.

# Chapter 20
# Cerebellar Hemorrhage

## Carlos S. Kase

Cerebellar hemorrhage treated by surgical drainage was first described by Ballance[1] in 1906. He reported the case of a 12-year-old-boy who sustained a left cerebellar hemorrhage following an episode of head trauma two months previously. He then developed headache, dizziness, vomiting, and gait ataxia, left limb ataxia, horizontal nystagmus to the left, paresis of conjugate gaze to that side and, possibly, papilledema. The patient made a good recovery after posterior fossa surgery with drainage of a left cerebellar clot. Ballance commented on several useful clinical points: he noted that the patient's dizziness was associated with a sensation of objects in the room moving across from his left to his right side; because of secondary pressure of the cerebellar hematoma on the lateral pons, he remarked on the diagnostic value of weakness of conjugate gaze and horizontal nystagmus toward the side of the lesion; he stated that in cases of cerebellar hemorrhage, the vessel most liable to rupture would be the superior cerebellar artery; finally, based on the good results achieved with surgical evacuation of the hematoma, he made a generalization about the value of surgery for "sufferers from intracranial disease." Since this concise and lucid early description of some aspects of cerebellar hemorrhage, a considerable amount of literature has been devoted to the precise delineation of the mechanisms, clinical features, and course of cerebellar hemorrhage (Figure 20.1), as well as its treatment and, more recently, the contribution of imaging studies to its diagnosis and management.

## Frequency

The frequency of cerebellar hemorrhage in autopsy series had been reported as 0.27%,[2] 0.38%,[3] and 0.44%[4] of all autopsies, and between 5% and 13% of intracranial hemor-

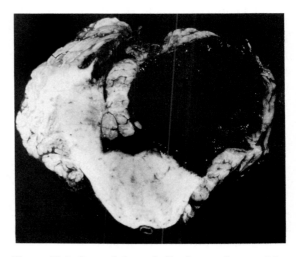

**Figure 20.1.** Large left cerebellar hemorrhage, with pressure effect on the pontine tegmentum. (Courtesy of Jorge F. Tapia, M.D., Catholic University, Santiago, Chile.)

rhages.[2-7] Mitchell and Angrist[3] found, among 3881 autopsies that yielded 151 "spontaneous intracranial hemorrhages," fifteen patients (13%) with hemorrhage in the cerebellum. These authors commented on the fact that cerebellar hemorrhage "tends to be more rapidly fatal than cerebral hemorrhage and produces a more variable clinical syndrome." A similar conclusion with regard to the low value of abnormal cerebellar findings for the diagnosis was reached by Dinsdale,[2] after analyzing fifty-two cases of fatal cerebellar hemorrhage, and by Hyland and Levy[5] in a series of thirty-one cases studied postmortem. The recurring theme of high mortality and unreliability of the clinical syndrome was common to most early autopsy series of cerebellar hemorrhage.[2-6] The latter view was even carried into clinical series, notably that of McKissock et al.,[8] which included twenty-six cases of cerebellar hemorrhage (a frequency of 8%) among a total of 308 patients with "primary" intracerebral hemorrhage (ICH), along with eight cases "due to vascular anomalies," for a total of thirty-four patients referred to their neurosurgical department. Although the analysis of their series did not contribute useful data regarding the clinical diagnosis of this condition, as they relied primarily on the results of posterior fossa imaging studies (vertebral angiography, ventriculography) for the diagnosis,[8,9] they documented the value of prompt surgical intervention by craniotomy as opposed to ventricular tapping or drainage, in improving its prognosis. Further reports of the difficulties in the clinical diagnosis of cerebellar hemorrhage (and infarction) followed into the late 1960s and mid-1970s,[10-12] prior to the widespread availability of computed tomography (CT). However, large clinical series at the time[13-15] were able to identify physical examination features that reliably allowed the clinical diagnosis of cerebellar hemorrhage, at the same time defining patterns of clinical evolution and outcome that resulted in better-defined therapeutic approaches to this condition. More recently, the introduction of CT and magnetic resonance imaging (MRI)

have made possible the immediate documentation of cerebellar hematomas, as well as the definition of a number of associated anatomical features that, in conjunction with the clinical picture, are useful in selecting the appropriate treatment, surgical or conservative, for cerebellar hemorrhage.

## Mechanism of Hemorrhage

The mechanism of cerebellar hemorrhage is considered to be predominantly hypertension, and old series[2,4,5,8,13,16] reported this cause in 60% to 90% of the cases, the remainder being attributed to vascular malformations, blood dyscrasias, or unknown mechanisms. In more modern series[7,14,15,17,18] anticoagulation and blood dyscrasias account for an increasing proportion of the cases (Figure 20.2 and Table 20.1), the former probably reflecting the current widespread use of warfarin anticoagulation in the management of vascular disease. Among the nonhypertensive causes of cerebellar hemorrhage, vascular malformations have been found in 4% to 17.5% of patients,[8,14,17,19] a condition that generally affects younger individuals,[5,14,20-22] including children,[23] as opposed to the predominant age distribution in the 60s and 70s for cases due to hypertension[2,8,14,17,19,24] (see Figure 20.2). The vascular malformations described in patients with cerebellar hemorrhage have been evenly distributed between arteriovenous and venous types,[5,20,23] and their locations appear to be random, the medially-placed lesions in the vermis and adjacent to the fourth ventricle being as common as those located more laterally in the cerebellar hemispheres. However, since the hypertensive varieties appear to originate most often in the vicinities of the dentate nucleus,[2-5,7,13,14,16] most commonly as a result of rupture of branches of the superior cerebellar artery,[1,13,16] the finding of a peripherally located hemispheric cerebellar ICH should raise the suspicion of a different mechanism,[2] especially a vascular malformation in individuals younger than age 60 (Fig-

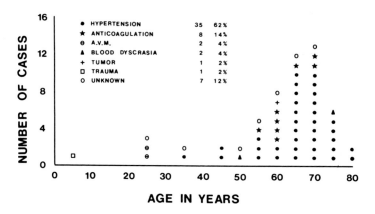

**Figure 20.2.** Mechanism and age distribution of fifty-six patients with cerebellar hemorrhage (Reprinted from Ott KH, Kase CS, Ojemann RG, et al. Cerebellar hemorrhage: diagnosis and treatment: a review of 56 cases. Arch Neurol 1974;31:160–167, with permission.)

ure 20.3). Mass lesions that cause cerebellar hemorrhage have usually been metastases,[7,17] but rare instances of hemangioblastoma[25] and even an abscess of otitic origin[26] have been described. Hemangioblastomas appear as enhancing nodules at the periphery of the acute ICH on contrast CT scan, and posterior circulation angiography shows tumor "stain" at the site of the hemispheric tumors.[25] A single patient with a hemorrhage in an area of deep cerebellar calcification has been reported,[27] in which histological examination of the biopsy specimen failed to show a causative vascular lesion, only documenting

heavy calcium deposits in vessel walls near the hematoma.

## Clinical Presentation

The clinical picture of cerebellar hemorrhage has been the subject of much interest and debate, in regard to the value and specificity of the presenting symptoms and signs for the diagnosis. In pre-CT series, the main emphasis was on the search for a combination of clinical features that would reliably diagnose cerebellar hemorrhage, allowing for

**Table 20.1.** Mechanisms of Cerebellar Hemorrhage

| Mechanism | Ott et al.[14] No. Cases (%) (N = 56) | Brennan and Bergland[15] No. Cases (%) (N = 12) | Dunne et al.[8] No. Cases (%) (N = 75) | Gilliard et al.[17]* No. Cases (%) (N = 39) |
|---|---|---|---|---|
| Hypertension | 35 (62%) | 8 (66%) | 39 (52%) | 23 (59%) |
| Anticoagulation | 8 (14%) | 3 (25%)† | 7 (9.3%) | 3 (7.5%) |
| Blood dyscrasia | 2 (4%) | — | 2 (2.7%) | — |
| Vascular malformation | 2 (4%) | — | 1 (1.3%) | 7 (18%) |
| Tumor | 1 (2%) | — | 3 (4%) | 1 (3%) |
| Trauma | 1 (2%) | — | — | — |
| Other | — | — | 1 (1.3%)‡ | 3 (7.5%) |
| Unknown | 7 (12%) | 1 (9%) | 22 (29.4%) | 6 (15%) |

*The total number of patients exceeds 39 because of combined mechanisms in four.
†Two patients on anticoagulants; a third patient had elevated PT in the setting of an intestinal malabsorption syndrome.
‡One patient (1.3%) was labeled as having cerebellar hemorrhage as a result of cerebral embolism.

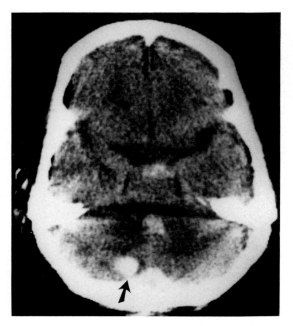

A

**Figure 20.3.** Peripheral hemispheric cerebellar hemorrhage due to ruptured vascular malformation. (A) CT scan without contrast showing small, peripherally located left cerebellar hemorrhage (arrow), and blood in the fourth and third ventricles. (B) Pathology specimen with acute left paravermian hemispheric hemorrhage. (C) Histological section with multiple dilated, malformed sulcal and pial blood vessels, with both arterial (long arrow) and venous (short arrows) components, corresponding to an arteriovenous malformation. (H&E, ×25.)

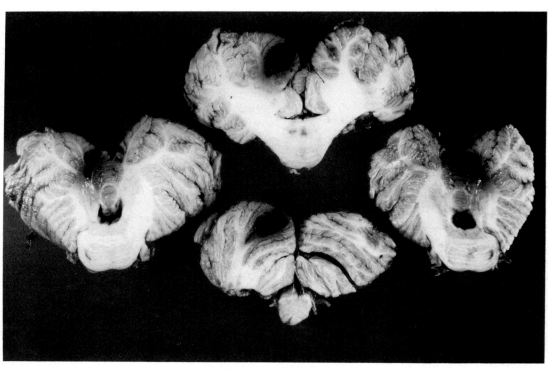

B

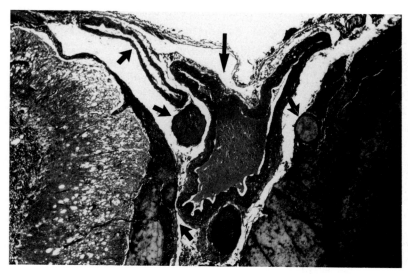

C

prompt selection of patients for emergency surgical therapy, without the concern about delaying proper treatment while performing time-consuming imaging studies.[13-15] Since the introduction of CT in the mid-1970s, prompt diagnosis has been greatly facilitated, and the focus of early evaluation has shifted to the use of imaging and clinical data in combination for the early selection of patients for either surgical or nonsurgical management.[28-32]

The characteristic *symptoms at onset* of cerebellar hemorrhage include headache, vertigo, vomiting, and inability to stand and walk. Headache is reported by about 60% to 75% of the patients,[7,14,18,19,24] and is generally described as bilateral occipital or frontal in location, although occasional examples of localized ocular or retro-ocular pain ipsilateral to the hemorrhage[14] cause initial diagnostic difficulties. The following example illustrates this unusual type of headache in the setting of an otherwise minimally symptomatic cerebellar hemispheric hemorrhage:

A 69-year-old man with a history of alcoholism presented to the emergency room because of left occipital pain radiating to his left eye. He had been well until the previous afternoon,

when he had the sudden onset of sharp pain in the left occipital area with radiation into the left orbit, described as "pain behind and around the eye." He denied associated nausea, vomiting, loss of consciousness, visual symptoms, or weakness. Upon awakening the next day he had persistent headache in the same location, and complained of nausea and of being unsteady on his feet. On arrival in the Emergency Room, he was alert and oriented, with intact speech, horizontal nystagmus in both directions of gaze, full abduction of both eyes, and limited adduction OS. There was no limb weakness, and sensory examination was normal. He had no dysmetria or dysdiadochokinesis. No gait ataxia was present, but he felt unsteady, and he had difficulty performing tandem gait. The plantar reflexes were flexor bilaterally.

Head CT showed a 2.5 × 3 cm area of increased attenuation consistent with hemorrhage in the inferior portion of the left cerebellar hemisphere, with slight mass effect on the fourth ventricle (Figure 20.4). Follow-up examination with detailed testing of cerebellar function revealed no changes from admission. A repeat CT scan with intravenous contrast showed no areas of enhancement. Three days after admission he had chest pain associated with trigeminy, respiratory distress, and hypotension unresponsive to pressors. He died four days after ICH onset. An autopsy was not performed.

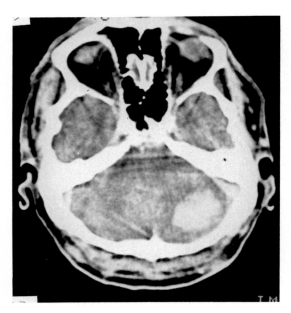

**Figure 20.4.** CT scan of left cerebellar hemorrhage, peripherally located in the hemisphere with partial obliteration of the fourth ventricle (Courtesy of James A. D. Otis, M.D., and Geoffrey L. Ahern, M.D., Boston VA Medical Center, Boston, MA.)

Frontal and orbital headache probably results from mechanical distortion of the tentorium by the hemorrhage,[10] its pattern of radiation being due to the innervation of the upper surface of this structure by recurrent fibers from the ophthalmic division of the trigeminal nerve.[33]

A more common presenting sign of cerebellar hemorrhage is vomiting, being the leading symptom in several reported series.[2,13,14,24] Vertigo is the next most common symptom, present in 40% to 60% of the cases.[7,14,18,19,24] The latter has been rarely described in detail, patients occasionally reporting rotation of the environment from affected to unaffected side,[1,14] others showing immediate vertigo and vomiting upon minimal head motion, at times vomiting clearly preceding the onset of vertigo.[34] An equally dramatic and diagnostically useful feature of cerebellar hemorrhage is the sudden development of inability to stand and walk. Fisher et al.[13] stressed the constancy of this finding in their cases, and Ott et al.[14] found it in thirty of thirty-two (93%) of their patients who were specifically questioned about this symptom. Others have reported inability to stand in about 40% of the patients,[19,24] and unsteadiness of gait in 87% of patients whose level of consciousness at presentation allowed the reporting of symptoms at onset.[7] A list of symptoms at onset of cerebellar hemorrhage is shown in Table 20.2.

The *findings on neurologic examination* in patients with cerebellar hemorrhage have generated much debate in clinical series. Fisher et al.[13] were the first to delineate the clinical features of this condition, pointing to the diagnostic value of oculomotor abnormalities, in particular ipsilateral horizontal gaze palsy

**Table 20.2.** Symptoms at Onset of Cerebellar Hemorrhage

| | Series | | |
|---|---|---|---|
| Symptom | Ott et al.[14] No. Cases (%) (N = 44) | Dunne et al.[7] No. Cases (%) (N = 48) | Gerritsen van der Hoop et al.[24] No. Cases (%) (N = 22) |
| Headache | 32 (73%) | 28 (58%) | 16 (72%) |
| Vertigo/dizziness | 24 (55%) | 30 (62%) | 13 (59%) |
| Nausea/vomiting | 42 (95%) | 33 (69%) | 17 (77%) |
| Loss of consciousness | 6 (14%) | 14 (29%) | 2 (9%) |
| Gait imbalance/inability to stand | 30/32 (93%)* | 42 (95%) | 9 (40%) |
| Dysarthria | 14 (32%) | — | 5 (22%) |

*Only 32 patients were questioned about this symptom.

and sixth nerve palsy (or "pseudopalsy"), involvement of other pontine cranial nerves, limb hemiataxia, and gait ataxia, in the absence of hemiplegia or hemiparesis. In addition, other uncommon but clinically useful signs included involuntary closure of one eye, which was subsequently shown to be either ipsilateral or contralateral to the hemorrhage,[35] and skew deviation with the ipsilateral eye being depressed.[13] Ocular "bobbing," a sign generally seen in the setting of pontine hemorrhage or infarction,[36] can occasionally occur in patients with cerebellar hemorrhage.[13,14,37] In rare instances, small cerebellar hemorrhages presenting with minimal symptoms have shown combinations of deficits characteristic of some of the "lacunar syndromes," including the "dysarthria–clumsy hand" syndrome[38] and "ataxic hemiparesis."[39] The former resulted from a small, deep paramedian cerebellar hemorrhage,[38] while the latter was due to the simultaneous occurrence of two small hemorrhages, one posterior capsular, the other a contralateral deep cerebellar hemorrhage.[39]

The clinical signs were further analyzed by Ott et al.,[14] who found a consistent clinical pattern in thirty-eight noncomatose patients admitted with cerebellar hemorrhage (Table 20.3). They documented a high frequency of cerebellar signs, including gait ataxia (78%), truncal ataxia (65%), and ipsilateral limb ataxia (65%), along with ipsilateral peripheral facial palsy (61%), horizontal gaze palsy (54%), horizontal nystagmus (51%), depressed corneal reflex (30%), and miosis (30%). Findings that were notably absent were subhyaloid hemorrhages, third or fourth nerve palsies, and hemiplegia, while hemiparesis was present in four (11%) patients, a deficit explained by cerebral hemispheric stroke in three, the paresis being only transient in the setting of cerebellar ataxia of the same limbs in the other patient. Based on these findings, they[14] suggested that the clinical triad of ipsilateral limb ataxia, horizontal gaze palsy, and peripheral facial palsy was a reliable formula for the diagnosis of cerebellar hemorrhage, since at

**Table 20.3.** Clinical Findings on Admission in Thirty-eight Noncomatose Patients with Cerebellar Hemorrhage

| Sign | No. of Cases (Sign Present/ No. Pts. Tested) | % |
|---|---|---|
| Nuchal rigidity | 14/35 | 40 |
| Dysarthria | 20/32 | 62 |
| Subhyaloid hem. | 0/34 | 0 |
| Resp. irregularity | 6/28 | 21 |
| CN abn. | | |
| 3rd, 4th n. palsy | 0/36 | 0 |
| 6th n. palsy | 10/36 | 28 |
| Corneal hyporeflexia | 10/33 | 30 |
| 7th n. palsy | 22/36 | 61 |
| Absent gag reflex | 6/30 | 20 |
| Skew deviation | 4/33 | 12 |
| Miosis | 11/37 | 30 |
| Nystagmus | 18/35 | 51 |
| Gaze palsy | 20/37 | 54 |
| Hemiparesis | 4/35 | 11 |
| Limb ataxia | 17/26 | 65 |
| Truncal ataxia | 11/17 | 65 |
| Gait ataxia | 11/14 | 78 |
| Babinski sign | 23/36 | 64 |

(From Ott KH, Kase CS, Ojemann RG, et al. Cerebellar hemorrhage: diagnosis and treatment: a review of 56 cases. Arch Neurol 1974;31:160–167. With permission.)

least two of the three signs were present in 73% of twenty-six patients who were tested for all three signs. The reliability of this syndrome was considered to be high enough to justify—in the pre-CT era—emergency surgical treatment of cerebellar hemorrhage diagnosed on clinical grounds, avoiding the performance of time-consuming radiological tests in these notoriously unstable patients.[14] Similar conclusions were reached by Brennan and Bergland's[15] analysis of their experience with twelve patients with cerebellar hemorrhage. However, other groups found such clinical data unhelpful for the clinical diagnosis of cerebellar hemorrhage.[7,12] Rosenberg and Kaufman's[12] series of thirty-three patients included thirteen who were correctly diagnosed on clinical grounds, but ten not suspected of having cerebellar hemorrhage were subsequently shown to have it ("false-negative" cases), and ten strongly suspected of having the diagnosis had other illnesses ("false-positive" cases), including ruptured aneurysms with adjacent hematoma, brainstem infarction, multiple sclerosis, and hypertensive encephalopathy. Their conclusion was that the clinical diagnosis was too unreliable to justify therapeutic decisions to be made in the absence of imaging studies that showed cerebellar hemorrhage.[12] Similarly, Dunne et al.[7] found a low clinical diagnostic accuracy of 23% in their analysis of sixty-two patients with proven cerebellar hemorrhage, the majority (58%) having been diagnosed by CT, and the remainder (19%) at autopsy. Finally, Gerritsen van der Hoop et al.[24] reached similar conclusions in the analysis of fourteen initially conscious patients with cerebellar hemorrhage, detecting only ipsilateral limb ataxia as a frequent (70%) clinical finding, whereas facial palsy (7%), gaze palsy (14%), and decreased corneal reflex (0%) were infrequent enough to be of no help in the diagnosis, which was based on CT scanning in their twenty-two patients.

## Radiological Diagnosis

In the pre-CT era, the diagnostic suspicion of cerebellar hemorrhage was generally followed by posterior fossa angiography and ventriculography which showed an avascular cerebellar mass, frequently with associated hydrocephalus.[40] Angiography revealed vascular displacements, generally of the posterior-inferior cerebellar artery and its vermian branches contralaterally, the inferior vermian veins contralaterally and posteriorly, and the ipsilateral superior cerebellar artery branches superiorly.[40] On rare occasions, ventriculography showed air filling the hematoma cavity in communication with the fourth ventricle.[41]

The sensitivity of the radiological diagnosis of cerebellar hemorrhage was dramatically changed with the introduction of CT, which permits the immediate diagnosis of

acute hemorrhage irrespective of its size (Figure 20.5), as well as the secondary effects of the hemorrhage on adjacent structures, including the ventricular system below and above the tentorium. On very rare occasions, an acute cerebellar ICH can be missed by CT because of a low hemoglobin level that results in an isodense or hypodense, rather than hyperdense, image. The hemoglobin value was 6.7 g%, with a hematocrit of 20%, in the patient with a hypodense acute cerebellar hematoma reported by Kasdon et al.[42] Except for this exceptional occurrence, CT is virtually 100% sensitive for the detection of acute ICH.

The early reporting of the value of CT in diagnosing cerebellar hemorrhage[14,29] was followed by the documentation of associated findings and their relationship to clinical course and outcome. Among the various anatomical features of cerebellar hemorrhage, the following are known to relate to clinical presentation and prognosis: (1) hematoma size, (2) hematoma location (hemispheric versus vermian), (3) presence of hydrocephalus, and (4) obliteration of the quadrigeminal cistern.

Hematoma *size* was related to outcome in the series of Little et al.,[30] who found a hematoma diameter of 3 cm or more associated with a progressive course leading to brainstem compression, whereas smaller hematomas were usually benign. The hematoma size was, in turn, directly correlated with the presence of hydrocephalus, found in all six patients with hematomas of 3 cm or more, and in none of the four with hematomas smaller than 3 cm. Similar relationships to outcome have been found with measurements of area[31] (as measured on the CT slice containing the hematoma of largest size) or volume[43] of cerebellar hematomas.

The *location* of the hematoma (Figure 20.6) has an impact on clinical presentation and prognosis: paramedian (dentate nucleus) or laterally-placed hematomas are more likely to present with the classical features of unilateral cerebellar and pontine deficits on examination, whereas midline, vermian hema-

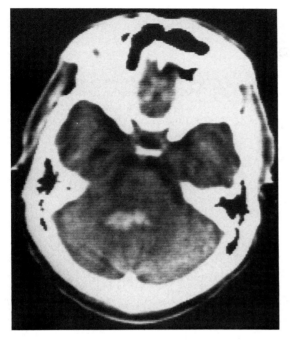

A

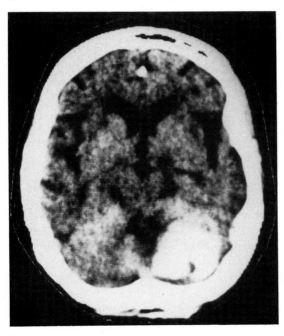

B

**Figure 20.5.** Variability in size of cerebellar hemorrhage, showing the wide spectrum between tiny examples with minimal symptomatology (A) and massive ones that involve most of the hemisphere (B).

tomas are frequently difficult to separate clinically from primary pontine hemorrhage.[14,18,44,45] The clinical and CT features of six of our patients with vermian cerebellar hemorrhage are shown in Table 20.4. These patients were generally hypertensive, and presented clinically with either the acute onset of coma or the rapid development of coma after a short period of gradually declining level of consciousness. In the latter situation, findings that preceded the onset of coma included an isolated sixth nerve palsy in one (patient D) and gait ataxia in another (patient E), but neither presented with unilateral limb ataxia, horizontal gaze palsy, or facial palsy at that stage. Pupillary size at onset was uniformly in the miotic range (1 to 2 mm) and with preservation of light reflex, becoming subsequently dilated (8 mm) and fixed in patient F after a cardiorespiratory arrest. One patient (patient A) had hyperthermia of 103°F on admission, which rose to 107°F four hours prior to death. Two patients were described as having "generalized tonic-clonic seizures," in one instance further characterized as "synchronous jerking of arms and legs" (patient A), in the setting of severe hyperthermia. The occurrence of seizure-like activity in patients with catastrophic brainstem lesions has been commented on by Ropper,[46] who reported the presence of "jerking" limb movements in patients with basilar artery occlusion and brainstem/cerebellar infarcts primarily affecting the pons, and interpreted them as accompaniments of acute decerebration rather than true convulsions. Similar phenomena are observed in pontine hemorrhage.[44]

The following example illustrates the presentation of a midline (vermian) cerebellar hemorrhage (corresponding to patient B in Table 20.4):

A 48-year-old hypertensive woman was found stuporous and lying on the floor at her home. On initial examination her blood pressure was 270/110, she was stuporous, without response to verbal stimuli, but had spontaneous movements of the limbs. The pupils were 2 to 3 mm in diameter, weakly reactive to light. Ocu-

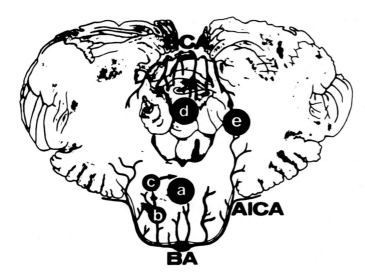

**Figure 20.6.** Sites of origin of pontine and cerebellar hemorrhage. The vermian (d) and hemispheric (e) forms of cerebellar hemorrhage and their arteries of origin are shown. Abbreviations: SCA = superior cerebellar artery, AICA = arterior-inferior cerebellar artery, BA = basilar artery. (From Kase CS, Caplan LR. Hemorrhage affecting the brainstem and cerebellum. In: Barnett HJM, Mohr JP, Stein BM, et al. (eds): Stroke: Pathophysiology, Diagnosis and Management. New York: Churchill Livingstone, 1986, with permission.)

locephalic reflexes were absent. The face moved symmetrically. The deep tendon reflexes were normal, and the plantar responses were absent. CT revealed a midline cerebellar hematoma (Figure 20.7B) with extension into the fourth ventricle, third ventricle, and frontal horns of the lateral ventricles. A slight degree of hydrocephalus was present. Following the CT she became comatose and apneic, and was intubated and started on mechanical ventilation. She was deeply comatose, without response to painful stimuli, with equal and unreactive pupils, absent oculomotor responses to the doll's eyes maneuver and ice-water calorics, and absent corneal reflexes bilaterally. She expired fourteen hours after the onset of her illness.

The six patients had generally large vermian hematomas on CT or at autopsy, invariably showing extension of the hemorrhages

**Table 20.4.** Clinical and CT Findings in Six Patients with Midline Cerebellar Hemorrhage

| | Patients | | | | | |
|---|---|---|---|---|---|---|
| Findings | A | B | C | D | E | F |
| Age/sex | 44/M | 48/F | 34/M | 67/M | 41/F | 66/F |
| BP | | | | | | |
|   History hypertension | Y | Y | N | Y | Y | Y |
|   BP on admission | 300/160 | 270/110 | 130/90 | ND | 230/140 | 180/100 |
| Type of onset | Abrupt | Abrupt | Gradual | Gradual | Gradual | Abrupt |
| Clinical features | | | | | | |
|   LOC at onset | Y | Y | N | N | N | Y |
|   Seizures | Y | N | Y | N | N | N |
|   Respiratory abn. | Y | Y | Y | Y | N | Y |
|   CN function | Absent | Absent | Absent | 6th n. palsy | Normal | Absent |
|   Decerebrate post. | Y | N | Y | N | N | Y |
|   Gait ataxia | ? | ? | ? | N | Y | ? |
| Outcome | Died | Died | Died | Died | Survived; operated | Died |

Abbreviations: M = male, F = female, Y = yes, N = no, ND = not done, BP = blood pressure, LOC = loss of consciousness, CN = cranial nerve, n. = nerve, ? = untestable, post. = posturing, abn. = abnormalities

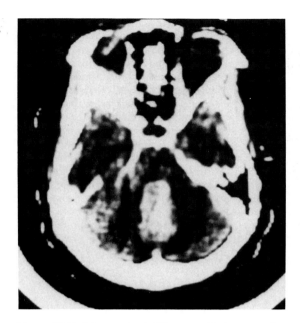

**Figure 20.7.** Noncontrast CT scan with large acute vermian cerebellar hemorrhage.

into the fourth ventricle, with either direct extension into or compression necrosis of, the dorsal aspect of the pons (Figure 20.8). These features result in these hematomas frequently being diagnosed clinically as primary pontine hemorrhages. The outcome is usually fatal, unless emergency surgery can be performed before the development of coma with signs of bilateral brainstem dysfunction (as in our patient E). The occasional patients who have an intermediate hematoma location, both vermian and paramedian in one cerebellar hemisphere, tend to behave as vermian hematomas, suggesting that they either originate in or rapidly extend into, the cerebellar vermis.

The presence of *hydrocephalus* is frequent, and has prognostic significance in cerebellar hemorrhage. It relates to both size and location of ICH, the vermian and large hemispheric hematomas showing hydrocephalus in virtually 100%,[18,31] and 70% to 90%[18,19,24,30] of the cases, respectively. Gilliard et al.[17] found hydrocephalus in four of twelve (33%) hematomas of 3.5 cm or less in diameter,

whereas eighteen of twenty-six (69%) hematomas larger than 3.5 cm had associated hydrocephalus. In addition, these authors correlated hydrocephalus with hematoma location, finding a higher frequency of it in median-paramedian hematomas (in twelve of fifteen cases, or 80%), as compared with lateral ones (in twelve of twenty-five cases, or 48%). Similarly, Auer et al.[47] found hydrocephalus in 75% of their sixteen patients, and Salazar et al.[32] documented moderate to severe hydrocephalus in seven of their fifteen patients (47%) with hematoma sizes between 2.3 and 5.5 cm; their four cases with severe hydrocephalus had all hematomas of 4 cm or more in diameter.

The CT finding of *obliteration of the quadrigeminal cistern* was reported by Taneda et al.[48] as a sign of rostral displacement of the vermis by the mass effect of the cerebellar hemorrhage, a finding that correlated with the presence of hydrocephalus: all sixteen (100%) patients with total cisternal obliteration had hydrocephalus, as compared with twelve of sixteen (75%) with partial, and eighteen of forty-three (42%) with no cisternal compression. These two features in turn determined prognosis and management.

## Clinical Course and Management

Since the early descriptions of cerebellar hemorrhage,[3–5,8,11,13,14,16,49,50] a notorious tendency to either sudden onset with rapid deterioration or unexpected abrupt decompensation after an initially stable course was observed. On the other hand, early studies[2] also suggested that cerebellar hemorrhage can have a benign course, with clinical recovery without surgical therapy, a feature now widely-documented in the literature.[14,24,51–54] In the series of Ott et al.,[14] among forty-three initially noncomatose patients, nine (21%) developed coma within three hours of onset, a subacute group of twenty-five patients (58%) deteriorated between three and one-half hours and thirteen and one-half days after onset, and nine (21%)

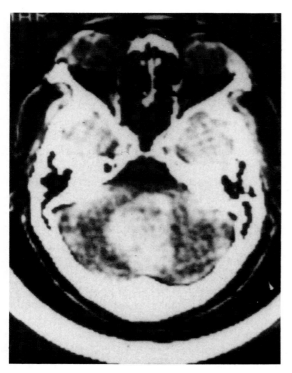

A

**Figure 20.8.** Anatomical features of six cases of midline (vermian) cerebellar hemorrhage. The letters correspond to the patients listed in Table 20.4. (A) Large median-paramedian hemorrhage. (B) Strictly vermian hemorrhage (corresponding to patient description Figure 20.7). (C) Vermian hemorrhage with compression of the pontine tectum (From Kase CS, Caplan LR. Hemorrhage affecting the brainstem and cerebellum. In: Barnett HJM, Mohr JP, Stein BM, et al. (eds): Stroke: Pathophysiology, Diagnosis and Management. New York: Churchill Livingstone, 1986, with permission.) (D) Large vermian hemorrhage communicating with the fourth ventricle. (E) Large vermian-paravermian hemorrhage. (F) Large midline hemorrhage involving the whole vermis and extending into the pontine tegmentum on the right (Courtesy of Flaviu C. A. Romanul, M.D., Boston University Medical Center, Boston, MA.)

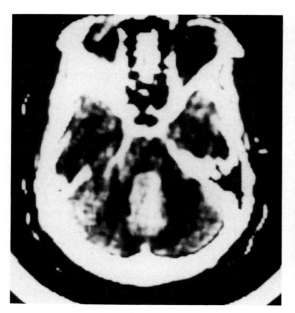

B

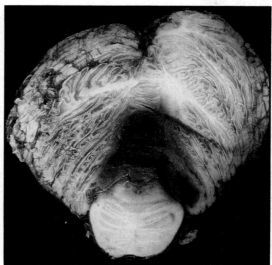

C

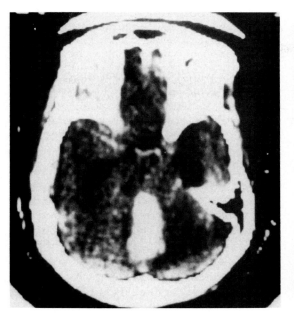

D

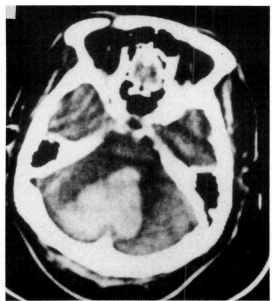

E

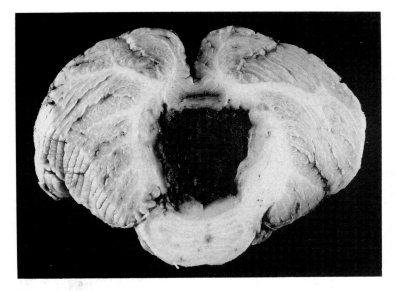

F

had a benign course (Figure 20.9). Approximately 50% of those who deteriorated to coma did so within forty-eight hours from onset,[14] whereas in Dunne et al.'s[7] series eighteen of twenty (90%) who deteriorated into stupor or coma underwent the clinical change even faster, within thirty-six hours from onset (Figure 20.10). This frequently-

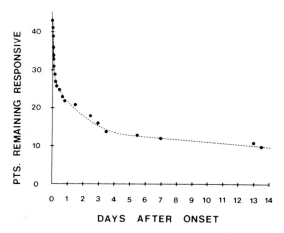

**Figure 20.9.** Development of coma in forty-three noncomatose patients with cerebellar hemorrhage as a function of time from onset of symptoms (From Ott KH, Kase CS, Ojemann RG, et al. Cerebellar hemorrhage: diagnosis and treatment: a review of 56 cases. Arch Neurol 1974;31:160–167, with permission.)

unstable clinical course in cerebellar hemorrhage could not be correlated with predictive clinical features at presentation,[14] as disturbing examples of precipitous development of coma after stable hospital course were reported,[14] at times even after prolonged stabil-

ity.[55] These observations were further qualified by showing that vital prognosis became hopelessly poor once coma ensued, with a mortality figure of 95% in the series of Ott et al.,[14] the examples of survival and good functional outcome after emergency surgery in comatose patients being actually exceptional.[13,14,19,56] However, these mortality figures were dramatically improved with surgical treatment, particularly in patients who were either alert or drowsy, as opposed to stuporous or comatose, preoperatively (Table 20.5). The combined mortality figures were 17% for alert and drowsy patients, and 75% for those stuporous or comatose.[14] Furthermore, Ott et al.[14] determined that the low surgical mortality of alert and drowsy patients justified surgical therapy up to eight days from onset, while beyond that time the spontaneous mortality was lower than the surgical mortality, suggesting that nonsurgical treatment should be given to patients presenting that late in their course. These figures led to the recommendation of considering surgery for any patient with a diagnosis of cerebellar hemorrhage made within forty-eight hours, and probably as late as eight days from onset, particularly for those patients who are alert or drowsy at presentation.[14]

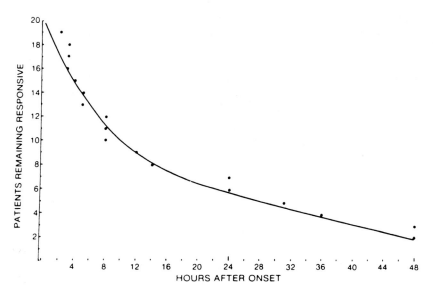

**Figure 20.10.** Time of onset of stupor and coma in twenty initially responsive patients with cerebellar hemorrhage as a function of time from onset (From Dunne JW, Chakera T, Kermode S. Cerebellar haemorrhage—diagnosis and treatment: a study of 75 consecutive cases. Quart J Med 1987;64:739–754, with permission.)

**Table 20.5.** Surgical Mortality According to Preoperative Mental Status

| Preoperative Status | No. | Died | % | |
|---|---|---|---|---|
| Alert | 2 | 0 | 0 | |
| | | | | 17% |
| Drowsy | 10 | 2 | 20 | |
| Stuporous | 4 | 2 | 50 | |
| | | | | 75% |
| Coma | 12 | 10 | 83 | |

(Modified from Ott KH, Kase CS, Ojemann RG, et al. Cerebellar hemorrhage: diagnosis and treatment: a review of 56 cases. Arch Neurol 1974;31:160–167.)

Following the introduction of CT, a number of authors reported the value of certain imaging parameters for predicting outcome and directing management of cerebellar hemorrhage. Little et al.[30] reported ten patients with cerebellar hemorrhage, six of whom showed progressive neurological deterioration, while the remaining four followed a benign course. These two patterns correlated with the finding of large hematomas (3 cm or more in diameter) in five of the six patients of the first group, while all four patients with benign course had hematomas smaller than 3 cm, without accompanying hydrocephalus. These CT features in turn correlated with treatment: all four patients with small hematomas remained clinically stable, showed progressive resolution of the hematomas, and survived with apparently minor residual deficits. Among the six patients with large hematomas and hydrocephalus, five underwent surgery for clot evacuation, with four surviving and subsequently regaining independent function. Subsequent series corroborated the value of these CT criteria in assisting therapeutic decisions: Theodore et al.[57] reported five patients with cerebellar hemorrhages of less than 3 cm in diameter, two of whom had hydrocephalus, who were successfully treated nonsurgically; Zieger et al.[43] reported better results with conservative than surgical treatment in patients with small hematomas (8 to 16 cm$^3$

in volume). Subsequently, Taneda et al.[48] added the CT criterion of obliteration of the quadrigeminal cistern, which results from upward displacement of the vermis secondary to mass effect from the hematoma, as a reliable indicator of clinical course and management. These authors reported seventy-five patients with cerebellar hemorrhage who were divided in three groups according to the degree of quadrigeminal cistern obliteration: grade I, corresponding to normal cisterns (forty-three patients); grade II, with partial compression of cisterns (sixteen patients); and grade III, with complete obliteration of cisterns (sixteen patients). In grade I patients the outcome was good in thirty-eight of forty-three (88%); eighteen of these patients had treatment for hydrocephalus, and fourteen underwent hematoma evacuation. Eleven of sixteen (69%) grade II patients had a good outcome, nine of whom had the hematoma evacuated within forty-eight hours from onset. Grade III patients had uniformly poor outcomes, with only one survivor among sixteen patients, despite hematoma evacuation within forty-eight hours from onset in eight patients and relief of hydrocephalus in two. These authors[48] and others[32,58] concluded that quadrigeminal cistern obliteration is a useful additional parameter to guide therapy, since it can help to separate the patients with benign course (grade I) who have good outcome (probably irrespective of treatment modality used), from those with poor prognosis (grade III) who do not benefit from heroic surgical measures, and from the intermediate ones (grade II) who appear to benefit from early (within forty-eight hours from onset) hematoma evacuation.

Although the value of these CT criteria in predicting outcome and assisting in the therapeutic decisions is well established, there are exceptions in which patients with hematomas larger than 3 cm and with concomitant hydrocephalus[17,24,54] have done well without the need for surgical treatment. The therapeutic decision in these cases was based on an alert or drowsy level of consciousness on admission, which remained stable or improved throughout the subsequent course. These observations emphasize the fact that the selection of therapy in cerebellar hemorrhage is primarily dictated by clinical criteria, among which level of consciousness and, to a lesser extent, signs of pontine cranial nerve involvement are the most valuable parameters for deciding between conservative and surgical therapy. Our personal approach to the management of cerebellar hemorrhage is to maintain close clinical observation of patients who have a stable level of consciousness and small hematomas with or without hydrocephalus. However, we have a low threshold for recommending surgical evacuation of hematomas in the event of any new sign of declining level of consciousness or pontine cranial nerve dysfunction. For those patients who present with an already deteriorating level of consciousness, irrespective of the size and location of the hematoma or presence or absence of hydrocephalus, we recommend emergency surgical treatment.

The *choice of surgical procedure* in patients with cerebellar hemorrhage has been controversial. After early reports of poor results from needle aspiration of the hematoma or ventricular drainage procedures,[8,9] it became clear that better results were obtained by suboccipital craniotomy with wide exposure of the cerebellar hemisphere for adequate clot evacuation, followed by careful attention to hemostasis and intra- and postoperative blood pressure control.[14,59] The management with only treatment of hydrocephalus by ventricular drainage, without clot evacuation, was felt to be unsafe because of the potential risk of upward cerebellar transtentorial herniation in the face of an unresected posterior fossa mass.[18,24,59] These concerns were disregarded by others,[48,60–63] who reported excellent results with ventricular drainage alone in the treatment of cerebellar hemorrhage with hydrocephalus.[64] This led Shenkin and Zavala[62] to propose that hematoma drainage is unnecessary in cerebellar hemorrhage, and management of hydrocephalus by ventricular drainage should be

the only treatment, stating that "when hydrocephalus develops . . . the state of consciousness is compromised and life is threatened." This view has been contested by Gerritsen van der Hoop et al.,[24] who argued that fatal outcome relates to hematoma size rather than presence of hydrocephalus, the latter considered to "accompany" rather than cause death. Others[18,19,47,65] have shown better outcomes with suboccipital craniotomy and hematoma evacuation than with ventricular drainage alone, at times patients requiring hematoma drainage after an unsuccessful ventriculostomy. However, it is apparent that, to some extent, there is a selection bias in the choice of therapy, since ventricular drainage alone is frequently performed as a palliative measure in either severely compromised patients or those who are poor surgical risks.[19,63] This controversy is likely to continue as there are no data available on the prospective comparison of postoperative results in patients randomly assigned to one or the other form of therapy. Our approach is to favor suboccipital craniotomy and hematoma evacuation in patients with deteriorating level of consciousness and large hematomas with or without hydrocephalus, using ventriculostomy only as an emergency procedure in rapidly decompensating patients with acute hydrocephalus, while preparations for posterior fossa craniotomy are underway.

The novel surgical approach of CT-guided stereotactic fibrinolysis of cerebellar hematomas has been recently reported by Mohadjer et al.[66] This technique involves the stereotactic puncture of the hematoma, followed by insertion of a 2-mm diameter silicone catheter into the hematoma cavity, for instillations of urokinase (5,000 units in 5 ml of saline solution) at 6- to 8-hour intervals, over a two-day treatment period. Their results were encouraging, with only one death (due to pulmonary embolism) in the postoperative period among fourteen treated patients, and two late deaths from unrelated causes (at six and eighteen months after the procedure). The remaining eleven patients were in good neurological condition and independent after an average follow-up period of nineteen months. Although the preoperative hematoma diameters or volumes were not provided, this group of patients had substantial neurological deficits preoperatively, as judged by the mean Glasgow Coma Scale of 9.3, which improved by three to five points in all patients postoperatively. One CT illustration shows a median-paramedian hematoma of moderate size, with effacement and shift of the fourth ventricle, and compression of basal cisterns, which appears completely removed on a CT scan performed four days after surgery, with better visualization of the fourth ventricle and basal cisterns. This promising form of therapy of ICH certainly deserves further testing in larger clinical series.

# References

1. Ballance HA. Case of traumatic hemorrhage into the left lateral lobe of the cerebellum, treated by operation, with recovery. Surg Gynecol Obstet 1906;3:223–225.
2. Dinsdale HB. Spontaneous hemorrhage in the posterior fossa: a study of primary cerebellar and pontine hemorrhages with observations on their pathogenesis. Arch Neurol 1964;10: 200–217.
3. Mitchell N, Angrist A. Spontaneous cerebellar hemorrhage: report of fifteen cases. Am J Pathol 1942;18:935–953.
4. Rey-Bellet J. Cerebellar hemorrhage: a clinicopathologic study. Neurology 1960;10:217–222.
5. Hyland HH, Levy D. Spontaneous cerebellar hemorrhage. Can Med Assoc J 1954;71:315–323.
6. Fang HCH, Foley JM. Hypertensive hemorrhages of the pons and cerebellum. Arch Neurol Psychiat 1954;72:638–639.
7. Dunne JW, Chakera T, Kermode S. Cerebellar hemorrhage—diagnosis and treatment: a study of 75 consecutive cases. Quart J Med 1987;64:739–754.
8. McKissock W, Richardson A, Walsh L. Spontaneous cerebellar haemorrhage: a study of 34 consecutive cases treated surgically. Brain 1960;83:1–9.
9. Richardson AE. Spontaneous cerebellar hemorrhage. In: Vinken PJ, Bruyn GW, eds. Handbook of Clinical Neurology. Vol. 12. Amsterdam: North-Holland, 1972;54–67.
10. Norris JW, Eisen AA, Branch CL. Problems in cerebellar hemorrhage and infarction. Neurology 1969;19:1043–1050.
11. Abud-Ortega AF, Rajput A, Rozdilsky B. Observations in five cases of spontaneous cerebellar hemorrhage. Can Med Assoc J 1972;106: 40–42.
12. Rosenberg GA, Kaufman DM. Cerebellar hemorrhage: reliability of clinical evaluation. Stroke 1976;7:332–336.
13. Fisher CM, Picard EH, Polak A, et al. Acute hypertensive cerebellar hemorrhage: diagnosis and surgical treatment. J Nerv Ment Dis 1965;140:38–57.
14. Ott KH, Kase CS, Ojemann RG, et al. Cerebellar hemorrhage: diagnosis and treatment: a review of 56 cases. Arch Neurol 1974;31:160–167.
15. Brennan RW, Bergland RM. Acute cerebellar hemorrhage: analysis of clinical findings and outcome in 12 cases. Neurology 1977;27: 527–532.
16. Freeman RE, Onofrio BM, Okazaki H, et al. Spontaneous cerebellar hemorrhage: diagnosis and surgical treatment. Neurology 1973;23: 84–90.
17. Gilliard C, Mathurin P, Passagia JG, et al. L'hématome spontané du cervelet. Neurochirurgie 1990;36:347–353.
18. Philippon J, Rivierez M, Nachanakian A, et al. Hémorragies cérébelleuses: confrontations clinicotopographiques et indications thérapeutiques. Neurochirurgie 1983;29:381–386.
19. Labauge R, Boukobza M, Zinszner J, et al. Hématomes spontanés du cervelet: vingt-huit observations personnelles. Rev Neurol 1983;139: 193–204.
20. Odom GL, Tindall GT, Dukes HT. Cerebellar hematoma caused by angiomatous malformations: report of four cases. J Neurosurg 1961;18:777–782.
21. Kawasaki N, Uchida T, Yamada M, et al. Conservative management of cerebellar hemorrhage in pregnancy. Int J Gynecol Obstet 1990;31:365–369.
22. Hollin SA, Decker RE, Gross SW. Spontaneous cerebellar hematomas. Mt Sinai J Med 1974;41:396–406.
23. Erenberg G, Rubin R, Shulman K. Cerebellar haematomas caused by angiomas in children. J Neurol Neurosurg Psychiat 1972;35: 304–310.

24. Gerritsen van der Hoop R, Vermeulen M, et al. Cerebellar hemorrhage: diagnosis and treatment. Surg Neurol 1988;29:6–10.

25. Matsumura A, Maki Y, Munekata K, et al. Intracerebellar hemorrhage due to cerebellar hemangioblastoma. Surg Neurol 1985;24:227–230.

26. Jamjoom AB, Atasoy M, Coakham HB. Spontaneous haemorrhage in a cerebellar abscess: a unique complication. Brit J Neurosurg 1990;4:231–236.

27. Kawakami Y, Nakao Y, Tabuchi K, et al. Bilateral intracerebellar calcification associated with cerebellar hematoma: case report. J Neurosurg 1978;49:744–748.

28. Pressman BD, Kirkwood JR, Davis DO. Posterior fossa hemorrhage: localization by computerized tomography. JAMA 1975;232:932–933.

29. Müller HR, Wüthrich R, Wiggli U, et al. The contribution of computerized axial tomography to the diagnosis of cerebellar and pontine hematomas. Stroke 1975;6:467–475.

30. Little JR, Tubman DE, Ethier R. Cerebellar hemorrhage in adults: diagnosis by computerized tomography. J Neurosurg 1978;48:575–579.

31. Turner DA, Howe JF. Cerebellar hemorrhage as evaluated by computerized tomography. West J Med 1982;136:198–202.

32. Salazar J, Vaquero J, Martinez P, et al. Clinical and CT scan assessment of benign versus fatal spontaneous cerebellar haematomas. Acta Neurochir 1986;79:80–86.

33. Feindel W, Penfield W, McNaughton FL. The tentorial nerves and localization of intracranial pain in man. Neurology 1960;10:555–563.

34. Kubo T, Sakata Y, Sakai S-I, et al. Clinical observations in the acute phase of cerebellar hemorrhage and infarction. Acta Otolaryngol 1988(suppl);447:81–87.

35. Messert B, Leppik IE, Sato S. Diplopia and involuntary eye closure in spontaneous cerebellar hemorrhage. Stroke 1976;7:305–307.

36. Fisher CM. Ocular bobbing. Arch Neurol 1964;11:543–546.

37. Bosch EP, Kennedy SS, Aschenbrener CA. Ocular bobbing: the myth of its localizing value. Neurology 1975;25:949–953.

38. Roy EP, Keefover RW, Riggs JE, et al. Dysarthria-clumsy hand syndrome and cerebellar hemorrhage. Ann Neurol 1987;21:415–416 (letter).

39. Verstichel P, Riss JM, Raybaud C, et al. Hémiparesie ataxique et hématomes simultanés sus et sous-tentoriels. Rev Neurol 1991;147:671–673.

40. Massie JD, Haussen S, Gerald B. Angiography of cerebellar hemorrhage secondary to hypertension. Am J Roentgenol Rad Ther Nucl Med 1975;123:22–26.

41. Puljic S, Zingesser LH, Kozic Z. Cerebellar hemorrhage: unusual ventriculographic findings. Neurology 1977;27:672–674.

42. Kasdon DL, Scott RM, Adelman LS, et al. Cerebellar hemorrhage with decreased absorption values on computed tomography: a case report. Neuroradiology 1977;13:265–266.

43. Zieger A, Vonofakos D, Steudel WI, et al. Nontraumatic intracerebellar hematomas: prognostic value of volumetric evaluation by computed tomography. Surg Neurol 1984;22:491–494.

44. Kase CS, Caplan LR. Hemorrhage affecting the brain stem and cerebellum. In: Barnett HJM et al., eds. Stroke: Pathophysiology, Diagnosis, and Management. Vol. 1. New York: Churchill Livingstone, 1986;621–641.

45. Chadduck WM, Loar CR. Cerebellar hemorrhage and CT scanning. Va Med 1978;105:854–857.

46. Ropper AH. "Convulsions" in basilar artery occlusion. Neurology 1988;38:1500–1501.

47. Auer LM, Auer T, Sayama I. Indications for surgical treatment of cerebellar haemorrhage and infarction. Acta Neurochir 1986;79:74–79.

48. Taneda M, Hayakawa T, Mogami H. Primary cerebellar hemorrhage: quadrigeminal cistern obliteration on CT scans as a predictor of outcome. J Neurosurg 1987;67:545–552.

49. Sypert GW. Cerebellar hemorrhage and infarction. Compr Ther 1977;3:42–47.

50. Vincent FM. Cerebellar hemorrhage. Minn Med 1976;59:453–458.

51. Heiman TD, Satya-Murti S. Benign cerebellar hemorrhages. Ann Neurol 1978;3:366–368.

52. Feijoo De Freixo M, Jimenez Garcia M, Galdos Alcelay L. Cerebellar hemorrhage: nonsurgical forms. Ann Neurol 1979;6:84 (letter).

53. Melamed N, Satya-Murti S. Cerebellar hemorrhage: a review and reappraisal of benign cases. Arch Neurol 1984;41:425–428.

54. Bogousslavsky J, Regli F, Jeanrenaud X. Benign outcome in unoperated large cerebellar hemorrhage: report of 2 cases. Acta Neurochir 1984;73:59–65.

55. Brillman J. Acute hydrocephalus and death one month after non-surgical treatment for acute cerebellar hemorrhage: case report. J Neurosurg 1979;50:374–376.

56. Yoshida S, Sasaki M, Oka H, et al. Acute hypertensive cerebellar hemorrhage with signs of lower brainstem compression. Surg Neurol 1978;10:79–83.

57. Theodore WH, Striar J, Burger A. Nonsurgical treatment of cerebellar hematoma. Mt Sinai J Med 1979;46:328–332.

58. Waidhauser E, Hamburger C, Marguth F. Neurosurgical management of cerebellar hemorrhage. Neurosurg Rev 1990;13:211–217.

59. Heros RC. Cerebellar hemorrhage and infarction. Stroke 1982;13:106–109.

60. Greenberg J, Skubick D, Shenkin H. Acute hydrocephalus in cerebellar infarct and hemorrhage. Neurology 1979;29:409–413.

61. Seelig JM, Selhorst JS, Young HF, et al. Ventriculostomy for hydrocephalus in cerebellar hemorrhage. Neurology 1981;31:1537–1540.

62. Shenkin HA, Zavala M. Cerebellar strokes: mortality, surgical indications, and results of ventricular drainage. Lancet 1982;2:429–432.

63. Firsching R, Frowein RA, Thun F. Intracerebellar haematoma: eleven traumatic and non-traumatic cases and a review of the literature. Neurochirugia 1987;30:182–185.

64. Rousseaux M, Lesoin F, Combelle G, et al. Intérêt et limites de la dérivation ventriculaire isoleé dans les hématomes cérébelleux non traumatiques. Neurochirurgie 1984;30:41–44.

65. Lui T-N, Fairholm DJ, Shu T-F, et al. Surgical treatment of spontaneous cerebellar hemorrhage. Surg Neurol 1985;23:555–558.

66. Mohadjer M, Eggert R, May J, et al. CT-guided stereotactic fibrinolysis of spontaneous and hypertensive cerebellar hemorrhage: long-term results. J Neurosurg 1990;73:217–222.

# Chapter 21
# Midbrain and Medullary Hemorrhage

## Carlos S. Kase

Nontraumatic hemorrhages in the brainstem are for the most part pontine in location.[1] The latter are estimated to account for at least 75% of brainstem hematomas, while the midbrain site accounts for over 20% of the cases, the few remaining examples being of the rare medullary variety.[2]

The early literature reports of hemorrhages in the midbrain and medulla were prompted by their clinical diagnosis and successful surgical evacuation. In the last decade or so, with the advent of computed tomography (CT) and magnetic resonance imaging (MRI), a number of reports have helped delineate the clinical and anatomical features of these unusual sites of brainstem hemorrhage.

## Midbrain Hemorrhage

Hemorrhage into the midbrain is most commonly a secondary phenomenon, resulting from either extension from an adjacent site, as in downward extension of thalamic intracerebral hemorrhage (ICH) (Figure 21.1A) or, less commonly, upward extension of a pontine hemorrhage (Figure 21.1B), or as Duret's hemorrhages secondary to mass lesions in the supratentorial compartment (Figure 21.1C). Primary spontaneous, nontraumatic, midbrain hemorrhages are rare, their frequency being estimated as 1.1% of

cases of ICH.[3] This rarity of midbrain hemorrhage is also encountered in large autopsy series of ICH (Table 21.1).

In *clinical series*, midbrain hemorrhage has been studied in great detail, and clinicoradiological correlations have been established. The first detailed description of midbrain hemorrhage was that of L'Hermitte,[9] who reported five patients diagnosed on the basis of the clinical presentation and the hemorrhagic/xanthochromic character of the cerebrospinal fluid (CSF). Although each case was not described in detail, the analysis of the group allowed him to comment on the main features of the syndrome of tegmental midbrain ICH, as follows: (1) ophthalmological abnormalities: they were consistently present, and included various combinations of Parinaud's syndrome (paralysis of upgaze, pupils with light-near dissociation, convergence-retraction nystagmus), skew deviation, loss of pupillary reactivity, Horner's syndrome, and third nerve paralysis with or without pupillary involvement; (2) "sleep disturbances:" he pointed out that patients frequently would appear to be deeply asleep or lethargic (leading to "unaware physicians confusing it with coma") but able to answer questions after repeated verbal or cutaneous stimulation; (3) hallucinations: he described in detail the phenomena of "peduncular" hallucinations, and commented that they do not occur immediately after the ictus,

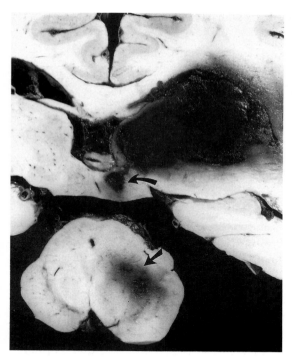

**Figure 21.1.** Patterns of secondary midbrain hemorrhage. (A) Left thalamic hemorrhage with direct extension into the midbrain tectum (curved arrow) and further downward dissection into the tegmentum (arrow) (Courtesy of J. P. Mohr, M.D., Neurological Institute, New York.) (B) Massive pontine hemorrhage (lower section) with upward extension into the midbrain (upper section), which is virtually replaced by acute hemorrhage. (C) Large median and paramedian (Duret's) midbrain hemorrhages in patient with massive supratentorial ICH and absent brainstem function.

A

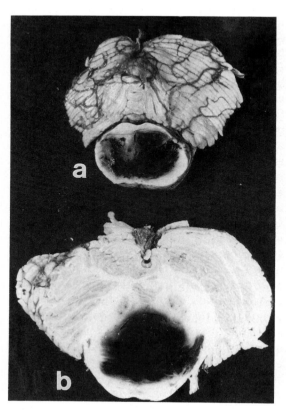

B

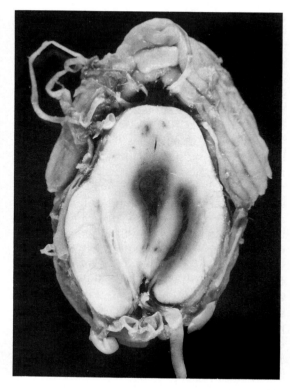

C

**Table 21.1.** Cases of Midbrain Hemorrhage in Autopsy Series of ICH

| Author | Site of ICH | No. of ICH Cases | No. of Midbrain ICH |
|---|---|---|---|
| Bottinelli et al.[4] | Brainstem | 25 | 1 |
| Collomb et al.[5] | Brainstem | 36 | 1 |
| Dinsdale[6] | Post. fossa | 82 | 0 |
| Freytag[7] | All sites, hypertensive | 393 | 0 |
| Boudouresques et al.[8] | All sites | 318 | 0* |

*In 5 of 14 cases with brainstem hematomas, there was midbrain extension of a pontine hemorrhage, but no primary, isolated instances of midbrain ICH.

but rather several days later; the hallucinations were described as being predominantly in the visual sphere, at times experienced during daytime, but especially occurring in the evening and night; the patients reported seeing "animated human beings or animals, that parade without noise in front of their amazed eyes;" the animals were at times domestic, "like cats, hens with dilated pupils reflecting a magnetic glow," at others "snakes, eels, or disgusting beasts," while at other times they were "strange animals or individuals of bizarre appearance that possessed the unique faculty of walking through walls or invading the patient's room in order to play comedies;" at times, "the scene becomes further animated by the figures grouping and mixing with each other, the space being filled by a fantasmagory that plunges the patient in a legitimate state of stupefaction, while at other times it is like a dream, leaving him indifferent or even amused at the performance being offered to him;" (4) motor deficits: hemiplegia was infrequent, since it occurred in only one of his patients, and three others had transient hemiparesis of a few days' duration; (5) difficulties in motor coordination: in contrast to hemiplegia or hemiparesis, these were prominent features in his cases, in the form of cerebellar ataxia affecting either all four limbs or those opposite the hemorrhage, resulting in severe gait ataxia and cerebellar action tremor, and only exceptionally with "transient unilateral rhythmic spontaneous tremor of the hand and fingers"; (6) lack of sensory abnormalities: none of the patients developed sensory deficits, paresthesias, or pain. L'Hermitte

noted the usually regressive course of midbrain ICH, in contrast with the generally held view of high mortality from this condition; his patients evolved with gradual disappearance of their lethargy, hallucinations, and ophthalmoplegia, generally being left with deficits of equilibrium and motor coordination.

In a classic paper, Scoville and Poppen[10] reported the case of a 44-year-old woman who had two episodes of bleeding into the left basis pedunculi. The second event led to right hemiplegia, bilateral supranuclear facial palsy, pinpoint pupils, slight bilateral palpebral ptosis, and absent extraocular movements (EOM). She had the successful evacuation of a clot located in the left basis pedunculi; there was no mention of histological study of the surgical specimen. The patient was able to walk within one month from the operation, despite residual right hemiparesis and ataxia; a right homonymous hemianopia resulted from a left occipital lobectomy performed to allow access to the left cerebral peduncle. Her main deficits at six years after surgery included a "faint rhythmic tremor" of the right arm, and scanning dysarthria, and she was described as leading a normal life. The authors' interpretation of the clinicoanatomical correlations implicated involvement of the medial lemniscus (with contralateral hemianesthesia), corticospinal tract (contralateral hemiplegia), corpora quadrigemina and third nerve nuclei (loss of EOM), supranuclear facial and bulbar fibers (bilateral facial weakness, unilateral weakness of the palate, dysarthria), red nucleus (delayed contralateral tremor), and superior cerebellar peduncle (bilateral, right more than left, limb ataxia). Almost 30 years after that report, La Torre et al.[11] described a 38-year-old woman who developed headache, bilateral sixth nerve palsy, upgaze palsy leading to paralysis, papilledema, and drowsiness that evolved into coma. She had a hematoma of the quadrigeminal plate, which was surgically drained. At surgery, a "cryptic vascular malformation" was described under the operating microscope, but no documentation of such lesion followed histological examination of the wall of the hematoma. She made an excellent recovery so that neurological examination at seven months after surgery was normal. Humphreys[12] reported the first case of successful drainage of a midline hematoma documented by CT in a child. The patient, a 10-year-old boy, presented with headache, vomiting, and inability to stand and walk, with physical findings of right hemiparesis and bilateral Babinski signs, with stupor that rapidly progressed to coma and right-sided decerebrate posturing. The hematoma was drained through a direct pedunculotomy, after an initial unsuccessful attempt at drainage through the floor of the fourth ventricle. Histological examination of the removed tissue showed "dilated thin-walled vessels," but no evidence of vascular malformation or tumor. The child recovered well, and was back to normal life, his only neurological sequela being mild weakness of the right superior oblique muscle.

More recently, Durward et al.[13] described two patients with midbrain hemorrhage: Case 1, a 71-year-old man, developed sudden inability to stand and to open the eyes, along with bilateral internuclear ophthalmoplegia (INO), pupils of 5 to 6 mm in diameter and unreactive to light, absent vertical eye movements, and dysphagia; CT showed a 1-cm hematoma of the ventral tegmentum of the midbrain, which caused progressive hydrocephalus requiring placement of a ventriculoperitoneal shunt, followed by improvement, but with residual paralysis of vertical gaze, bilateral INO, pupils with absent light reflex, and gait instability; he had a normal angio-gram, and the mechanism of the hemorrhage was thought to be hypertension. Case 2, an 18-year-old man, developed headache, diplopia, and left leg weakness, with physical findings of right third nerve paralysis, right fourth nerve palsy, and mild left hemiparesis. CT showed a 2 × 2.5 cm hematoma in the right side of the midbrain. Cerebral angiography revealed an avascular midbrain mass, which was drained surgically after the patient deteriorated clinically, with development of paralysis of all movements of the right eye and adduction of the left eye, the latter showing only minimal residual abduction; the surgical specimen histologically showed a small arteriovenous malformation (AVM) as the mechanism of the hemorrhage; he was left with sequelae of right sixth nerve palsy, dysarthria, left-sided ataxia, and gait imbalance. Roig et al.[3] reported three cases of midbrain hemorrhage, one (Case 1) presenting with sudden right hemiparesis and hemifacial paresthesias, along with complete right ophthalmoplegia, in a patient who had a predominantly dorsal midbrain ICH located to the right of the midline. After approximately one month, the patient developed a "rubral" tremor of the left limbs, being labeled as an example of Benedikt's syndrome.[14] Case 2 presented with complete right ophthalmoplegia, bilateral upgaze palsy, dysarthria, and left hemiparesis, due to a small hemorrhage in the midline tegmentum. This patient developed, on day 3, transient prominent and bizarre visual ("peduncular") hallucinations, and she had right ophthalmoplegia and upgaze palsy as sequelae when tested five months after the event. Case 3 developed sudden coma, and on examination he had a left third nerve palsy, midposition pupils that were unreactive to light, and bilateral Babinski signs, from a small hemorrhage in the ventral midbrain. After one month his eyes remained open, but showed no ocular pursuit movements and he had only "weak responses to pain." He died several months later without further neurological changes. Morel-Maroger et al.[15] reported the case of a 71-year-old hypertensive man who suddenly lost consciousness and three hours later awoke with confusion, diffuse headache, and vomiting, along with vertigo, left hemiparesis, and vertical diplopia; on examination he had left hemiparesis, complete extrinsic right third nerve paralysis without anisocoria, and a right cerebellar syndrome, with preserved alertness. CT scan showed a 12 × 16 mm basal-tegmental hematoma in the right cerebral peduncle, with slight supratentorial hydrocephalus but without ventricular extension of the hemorrhage. His clinical course was benign, with gradual disappearance of the cerebellar ataxia, diplopia, and hemiparesis.

Sand et al.[16] reported three cases of midbrain hemorrhage in a dorsal location diagnosed by CT or MRI; all cases had sudden onset, and two presented with features of the dorsal midbrain syndrome of Parinaud's in the setting of small rostral tectal hemorrhages, while the third patient had a more caudal tectal hemorrhage that produced a bilateral fourth nerve palsy. The authors postulated two distinct syndromes of small dorsal mesencephalic hemorrhages, a rostral, superior collicular one with Parinaud's syndrome, and a caudal, inferior collicular one with bilateral fourth nerve palsy. In either instance, unilateral or bilateral Horner's syndrome occurred as a result of central oculosympathetic paralysis. The mechanism of the hemorrhages in the three normotensive patients with normal cerebral angiograms could not be determined, and it was assumed to be the rupture of "cryptogenic arteriovenous malformations." Weisberg[17] reported six normotensive patients with midbrain ICH, all of whom presented with sudden onset of headache and vomiting, and physical examination showed impaired upward gaze and pupils that were poorly reactive to light but with preserved near-reflex in the two patients who were responsive enough to be tested for this reflex. One alcoholic patient had transient bizarre visual hallucinations during the first week after the stroke. All patients had normal cerebral angiograms, and all were left

with pupillary and upgaze abnormalities as sequelae. de Mendonça et al.[18] reported an autopsy case of a 70-year-old hypertensive woman who developed inability to open her eyes while active, on physical examination being alert and oriented but with complete bilateral ptosis, dilated pupils unreactive to light, upward gaze paralysis, absent convergence-accommodation, and mild right hemiparesis. She worsened after admission, developing stupor, complete bilateral ophthalmoplegia, and absent oculocephalic and vestibulo-ocular reflexes. She died five weeks after onset from a myocardial infarction, and autopsy showed a large midline tegmental mesencephalic hematoma, without a clear local cause on histological examination.

The clinical details of these cases, some of which are summarized in Table 21.2, conform to the "classic" presentation of mesencephalic hemorrhage. Its characteristic features include sudden onset with prominent headache and frequent vomiting; Parinaud's syndrome in rostral tectal hemorrhages, and bilateral fourth nerve palsy in caudal tectal hemorrhages; unilateral or bilateral palpebral ptosis; and variable occurrence of Horner's syndrome, hemiataxia, or "rubral" tremor, depending on the degree of ventral extension of hematomas that tend to be predominantly tectal in location. The following example corresponds to the "classic" presentation of primary midbrain hemorrhage:

A 51-year-old hypertensive man suddenly developed diffuse headache and "dizziness," followed by a fall with inability to stand back up or to open his eyes; he was able to follow commands and respond to questions appropriately, with dysarthria. On first examination, BP was 300/150; he was responsive, but dysarthric, with complete bilateral ptosis, absent EOM on the right except for full abduction, with traces of upward movement and adduction on the left, with preserved abduction, pupils of 6 mm. on the right and 5 mm. on the left and unreactive to light, but with preserved near-reflex; facial and limb strength were normal, and the plantar reflexes were extensor bilaterally. CT showed a large midline mesencephalic hemorrhage

**Table 21.2.** Primary Midbrain Hemorrhage: Cases from the Literature with Detailed Clinical Information

| Author | Clinical Presentation | CT/MRI | Outcome | Cause of ICH |
|---|---|---|---|---|
| Durward et al.[13] (2 cases) | *Case 1*: inability to walk, bilat. 3rd n. palsy, bulbar paresis | Hematoma tegmentum, hydrocephalus | Shunt, survived | Hypertension |
| | *Case 2*: HA, R 3rd n. palsy, L hemiparesis | Hematoma R side | Operated, survived | AVM |
| Roig et al.[3] (3 cases) | *Case 1*: R 3rd n. palsy, L sensory loss & ataxia | Hematoma R tegmentum | Survived | Hypertension |
| | *Case 2*: R 3rd n. palsy, L hemiparesis | Hematoma R tegmentum | Survived | Hypertension |
| | *Case 3*: L 3rd n. palsy, coma, pupils unreactive to light | Hematoma in midline, rostral tegmentum | Died | Unknown |
| Morel-Maroger et al.[15] | HA, LOC, R 3rd n. palsy, L hemiparesis, R ataxia | Hematoma R sup. cerebellar peduncle | Survived | Hypertension |
| Sand et al.[16] (3 cases) | *Case 1*: HA, dizziness, ↓ vert. gaze, convergence-retraction nyst.; light-near dissociation | Hemorrhage R tectum | Survived | Unknown |
| | *Case 2*: Dysarthria, inability to stand; up & down gaze palsy, bilat., R hemiparesis | Hemorrhage L tectum, hydrocephalus | Survived | Unknown |
| | *Case 3*: Diplopia, unsteady gait & R hand incoordination, bilat. 4th n. palsy, L Horner's, bilat. limb ataxia | Hemorrhage L tectum | Survived | Unknown |
| Weisberg[17] (6 cases) | All normotensive, with HA, vomiting; all with ↓ up-gaze, poor pupillary reflexes; ptosis in 3/6 | Ovoid, nonenhancing hematomas; hydrocephalus in all | All 6 survived | Unknown in all 6 |
| de Mendonça et al.[18] | Bilat. ptosis, midriatic pupils unreactive to light, absent vert. gaze, R hemiparesis | Large tegmental hematoma with ventricular extension | Died | Unknown, ? hypertensive |

Abbreviations: R = right, L = left, HA = headache, LOC = loss of consciousness, vert. = vertical, ↓ = decreased, nyst. = nystagmus, bilat. = bilateral, pts. = patients, movts. = movements, n. = nerve, AVM = arteriovenous malformation.

rhage involving the tectum and tegmentum, and extending into the third and lateral ventricles, with moderate dilatation of the temporal horns of the lateral ventricles (Figure 21.2). He developed a slight increase in the degree of hydrocephalus, but at the time of transfer to a rehabilitation facility his ophthalmoplegia was partially improved, with traces of vertical motion bilaterally and persistent palpebral ptosis and loss of pupillary reactivity to light.

This case exemplifies the typical presentation of mesencephalic hemorrhage, which has been described as being predominantly dorsal in location,[3,13–17,19] either in the midline[3,12,13,18] or lateralized,[3,10,13,15,17,19] generally associated with good vital prognosis,[9,17,19,20,21] with uniformly normal cerebral angiograms,[3,12,15,17] and mechanism that is either hypertensive[3,13,18] or unknown,[3,10,12,15,17] with only rare examples of documented AVM.[11,13] The diagnosis of this

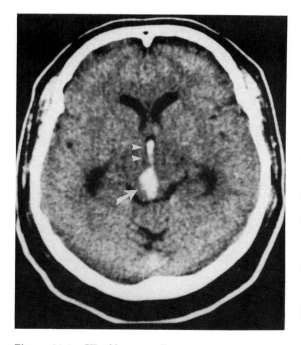

**Figure 21.2.** CT of large midline tectal and tegmental mesencephalic hemorrhage (arrow) with extension into the third ventricle (arrowheads) and early hydrocephalus with dilatation of the temporal horns of the lateral ventricles.

condition has been greatly facilitated by the availability of CT (Figure 21.3A) and, especially, MRI, as the latter allows precise localization of the ICH by its visualization in axial as well as sagittal planes (Figure 21.3B and C).

### Clinical Variants of Midbrain Hemorrhage Produced by Small, Partial Hematomas

#### Partial Ophthalmoplegia

A number of variants of ophthalmoplegia have been reported in patients with midbrain ICH. Unilateral involvement of the third cranial nerve is common, and it has been described in several combinations: (1) *Weber's syndrome:* a unilateral paralysis of the third nerve with contralateral hemiplegia is more often the result of tegmental and basal midbrain infarction in a paramedian distribution,[22] but occasional examples of unilateral midbrain hemorrhage have produced the syndrome.[15,23] The degree of motor involvement has generally been of hemiparesis rather than hemiplegia, but the unilateral third nerve involvement has been complete, reflecting the full compromise of the third nerve fascicles on their way to exiting ventrally in the pes pedunculi. (2) *Nuclear third nerve ophthalmoplegia and contralateral gaze palsy:* an unusual combination of ipsilateral complete third nerve paralysis, contralateral horizontal gaze palsy, and "ocular tilt reaction" occurred in a patient with a median–right paramedian mesencephalic hemorrhage.[24] The nuclear third nerve lesion produced complete extrinsic and pupillary paralysis ipsilaterally, with contralateral paresis of superior rectus function, but an added component of ipsilateral fascicular third nerve involvement was suggested by the presence of unilateral, rather than bilateral, ptosis. The partial contralateral horizontal gaze palsy, confirmed by electrooculographic recordings, was thought to be due to compromise of descending cortioco-

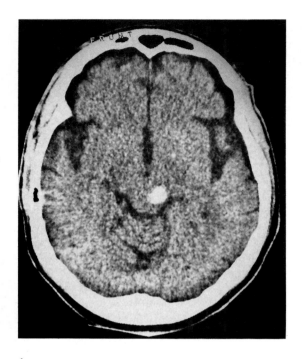

**Figure 21.3.** (A) Noncontrast CT scan with sharply demarcated acute hemorrhage in the right midbrain tegmentum. Axial (B, spin-echo sequence, TR/TE = 3350/20 msec) and midsagittal (C, T1-weighted sequence, TR/TE = 350/15 msec) of same patient, showing increased signal corresponding to the acute hematoma and mild surrounding edema (arrow).

A

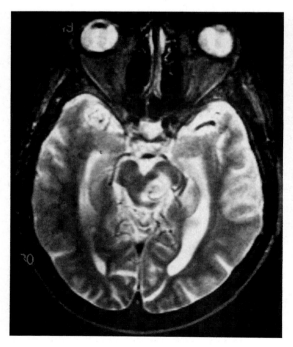

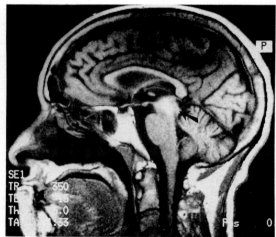

C

B

pontine "oculogyric" tracts above their decussation. (3) *Partial unilateral third nerve involvement:* a syndrome of partial "pupil-sparing" oculomotor palsy was described by Fleet et al.[25] in a patient with a tiny (5-mm diameter), presumably hypertensive hemorrhage in the left midbrain tegmentum. The mechanism of the partial involvement of the left third nerve was thought to be fascicular rather than nuclear, since the patient had no palpebral ptosis contralaterally, where the superior rectus function was also spared, both elements arguing against a nuclear lesion. The likelihood of partial involvement of third nerve fibers, with pupillary sparing, in a fascicular lesion was interpreted as due to the degree of anatomical dispersion of the third nerve fibers as they run ventrally from the third nerve nucleus, allowing for partial sparing of the relatively pressure-resistant smaller pupillomotor fibers.[26] On the other end of the spectrum of partial third nerve involvement, Shuaib et al.[27] described the unique case of a 35-year-old woman who developed sudden, recurrent headaches, and had an isolated unilateral mydriatic (8-mm diameter) pupil without response to light, with intact EOM and no signs of long-tract involvement on neurological examination. On CT, a midbrain ICH was strictly unilateral and ventral (basis pedunculi) in location. Following gradual resolution of the hemorrhage, the patient had normalization of pupillary size and reactivity within one month from the onset of symptoms. (4) *Partial oculomotor nuclear lesions:* a small unilateral tectal-tegmental hemorrhage produced bilateral palpebral ptosis and isolated ipsilateral inferior rectus weakness, without elements of Parinaud's syndrome or pupillary changes, with an otherwise normal neurologic examination.[28] The isolated neuro ophthalmologic features in this patient were interpreted as due to injury to the caudal midline cell group of the oculomotor nuclear complex, with involvement of the single midline levator palpebrae and adjacent inferior rectus subnuclei.[28] The patient recovered

fully in two months, and cranial MRI three months later was normal. (5) *Bilateral fourth nerve palsy:* in addition to the case (Patient 3) reported by Sand et al.,[16] bilateral fourth nerve palsy was reported in a patient with a 10-mm unilateral hematoma in the midbrain tegmentum-tectum.[29] The combination with unilateral involvement of the spinothalamic tract resulted in the additional finding of contralateral thermoanalgesia. The patient survived the event, but was left with residual contralateral hypesthesia to pain and temperature, as well as diplopia on downgaze. CT scan and MRI after five and eleven weeks from onset, respectively, were normal.

### Brainstem Sensory Syndromes

Small hemorrhages located unilaterally in the midbrain tegmentum have presented with isolated contralateral sensory syndromes, including *"pure sensory stroke,"*[30,31] one of the classic syndromes found in patients with lacunar infarcts in the sensory nucleus of the contralateral thalamus.[32] Tuttle and Reinmuth[30] described a 52-year-old hypertensive man who suddenly complained of subjective feelings of "numbness" and "tingling" in the right limbs, without detectable sensory deficits on examination, except for his reporting a "numb" feeling with light stroking of the right limbs, and a patch of dysesthesia behind the right ear. CT showed a small (0.5-cm) hematoma in the left dorsolateral aspect of the midbrain. He was left with persistent paresthesias of the right limbs. Azouvi et al.[31] reported a patient who developed loss of pain and temperature sensation over the entire left side of his body, with normal touch, vibration, joint position sense, graphesthesia, and stereognosis. CT documented a 7-mm diameter midbrain hemorrhage located in the right dorsal tegmentum. The authors correlated the dissociated thermoanalgesia with involvement of the dorsal spinothalamic tract, with sparing of the more anteriorly located medial lemniscus.[31] An even more restrictive form of sensory syndrome, the *"cheiro-oral syndrome,"* was described by Ono and Inoue[33] in a patient with a small left tegmental midbrain hemorrhage. The features of the syndrome, including sensory symptoms involving the corner of the mouth and the palm of the hand on the same side, are generally correlated with small lesions, usually infarcts, limited to the medial aspect of the posterolateral ventral (VPL) and the lateral aspect of the posteromedial ventral (VPM) thalamic nuclei.[34,35] Ono and Inoue's patient suddenly developed "numbness" of the corner of the mouth and the palm of the hand on the right side, along with slight right arm weakness and a sensory abnormality (decreased pain and temperature sensation) restricted to the right side of the face, without other sensory defects. They interpreted the sensory defect as due to involvement of the medial lemniscus, with interruption of fibers projecting to those thalamic nuclei (medial VPL, lateral VPM) that are often affected in the more common cases of "cheiro-oral" syndrome of thalamic origin.

### Long-Tract Involvement without Ophthalmoplegia

On rare occasions, small midbrain hematomas in basal locations result in involvement of long tracts, without concomitant ophthalmoplegia (Figure 21.4). Fingerote et al.[36] reported a 30-year-old normotensive woman who developed severe right occipital headache, followed by left hemiparesis and left-sided dysmetria, with gait instability, but without abnormalities of cranial nerves or sensory functions. On CT, she had a small right-sided basal midbrain ICH. Sano[37] reported a 35-year-old woman who presented with left hemiplegia, and remained alert and without ophthalmoplegia, in the setting of a large right basal peduncular hemorrhage. At operation, areas "suggestive of cryptic angiomatous malformation" were described in the cavity wall, but there was no mention of histological study. The patient made a good recovery.

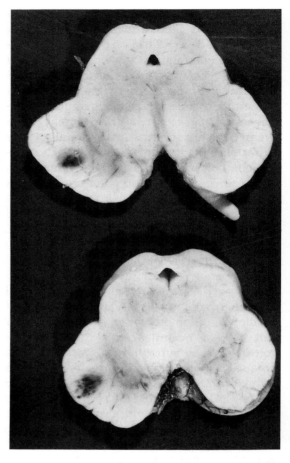

**Figure 21.4.** Small hemorrhage limited to the right pes pedunculi, clinically presenting with left hemiparesis, without ophthalmoplegia.

### Oculomotor Deficits and Retrograde Amnesia

A single case of midbrain ICH associated with retrograde amnesia was reported by Mehler and Ragone.[38] The patient, a 48-year-old normotensive alcoholic man, developed generalized throbbing headache, unsteady gait, "slurred" speech, and right eyelid droop, along with retrograde amnesia covering a 12 to 15 year span. On examination he was alert and oriented, with paresis of upgaze, convergence-retraction nystagmus, small pupils that were sluggishly reactive to light, and right ptosis, along with left arm weakness and incoordination, with a tendency to fall to the left on walking. CT revealed a hematoma in the right side of the midbrain ventrally, with intraventricular and posterior thalamic extension. The unusual retrograde amnesia was explained by involvement of the mesencephalic reticular activating system,[38] although a role for the posterior thalamic extension of the hemorrhage is possible as well, since hemorrhagic lesions in that area have been described in association with sometimes prolonged amnestic syndromes.[39]

### Hypothalamic Extension of Midbrain Hemorrhage

Although hypothalamic extension of midbrain ICH has been described on CT,[36] clinical features of diencephalic involvement are exceptionally rare. Riser et al.[40] described a 58-year-old woman with history of recurrent headaches and "asthenia," who developed features of abulia and mutism, without involvement of cranial nerves or long tracts, followed by abrupt onset of hyperthermia (up to 41.5°C) and coma. On pathological examination, a fresh hematoma was present in the tegmentum of the pons and midbrain bilaterally, extending into the posterior hypothalamus. Histological studies suggested an "angiomatous vascular malformation," based on abundant local capillary vascularity; vessels showed extensive connective tissue proliferation of the walls and endothelial thickening.

## Medullary Hemorrhage

Primary hemorrhage into the substance of the medulla oblongata is uncommon, since most instances of bleeding into this area of the brainstem represent the downward extension of hematomas that originated in the pons (Figure 21.5). In the latter situation, the clinical picture is variable, and is characterized by a combination of generally unilateral pontine and medullary signs, as the hematomas tend to remain confined to one half of the brainstem.

The *clinical features* of primary medullary ICH have been delineated in a handful of well-studied cases (Table 21.3). Kempe[41] described the case of a 25-year-old man who developed nausea, vomiting, vertigo, and hiccups; on examination he had gait imbalance with veering to the left, bilateral horizontal nystagmus (predominating to the left), left facial hypesthesia with facial palsy, decreased hearing, and absent gag reflex, along with left hemiparesis and decreased sweating of the left side of the body, with sparing of the face. At surgery, a hematoma was drained from the left dorsolateral medulla; histological examination of the specimen disclosed no evidence of vascular malformation or tumor. The patient's only residual sequela was left arm dysmetria. The author speculated that "although microscopic examination . . . did not reveal any vascular structure . . . (the hemorrhage) was the result of a small vascular malformation destroying itself at the time of rupture. . . ." Mastaglia et al.[42] reported two cases of medullary hemorrhage, the first (Case 1) being purely medullary in location, the other (Case 2) representing an example of right basal pontine ICH with medullary extension. Case 1, a 48-year-old hypertensive woman on oral anticoagulants (phenindione) for history of angina pectoris, developed unilateral headache, vomiting, and "numbness over the right eye," after a last recorded prothrombin time of 25 seconds (with a control value of 13 seconds) nine days before stroke onset. Her examination showed left arm ataxia and slight hemiparesis, without sensory defects, with normal cranial nerve function. At autopsy, a recent hemorrhage of maximal diameter of 6 mm was present in the left central-ventral aspect of the medulla, with downward extension into the cervical cord. Histological examination failed to reveal a vascular malformation or other type of local pathology to account for the ICH, but the walls of many arterioles and small arteries

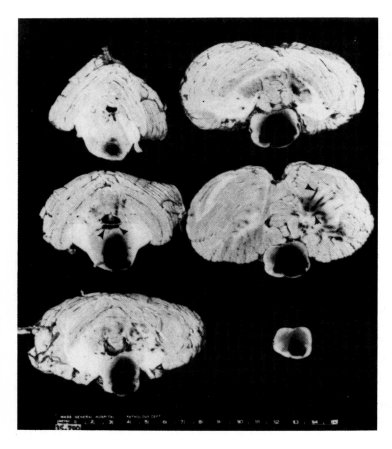

**Figure 21.5.** Medullary hemorrhage as downward extension of pontine hemorrhage. Extensive hemorrhage in the medulla (slices on right side) due to downward extension of hemorrhage originated in a pontine cavernous angioma (slices on left side). Arrowheads point to multiple associated telangiectases of the pons and cerebellum. (From Roberson GH, Kase CS, Wolpow ER. Telangiectases and cavernous angiomas of the brainstem: "cryptic" vascular malformations. Neuroradiology 1974;8:83–89. With permission.)

had extensive hyalinization of the media, at times also extending into the intima. Case 2, an 87-year-old woman, was found unconscious at a convalescent home, and physical examination showed drowsiness but with sustained ability to arouse and follow commands, with inability to speak, right conjugate gaze paralysis, right facial palsy, absent palatal movement and gag reflex and swallowing ability, left hemiparesis and limb ataxia, with intact sensory examination. She remained dysarthric and with marked dysphagia, and died three weeks after stroke onset. Autopsy revealed a right basal pontine hemorrhage with extension into the ipsilateral upper medulla, the latter involving the pyramid and the medial aspect of the inferior olivary nucleus. Microscopic examination showed homogeneous changes in the media

of arterioles and small arteries, but no evidence of a vascular malformation or tumor. The authors commented on the rarity of primary medullary ICH, and speculated that the relatively higher frequency of pontine hemorrhage could be due to the fact that microaneurysms are common in the pons, which is supplied by long basilar penetrating arteries, branches that are not present in the medulla. In support of this view, they cited the lack of documentation of microaneurysms in the medulla in the anatomical study of Cole and Yates.[43]

Plum and Posner,[44] in discussing the absence of coma in destructive medullary lesions, described a 62-year-old woman who had had an episode of hemiparesis with loss of deep sensory modalities on the right side twenty-five years previously, and presented

**Table 21.3.** Primary Medullary Hemorrhage: Cases from the Literature

| Author | Clinical Presentation | Outcome | Cause |
|---|---|---|---|
| Kempe[41] | L ↓ hearing, HA, vomit., vertigo, hiccups, nyst., ↓ pin & paresis L face | Operated, survived | Unknown |
| Mastaglia et al.[42] (Case 1) | Ataxia & ↓ JPS L limbs, numbness R limbs | Died; hematoma L pyramid & cervical cord | Anticoagulants, hypertension |
| Plum and Posner[44] | R vocal cord & 12th n. paralysis | Died; hematoma R medial & lateral tegmentum | AVM |
| Arseni and Stanciu[45] | *Case 1:* HA, gait imbalance, R dysmetria; paresis L 3rd & 6th n.; horiz. & vert. nyst.; dysphonia & dysphagia, R hemiparesis, L facial paralysis | Operated, survived | Unknown |
| | *Case 2:* Dizziness, HA, vomit., L ataxia & hemiparesis; L 5th n. palsy, nyst., dysphonia, dysphagia | Operated, survived | Unknown |
| Morel-Maroger et al.[15] | Dysphagia, L 7th, 10th, 12th n. palsy, Horner's; ↓ hearing, paresthesias R limbs | Survived (CT: L tegmental hematoma) | Hypertension |
| Neumann et al.[46] | HA, vertigo, dysphagia, dysarthria; R Horner's 5th n. palsy, ↓ palatal motion & gag, tongue paresis; R hemiparesis | Died; hematoma R rostral dorsolateral medulla | Unknown |
| Hommel et al.[47] | R leg weakness, vomit. inability to stand or sit, with R lateropulsion | Survived (CT: hematoma R medullary tegmentum) | Unknown |
| Cappa et al.[48] | Gait imbalance, vomit., vertigo; L 6th, 7th n. palsy L-beating nyst.; dysphonia, dysphagia, L arm ataxia, R-sided hemihypalgesia | Survived (CT: hematoma L dorsolateral medulla) | Unknown |
| Biller et al.[49] | HA, dizziness, L paresthesias; bilat. horiz. nyst., paralysis R palate & vocal cords, absent gag, R tongue paresis; truncal ataxia | Survived (MRI: R medullary hemorrage) | Hypertension |
| Shuaib[56] | LOC, vertigo, vomit., dysarthria, dysphagia; paralysis L conjugate gaze, L 5th n. palsy, L hemiparesis, ↓ pain & temp. R limbs; resp. arrest | Survived (CT: pontomedullary hemorrhage) | Unknown |
| Rousseaux et al.[53,57] | HA, somnolence; pulmonary edema; upbeat, downbeat nyst.; pharyngeal & lingual paresis, gait imbalance | Operated, survived (MRI: dorsomedial medullary hemorrhage) | Unknown |

Abbreviations: R = right, L = left, HA = headache, JPS = joint position sense, ↓ = decreased, vomit. = vomiting, nyst. = nystagmus, bilat. = bilateral, LOC = loss of consciousness, temp. = temperature, horiz. = horizontal, resp. = respiratory, n. = nerve, AVM = arteriovenous malformation.

with the new onset of right vocal cord paralysis and atrophy of that half of the tongue, followed by slowly progressive unsteadiness of gait and worsening right hemiparesis, with the addition of dysphagia prior to hospital admission. Her examination showed a preserved state of alertness, up-beating nystagmus on upward gaze, left facial hypesthesia, right pharyngeal, palatal and lingual weakness, right hemiparesis with decreased deep sensory modalities ipsilaterally and hypalgesia contralaterally. Because of respiratory failure, she was intubated and connected to a respirator. CSF examination showed xanthochromia. Her course was characterized by progressive loss of motor function in all four limbs, and development of ocular "bobbing" prior to death. Autopsy showed an AVM in the right lateral medulla associated with a large hemorrhage that extended up into the ponto-medullary junction. Arseni and Stanciu[45] reported two cases of medullary hemorrhage that were treated surgically, with survival: Case 1, a 43-year-old woman, had a history of episodic dizziness for six months, followed by an episode of headache, oral-lingual paresthesias, and loss of consciousness from which she recovered, to again develop severe headache, with gait instability and diplopia, prior to hospital admission; her examination disclosed "right dysmetria, positive Romberg sign with falling backwards, paresis of left third and sixth cranial nerves, horizontal and vertical nystagmus, and neck rigidity." She subsequently developed dysphonia and dysphagia, inability to get out of bed, right hemiparesis, left hemihypalgesia, loss of deep sensory modalities on the right side, and left peripheral facial paralysis. CSF was hemorrhagic. At surgery, an intramedullary hematoma was drained through the floor of the fourth ventricle. Case 2, a 40-year-old woman, developed one month before admission sudden occipital headache, dizziness, and vomiting, followed by paresthesias of the right limbs, symptoms that improved partially before recurring two weeks later, with the addition of dysphagia and gait im-

balance. On examination she had slight left hemiparesis with hemihypalgesia and limb and gait ataxia, with horizontal nystagmus, dysphonia, and dysphagia. At operation a left-sided medullary hematoma was drained through the floor of the fourth ventricle. Both patients survived with residual gait imbalance, with disappearance of the dysphagia and dysphonia. Morel-Maroger et al.[15] described a 56-year-old hypertensive man who developed the abrupt onset of dysphagia due to left palatal-pharyngeal paralysis, along with left facial, hypoglossal, and vocal cord paralysis, hypoacusis, Horner's syndrome, and right-sided hemiparesthesias. CT demonstrated an 8-mm hemorrhage of the left lateral medulla with extension to the basal pons. The patient had made a full recovery when tested five months after stroke onset, when follow-up CT was also normal. Neuman et al.[46] recently reported a case of a 33-year-old hypertensive man who developed sudden headache and a fall without loss of consciousness, along with vertigo, dysarthria, hoarseness, and dysphagia. On examination, blood pressure was 170/130, he was intermittently lethargic, with right Horner's syndrome, decreased facial sensation and corneal reflex, decreased facial and palatal motility, and gag reflex, as well as tongue deviation to that side, with slight right hemiparesis and normal coordination. He developed obstructive hydrocephalus requiring ventriculostomy and shunting, and ventilatory support was necessary after he became apneic. He died twenty-seven days after stroke onset, and autopsy revealed a hematoma in the right rostral dorsolateral medulla and inferior cerebellar peduncle, with histological findings of hyaline thickening of the walls of small medullary arteries, without evidence of vascular malformation or tumor. Hommel et al.[47] documented the unusual occurrence of a hypertensive 65-year-old man who developed a small right tegmental medullary ICH associated with marked ipsilateral lateropulsion on standing and sitting up. This disorder of stance occurred in the face of lack of hemiparesis, hemiataxia, vertigo, or involvement of cranial nerves, the only additional feature of the case having been transient obstructive hydrocephalus. The course was benign, with restoration of ambulation without assistance by three months after stroke onset, at which time follow-up CT showed normal ventricular size. Cappa et al.[48] reported the case of a 44-year-old woman who suddenly developed a lateral medullary syndrome, with gait unsteadiness, vertigo, and vomiting, with findings of left sixth nerve palsy, facial weakness, and horizontal nystagmus, along with dysphonia, dysarthria, and dysphagia, hiccups, left-sided limb ataxia, and right-sided hemihypalgesia involving the limbs and face. CT documented a small hematoma in the left dorsolateral aspect of the medulla; her course was benign, and one month after stroke onset the cranial nerve deficits had cleared, and she was left with left-beating nystagmus and right-sided hemihypalgesia.

Biller et al.[49] documented in detail the case of a 72-year-old hypertensive woman who developed sudden occipital headache, postural dizziness, left hemibody paresthesias, and dysarthria, with physical findings of bilateral horizontal nystagmus, paralysis of the right palate and vocal cord, absent gag reflex, and tongue deviation to the right, with truncal ataxia (leaning to the right), and normal corneal and facial sensation. MRI showed a right medullary hemorrhage, extending from the pontomedullary junction to the caudal medulla. The patient developed transient respiratory difficulties that required intubation, and survived the hemorrhage with gradual resolution of her deficits, her only sequela being right hypoglossal palsy. The authors emphasized the value of MRI in the diagnosis of brainstem hemorrhages, due to the potential difficulties in diagnosing them with CT scan in view of the frequent image degradation by the intrapetrous beam-hardening artifact.[49] They also pointed out that among fourteen patients reported in the literature, 50% had been fatal, close to 30% (four cases[44,50-52]) were due to vascular malformations, and over 50% of them had

no documented mechanism. With regard to treatment, a number of patients with primary medullary[41,45,46,52,53] and with ponto-medullary[54,55] hemorrhages have been treated with surgical resection of the hematoma, and the results have been surprisingly good, with survival of all seven patients thus treated. Further patients have been recently reported by Shuaib[56] and Rousseaux et al.[53,57] The latter authors reported the case of a 21-year-old normotensive woman with a small dorsomedial medullary hemorrhage characterized by sudden occipital headache at onset, followed by somnolence, tachycardia, and pulmonary edema; her physical findings included small, reactive pupils and upbeating vertical nystagmus. Following surgical drainage of a medial medullary hematoma, she was left with bilateral pharyngeal and lingual palsy, and gait imbalance. She also initially had up-beating vertical nystagmus in the primary position (which increased in amplitude with upgaze), and down-beating nystagmus on downgaze which changed two and a half months after the hemorrhage to down-beating nystagmus on primary position and downgaze, and up-beating nystagmus in upgaze. The patient was left with persistent bilateral lingual atrophy as sequela, reflecting suspected bilateral damage to the hypoglossal nuclei. The peculiar course of the vertical nystagmus was interpreted as secondary to injury to the superior vestibular nuclei and the medial longitudinal fasciculi causing, respectively, the initial predominantly up-beating nystagmus and the subsequent down-beating nystagmus.[57]

The following represents a typical example of primary medullary hemorrhage:

A 54-year-old man presented with a one-day history of dizziness, imbalance and dysarthria. He was well until the night of admission when he developed dizziness on getting up to go to the bathroom along with marked unsteadiness, being unable to walk without assistance. The following morning he awoke with severe vertigo, and later developed dysarthria and dysphagia. On physical examination he was alert, oriented and cooperative, with hoarseness and moderate dysarthria. Pupils were 4 mm on the right, 3 mm on the left, with mild bilateral ptosis. EOMs were full, with spontaneous upbeating vertical nystagmus in primary gaze which persisted in all directions of gaze, but diminished with downgaze. Corneal reflexes were equal and brisk. Facial sensation was intact to light touch and pinprick. There was slight flattening of the right nasolabial fold. Hearing was intact. Gag reflex was diminished bilaterally and the palate deviated slightly to the left. The tongue deviated to the right and protruded only about 1 to 2 cm, with bilateral weakness on lateral movements. On motor testing there was no drift, and strength was 5/5, with normal tone. Slight dysmetria of the upper limbs was present, left greater than right. Gait was wide-based and ataxic, with positive Romberg sign, falling to the right. Sensation was normal to light touch, pinprick, joint position sense and vibration. Reflexes were 2+ and equal, and plantar reflexes were flexor.

CT scan, with and without contrast, showed a 1 × 1 cm hemorrhage to the right of the midline in the tegmentum of the medulla (Figure 21.6). Vertebral angiography revealed no abnormality.

During his hospital course he became more steady and less ataxic, and his speech and swallowing gradually improved. The nystagmus improved, and by one month from onset it had disappeared. The tongue was still weak, the palate elevated deviated to the left, and there was still mild dysarthria and hoarseness, and left-sided dysmetria.

From the analysis of the cases reported in the literature, it is apparent that medullary hemorrhage is virtually always unilateral, either tegmental or basal, and is rarely restricted to the dorsolateral region, thus explaining the rarity of Wallenberg's syndrome as its presentation.[48] Most published cases have had horizontal nystagmus, ipsilateral facial hypesthesia, limb ataxia and gait imbalance, along with palatal weakness, dysphonia and dysphagia,[41,44-46,48,56] less common features being ipsilateral Horner's syndrome[15,46] and contralateral hemihypalgesia.[15,44,45,48,49] The two most common fea-

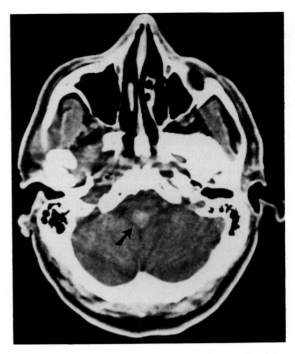

**Figure 21.6.** Noncontrast CT scan with dorsal medullary hemorrhage (arrow) (Courtesy of Donna Gabuzda, M.D., Dana Farber Institute, Boston, MA.)

tures that separate the presentation of medullary ICH from Wallenberg's syndrome are the frequency of contralateral hemiparesis[41-46,56] and ipsilateral hypoglossal palsy,[15,44,46,49,53] indicative of hemorrhages that extend both ventrally and medially, respectively, from the area of the dorsolateral medulla.

In the majority of these cases the mechanism is unknown.[20,58] The already mentioned four cases due to ruptured vascular malformations, along with five presumably hypertensive ones (one also receiving an oral anticoagulant, an association also briefly mentioned in a report of anticoagulant-related hemorrhages by Barron and Fergusson[59]) and a single instance of fatal bleeding into a syringobulbia cavity,[60] leaves ten of seventeen reported cases (59%) unexplained. This probably represents the highest frequency of instances of unknown mechanism among the various anatomical sites of ICH.

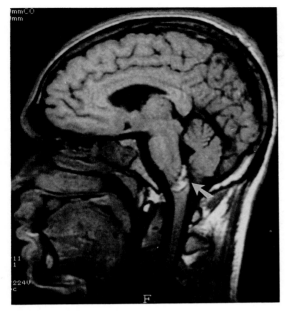

A

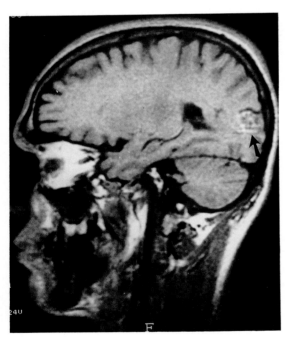

B

**Figure 21.7.** MRI (TR/TE = 600/25 msec) of acute medullary hemorrhage (arrow) (A), with an associated cavernous angioma of the occipital lobe (arrow) (B) (Courtesy of Dr. Fernando Barinagar-rementería, Mexico City, Mexico.)

On occasion, the finding of a concomitant cavernous angioma suggests the rupture of that type of malformation as the possible cause of a medullary hemorrhage (Figure 21.7). Other mechanisms of ICH, such as bleeding into a tumor, sympathomimetic drug effect, or the age-related cerebral amyloid angiopathy,[61] have not been described in medullary hemorrhage, in the latter situation undoubtedly as a result of the distribution of the angiopathy, which tends to spare the brainstem.[62]

## References

1. Kase CS, Caplan LR. Hemorrhage affecting the brainstem and cerebellum. In: Barnett HJM, et al., eds. Stroke: Pathophysiology, Diagnosis, and Management. New York: Churchill Livingstone, 1986;621–641.
2. Le Coz P, Woimant F, George B, et al. Aspects cliniques et évolutifs des hématomes circonscrits du tronc cérébral: apport du scanner X. Rev Neurol 1986;142:52–60.
3. Roig C, Carvajal A, Illa I, et al. Hémorragies mésencéphaliques isolées: trois cas diagnostiqués par tomodensitométrie. Rev Neurol 1982;138:53–61.
4. Bottinelli MD, Purriel JA, Medoc J, et al. Hemorragia primitiva espontánea del tronco cerebral: estudio clínico anatómico. Acta Neurol Latinoamer 1969;15:154–179.
5. Collomb H, Dumas M, Girard P-L, et al. Hémorragies primitives du tronc cérébral: étude anatomique et clinique de 36 cas. Rev Neurol 1973;129:185–210.
6. Dinsdale HB. Spontaneous hemorrhage in the posterior fossa: a study of primary cerebellar and pontine hemorrhages with observations on their pathogenesis. Arch Neurol 1964;10:200–217.
7. Freytag E. Fatal hypertensive intracerebral haematomas: a survey of the pathological anatomy of 393 cases. J Neurol Neurosurg Psychiat 1968;31:616–620.
8. Boudouresques G, Hauw JJ, Escourolle R. Etude anatomique de 318 hémorragies intraparenchymateuses de l'adulte. Rev Neurol 1979;135:845–865.
9. L'Hermitte J. Les hémorragies des pédoncules cérébraux: étude clinique. Presse Med 1942; 50:625–626.

10. Scoville WB, Poppen JL. Intrapeduncular hemorrhage of the brain: successful operative approach, with evacuation of clot and a seven and one-fourth year observation period. Arch Neurol Psychiat 1949;61:688–694.

11. La Torre E, Delitala A, Sorano V. Hematoma of the quadrigeminal plate: case report. J Neurosurg 1978;49:610–613.

12. Humphreys RP. Computerized tomographic definition of mesencephalic hematoma with evacuation through pedunculotomy: case report. J Neurosurg 1978;49:749–752.

13. Durward QJ, Barnett HJM, Barr HWK. Presentation and management of mesencephalic hematoma: report of two cases. J Neurosurg 1982;56:123–127.

14. Benedikt M. Tremblement avec paralysie croisée du moteur oculaire commun. Bull Méd 1889;3:547–548.

15. Morel-Maroger A, Metzger J, Bories J, et al. Les hématomes bénins du tronc cérébral chez les hypertendus artériels. Rev Neurol 1982;138:437–445.

16. Sand JJ, Biller J, Corbett JJ, et al. Partial dorsal mesencephalic hemorrhages: report of three cases. Neurology 1986;36:529–533.

17. Weisberg LA. Mesencephalic hemorrhages: clinical and computed tomographic correlations. Neurology 1986;36:713–716.

18. de Mendonça A, Pimentel J, Morgado F, et al. Mesencephalic hematoma: case report with autopsy study. J Neurol 1990;237:55–58.

19. Zuccarello M, Iavicoli R, Pardatscher K, et al. Primary brain stem haematomas: diagnosis and treatment. Acta Neurochir 1980;54:45–52.

20. Shuaib A. Benign brainstem hemorrhage: a brief review. J Stroke Cerebrovasc Dis 1991;1:146–151.

21. Brismar J, Hindfelt B, Nilsson D. Benign brainstem hematoma. Acta Neurol Scand 1979;60:178–182.

22. Bogousslavsky J. Syndromes oculomoteurs résultant de lésions mésencéphaliques chez l'homme. Rev Neurol 1989;145:546–559.

23. Shuaib A, Murphy W. Mesencephalic hemorrhage and third nerve palsy. J Comput Tomogr 1987;11:385–388.

24. Nighoghossian N, Vighetto A, Trouillas P. Syndrome nucléaire du nerf moteur oculaire commun et réaction d'inclinaison oculaire: par hématome mésencéphalique. Rev Neurol 1991;147:676–679.

25. Fleet WS, Rapcsak SZ, Huntley WW, et al. Pupil-sparing oculomotor palsy from midbrain hemorrhage. Ann Ophthalmol 1988;20:345–346.

26. Nadeau SE, Trobe JD. Pupil sparing in oculomotor palsy: a brief review. Ann Neurol 1983;13:143–148.

27. Shuaib A, Israelian G, Lee MA. Mesencephalic hemorrhage and unilateral pupillary deficit. J Clin Neuro-ophthalmol 1989;9:47–49.

28. Stern LZ, Bernick C. Spontaneous, isolated, mesencephalic hemorrhage. Neurology 1986;36:1627 (letter).

29. Dussaux P, Plas J, Brion S. Parésie bilatérale du muscle grand oblique, par hématome de la calotte mésencéphalique. Rev Neurol 1990;146:45–47.

30. Tuttle PV, Reinmuth OM. Midbrain hemorrhage producing pure sensory stroke. Arch Neurol 1984;41:794–795.

31. Azouvi P, Tougeron A, Hussonois C, et al. Pure sensory stroke due to midbrain haemorrhage limited to the spinothalamic pathway. J Neurol Neurosurg Psychiat 1989;52:1427–1428.

32. Fisher CM. Pure sensory stroke involving face, arm, and leg. Neurology 1965;15:76–80.

33. Ono S, Inoue K. Cheiro-oral syndrome following midbrain haemorrhage. J Neurol 1985;232:304–306.

34. Garcin R, Lapresle J. Syndrome sensitif de type thalamique et à topographie chéiro-orale par lésion localisée du thalamus. Rev Neurol 1954;90:124–129.

35. Garcin R, Lapresle J. Deuxième observation personnelle de syndrome sensitif de type thalamique et à topographie chéiro-orale par lésion localisée du thalamus. Rev Neurol 1960;103:474–481.

36. Fingerote RJ, Shuaib A, Brownell AKW. Spontaneous midbrain hemorrhage. South Med J 1990;83:280–282.

37. Sano K. Spontaneous brain stem haematoma. Neurosurg Rev 1983;6:71–77.

38. Mehler MF, Ragone PS. Primary spontaneous mesencephalic hemorrhage. Can J Neurol Sci 1988;15:435–438.

39. Stein RW, Kase CS, Hier DB, et al. Caudate hemorrhage. Neurology 1984;34:1549–1554.

40. Riser M, Géraud J, Rascol A, et al. Hémorragie méso-diencéphalique, avec troubles du la conscience et coma terminal. Rev Neurol 1957;96:252–256.

41. Kempe LG. Surgical removal of an intramedullary haematoma simulating Wallenberg's

syndrome. J Neurol Neurosurg Psychiat 1964; 27:78–80.

42. Mastaglia FL, Edis B, Kakulas BA. Medullary haemorrhage: a report of two cases. J Neurol Neurosurg Psychiat 1969;32:221–225.

43. Cole FM, Yates PO. The occurrence and significance of intracerebral micro-aneurysms. J Path Bact 1967;93:393–411.

44. Plum F, Posner JB. The Diagnosis of Stupor and Coma. Third edition. Philadelphia: FA Davis, 1980;29–30.

45. Arseni C, Stanciu M. Primary haematomas of the brain stem. Acta Neurochir 1973;28: 323–330.

46. Neumann PE, Mehler MF, Horoupian DS. Primary medullary hypertensive hemorrhage. Neurology 1985;35:925–928.

47. Hommel M, Borgel F, Gaio JM, et al. Latéropulsion ipsilatérale isolée par hématome bulbaire. Rev Neurol 1985;141:53–54.

48. Cappa SF, Riva M, Sterzi R, et al. Brain-stem haematoma with complete recovery. J Neurol 1985;232:352–353.

49. Biller J, Gentry LR, Adams HP, et al. Spontaneous hemorrhage in the medulla oblongata: clinical MR correlations. J Comput Assist Tomogr 1986;10:303–306.

50. Bergman PS. Hemangioma of the pons: case report and review of the literature. J Mt Sinai Hosp 1950;17:119–131.

51. Bosch K, Janssen W. Plötzlicher Tod durch intramedulläres Hämangiom. Dtsch Z ges Gerichtl Med 1962;52:571–577.

52. Cohen HCM, Tucker WS, Humphreys RP, et al. Angiographically cryptic histologically verified cerebrovascular malformations. Neurosurgery 1982;10:704–714.

53. Rousseaux M, Griffie G, Dhellemmes P, et al. Hématome bulbaire postéro-médian d'évolution favorable: étude de la dysautonomie. Rev Neurol 1988;144:481–488.

54. Obrador S, Dierssen G, Odoriz BJ. Surgical evacuation of a pontine-medullary hematoma: case report. J Neurosurg 1970;33:82–84.

55. Martin P, Noterman J. L'hématome bulboprotubérantiel opérable. Acta Neurol Belg 1971; 71:261–268.

56. Shuaib A. Benign brainstem hemorrhage. Can J Neurol Sci 1991;18:356–357.

57. Rousseaux M, Dupard T, Lesoin F, et al. Upbeat and downbeat nystagmus occurring successively in a patient with posterior medullary haemorrhage. J Neurol Neurosurg Psychiat 1991;54:367–369.

58. Barinagarrementería F, Cantú C. Spontaneous medullary hemorrhage: features related to prognosis. J Stroke Cerebrovasc Dis 1992;2 [suppl 1]:119 (abstract).

59. Barron KD, Fergusson G. Intracranial hemorrhage as a complication of anticoagulant therapy. Neurology 1959;9:447–455.

60. Roig C, Lopez-Pousa S, Ferrer I. Bleeding in syringobulbia: a fatal complication. Eur Neurol 1982;21:189–193.

61. Kase CS. Intracerebral hemorrhage: nonhypertensive causes. Stroke 1986;17:590–595.

62. Vinters HV, Gilbert JJ. Cerebral amyloid angiopathy: incidence and complications in the aging brain. II. The distribution of amyloid vascular changes. Stroke 1983;14:924–928.

# PART FOUR
## Prognosis and Treatment: An Overview

# Chapter 22
# Prognosis and Treatment of Patients with Intracerebral Hemorrhage

## Carlos S. Kase and Robert M. Crowell

The prognosis and treatment of the various anatomical sites of intracerebral hemorrhage (ICH) have already been discussed in detail in the corresponding chapters. This chapter provides an overview of these two aspects of ICH, with an emphasis on general prognostic features, the prevention and management of raised intracranial pressure (ICP), the indications for surgical and nonsurgical management, and novel approaches to the surgical management of ICH.

## Prognosis

The incidence and outcome figures in patients with ICH have varied substantially in recent decades. The incidence rates of ICH showed a significant and sustained decline in the population of Rochester, Minnesota, when they were calculated for four consecutive eight-year intervals between 1945 and 1976[1] (Figure 22.1). This decline in incidence was attributed to improved control of risk factors for ICH, especially hypertension. A transient increase in incidence during the period between 1961 and 1968 was attributed to a large number of hemorrhages in patients on long-term anticoagulant treatment, coinciding with "the period of peak enthusiasm for the use of anticoagulants for all diagnoses."[1]

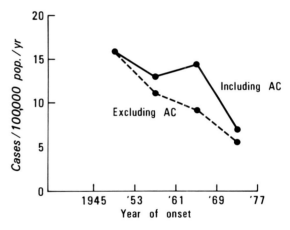

**Figure 22.1.** Decline in incidence of ICH in Rochester, Minnesota, 1945 through 1976. AC = anticoagulant therapy at onset of ICH. (Reprinted from Furlan AJ, Whisnant JP, Elveback LR. The decreasing incidence of primary intracerebral hemorrhage: a population study. Ann Neurol 1979;5:367–373, with permission.)

In a subsequent study from the same institution (Mayo Clinic), but encompassing the period between 1975 and 1979, Drury et al.[2] showed an *increase* in the incidence of ICH, attributed to the introduction of computed tomography (CT) in 1973. This resulted in improved case ascertainment by the inclusion of patients with small ICHs, which in the pre-

467

CT era would have likely been diagnosed as cerebral infarcts. This interpretation was further supported by a marked improvement in thirty-day survival rates in patients with ICH, from 8% during the period 1945 to 1976[1] to 42% during the period 1975 to 1979,[3] a change that was also attributed to the inclusion of CT-diagnosed small hematomas, which have a better prognosis.[2,3] Similar changes in incidence and prognosis of ICH in relation to the introduction of CT were recently reported by Rowe et al.[4]

## Mortality

Improved mortality figures are an almost uniform finding in modern series, in comparison with the old, pre-CT series that relied on autopsy data and on the clinical diagnosis of the larger hemorrhages, biasing the samples toward the larger, more severely symptomatic and often fatal ICHs (Table 22.1). The mortality rates in the pre-CT series were between 58% and 92%,[1,5,6] whereas those in the post-CT area range between 20% and 56%. The substantial disparities in mortality rates among modern series are in part due to the use of different time periods of estimation of mortality. In some series the time period was not provided,[8] other authors used thirty-day,[11,14,16,20,22,23] sixty-day,[19] six-month,[21] or one-year[18] rates; others referred only to "in hospital"[7,12,15] or "acute"[9,17] mortality, while other figures reflected early mortality, within sixteen days[10] or fourteen days[13] from onset. Although these disparities make comparisons among series difficult, the figures nevertheless illustrate a substantial overall reduction in mortality rates in modern, post-CT series.

## Long-term Prognosis

In contrast with the abundant data on short-term outcome and mortality, relatively little information is available on the long-term prognosis of ICH. Among the seventy pa-

**Table 22.1.** Mortality Figures in Old (Pre-CT) and Recent (Post-CT) Series of ICH*

| Author | No. Pts. ICH | Mortality No. Pts. (%) |
|---|---|---|
| *Pre-CT* | | |
| Furlan et al.[1] | 142 | 130 (92%) |
| McKissock et al.[5] | 244 | 181 (74%) |
| McKissock et al.[6] | 180 | 104 (58%) |
| *Post-CT* | | |
| Douglas and Haerer[7] | 70 | 28 (40%) |
| Nath et al.[8] | 244 | 66 (27%) |
| Steiner et al.[9] | 42 | 11 (26%) |
| Helweg-Larsen et al.[10] | 53 | 14 (26%) |
| Silver et al.[11] | 106 | 59 (56%) |
| Dixon et al.[12] | 100 | 23 (23%) |
| Portenoy et al.[13] | 112 | 52 (46%) |
| Fieschi et al.[14] | 104 | 31 (30%) |
| Bogousslavsky et al.[15] | 109 | 22 (20%) |
| Tuhrim et al.[16] | 94 | 32 (34%) |
| Omae et al.[17] | 223 | 56 (25%) |
| Westling et al.[18] | 28 | 11 (39%) |
| Gras et al.[19] | 238 | 107 (45%) |
| Bamford et al.[20] | 66 | 34 (52%) |
| Daverat et al.[21] | 166 | 71 (43%) |
| Fogelholm et al.[22] | 158 | 80 (51%) |
| Franke et al.[23] | 157 | 68 (43%) |

Abbreviations: CT = computerized tomography, No. = number, pts. = patients.

*Mortality rates correspond to variable periods after onset of ICH in the different series; see text for explanation.

tients with hypertensive ICH reported by Douglas and Haerer,[7] forty-two survived the acute phase, but seven of them subsequently died of noncerebrovascular causes over a 2½-year follow-up period. Among the remaining thirty-five patients, thirty-two (91%) were ambulatory at follow-up, and five of them had returned to work. There were no instances of recurrent ICH. The authors concluded that patients who survived the acute phase of ICH had a relatively good functional prognosis, thus "deserving aggressive medical care and rehabilitation efforts." Similarly, Steiner et al.[9] reported that 55% of the thirty-one patients in their series who survived the acute stage of the ICH "returned to previous activity." Helweg-Larsen et al.[10] documented a normal neurological examination in 50% and ability to resume their previous work in 41% of the patients who survived the acute phase of the ICH and the 7- to 62-month follow-up period. Portenoy et al.[13] and Omae et al.[17] reported that 37% of the survivors of ICH were functionally independent at follow-up, whereas Fieschi et al.[14] found 49% of the survivors independent at one year of follow-up. The latter authors reported no instances of rebleeding in the group of sixty-nine one-year survivors. Functional independence was achieved by 28% of sixty-day survivors in the series of Gras et al.,[19] while 49% had moderate handicap and 23% required frequent or permanent assistance in their activities. Daverat et al.[21] reported functional independence in sixty-nine of ninety-five (73%) patients who were alive six months after the ICH. In a population study in central Finland, Fogelholm et al.[22] found a high mortality rate (51%) at thirty days from onset of ICH, but 51% of the survivors were independent in activities of daily living after a median follow-up of thirty-two months. These authors found that the rates of subsequent mortality after the first month from ICH onset were not different from those of age- and sex-matched members of the population. A similar conclusion was reached by Franke et al.,[23] who found high early mortality (24% within two days from onset of ICH), but equal survival rates and functional levels at one year in 120 survivors from ICH in comparison with an equal number of matched patients with cerebral infarction. These data contrast with those of Helweg-Larsen et al.,[10] who found an excess mortality in ICH survivors in comparison with an age-matched normal population, but the number of patients included in their series was too small to allow accurate calculation of the death risk.

These figures on mortality and long-term outcome in ICH give a general picture of high mortality during the acute phase, especially within days after onset, followed by a relatively good functional prognosis on long-term follow-up. The latter does not appear to be different for survivors of ICH when compared with patients with cerebral infarction.[23] The issue of whether there is excess mortality in ICH survivors in comparison with the general population has not been yet fully clarified.[10,22]

### Predictors of Outcome

A great deal of research into the prognosis of ICH has been devoted to the identification of early clinical and CT features that might predict outcome, both vital and functional. The various studies have analyzed a large number of clinical features (prior history, general physical and neurological examinations) and CT parameters in order to determine their contribution to prognosis, as well as their possible interaction, the latter resulting in the creation of various models for the determination of prognosis in ICH.

The most consistent and reliable clinical predictor of outcome in ICH is the *level of consciousness* at presentation or in the early hours after onset. Coma at presentation carries a mortality that is virtually 100%, except for the occasional patient who survives immediate surgical evacuation of the clot. Lesser degrees of compromised alertness are closely correlated with outcome as well. Most modern series have evaluated this factor by using the Glasgow Coma Scale (GCS),[24] a numerical scoring instrument designed for the evaluation of patients with head injuries, that has also proven useful in the assessment of level of consciousness in stroke patients.[25] The level of consciousness,[7,9,10] generally measured by the admission GCS,[8,12–14,16,21,23] has been closely correlated with both early[8,13,23] and thirty-day[14–16] mortality (Figure 22.2), as well as with mortality at six months after ICH onset.[21] A closely related factor, *hematoma size* on admission CT, has shown a similarly high predictive value for mortality in ICH (Figure 22.3). One study only[9] found mortality to be unaffected by size of ICH. Since level of consciousness and size of hematoma are closely interdependent vari-

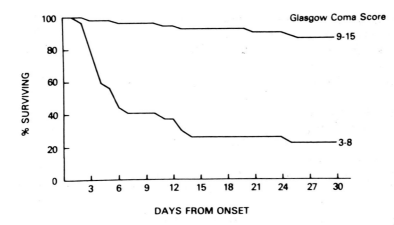

**Figure 22.2.** Survival curves after thirty days from ICH onset, in relation to Glasgow Coma Score at presentation with ICH. (Reprinted from Tuhrim S, Dambrosia JM, Price TR, et al. Prediction of intracerebral hemorrhage survival. Ann Neurol 1988;24:258–263. With permission.)

ables, both factors are significant predictors of outcome in studies that have used univariate analysis.[13,14,16,21,23] With multivariate analysis, most series have found one or both of these factors, GCS and hematoma size, to be highly predictive of outcome.[12,13,16,21,23] The correlation between hematoma volume and mortality is particularly close in supratentorial hematomas[22] (Figure 22.4), a correlation that applies to functional outcome as well.[12–14,21,26] In some studies of supratentorial ICH[27] or ICH in general,[10,23] measurements of hematomas suggest that a critical volume of 40 to 50 cm³ separates patients between bad and good prognostic groups, with volumes above and below that figure, respectively. Mass effect, a factor closely related to

hematoma size, either measured simply as midline shift[8] or more precisely as pineal gland calcification displacement of 3 mm or more,[23] has also been correlated closely with outcome. Other CT features, in particular *intraventricular extension* of the ICH, have been less uniformly found to contribute independently to outcome, in one series[28] even showing no relationship to outcome. This seems to relate primarily to the fact that ventricular extension of the ICH has different prognostic implications depending on the site of the initial intraparenchymal hemorrhage that secondarily extends into the ventricular system. In some series,[7–9] ventricular extension in general, irrespective of hematoma location, carried a mortality of 45% to 75%, in

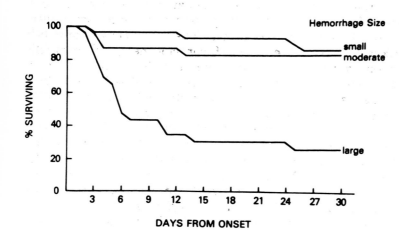

**Figure 22.3.** Survival curves after thirty days from ICH onset, in relation to hematoma size as measured in admission CT. (Reprinted from Tuhrim S, Dambrosia JM, Price TR, et al. Prediction of intracerebral hemorrhage survival. Ann Neurol 1988;24:258–263. With permission.)

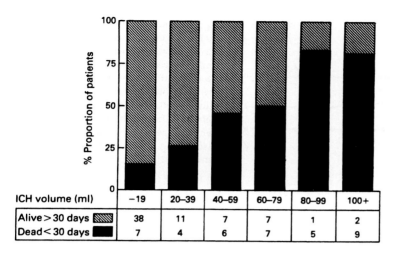

**Figure 22.4.** Mortality after thirty days from onset in patients with supratentorial ICH in relation to hematoma volume. (Reprinted from Fogelholm R, Nuutila M, Vuorela A-L. Primary intracerebral haemorrhage in the Jyväskylä region, Central Finland 1985–89: incidence, case fatality rate, and functional outcome. J Neurol Neurosurg Psychiat 1992;55:546–552. With permission.)

comparison with only 9% to 21% for patients without that feature on initial CT. In the series of Daverat et al.,[21] intraventricular extension of the hematoma was a strong predictor of mortality at one month after onset. Others[10,26] found this factor to be a poor prognostic sign only in putaminal and thalamic hemorrhages, while it had no predictive value in patients with caudate hemorrhage.[26] The latter data may reflect in part the effect of hematoma size, rather than ventricular extension per se, in mortality after ICH. Since the lateral putaminal hemorrhages need to attain a large size in order to communicate with the medial ventricular system, hematoma size may be the actual factor that conditions outcome, a view supported by the comparatively lower mortality rates of caudate ICH, which virtually always drains into the adjacent ventricular system[29] by virtue of its medial location, despite the generally small size of the parenchymal hematomas. In a detailed quantitative analysis of ventricular extension in a series of forty-seven patients with forty-eight supratentorial hemorrhages, Young et al.[30] found that the volume of intraventricular blood was a determinant of prognosis, as all but one patient with more than 20 cm[3] of ventricular blood died, irrespective of the site of origin of the intraparenchymal hematoma. The associated feature of hydrocephalus also correlated with poor outcome,

but its independent contribution and importance were questionable, as judged by a lack of improvement in prognosis in patients who underwent ventricular drainage for the treatment of hydrocephalus.[30]

A number of other clinical features that have been assessed in relation to prognosis have shown weaker correlations, although some have been retained as good predictors in models derived from multivariate analysis. *Age* has not been correlated with mortality in some series,[9,10] whereas increasing age (over age 69) has been associated with poor prognosis in others,[14] in particular with regard to long-term (six to thirty-two months) prognosis[21–23] (Figure 22.5). Other factors have been measured in only limited numbers of studies, and the following have been found to correlate with prognosis: *systolic blood pressure,*[13,16,26] *pulse pressure,*[16] *gaze palsies*[10,16,23] and *motor deficits*[16,21,23] *PO₂* on initial arterial blood gases,[12] *ECG changes,*[12] *blood glucose* on admission,[23] and *neurological deterioration* after onset.[8,16] Some of these features, along with the highly correlated clinical and CT criteria detailed above, have been incorporated into models generated by logistic regression techniques of multivariate analysis that have a high predictive value for early (two,[23] fourteen,[13] or thirty[16] days from onset) mortality in ICH. Portenoy et al.[13] identified the GCS, hematoma size, and in-

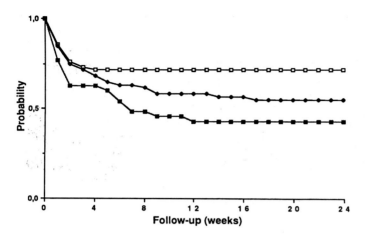

**Figure 22.5.** Survival curves after six months from supratentorial ICH onset according to age group. Empty squares: under 60 years; diamonds: 60 to 69 years; solid squares: over 69 years. (Reprinted from Daverat P, Castel JP, Dartigues JF, et al. Death and functional outcome after spontaneous intracerebral hemorrhage: a prospective study of 166 cases using multivariate analysis. Stroke 1991;22:1–6. With permission.)

traventricular extension of the hemorrhage as strong predictors of outcome. Tuhrim et al.[16] incorporated the GCS, systolic blood pressure, pulse pressure, gaze palsies, severity of weakness, signs of brainstem-cerebellar deficits, worsening after onset, and hemorrhage size into a model that correctly predicted survival or death at thirty days in 92% of patients. The predictive value of probability of thirty-day survival as a function of the variables included in the model is shown in Figure 22.6. Franke et al.[23] found that the risk of death within two days of ICH onset was determined by pineal calcification displacement of 3 mm or more, admission blood glucose of 8 mmol per liter or more, eye and motor score of eight or less on the GCS, and hematoma volume of 40 cm$^3$ or more.

These data on early features predictive of short-term and long-term outcome in ICH are valuable not only in clinical practice for assessing the prognosis during the acute stage in individual patients, but also in the planning of prospective studies intended to analyze the value of therapeutic measures in ICH. These clinical and CT features should

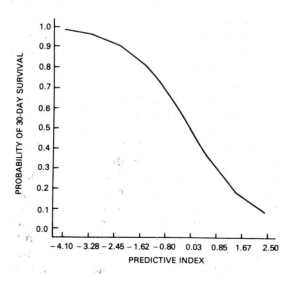

**Figure 22.6.** Probability of thirty-day survival as a function of the predictive index derived from model for survival in ICH. (Reprinted from Tuhrim S, Dambrosia JM, Price TR, et al. Prediction of intracerebral hemorrhage survival. Ann Neurol 1988;24:258–263. With permission.)

permit the stratification of patients into various prognostic categories at the time of entry into a therapeutic trial, in order to allow for the assessment of the effect of a given treatment modality on outcome, within clinically homogeneous groups of patients.

## Treatment

The modern management of patients with ICH involves a variety of aspects, including the prevention and treatment of raised ICP, the choice between surgical and nonsurgical approaches, and the eventual use of novel surgical techniques. Since there is still a remarkable paucity of prospective controlled clinical trials in this area, most therapeutic decisions have to be individualized, taking into consideration variables such as the site and size of the hematoma, the mechanism of ICH, and the presence of accompanying systemic complications.[17]

### Control of Intracranial Pressure

ICP varies directly in relation to the volume of the intracranial contents that include brain volume, CSF volume, and cerebral blood volume (CBV). In the presence of a cerebral mass lesion such as ICH, the increased brain volume may result in raised ICP, unless a concomitant reduction in the volume of the other compartments takes place, either physiologically or through therapeutic intervention. The management of raised ICP in patients with ICH largely depends on the manipulation of the various parameters that determine ICP.

ICP can be increased purely as a result of the presence of a hematoma, or there can be additional contributors to raised ICP. Both need to be treated vigorously. The features that further raise ICP in patients with intracranial mass lesions include fever, hypoxia, hypertension, seizures, and transient or persistent elevations of intrathoracic pressure.[31]

*Hyperthermia* increases the cerebral metabolic rate and cerebral blood flow (CBF), resulting in increased ICP. The immediate and effective control of hyperthermia with the use of cooling blankets and antipyretics is mandatory in patients with mass lesions and already elevated ICP. Conversely, hypothermia reduces the brain metabolic rate, by as much as 50% at a body temperature of 30°C.[32] However, no therapeutic value of induced hypothermia following acute brain vascular injuries has been demonstrated.[31] *Hypoxia* is a potent stimulus for increase in CBF and CBV, resulting in raised ICP in patients with poor intracranial compliance.[33] The maintenance of adequate oxygenation, attaining levels of $Po_2$ of 100 to 150 mm Hg, should be the aim in patients with ICH.[31]

*Hypertension* in the face of an acute brain injury contributes to increased ICP by increasing the cerebral perfusion pressure (CPP) and promoting brain edema. Conversely, excessive correction of hypertension with resulting hypotension can result in cerebral ischemia and further brain damage. The blood pressure (BP) should be maintained within the extreme levels of harmful hypertension and hypotension, but precise guidelines for BP control are unfortunately not available.[31] A normal and desirable CPP (which is calculated using the formula: $CPP = MAP - ICP$, where MAP is the mean arterial pressure), should be in the 50 to 60 mm Hg range.[31] The main issue regarding BP control in patients with ICH relates to the need and intensity of BP control in the face of hypertension that in part may be secondary to increased ICP (the "Cushing's phenomenon"). Ideally, hypertension will subside to some extent with the rapid control of raised ICP, but if hypertension persists and is associated with increased CPP (85 to 100 mm Hg), pharmacological treatment is indicated.[31] The antihypertensives that are primarily peripheral vasodilators, such as nitroprusside, hydralazine, nitroglycerine, verapamil, and nicardipine, have the inconvenience of also being cerebral vasodilators, thus theoretically leading to increased ICP in patients with poor intracranial compliance.[34] Still, nitroprusside is widely used in patients with intracranial catastrophes and severe hypertension, despite its unpredictable effect on ICP, because of the ease of administration and titration, and its rapid and reliable control of BP.[31] Other agents, such as the alpha- and beta-blocking agent labetalol, in combination with diuretics (furosemide), are recommended for the treatment of hypertension in previously normotensive individuals.[31] No specific BP guidelines are available for the treatment of previously hypertensive patients, a common situation in those with ICH. We have empirically adopted a policy of active BP control in patients with levels of hypertension of 180/100 or more, irrespective of their previous normotensive or hypertensive status.

*Seizures* can occur in patients with acute ICH, especially in those with lobar ICH,[27] usually at the time of stroke onset. The rare occurrence of subsequent seizures is associated with transiently increased CBF, CBV, and ICP, even in paralyzed patients.[35] The seizures should be treated promptly, with the immediate use of intravenous diazepam, followed by loading doses of either phenytoin or phenobarbital. Recalcitrant status epilepticus, a very rare event, may require the use of anesthetic doses of thiopental.[31] *Elevations in intrathoracic pressure* can result in marked

transient increases in ICP, in situations of therapeutic use of positive end-expiratory pressure (PEEP), endotracheal suctioning and coughing, and chest therapy.[31] Awareness and control of these factors in patients with ICH and raised ICP are of great importance in the management of the acute phase of the illness.

The specific measures to control the raised ICP itself are effective in acutely decreasing ICP, and are generally associated with an improved outcome. These include controlled hyperventilation, diuretic therapy, corticosteroids, and high-dose barbiturate therapy. The parameters of administration, advantages, and limitations of these therapies are outlined in Table 22.2. *Hyperventilation* rapidly reduces ICP by inducing cerebral vasoconstriction secondary to hypocarbia.[35] This vascular response occurs in normal brain areas, since those affected by an acute vascular injury suffer an early loss of vascular reactivity and cerebral autoregulation. An effective level of hyperventilation should aim for a $P_{CO_2}$ in the range of 28 to 35 mm Hg initially, subsequently in the 25 to 30 mm Hg range if the ICP continues to be elevated.[31] The value of this form of therapy for raised ICP after the initial hours of treatment is questionable, as compensatory mechanisms within the CNS tend to overcome the vasoconstrictive effect of serum hypocarbia.[31] The greatest effect of hyperventilation on ICP occurs within the

**Table 22.2.** Major Therapies for Acutely Raised ICP

| Treatment | Dose | Advantages | Limitations |
|---|---|---|---|
| Hypocarbia | $P_{CO_2}$ 25–33 mm Hg, RR 10–16/min | Immediate onset, well tolerated | Hypotension, short duration |
| Osmotic diuresis | Mannitol, 0.5–1 g/kg | Rapid onset, titrable, predictable | Hypotension, hypokalemia, short duration |
| Barbiturates | Pentobarbital, 1.5 mg/kg | Mutes BP and respiratory fluctuations | Hypotension, small fixed pupils, long duration |

Abbreviations: ICP = intracranial pressure, RR = respiratory rate, BP = blood pressure. (From Ropper AH. Treatment of intracranial hypertension. In Ropper AH (ed): Neurological and Neurosurgical Intensive Care, 3rd edition. New York: Raven Press, 1993, pp. 29–52. With permission.)

few hours that follow its institution, and thus hyperventilation is highly effective and valuable in situations of acute decompensation with impending cerebral herniation or midline displacement in patients with ICH.

*Osmotic diuretics*, such as mannitol, are also a rapid and reliable way of lowering ICP. Their effect is primarily through shifting of water from the brain substance into the intravascular space, although a small additional beneficial effect may occur by a reduction in CSF production and volume.[31] Their main complications are electrolytic disturbances, mainly hypokalemia, and profound serum hyperosmolarity with renal failure. A "rebound" of raised ICP after the withdrawal of osmotic agents has been described, but it is considered rare and usually without clinical consequence.[31]

*Corticosteroids* have a limited and controversial role in the treatment of raised ICP. Although they are valuable in reducing peritumoral edema in patients with metastatic or primary brain tumors,[36] their effect in the treatment of acute stroke patients has been disappointing.[37,38] In supratentorial ICH, Poungvarin et al.[39] conducted a randomized double-blind trial on the effect of dexamethasone on survival in ninety-three patients. The comparison of dexamethasone (10 mg initial dose, then 5 mg every six hours for six days, 5 mg every twelve hours for two days, and 5 mg for one day) with placebo showed no differences in mortality between the two groups after twenty-one days from onset, and the rate of complications (infections, complications of diabetes) was significantly higher in the dexamethasone-treated patients than in the controls. This result from an interim analysis led to early termination of the trial because of a significantly poorer outcome in the dexamethasone-treated patients. In patients who had GCS of 8 or more at entry, mortality at seven days was significantly lower in treated patients than in controls, but no differences in mortality were found at twenty-one days after onset. These data suggest that dexamethasone is not a useful agent in the treatment of acute ICH, although some

authors recommend its use during the first week after ICH onset.[31]

*High-dose intravenous barbiturates* are effective agents for the reduction of CBF and metabolism, with a concomitant decline in ICP.[40] The most commonly used agent for the purpose of reducing increased ICP is thiopental, at a dose of 1 to 5 mg per kg. The main drawbacks of this therapy are the possible induction of hypotension and the marked effects on neurologic function, including brainstem reflexes, that render the clinical neurological examination impossible to follow. Furthermore, it is still unclear whether such a drastic therapeutic measure is actually followed by an improved clinical outcome in acute stroke patients.[31]

### Continuous Intracranial Pressure Monitoring

The use of continuous monitoring of ICP in patients with ICH has contributed to a better understanding of the course and significance of this feature during the evolution of ICH. Janny et al.[41] reported in 1978 the results of continuous ICP monitoring with a ventricular catheter in seventeen patients with ICH. In the majority of them (twelve patients), the highest levels of increased ICP were recorded early in their course, with subsequent gradual decline in ICP until normalization in twenty to thirty days. They concluded that ICH acts as an expanding mass with intracranial hypertension only in its early stages, its subsequent morbidity being the result of tissue destruction by the ICH rather than the effect of raised ICP. They suggested that continuous ICP monitoring is a valuable tool in the management of patients with ICH, in particular as a measure indicative of the need to subject patients to surgical drainage of the ICH, in patients in whom the initially raised ICP fails to decline with the use of maximal medical therapy. These initial observations were subsequently tested by the authors in larger groups of patients. Papo et al.[42] analyzed the ICP pattern in sixty-six patients with supratentorial ICH who had ICP monitored by intraventricular catheter, and found an inconsistent correlation between ICP and level of consciousness, in relationship to outcome. At the two extremes of ICP the correlation of level of consciousness was good, in that patients who were alert had normal or slightly elevated ICP (20 mm Hg or less), whereas those in coma had markedly elevated ICP (greater than 30 mm Hg) that was resistant to treatment measures and resulted in high mortality. In patients with intermediate levels of ICP, the correlation with level of consciousness was poor, and the authors concluded that patient outcome could not be correlated well with the measured ICP values.[42] The twenty-two patients who had surgical drainage of ICH on the basis of their clinical and ICP parameters had the same mortality (32%) as the forty-four patients treated nonsurgically (29%). However, these two groups are difficult to compare, since it is apparent that the surgical patients were sicker than the nonsurgical ones by virtue of their level of consciousness and ICP pattern. In addition, the operations were performed at different intervals from ICH onset (within seventy-two hours, between days four and twenty-five), again making comparisons of outcome meaningless, since vital prognosis is markedly improved in patients who survive ICH for as long as two or three weeks from onset. In a third report, Janny et al.[43] analyzed a group of sixty patients with ICH, and found a closer correlation between level of consciousness and ICP than in previous studies: in forty-two patients who were either alert or stuporous, mean ICP was in the 22.2 mm Hg and 25.3 mm Hg range, respectively, whereas eighteen comatose patients had a mean ICP of 37 mm Hg. Again, outcome and ICP correlated poorly, as they detected normal or only slightly elevated ICP in seventeen of the twenty-six patients who died, the ICP being clearly elevated in only nine patients, when measured close to the time of their demise. They concluded that in most of the fatal outcomes, "intracranial hypertension was not the immediate cause of death."[43] Similar observations were reported by Duff et al.,[44] who monitored twelve consecutive patients with supratentorial ICH via an epidural fiberoptic ICP sensor, all of them managed nonsurgically, with osmotic diuretics, intermittent hyperventilation, and fluid restriction, without the use of corticosteroids. They measured both ICP and CPP, attempting to maintain the latter at 50 mm Hg or higher. The treatment program used was able to maintain the CPP above 50 mm Hg in all patients, and surgical evacuation of hematomas was not performed in any patient. There was only one death in a patient who had a myocardial infarction while at home and ambulatory, two months after discharge. These authors aimed at ICP reductions below 40 mm Hg, a figure that is substantially higher than normal (15 to 20 mm Hg), but in their experience being often observed in alert patients, thus disagreeing with those who maintain that the goal of treatment should be an ICP of 20 mm Hg or less.[31] Duff et al.[44] concluded that the treatment of elevated ICP based on continuous monitoring of ICP and CPP "can improve the outcome of conservatively treated patients" with supratentorial ICH.

The experience reported by Ropper and King[45] on the ICP monitoring of ten consecutive *comatose* patients with supratentorial ICH led them to reach somewhat different conclusions. Using a subarachnoid screw device for ICP monitoring, along with hyperventilation, mannitol, dexamethasone, and high-dose barbiturates (the latter in four patients) they found that all four patients who remained with ICP consistently above 20 mm Hg and did not undergo surgical evacuation of the hematoma died. The three patients with similar ICP recording patterns who underwent surgery survived. One of them died one month later from sepsis and metastatic cancer. These authors found no correlation between the initial ICP measurements and subsequent ICP course and outcome, as previously reported by Janny et al.[41] and Papo et al.[42] This poor predictive value of the initial ICP measurements and the clinical features (GCS, clinical signs), along with the improved results in patients subjected to surgery based on ICP measurements, led Ropper and King to conclude that continuous ICP measurement in comatose patients with supratentorial ICH is a valuable tool in the decision to subject these critically ill patients to surgical drainage of the hematoma.[45]

In conclusion, the management of raised ICP is one major aspect of the treatment of ICH, and it can be achieved most effectively by the use of hyperventilation and osmotic diuretics. The results of surgical drainage of hematomas, as guided by the data generated by continuous monitoring of ICP, need to be further evaluated in regard to outcome, in comparison with patients subjected to less intensive treatment of ICP.

### Choice between Surgical and Nonsurgical Treatment

The issue of surgical or nonsurgical treatment of patients with ICH continues to be controversial. This is largely the result of a paucity of prospective randomized treatment trials, and most of the opinions on the subject have been based on clinical series with various types of biases.[46,47]

The early experience reported by McKissock et al.[5] in 1959, prior to the introduction of CT, showed that surgical treatment by craniotomy of a large group of patients (N = 208) was followed by very high mortality (106 of 208, or 51%) within three weeks after operation. Since that series included only a surgical group without a nonsurgically-treated comparison group, McKissock et al.[6] subsequently conducted the first pre-CT era controlled randomized trial of surgical versus nonsurgical treatment of supratentorial ICH. Despite the obvious limitations imposed by the lack of modern imaging characterization of the features of the hematomas (size, precise location) that are now known to influence outcome, this was a well-designed and well-conducted trial that showed no differences in outcome between the two groups.

The 180 patients, ninety-one treated nonsurgically and eighty-nine treated by surgery, were comparable in regard to baseline characteristics, and the majority of them were treated within forty-eight hours from ICH onset. The mortality rates were not different for the two groups, 51% (46 of 91 patients) for the nonsurgical group and 65% (58 of 89 patients) for the surgical group. Similarly, the levels of functional disability on follow-up were essentially the same for both groups (Table 22.3). They also found that patients with lobar hematomas fared better than those with basal ganglionic or thalamic hemorrhages, but in neither group was surgery superior to nonsurgical treatment. A clinical profile that suggested an improved outcome was that of nonsurgically-treated hypertensive women without midline displacement by angiography. The authors suggested that this, and other possible determinants of outcome, such as the timing of operation, had to be further tested in prospective studies.

During the following decade, still prior to the introduction of CT, six uncontrolled studies addressed the issue of surgical treatment of ICH.[48-53] Cuatico et al.[48] reported 102 patients treated surgically, with a remarkably low mortality of 8%. However, it is not possible to determine from that report what was the distribution of patients by degree of preoperative clinical severity, or what were the criteria for the selection of surgical therapy,

**Table 22.3.** Outcome after Surgical versus Conservative Treatment of Intracerebral Hemorrhage, Randomized Clinical Trial

| Outcome | Treatment | |
|---|---|---|
| | Conservative (N = 91) | Surgical (N = 89) |
| Full recovery | 11 (12%) | 10 (11%) |
| Partial disability | 20 (22%) | 8 (9%) |
| Total disability | 14 (15%) | 13 (15%) |
| Dead | 46 (51%) | 58 (65%) |

(From McKissock W, Richardson A, Taylor J. Primary intracerebral haemorrhage: a controlled trial of surgical and conservative treatment in 180 unselected cases. Lancet 1961;2:221-226. With permission.)

other than stating that "urgency of operative intervention" was determined by a deteriorating neurologic condition. These authors also commented on a more favorable outcome in operated patients with lobar ("medullary," in their terminology) hematomas than in those with deep "nuclear" hemispheric hemorrhages.[48] Cook et al.[49] reported their experience with fifty-seven surgically-treated patients with supratentorial ICH and, not unexpectedly, documented the best results in patients who had preoperative less severe deficits and who were clinically stable or improving. They properly pointed out the biases inherent to selected surgical series, by showing that only one-third of the patients were in a poor preoperative prognostic category, and by wondering about the eventual outcome of those in the better prognostic group, should they have been treated nonsurgically (". . . among the patients with the more favorable results after surgical intervention are those who might have recovered spontaneously."[49]) Luessenhop et al.[50] reported sixty-four patients with supratentorial ICH, thirty-seven of whom were subjected to craniotomy, which was performed within the first twenty-four hours in all but two patients. Twelve of these thirty-seven operated patients died, for a mortality of 32%, whereas twelve of twenty-seven (44%) nonoperated patients died (Table 22.4). Decisions regarding surgery were based on the judgment of the surgeon as guided by the clinical evaluation of each patient. They also observed much lower mortality rates in patients with lobar (11%) than with deep basal ganglionic (92%) hemorrhages, which had operative mortalities of 4% and 89%, respectively.[50] Based on the postmortem study of twelve of their operated patients, they determined that the main cause of postoperative morbidity and mortality was reaccumulation of the hematoma. Paillas and Alliez,[51] in a larger series of 250 surgical patients, reported a thirty-day mortality rate of 36% in a group that had similar numbers of patients with lobar (106 patients) and deep (129 patients) hemorrhages. The selection biases in

**Table 22.4.** Mortality in Surgical and Nonsurgical Patients, Nonrandomized Clinical Series

| Group | Treatment | | | |
| | Surgical | | Nonsurgical | |
| | Survived | Died | Survived | Died |
|---|---|---|---|---|
| 1 | 0 | 0 | 7 | 0 |
| 2 | 22 | 2 (8%) | 8 | 1 (12%) |
| 3 | 3 | 10 (77%) | 0 | 11 (100%) |
| TOTAL | 25 | 12 (32%) | 15 | 12 (44%) |

Group 1: alert or drowsy; minor motor deficit; normal pupils; normal respirations.
Group 2: drowsy or stuporous, with purposeful response to pain; mild paresis to complete hemiplegia; normal to small and reactive pupils; eupneic or dyspneic.
Group 3: unresponsive to voice, with decorticate or decerebrate response to pain; unilateral or bilateral decorticate or decerebrate, with bilateral Babinski signs; unilateral mydriasis, or midposition and fixed pupils, or disconjugate eye movements with head turning; eupneic to apneic.
(From Luessenhop AJ, Shevlin WA, Ferrero AA, et al. Surgical management of primary intracerebral hemorrhage. J Neurosurg 1967;27:419–427. With permission.)

the series included the authors' "greater reluctance to operate on patients over 60" (only 45 of the 250 patients, or 18%, were in that age group), and a tendency to delay surgery (61 of the 250 patients, or 24%, were operated on before day 5, whereas 75, or 30%, were operated on between days 5 and 10, and 114, or 46%, were operated on after day 10). The postoperative results in these three groups, with mortalities of 54%, 30%, and 29%, respectively, led the authors to state that "between the fifth and tenth day seems to be the most favorable time to operate as the initial vegetative storm has subsided and a temporary remission phase has begun, which one must not let pass."[51] This surgical approach certainly takes advantage of the natural history of ICH, with improved prognosis for those who survive the initial forty-eight hours of illness,[11] a form of "Darwinian test" of survival after a catastrophic event. Pásztor et al.[52] analyzed the results in a series of 156 patients with supratentorial ICH, who had a 17% operative mortality. However, 136 patients (87%) were operated on after day 4 from onset, eighty-seven of them (56% of the total group) after two weeks from onset. As expected, the number of comatose or stuporous patients at the time of operation declined from 65% (thirteen of twenty patients) for those operated within three days from onset, to 16% (eight of fifty patients) for those operated between two and four weeks from onset, and 11% (four of thirty-seven patients) for those operated after one month had passed from ICH onset. The surgical mortality for the latter group was 3% (one of thirty-seven patients).

Kaneko et al.[53] are proponents of the *early* surgical drainage of ICH, based on their initial experience with thirty-eight patients with putaminal hemorrhage who had microsurgical clot evacuation within seven hours of ICH onset. The mortality in this series was 8% (three of thirty-eight patients), and they attributed their success to the ability to surgically obliterate the bleeding artery, usually identified as "a branch of the lenticulostriate artery of a diameter of approximately 200 to 400 $\mu$," thus preventing the reaccumulation of the hematoma.[53] In addition, they believe that early surgery offers the advantage of clot removal *before* the full development of cerebral edema, a feature that they related to the improved outcome in their series. On admission, twenty-three patients were described as "stuporous," twelve as "semicomatose," and three as "lethargic." The outcome of the thirty-five survivors was good, with "complete functional recovery" or "mild functional deficit" in sixteen of them. Based on this experience, Kaneko et al. stated that "all cases except those in deep coma or decerebrate rigidity are candidates for surgery," and "in mild cases with only lethargy . . . early surgery is still indicated for better recovery of function."[53]

Following the introduction of CT, refinements in the diagnosis of variables related to the hematoma itself have stimulated further attempts at defining subgroups of patients that may benefit from surgical drainage of the ICH, and evaluating the results of surgical and nonsurgical treatment of comparable groups of patients. The large series of Kanaya et al.[54] analyzed retrospectively 410 patients who had surgical drainage of a putaminal hemorrhage and 204 patients treated nonsurgically. There were no differences in outcome in patients described as "alert or confused" or "somnolent" on one hand, and in patients who were in either "semicoma with herniation signs" or coma, on the other, suggesting that surgery is not a therapeutic option for putaminal hemorrhage patients at both ends of the spectrum of neurologic severity. In the intermediate groups, those of patients described as either "stuporous" or "semicomatose without herniation signs" the surgical mortality was 18%, in comparison with 52% for patients treated nonsurgically (Table 22.5). In addition, functional outcome at six months was better in surgically-treated patients than in those treated nonsurgically, a difference that was significant for patients in the group labeled as "stuporous" and in "semicoma without herniation signs" (the latter signs defined as "unilateral or bilateral mydriasis without reactivity to light and unilateral or bilateral decorticate or decerebrate rigidity"). These authors also found better results with surgical than nonsurgical treatment in patients with putaminal hemorrhages that extended into the posterior limb of the internal capsule (with or without involvement of the anterior limb as well). Kanaya et al.[54] concluded that patients with putaminal hemorrhage who were alert or somnolent should receive nonsurgical treatment, whereas those with a more severely depressed level of consciousness should be treated surgically. In comatose patients, they stated that surgical treatment is not expected to improve the functional outcome, but "just . . . preserving life." These encouraging results from a retrospectively analyzed series were also found in a large series reported by Kaneko et al.,[55] using their recommended "ultra-early" (within seven hours from onset) operation on patients with putaminal hemorrhage. These

**Table 22.5.** Correlation between Neurological Grading and Outcome, Six Months after Surgical or Nonsurgical Treatment

| Clinical Grade | Treatment | No. Pts. | No. Deaths | Mortality |
|---|---|---|---|---|
| Alert or confused | Medical | 61 | 3 | 4.9% |
| | Surgical | 37 | 1 | 2.7% |
| Somnolent | Medical | 58 | 9 | 15.5% |
| | Surgical | 107 | 10 | 9.3% |
| Stuporous | Medical | 38 | 20 | 52.6% |
| | Surgical | 107 | 19 | 17.8% |
| Semicoma without herniation signs | Medical | 12 | 7 | 58.3% |
| | Surgical | 85 | 24 | 28.2% |
| Semicoma with herniation signs | Medical | 6 | 6 | 100.0% |
| | Surgical | 42 | 24 | 57.1% |
| Deep coma | Medical | 29 | 29 | 100.0% |
| | Surgical | 32 | 28 | 87.5% |

(From Kanaya H, Yukawa H, Itoh Z, et al. Grading and the indications for treatment in ICH of the basal ganglia cooperative study in Japan. In Pia HW, Longmaid C, Zierski J (eds): Spontaneous Intracerebral Haematomas: Advances in Diagnosis and Therapy. Heidelberg: Springer-Verlag, 1980, pp. 268–274. With permission.)

authors reported the results in 100 patients treated surgically who were either "stuporous" (GCS scores of 10 to 12) or "semicomatose" (GCS scores of 6 to 9), and who usually had on CT hematomas of more than 20 to 30 cm$^3$ in volume, with more than 5 mm of midline shift. Patients with "mild symptoms" and those in coma with decerebrate rigidity (GCS scores of 5 or below) were treated nonsurgically. The surgical mortality was remarkably low at 7%, and the long-term outcome was highly satisfactory as 89% of the 93 survivors were ambulatory six months after surgery (Table 22.6). After ten years of follow-up, twelve of the ninety-three patients (13%) had a recurrent ICH, which was fatal in ten of them, and associated with poor control of hypertension in eight. These results should be

**Table 22.6.** Correlation between Clinical Grade on Admission and Functional Outcome at Six Months after Ultra-early Operation

| Clinical Grade | No. Pts. | Functional Recovery Class* | | | | | No. Deaths |
|---|---|---|---|---|---|---|---|
| | | 1 | 2 | 3 | 4 | 5 | |
| Alert or confused | 0 | | | | | | |
| Somnolent | 10 | 5 | 2 | 2 | | | 1 |
| Stuporous | 68 | 9 | 27 | 25 | 4 | | 3 |
| Semicoma without herniation signs | 18 | 1 | 6 | 5 | 4 | 2 | 0 |
| Semicoma with herniation signs | 4 | | | 1 | | | 3 |
| Deep coma | 0 | | | | | | |
| Total | 100 | 15 | 35 | 33 | 8 | 2 | 7 |

*Functional recovery class:
Class 1: full recovery to social life.
Class 2: independent home life with self-care.
Class 3: dependent home life, usually ambulatory with cane.
Class 4: bedridden but conscious.
Class 5: vegetative state.
(From Kaneko M, Tanaka K, Shimada T, et al. Long-term evaluation of ultra-early operation for hypertensive intracerebral hemorrhage in 100 cases. J Neurosurg 1983;58:838-842. With permission.)

interpreted with caution, since there was no control group treated nonsurgically, and the preoperative level of consciousness was relatively good for the group, as 78% of the patients were described as "stuporous" or "lethargic" (GCS scores of 10 to 13), and only 22% were in the "semicoma" group, with GCS scores of six to nine. The authors made the statement that this reflects the fact that "severely disturbed consciousness and cerebral herniation are relatively rare during the initial 7 hours" after putaminal ICH.[55] However, at least eighty-seven patients were excluded from surgery, forty-six of whom had initial GCS scores of nine of less.

Despite its limitations, the study of Kaneko et al.[55] stimulated others[56] to undertake a prospective randomized trial of surgical versus nonsurgical treatment of hypertensive putaminal hemorrhage. Batjer et al.[56] randomized patients to three treatment groups: (1) "best" medical management (BMM), including intubation and hyperventilation, osmotic diuretics and furosemide, dexamethasone, and appropriate treatment of hypertension and other medical complications (fever, hypoxia); (2) BMM plus ICP monitoring by frontal ventriculostomy, aimed at maintaining ICP below 20 mm Hg, with the use of medical therapy, at times with the addition of intermittent CSF drainage; and (3) surgical evacuation of the hematoma using microsurgical technique. They were able to randomize twenty-one patients (nine to BMM, four to BMM plus ICP monitoring, and eight to surgery), and an interim analysis showed dismal results in all treatment groups: fifteen patients (71%) had died or remained in a vegetative state at six months after treatment, and only four (19%) were at home and living independently. Although the small numbers of patients do not allow for valid statistical comparisons, the preliminary results were so poor that the trial was terminated. Although the GCS scores were not used to assess preoperative level of consciousness and hematoma volumes were not provided, it appears that the majority of the patients (fourteen of twenty-one, or

67%) were in an intermediate level of neurological involvement (judged by their motor deficits rather than by either descriptive or quantitative assessment of level of consciousness, neither of which was reported). The results of this trial are difficult to interpret, due to the incomplete characterization of the clinical and CT features of the treatment groups, and the small numbers of patients enrolled.

Other recent nonrandomized trials of surgical versus nonsurgical treatment of ICH have usually shown lack of superiority of one form of therapy over the other. Waga and Yamamoto[57] compared all eighteen patients with putaminal hemorrhage treated surgically during 1977, with all fifty-six patients treated nonsurgically between 1978 and 1980. The thirty-day mortality rate was 28% for the surgical group, and only 14% for the nonsurgical group, a statistically significant difference in favor of nonsurgical treatment. Furthermore, functional outcome at six months showed that 60% of patients had good outcomes (independent with minimal or no residual disability) in the nonsurgical group, as opposed to 31% in the surgical group. These results are difficult to interpret, since the two treatment groups were markedly different in size, nonrandomly selected, noncontemporaneous, and with marked differences in the preoperative level of consciousness between them; eight of the eighteen (44%) surgical patients were in poor clinical grades ("semicoma without herniation signs," "semicoma with herniation signs," "deep coma"), whereas only eleven of fifty-six (20%) were in those categories in the nonsurgical group (the remaining 80% being "stuporous," "somnolent," or "alert or confused"). This difference in initial clinical grading is surprising, since the study design indicated that the selection of treatment was not based on clinical or CT features, but rather on an arbitrary treatment decision assigned during two different time periods (1977 and 1978 to 1980).

Bolander et al.,[58] in a nonrandomized study of seventy-five patients with supratentorial ICH found no differences in mortality between the thirty-nine patients treated surgically and the thirty-five treated nonsurgically (mortality at three months, 13% and 20%, respectively), and the functional outcome after a mean follow-up of fifteen months (range, four to thirty-eight months) was not different between the groups (35% of good outcomes in the surgical group, 44% in the nonsurgical group). Although the surgical group was overall more severely affected than the nonsurgical group, as measured by initial level of consciousness, these results do not support a role for surgery in supratentorial ICH. However, Bolander et al.[58] found that patients with hematoma volumes of 40 to 80 cm$^3$ fared better in the surgical group (6% mortality), than in the nonsurgical group (25% mortality) (Table 22.7). However, the markedly different size of the two groups of patients (sixteen patients operated, four nonoperated) suggests a selection bias, possibly based on surgical risk or associated medical morbidity. Similar conclusions were reached by Volpin et al.[59] after the analysis of 132 patients with basal ganglionic and lobar hemorrhages. Based on initial clinical condition and hematoma volumes, they found no mortality among thirty-nine patients with volumes below 26 cm$^3$, all treated nonsurgically, whereas thirty-four comatose patients with hematoma volumes of 85 cm$^3$ or more (twenty-three treated surgically, eleven nonsurgically) had 100% mortality. In the intermediate group of fifty-nine patients with hematoma volumes between 26 and 85 cm$^3$, the twenty-seven who had surgery had a significantly better survival rate than the

thirty-two who were treated nonsurgically, a benefit that applied to the whole group as well as to those who were initially comatose. Although the study was not randomized and the number of patients included was small, the data suggested a benefit for operated patients with intermediate size hematomas and severely compromised level of consciousness, including those in coma.

Kanno et al.[60] analyzed the results of surgical treatment of 154 patients with various types of ICH and compared them with those of 305 patients treated nonsurgically. Among the 265 patients with putaminal hemorrhages, they found differences in outcome between the two groups that depended on the severity of the initial clinical picture and the degree of extension and mass effect of the hematoma on CT. As expected, those with large hematomas that displaced the midline and extended into the diencephalon and midbrain had poor outcomes irrespective of the form of treatment used; those with small hematomas with little mass effect and no ventricular extension did well irrespective of the treatment modality used; those in the intermediate category had slightly better outcomes after surgery, especially when performed within six hours from ICH onset. Similar conclusions were reached by Fujitsu et al.[61] based on the analysis of 180 patients with putaminal hemorrhage, sixty-nine treated surgically and 111 nonsurgically. They found that in patients with stable (nonprogressive) clinical conditions following ICH, surgery offered no benefit over nonsurgical treatment, a conclusion that also applied to patients who had either a slowly pro-

**Table 22.7.** Correlation between Hematoma Volume and Mortality

| Hematoma Volume | Surgical Treatment | | Nonsurgical Treatment | |
|---|---|---|---|---|
| | No. Pts. | Deaths (%) | No. Pts. | Deaths (%) |
| Small (<40 cm$^3$) | 11 | 0 | 24 | 1  (4%) |
| Medium (40–80 cm$^3$) | 16 | 1  (6%) | 4 | 1 (25%) |
| Large (>80 cm$^3$) | 5 | 4 (80%) | 5 | 5 (100%) |

(From Bolander HG, Kourtopoulos H, Liliequist B, et al. Treatment of spontaneous intracerebral haemorrhage: a retrospective analysis of 74 consecutive cases with special reference to computer tomographic data. Acta Neurochir 1983;67:19–28. With permission.)

gressive course or a fulminant course after admission. For those with a rapidly progressive course, surgical treatment was superior to nonsurgical treatment.

In a recent prospective clinical trial, Juvela et al.[62] randomized fifty-two patients with supratentorial ICH to surgical (twenty-six patients) or nonsurgical (twenty-six patients) treatment groups within forty-eight hours from ICH onset. Patients were enrolled if they had severely depressed level of consciousness (GCS score less than 9) and/or severe hemiparesis or dysphasia, and were admitted within twenty-four hours from ICH onset. The mean time from onset of symptoms of bleeding to operation was 14.5 hours (range, 6 to 48 hours). The mortality rates were the same for the two groups, both acutely and after long-term follow-up (Table 22.8). When patients were stratified according to their prerandomization clinical status, those "stuporous" or "semicomatose" with GCS scores of 7 to 10 fared better in the surgical group, but the numbers of patients in the groups were small (four surgical, five nonsurgical), and the quality of life of the five survivors (one nonsurgical, four surgical) was poor, all being totally disabled at one year after ICH. These authors found no differences in outcome in the surgical group

based on early or late operations during the initial twenty-four hours. Their conclusion, based on an overall mortality of 42% at six months and the poor quality of life in the survivors (irrespective of the treatment modality used), was that supratentorial ICH "should be treated conservatively."[62]

In conclusion, despite the large number of studies that have addressed the issue of surgical versus nonsurgical treatment of supratentorial ICH, it is still uncertain whether one treatment modality is superior to the other. Clearly, patients at both ends of the spectrum of severity, with either small hemorrhages and minimally depressed level of consciousness, or large hemorrhages and severely depressed level of consciousness, should be treated nonsurgically, an approach that usually results in good outcomes in the former group and dismal ones in the latter group. For those patients in the intermediate categories, a large prospective randomized multicenter trial with groups of patients categorized by initial clinical status and hematoma features (size, location, mass effect, ventricular extension) on CT should provide the much needed data required to make sound decisions in the management of these patients.

While uncertainties about the surgical indications of ICH remain, treatment decisions have to be made on individual patients. The following are some guidelines used by the authors in the management of patients with ICH: (1) when a brain hematoma threatens life, operative removal of the lesion should be considered, especially in a young person with ongoing clinical deterioration; (2) surgery is not recommended if there is massive hemorrhage with loss of brainstem function and lack of response to medical therapy; (3) certain hematoma sites, such as the cerebellum and the cerebral lobes, have generally better outcome with surgical intervention than others; and (4) diagnostic uncertainty as to the mechanism of the ICH at times favors exploratory operation, such as in the case of suspected tumor, AVM, or cavernous angioma.

**Table 22.8.** Cumulative Time from Hemorrhage to Death, Correlated with Type of Treatment

| Time after ICH | Type of Treatment | | Deaths | |
|---|---|---|---|---|
| | Nonsurgical (N = 26) | Surgical (N = 26) | No. | % |
| 0–4 days | 5 | 4 | 9 | 17 |
| 1 week | 8 | 8 | 16 | 31 |
| 1 month | 10 | 10 | 20 | 38 |
| 6 months | 10 | 12 | 22 | 42 |
| 12 months | 10 | 13 | 23 | 44 |
| 2 years | 11 | 14 | 25 | 48 |

(From Juvela S, Heiskanen O, Poranen A, et al. The treatment of spontaneous intracerebral hemorrhage: a prospective randomized trial of surgical and conservative treatment. J Neurosurg 1989;70:755–758. With permission.)

## Surgical Techniques

### Hematoma Evacuation

The standard operation is a craniotomy with careful removal of the hematoma, exposed through a cortical incision.[63] Supratentorial hemorrhages are usually removed with the patient in a supine or lateral position; cerebellar hematomas are evacuated in the prone position, and an occipital ventricular catheter is placed to relieve hydrocephalus. With the CT and MRI findings, there is usually no difficulty in localizing the hematoma; on occasion, problems in hematoma localization can be solved with the use of intraoperative ultrasound.

In the deteriorating patient, surgical treatment begins with maximal "medical decompression," using 100 g of intravenous mannitol, as well as hyperventilation. An arterial catheter is inserted, and BP is controlled. Direct exposure of the hematoma is needed for its removal, because the clot is usually too firm to aspirate. A cortical incision is performed in an appropriate noneloquent gyrus: the anterior superior temporal gyrus for temporal or putaminal lesions, the superior parietal lobule for parieto-occipital lesions, the superior frontal gyrus anterior to the motor strip for frontal lesions, and the vermis or paravermian area for cerebellar hematomas. A 2- to 3-cm cortisectomy is made with bipolar cautery and microscissors. Loupes and headlight permit satisfactory visualization. Deep exposure is greatly aided by self-retaining retractors (Figure 22.7). Evacuation of the hemorrhage is achieved with careful suction and irrigation. Sometimes a tumor forceps can extract a large, firm clot. The bulk of the hematoma is removed to achieve decompression, but the last adherent bits of the clot may be left behind, to avoid injury or bleeding from the wall of the cavity. Great care is taken to keep instruments, particularly the suction, away from the edematous white matter adjacent to the hematoma. Tissue suspicious for angioma, tumor, or other pathol-

ogy warrants careful microsurgical biopsy or excision. Hemostasis is achieved with bipolar cautery, and Surgicel is used to line the hematoma cavity. Hemostasis must be meticulous to avoid hematoma recurrence. The BP is raised for five to ten minutes to high-normal values in order to check hemostasis; this maneuver has allowed the visualization and control of additional bleeders in a number of cases. Great care must be taken to avoid frank hypertension, which can cause brain swelling. Closure is performed in routine fashion, almost always without a drain. For cerebellar hemorrhage with hydrocephalus, a ventricular catheter is left in place for a few days.

Postoperative care includes meticulous control of BP and use of corticosteroids to reduce brain edema. If antithrombotic agents such as aspirin are needed, they can be safely started after surgery with little increased risk of hematoma recurrence; data on safe timing for initiation of warfarin therapy are lacking, but it probably can be started one month after surgery without risk of intraparenchymal bleeding. Serum electrolytes and osmolarity are checked regularly, and in case of neurological deterioration CT is performed to detect recurrent hemorrhage or hydrocephalus. To prevent deep vein thrombosis and potentially fatal pulmonary embolus, perioperative pneumatic compression boots and subcutaneous heparin (5000 U twice a day) are utilized. To avert seizures, phenytoin (300 mg per day) is routinely given to patients with supratentorial hemorrhages; it is tapered gradually after six months of treatment if an EEG shows no epileptiform activity. In patients with symptomatic hydrocephalus, a ventriculoperitoneal shunt may be required.

### Ventriculostomy

When hydrocephalus or intraventricular hemorrhage is symptomatic, ventricular drainage is indicated. A ventricular drain is placed through a frontal burr hole, usually on the right, but at times on the left if that ventricle seems more likely to drain satisfac-

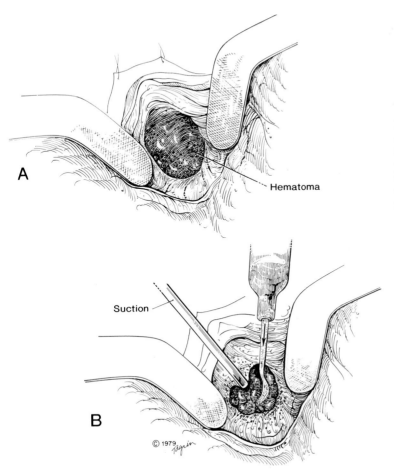

A

Hematoma

Suction

B

© 1979

**Figure 22.7.** Surgical technique for removal of intraparenchymal hematomas. (A) Exposure of hematoma with self-retaining retractors. (B) Removal of hematoma by suction. (Reprinted from Crowell RM, Ojemann RG, Ogilvy CS. Spontaneous brain hemorrhage: surgical considerations. In: Barnett HJM, Mohr JP, Stein BM, et al. (eds): Stroke: pathophysiology, diagnosis, and treatment, 2nd ed. New York: Churchill Livingstone, 1992, pp. 1169–1187. With permission.)

torily. Continuous drainage is established through a closed, sterile system, with the spillway set at 15 cm above the foramen of Monro. Within a few days, a decision is made regarding removal of the catheter or conversion to a ventriculoperitoneal shunt. Serial CT and a trial clamping of the drain may help make the decision. Oxacillin is given at a dose of 1 g every six hours intravenously as antibiotic prophylaxis while the drain is in place.

### Novel Approaches to the Surgical Therapy

In recent years, several new techniques have been developed for the surgical removal of intracerebral hematomas, in an attempt at minimizing the surgical trauma associated with conventional hematoma evacuation by craniotomy. In 1978, Backlund and von Holst[64] introduced a new instrument for the stereotactic evacuation of intracerebral hematomas. It consisted of a rotating drill and an aspiration cannula that were introduced through a burr hole into the center of the hematoma. Using this technique, they were able to remove about 70 cm$^3$ of an estimated 100cm$^3$ hematoma from the right temporoparietal area in a 55-year-old patient. His recovery was excellent, and he was able to return to his prior occupation ten months after the operation. This experience stimulated a number of surgeons, especially from Japan, to use this procedure in larger groups of patients. In most instances, stereotactic introduction of the drainage system was done under local anesthesia using CT guidance. CT was also used to follow the results of the operation. Some groups have used simple hematoma aspiration with irrigation,[65,66] while others[67,68] have performed the aspiration with the use of a fibrinolytic agent (urokinase) for the purpose of liquefying the clot prior to its removal. The procedure has been applied to patients with putaminal, thalamic, and lobar hematomas, and the results have been reported as usually satisfactory, with a low rate of postoperative complications. The duration of the procedure has been reported to be approximately two hours,[65] and the volume of hematoma removed has been estimated between 50% and 80% of the original mass.[66,68] With the addition of urokinase instillations (6000 IU in 3 to 5 cm$^3$ of saline) into the hematoma, it has been possible to gradually remove the hematoma over periods of several days, by repeating the procedure of urokinase instillation and hematoma suction every six to twelve hours, through a silicone tube that remains in place until the clot has been completely removed.[67] Experience with this technique is still preliminary. However, comparisons with hematoma removal by conventional craniotomy showed similar postoperative mortality, but with better functional outcome in patients who had the stereotactic aspiration procedure.[67] This has led to the suggestion that this technique could have a role in the surgical treatment of hematomas that are deep in location (thalamic, putaminal), and in patients who may be at too high risk for hematoma drainage through a conventional craniotomy under general anesthesia.[67] However, the potential for rebleeding after stereotactic drainage always exists, a complication that occurred in 7% (seven patients) of the ninety-seven patients reported by Niizuma et al.[68] Two of these patients required hematoma drainage by conventional craniotomy.

Auer et al.[69] reported preliminary results of the use of an endoscopic surgical technique for the removal of intracerebral hematomas. The procedure was performed with a "neuroendoscope" that was introduced into the hematoma by ultrasound-assisted stereotactic technique; the hematoma was subtotally evacuated under direct visual control via a miniature videocamera attached to the endoscope. Patients treated had putaminal, lobar, and thalamic hemorrhages. The best results were obtained in patients under age 60 who were either alert or somnolent preoperatively.

These new surgical techniques offer the hope that, in properly selected subgroups of patients, there will be an alternative to conventional craniotomy for the drainage of hemispheric ICH.[70] Still, their value will have to be established through large, multicenter, prospective randomized trials, with comparisons of stereotactic or endoscopic techniques with conventional craniotomy and nonsurgical treatment.[71]

## References

1. Furlan AJ, Whisnant JP, Elveback LR. The decreasing incidence of primary intracerebral hemorrhage: a population study. Ann Neurol 1979;5:367–373.
2. Drury I, Whisnant JP, Garraway WM. Primary intracerebral hemorrhage: impact of CT on incidence. Neurology 1984;34:653–657.
3. Garraway WM, Whisnant JP, Drury I. The changing pattern of survival following stroke. Stroke 1983;14:669–703.
4. Rowe CC, Donnan GA, Bladin PF. Intracerebral haemorrhage: incidence and use of computed tomography. Br Med J 1988;297:1177–1178.
5. McKissock W, Richardson A, Walsh L. Primary intracerebral haemorrhage: results of surgical treatment in 244 consecutive cases. Lancet 1959;2:683–686.
6. McKissock W, Richardson A, Taylor J. Primary intracerebral haemorrhage: a controlled trial of surgical and conservative treatment in 180 unselected cases. Lancet 1961;2:221–226.
7. Douglas MA, Haerer AF. Long-term prognosis of hypertensive intracerebral hemorrhage. Stroke 1982;13:488–491.

8. Nath FP, Nicholls D, Fraser RJA. Prognosis in intracerebral haemorrhage. Acta Neurochir 1983;67:29–35.

9. Steiner I, Gomori JM, Melamed E. The prognostic value of the CT scan in conservatively treated patients with intracerebral hematoma. Stroke 1984;15:279–282.

10. Helweg-Larsen S, Sommer W, Strange P, Lester J, Boysen G. Prognosis for patients treated conservatively for spontaneous intracerebral hematomas. Stroke 1984;15:1045–1048.

11. Silver FL, Norris JW, Lewis AJ, et al. Early mortality following stroke: a prospective review. Stroke 1984;15:492–496.

12. Dixon AA, Holness RO, Howes WJ, et al. Spontaneous intracerebral haemorrhage: an analysis of factors affecting prognosis. Can J Neurol Sci 1985;12:267–271.

13. Portenoy RK, Lipton RB, Berger AR, et al. Intracerebral haemorrhage: a model for the prediction of outcome. J Neurol Neurosurg Psychiat 1987;50:976–979.

14. Fieschi C, Carolei A, Fiorelli M, et al. Changing prognosis of primary intracerebral hemorrhage: results of a clinical and computed tomographic follow-up study of 104 patients. Stroke 1988;19:192–195.

15. Bogousslavsky J, Van Melle G, Regli F. The Lausanne Stroke Registry: analysis of 1,000 consecutive patients with first stroke. Stroke 1988;19:1083–1092.

16. Tuhrim S, Dambrosia JM, Price TR, et al. Prediction of intracerebral hemorrhage survival. Ann Neurol 1988;24:258–263.

17. Omae T, Ueda K, Ogata J, et al. Parenchymatous hemorrhage: etiology, pathology and clinical aspects. In: Vinken PJ, et al., eds. Handbook of clinical neurology. New York: Elsevier, 1989;287–331.

18. Westling B, Norrving B, Thorngren M. Survival following stroke: a prospective population-based study of 438 hospitalized cases with prediction according to subtype, severity and age. Acta Neurol Scand 1990; 81:457–463.

19. Gras P, Arveux P, Clavier I, et al. Étude rétrospective d'une série hospitalière de 238 hémorragies intracérébrales spontanées. Sem Hôp Paris 1990;66:1677–1683.

20. Bamford J, Dennis M, Sandercock P, et al. The frequency, causes and timing of death within 30 days of a first stroke: the Oxfordshire Community Stroke Project. J Neurol Neurosurg Psychiat 1990;53:824–829.

21. Daverat P, Castel JP, Dartigues JF, et al. Death and functional outcome after spontaneous intracerebral hemorrhage: a prospective study of 166 cases using multivariate analysis. Stroke 1991;22:1–6.

22. Fogelholm R, Nuutila M, Vuorela A-L. Primary intracerebral haemorrhage in the Jyväskylä region, Central Finland 1985–89: incidence, case fatality rate, and functional outcome. J Neurol Neurosurg Psychiat 1992; 55:546–552.

23. Franke CL, van Swieten JC, Algra A, et al. Prognostic factors in patients with intracerebral haematoma. J Neurol Neurosurg Psychiat 1992;55:653–657.

24. Teasdale G, Jennett B. Assessment of coma and impaired consciousness: a practical scale. Lancet 1974;2:81–83.

25. Kunitz SC, Gross CR, Heyman A, et al. The Pilot Stroke Data Bank: definition, design, and data. Stroke 1984;15:740–746.

26. Stein RW, Caplan LR, Hier DB. Outcome of intracranial hemorrhage: role of blood pressure and location and size of lesions. Ann Neurol 1983;14:132–133 (abstract).

27. Kase CS, Williams JP, Wyatt DA, et al. Lobar intracerebral hematomas: clinical and CT analysis of 22 cases. Neurology 1982;32:1146–1150.

28. de Weerd AW. The prognosis of intraventricular hemorrhage. J Neurol 1979;222:45–51.

29. Stein RW, Kase CS, Hier DB, et al. Caudate hemorrhage. Neurology 1984;34:1549–1554.

30. Young WB, Lee KP, Pessin MS, et al. Prognostic significance of ventricular blood in supratentorial hemorrhage: a volumetric study. Neurology 1990;40:616–619.

31. Ropper AH. Treatment of intracranial hypertension. In: Ropper AH, ed. Neurological and neurosurgical intensive care. Third edition. New York: Raven Press, 1993;29–52.

32. Vandam LD, Burnap TK. Hypothermia. N Engl J Med 1959;261:546–553, 595–603.

33. Siesjö BK, Carlsson C, Hägerdal M, et al. Brain metabolism in the critically ill. Crit Care Med 1976;4:283–294.

34. Marsh ML, Marshall LF, Shapiro HM. Neurosurgical intensive care. Anesthesiology 1977; 47:149–163.

35. Lassen NA. Control of cerebral circulation in health and disease. Circ Res 1974;34: 749–760.

36. Patchell RA, Posner JB. Neurologic complications of systemic cancer. Neurol Clin 1985; 3:729–750.

37. Norris JW. Steroid therapy in acute cerebral infarction. Arch Neurol 1976;33:69–71.

38. Norris JW, Hachinski VC. High dose steroid treatment in cerebral infarction. Br Med J 1986;292:21–23.

39. Poungvarin N, Bhoopat W, Viriyavejakul A, et al. Effects of dexamethasone in primary supratentorial intracerebral hemorrhage. N Engl J Med 1987;316:1229–1233.

40. Shapiro HM. Intracranial hypertension: therapeutic and anesthetic considerations. Anesthesiology 1975;43:445–471.

41. Janny P, Colnet G, Georget A-M, et al. Intracranial pressure with intracerebral hemorrhages. Surg Neurol 1978;10:371–375.

42. Papo I, Janny P, Caruselli G, et al. Intracranial pressure time course in primary intracerebral hemorrhage. Neurosurgery 1979;4:504–511.

43. Janny P, Papo I, Chazal J, et al. Intracranial hypertension and prognosis in spontaneous intracerebral haematomas: a correlative study of 60 patients. Acta Neurochir 1982;61:181–186.

44. Duff TA, Ayeni S, Levin AB, et al. Nonsurgical management of spontaneous intracerebral hematoma. Neurosurgery 1981;9:387–393.

45. Ropper AH, King RB. Intracranial pressure monitoring in comatose patients with cerebral hemorrhage. Arch Neurol 1984;41:725–728.

46. Ransohoff J, Derby B, Kricheff I. Spontaneous intracerebral hemorrhage. Clin Neurosurg 1970;18:247–266.

47. Ojemann RG, Heros RC. Spontaneous brain hemorrhage. Stroke 1983;14:468–475.

48. Cuatico W, Adib S, Gaston P. Spontaneous intracerebral hematomas: a surgical appraisal. J Neurosurg 1965;22:569–575.

49. Cook AW, Plaut M, Browder J. Spontaneous intracerebral hemorrhage: factors related to surgical results. Arch Neurol 1965;13:25–29.

50. Luessenhop AJ, Shevlin WA, Ferrero AA, et al. Surgical management of primary intracerebral hemorrhage. J Neurosurg 1967;27: 419–427.

51. Paillas JE, Alliez B. Surgical treatment of spontaneous intracerebral hemorrhage: immediate and long-term results in 250 cases. J Neurosurg 1973;39:145–151.

52. Pásztor E, Áfra D, Orosz É. Experiences with the surgical treatment of 156 ICH (1955-1977). In: Pia HW, et al., eds. Spontaneous intracerebral haematomas: advances in diagnosis and therapy. Heidelberg: Springer-Verlag, 1980; 251–257.

53. Kaneko M, Koba T, Yokoyama T. Early surgical treatment for hypertensive intracerebral hemorrhage. J Neurosurg 1977;46:579–583.

54. Kanaya H, Yukawa H, Itoh Z, et al. Grading and the indications for treatment in ICH of the basal ganglia (cooperative study in Japan). In: Pia HW, et al., eds. Spontaneous intracerebral haematomas: advances in diagnosis and therapy. Heidelberg: Springer-Verlag, 1980;268–274.

55. Kaneko M, Tanaka K, Shimada T, et al. Long-term evaluation of ultra-early operation for hypertensive intracerebral hemorrhage in 100 cases. J Neurosurg 1983;58:838–842.

56. Batjer HH, Reisch JS, Allen BC, et al. Failure of surgery to improve outcome in hypertensive putaminal hemorrhage: a prospective randomized trial. Arch Neurol 1990;47: 1103–1106.

57. Waga S, Yamamoto Y. Hypertensive putaminal hemorrhage: treatment and results: is surgical treatment superior to conservative one? Stroke 1983;14:480–485.

58. Bolander HG, Kourtopoulos H, Liliequist B, Treatment of spontaneous intracerebral hemorrhage: a retrospective analysis of 74 consecutive cases with special reference to computer-tomographic data. Acta Neurochir 1983;67: 19–28.

59. Volpin L, Cervellini P, Colombo F, et al. Spontaneous intracerebral hematomas: a new proposal about the usefulness and limits of surgical treatment. Neurosurgery 1984;15: 663–666.

60. Kanno T, Sano H, Shinomiya Y, et al. Role of surgery in hypertensive intracerebral hematoma: a comparative study of 305 nonsurgical and 154 surgical cases. J Neurosurg 1984;61:1091–1099.

61. Fujitsu K, Muramoto M, Ikeda Y, et al. Indications for surgical treatment of putaminal hemorrhage: comparative study based on serial CT and time-course analysis. J Neurosurg 1990;73:518–525.

62. Juvela S, Heiskanen O, Poranen A, et al. The treatment of spontaneous intracerebral hemorrhage: a prospective randomized trial of surgical and conservative treatment. J Neurosurg 1989;70:755–758.

63. Crowell RM, Ojemann RG, Ogilvy CS. Spontaneous brain hemorrhage: surgical consider-

ations. In: Barnett HJM, et al., eds. Stroke: pathophysiology, diagnosis, and management. Second edition. New York: Churchill Livingstone, 1992;1169–1187.

64. Backlund E-O, von Holst H. Controlled subtotal evacuation of intracerebral hematomas by stereotactic technique. Surg Neurol 1978; 9:99–101.

65. Tanizaki Y, Sugita K, Toriyama T, et al. New CT-guided stereotactic apparatus and clinical experience with intracerebral hematomas. Appl Neurophysiol 1985;48:11–17.

66. Tanikawa T, Amano K, Kawamura H, et al. CT-guided stereotactic surgery for evacuation of hypertensive intracerebral hematoma. Appl Neurophysiol 1985;48:431–439.

67. Matsumoto K, Hondo H. CT-guided stereotaxic evacuation of hypertensive intracerebral hematomas. J Neurosurg 1984;61:440–448.

68. Niizuma H, Otsuki T, Johkura H, et al. CT-guided stereotactic aspiration of intracerebral hematoma: result of a hematoma-lysis method using urokinase. Appl Neurophysiol 1985;48: 427–430.

69. Auer LM, Deinsberger W, Niederkorn K, et al. Endoscopic surgery versus medical treatment for spontaneous intracerebral hematoma: a randomized study. J Neurosurg 1989;70: 530–535.

70. Shields CB, Friedman WA. The role of stereotactic technology in the management of intracerebral hemorrhage. Neurosurg Clin NA 1992;3:685–702.

71. Kopitnik TA, Kaufman HH. The future: prospects of innovative treatment of intracerebral hemorrhage. Neurosurg Clin NA 1992;3: 703–707.

# Index

Page numbers followed by *t* and *f* indicate tables and figures, respectively.